Clinical Pediatric Neurology

Clinical Pediatric Neurology

A Signs and Symptoms Approach

Gerald M. Fenichel, M.D.

Professor and Chairman
Department of Neurology
Vanderbilt University School of Medicine
Nashville, Tennessee

**THIRD
EDITION**

W.B. SAUNDERS COMPANY
A *Harcourt Health Sciences Company*
St. Louis   Philadelphia   London   Sydney   Toronto

W.B. SAUNDERS COMPANY
A *Harcourt Health Sciences Company*

The Curtis Center
Independence Square West
Philadelphia, Pennsylvania 19106

Library of Congress Cataloging-in-Publication Data

Fenichel, Gerald M.
    Clinical pediatric neurology : a signs and symptoms approach /
Gerald M. Fenichel. — 3rd ed.
        p.   cm.
    Includes bibliographical references.
    ISBN 0-7216-6852-6
    1. Pediatric neurology.   I. Title.
    [DNLM: 1. Nervous System Diseases—in infancy & childhood.
    2. Nervous System Diseases—diagnosis.   WS 340 F333c 1997]
    RJ486.F46   1997
    618.92′8—dc20
    DNLM/DLC   96-16719

Every effort has been made by the authors, the editors, and the publisher of this book to ensure that dosage recommendations are precise and in agreement with the standards of practice accepted at the time of publication.

However, dosage schedules are changed from time to time in the light of accumulating clinical experience and continuing laboratory studies. This is most likely to occur in the case of recently introduced products.

We urge, therefore, that you check the package information data for the manufacturer's recommended dosage to be certain that changes have not been made in the recommended dose or in the contraindications for administration.

The Editors

CLINICAL PEDIATRIC NEUROLOGY   ISBN 0-7216-6852-6

Printed in the United States of America.

Last digit is the print number: 9   8   7   6   5   4

P R E F A C E

I've had the great pleasure during the 9-year history of this text to regularly receive letters and telephone calls from grateful neurologists who, having just learned that they passed the Pediatric Neurology portion of the Board Certification Examination, attribute their success to this book. People who fail the examination never call or write, nor am I encouraging such behavior, so the reader should know that data concerning this book's usefulness for Board preparation are anecdotal and incomplete. The real intent of the book is to provide an approach to the common presenting problems of children with disorders of the nervous system. The chapter titles have remained the same in all three editions because presenting complaints have remained the same. However, the reader will find considerable change in the content of the third edition as compared with the second. Not only are all the references new, but the approach to many complaints and diseases has changed.

The text remains a manual of practical information, much derived from my own experience. I have felt free to indicate my own biases concerning patient management in situations where a single standard of practice is not established.

I am grateful to the following colleagues who provided counsel: Kathryn Edwards (infectious disease), Mark T. Jennings (neuro-oncology), Patrick J.M. Lavin (neuro-ophthalmology), Thomas Davis (movement disorders), and Noel Tulipan (neurosurgery); to James Atkinson, who provided new photomicrographs of muscle biopsies and Theodore Larson III, who provided new MRI images, and to Mrs. Lester Tilley, who keeps my office running so that I have the opportunity to write.

Gerald M. Fenichel, M.D.
Nashville, Tennessee
1996

CONTENTS

1

Paroxysmal Disorders

Paroxysmal events are almost never witnessed by the diagnosing physician. The nature of the event must be surmised by listening to the eyewitness description offered by a family member or, even worse, to the second-hand description that the parent heard from the teacher. Most "spells" are not seizures, and epilepsy is not a diagnosis of exclusion. "Spells" seldom remain unexplained after being viewed. Because observation of the spell is critical to diagnosis, the event in question should be recorded on video tape. Most families either own or can borrow a video camera; even if the camera must be purchased, it is more cost effective than brain imaging studies, and at least the family has something useful to show for the expenditure.

In children the common causes of sudden and recurrent episodes of neurologic dysfunction that clear completely are epilepsy, syncope, and migraine. Less common causes are movement disorders, psychogenic disturbances, and some metabolic disorders. Episodic symptoms that last only seconds and cause no abnormal signs are rarely explained and usually do not warrant laboratory investigation. The differential diagnosis of paroxysmal disorders is somewhat different in the neonatal period, infancy, childhood, and adolescence, and is best presented by age groups.

Paroxysmal Disorders of Newborns

Seizures are the main paroxysmal disorder of the newborn. The challenge for the clinician is to differentiate seizure activity from normal neonatal movements and from pathologic movements caused by other mechanisms (Table 1-1).

APPROACH TO DIAGNOSIS

Seizure Patterns

Seizures in newborns, especially those who are premature, are poorly organized and difficult to distinguish from normal activity. Newborns with hydranencephaly or atelencephaly are capable of generating the full variety of neonatal seizure patterns. This supports the notion that seizures may arise from the brainstem as well as the hemispheres. Seizures arising in the brainstem may be confined there by the absence of myelinated pathways for propagation. For the same reason, seizures originating in one hemisphere are unlikely to spread beyond the contiguous cortex or to produce secondary bilateral synchrony.

Table 1-2 lists clinical patterns that have been associated with epileptiform discharges in newborns. This classification is useful but does not do justice to the rich variety of patterns actually observed or take into account that 50% of prolonged epileptiform discharges on the electroencephalogram (EEG) are not associated with visible clinical changes (Scher et al, 1993). Generalized tonic-clonic seizures do not occur. Many newborns suspected of having generalized tonic-clonic seizures are actually *jittery* (see Jitteriness, later on). Newborns paralyzed with pancuronium to assist mechanical ventilation pose a special problem in seizure identification. In this circumstance physicians may be alerted to

■ TABLE 1–1
Movements That Resemble Neonatal Seizures

Benign nocturnal myoclonus
Jitteriness
Nonconvulsive apnea
Normal movement
Opisthotonos
Pathologic myoclonus

■ TABLE 1–2
Seizure Patterns in Newborns

Apnea with tonic stiffening of body
Focal clonic movements of one limb or both limbs
 on one side
Multifocal clonic limb movements
Myoclonic jerking
Paroxysmal laughing
Tonic deviation of the eyes, upward or to one side
Tonic stiffening of the body

the possibility of seizures by the presence of rhythmic increases in systolic arterial blood pressure, heart rate, and oxygenation.

The term *subtle seizures* encompasses several different patterns in which tonic or clonic movements of the limbs are lacking. EEG monitoring has consistently failed to show that such movements are associated with epileptiform activity. One exception is tonic deviation of the eyes, which is almost always a seizure manifestation.

The definitive diagnosis of neonatal seizures requires EEG monitoring. This is best accomplished with split-screen 16-channel video-EEG, but an ambulatory EEG cassette capable of marking the time of events can also be used. Epileptiform activity in the newborn is usually widespread and can be detected even when the newborn is clinically asymptomatic.

Focal Clonic Seizures

CLINICAL FEATURES. Focal clonic seizures are characterized by repeated, irregular jerking movements affecting one limb or both limbs on one side. The movements are rarely sustained for long periods and they do not "march" as though spreading along the motor cortex. Focal clonic seizures in a full-term newborn who is otherwise alert and responsive suggests a cerebral infarction or hemorrhage. In newborns with states of decreased consciousness, focal clonic seizures may indicate a focal infarction superimposed on a generalized encephalopathy.

DIAGNOSIS. During the seizure, the EEG may show a unilateral focus of high-amplitude sharp waves adjacent to the rolandic fissure. The discharge can spread to involve contiguous areas in the same hemisphere and can be associated with unilateral seizures of the limbs and adversive movements of the head and eyes. The interictal EEG usually shows focal slowing or amplitude attenuation.

Newborns with focal clonic seizures should be evaluated immediately using non–contrast-enhanced computed tomography (CT) or ultrasound to look for intracerebral hemorrhage. If the CT scan is normal, contrast-enhanced CT or magnetic resonance imaging (MRI) should be done 3 days later to look for cerebral infarction. Ultrasound is not useful in detecting small cerebral infarctions.

Multifocal Clonic Seizures

CLINICAL FEATURES. In multifocal clonic seizures, migratory jerking movements are noted in first one limb and then another; facial muscles may be involved as well. The migration appears random and does not follow expected patterns of epileptic spread. Movements in one limb are sometimes prolonged, suggesting a focal rather than a multifocal seizure. The multifocal nature is detected later, when nursing notes are found to be contradictory concerning the side or the limb affected. Multifocal clonic seizures are a neonatal equivalent of generalized tonic-clonic seizures. They are ordinarily associated with severe, generalized cerebral disturbances, such as hypoxic-ischemic encephalopathy.

DIAGNOSIS. Multifocal epileptiform activity can usually be detected on a standard EEG. If epileptiform activity is not seen, a 24-hour monitor is recommended.

Myoclonic Seizures

CLINICAL FEATURES. Myoclonic seizures are characterized by brief, repeated extension and flexion movements of the arms, the legs, or all limbs. They constitute an uncommon seizure pattern in the newborn but their presence suggests severe, diffuse brain damage.

DIAGNOSIS. No specific EEG pattern is associated with myoclonic seizures in the newborn. Myoclonic jerks are often seen in babies born to drug-addicted mothers. Whether these movements are seizures, jitteriness, or myoclonus (discussed later) is not certain.

Tonic Seizures

CLINICAL FEATURES. Tonic seizures are characterized by extension and stiffening of the body, usually associated with apnea and upward deviation of the eyes. Tonic posturing without the other features is rarely a seizure manifestation. Tonic seizures are more common in premature than in full-term newborns and usually indicate structural brain damage rather than a metabolic disturbance.

DIAGNOSIS. Tonic seizures in premature newborns are often a symptom of intraventricular hemorrhage and are an indication for ultrasound study. Tonic posturing also occurs in newborns with forebrain damage, not as a seizure manifestation but as a disinhibition of brainstem reflexes. Prolonged disinhibition results in *decerebrate posturing,* an extension of the body and limbs associated with internal rotation of the arms, dilation of the pupils, and downward deviation of the eyes. Decerebrate posturing is often encountered as a terminal sign in premature infants with intraventricular hemorrhage caused by pressure on the upper brainstem (see Chapter 4).

Tonic seizures and decerebrate posturing must also be distinguished from *opisthotonos,* a prolonged arching of the back not necessarily associated with eye movements. Opisthotonos is probably caused by meningeal irritation and is seen in kernicterus, infantile Gaucher disease, and some aminoacidurias.

Apnea

CLINICAL FEATURES. An irregular respiratory pattern with intermittent pauses of 3 to 6 seconds, often followed by 10 to 15 seconds of hyperpnea, is regularly seen in premature infants. The pauses are not associated with significant alterations in heart rate, blood pressure, body temperature, or skin color. This respiratory pattern, termed *periodic breathing,* is caused by immaturity of the brainstem respiratory centers. The incidence of periodic breathing correlates directly with the degree of prematurity. Apneic spells are more common during active than quiet sleep.

Apneic spells of 10 to 15 seconds are detectable at some time in almost all premature and some full-term newborns. Apneic spells of 10 to 20 seconds are usually associated with a 20% reduction in heart rate. Longer episodes of apnea are almost invariably associated with a 40% or greater reduction in heart rate. The frequency of these apneic spells correlates with

brainstem myelination. Even at 40 weeks conceptional age, premature newborns continue to have a higher incidence of apnea than do full-term newborns. The incidence of apnea sharply decreases in all infants at 52 weeks conceptional age.

DIAGNOSIS. Apneic spells in otherwise normal-appearing newborns should be considered a sign of brainstem immaturity and not a pathologic condition. The brainstem auditory evoked response is useful in this regard. The interpeak latency between waves V and I is longer in premature infants with apnea than in those without apnea at the same conceptional age. Apnea is common when the interpeak latency is greater than 6 ms and decreases in frequency as latencies less than 5.6 ms are attained.

The sudden onset of apnea and states of decreased consciousness, especially in premature newborns, suggests an intracranial hemorrhage with brainstem compression. Immediate ultrasound examination is indicated.

Apneic spells are almost never a seizure manifestation unless they are associated with tonic deviation of the eyes, tonic stiffening of the body, or characteristic limb movements. The absence of bradycardia in association with prolonged apnea suggests the possibility of seizures.

Benign Nocturnal Myoclonus

CLINICAL FEATURES. Sudden jerking movements of the limbs during sleep occur in normal people of all ages (see Chapter 14). They appear primarily during the early stages of sleep as repeated flexion movements of the fingers, wrists, and elbows. The jerks are never consistently focal, are not stopped by gentle restraint, but end abruptly with arousal (Daoust-Roy and Seshia, 1992). When prolonged, they may be misdiagnosed as focal clonic or myoclonic seizures.

DIAGNOSIS. Nocturnal myoclonus can be distinguished from seizures and jitteriness because it occurs solely during sleep, it is not activated by a stimulus, and the EEG is normal.

TREATMENT. Treatment is not required. Anticonvulsant drugs may increase the frequency of myoclonus by causing sedation.

Jitteriness

CLINICAL FEATURES. Jitteriness or tremulousness is an excessive response to stimulation. Touch, noise, and especially motion produce low-frequency, high-amplitude shaking of the limbs and jaw. Jitteriness is commonly associated with a low threshold for the Moro reflex, but it can occur in the absence of any apparent stimulation and be confused with myoclonic seizures.

DIAGNOSIS. Jitteriness usually occurs in newborns with perinatal asphyxia, some of whom have seizures as well. It can be distinguished from seizures by EEG monitoring, by the absence of eye movements or alteration in respiratory pattern, and by the presence of stimulus activation. Jitteriness is also encountered in newborns of addicted mothers and in newborns with metabolic disorders.

TREATMENT. Reduced stimulation decreases jitteriness. However, newborns of addicted mothers require sedation to facilitate feeding and to decrease energy expenditure.

DIFFERENTIAL DIAGNOSIS OF SEIZURES

Seizures are a feature of almost all brain disorders in the newborn. The time of onset of the first seizure is very helpful in determining the cause (Table 1–3). Seizures occurring during the first 24 hours, and especially in the first 12 hours, are usually due to hypoxic-ischemic encephalopathy. Sepsis, meningitis, and subarachnoid hemorrhage are next in frequency, followed by intrauterine infection and trauma. Direct drug effects, intraventricular hemorrhage at term, and pyridoxine dependency are relatively rare causes of seizures.

During the period from 24 to 72 hours after birth, seizures are most commonly caused by intraventricular hemorrhage in premature newborns, by subarachnoid hemorrhage and cerebral contusion in large full-term newborns, and by sepsis and meningitis at all gestational ages. Focal clonic seizures in full-term newborns are usually caused by cerebral infarction, intracerebral hemorrhage, or venous thrombosis. Cerebral dysgenesis causes seizures at this time and remains an important cause of seizures throughout infancy. All other conditions are relatively rare. Newborns with metabolic disorders are usually lethargic and feed poorly before the onset of seizures.

After 72 hours, inborn errors of metabolism, especially aminoacidurias, become a more important consideration because protein and glucose feedings have been initiated. A battery of screening tests for metabolic disorders is outlined in Table 1–4. Herpes simplex infection is

■ TABLE 1–3

Differential Diagnosis of Neonatal Seizures by Peak Time of Onset

24 Hours

Bacterial meningitis and sepsis (see Chapter 4)
Direct drug effect
Hypoxic-ischemic encephalopathy
Intrauterine infection (see Chapter 5)
Intraventricular hemorrhage at term (see Chapter 4)
Laceration of tentorium or falx
Pyridoxine dependency
Subarachnoid hemorrhage

24 to 72 Hours

Bacterial meningitis and sepsis (see Chapter 4)
Cerebral contusion with subdural hemorrhage
Cerebral dysgenesis (see Chapter 18)
Cerebral infarction (see Chapter 11)
Drug withdrawal
Glycine encephalopathy
Glycogen synthase deficiency
Hypoparathyroidism-hypocalcemia
Idiopathic cerebral venous thrombosis
Incontinentia pigmenti
Intracerebral hemorrhage (see Chapter 11)
Intraventricular hemorrhage in premature newborns (see Chapter 4)
Pyridoxine dependency
Subarachnoid hemorrhage
Tuberous sclerosis
Urea cycle disturbances

72 Hours to 1 Week

Familial neonatal seizures
Cerebral dysgenesis (see Chapter 18)
Cerebral infarction (see Chapter 11)
Hypoparathyroidism
Idiopathic cerebral venous thrombosis
Intracerebral hemorrhage (see Chapter 11)
Kernicterus
Methylmalonic acidemia
Nutritional hypocalcemia
Propionic acidemia
Tuberous sclerosis
Urea cycle disturbances

1 Week to 4 Weeks

Adrenoleukodystrophy, neonatal (see Chapter 6)
Cerebral dysgenesis (see Chapter 18)
Fructose dysmetabolism
Gaucher disease type 2 (see Chapter 5)
GM_1 gangliosidosis type 1 (see Chapter 5)
Herpes simplex encephalitis
Idiopathic cerebral venous thrombosis
Ketotic hyperglycinemias
Maple syrup urine disease, neonatal
Tuberous sclerosis
Urea cycle disturbances

transmitted during delivery and does not become symptomatic until the second half of the first week. Among the conditions that cause early seizures and can also cause late seizures are cerebral dysgenesis, cerebral infarction, intrace-

■ TABLE 1–4
Screening for Inborn Errors of Metabolism That Cause Neonatal Seizures

Blood Glucose Low
Fructose 1,6-diphosphatase deficiency
Glycogen storage disease type 1
Maple syrup urine disease

Blood Calcium Low
Hypoparathyroidism
Maternal hyperparathyroidism

Blood Ammonia High
Argininosuccinic acidemia
Carbamyl phosphate synthetase deficiency
Citrullinemia
Methylmalonic acidemia (may be normal)
Multiple carboxylase deficiency
Ornithine transcarbamylase deficiency
Propionic acidemia (may be normal)

Blood Lactate High
Fructose 1,6-diphosphatase deficiency
Glycogen storage disease type I
Mitochondrial disorders
Multiple carboxylase deficiency

Metabolic Acidosis
Fructose 1,6-diphosphatase deficiency
Glycogen storage disease type I
Maple syrup urine disease
Methylmalonic acidemia
Multiple carboxylase deficiency
Propionic acidemia

Urine Ferric Chloride or Dinitrophenylhydrazine
Maple syrup urine disease

No Rapid Screening Test
Adrenoleukodystrophy, neonatal form
Glycine encephalopathy
Glycogen synthase deficiency
Infantile GM_1 gangliosidosis type 1

rebral hemorrhage, and familial neonatal seizures.

Hypoxic-Ischemic Encephalopathy

Asphyxia at term is almost always an intrauterine event, and hypoxia and ischemia occur together; the result is hypoxic-ischemic encephalopathy (HIE). Acute total asphyxia usually leads to death from circulatory collapse. Affected fetuses are stillborn or die in the perinatal period. Occasional survivors are born comatose and have evidence of cranial nerve dysfunction. The usual mechanism of HIE in surviving full-term newborns is partial, prolonged asphyxia. The fetal circulation accommodates to reductions in arterial oxygen by maximizing blood flow to the brain, and to a lesser extent the heart, at the expense of other organs.

Clinical experience indicates that the fetus may be subjected to considerable hypoxia without brain damage developing. The incidence of cerebral palsy among full-term newborns with a 5-minute Apgar score of 0 to 3 is only 1% if the 10-minute score is 4 or higher. Any episode of hypoxia sufficiently severe to cause brain damage also causes derangements in other organs. Newborns with mild HIE always have a history of irregular heart rate and usually pass meconium. Those with severe HIE may have lactic acidosis, elevated serum concentrations of hepatic enzymes, enterocolitis, renal failure, and fatal myocardial damage.

CLINICAL FEATURES. Mild HIE is relatively common. The newborn is lethargic but not unconscious immediately after birth. Other characteristic features are jitteriness and sympathetic overactivity (tachycardia, dilatation of pupils, and decreased bronchial and salivary secretions). Muscle tone is normal at rest, tendon reflexes are normoreactive or hyperactive, and ankle clonus is usually elicited. The Moro reflex is complete, and repetitive extension and flexion movements are generated by a single stimulus. Seizures are not an expected feature, and their occurrence suggests concurrent hypoglycemia or the presence of a second condition.

Symptoms diminish and disappear during the first few days, although some degree of overresponsiveness may persist. Newborns with mild HIE are believed to recover normal brain function completely. They are not at greater risk for later epilepsy or learning disabilities.

Newborns with severe HIE are stuporous or comatose immediately after birth, and respiratory effort is usually periodic and insufficient to sustain life. Seizures begin within the first 12 hours. Hypotonia is severe, and tendon reflexes, the Moro reflex, and the tonic neck reflex are absent as well. Sucking and swallowing are depressed or absent, but the pupillary and oculovestibular reflexes are present. Most have frequent seizures, which may only be appreciated on EEG, that progress to status epilepticus. The response to anticonvulsant drugs is usually incomplete. Generalized increased intracranial pressure develops between 24 and 72 hours of age. This is characterized by coma, bulging of the fontanelles, loss of pupillary and oculovestibular reflexes, and respiratory arrest.

The newborn may die at this time or may remain stuporous for several weeks. The encephalopathy begins to subside after the third day, and seizures decrease in frequency and eventually stop. Jitteriness is common as the child becomes arousable. Tone increases in the limbs during the succeeding weeks. Neurologic sequelae are expected in newborns with severe HIE who remain comatose for more than a week.

DIAGNOSIS. EEG and CT are helpful in determining the severity and prognosis of HIE. In mild HIE the EEG background rhythms are normal or lacking in variability. In severe HIE the background is always abnormal and shows suppression of background amplitude. The degree of suppression correlates well with the severity of HIE. The worst case is a flat EEG or one with a burst-suppression pattern. A bad outcome is invariable if the amplitude remains suppressed for 2 weeks or a burst-suppression pattern is present at any time. Epileptiform activity may also be present but is less predictive of outcome than is background suppression.

Two to 4 days after injury, CT shows the cerebral edema of severe HIE as a diffuse decrease in tissue attenuation. Repeat CT or MRI after 1 month shows the full extent of injury.

TREATMENT. The management of HIE in newborns requires immediate attention to derangements in several organs and correction of acidosis. No therapeutic regimen has proved effective in treating the encephalopathy, although many new approaches seem promising (Palmer and Vannucci, 1993). Nevertheless, clinical experience and some studies indicate that control of seizures, maintenance of adequate ventilation and perfusion, and prevention of fluid overload increase the chance of a favorable outcome. Intracranial pressure may be lessened by the simple procedure of elevating the head to 30 degrees and reducing fluids by 10%.

The use of phenobarbital to treat seizures in newborns is detailed in a separate section. If high dosages of phenobarbital prove ineffective, other drugs are unlikely to be successful. Seizures usually cease spontaneously during the second week, and anticonvulsants should be stopped after a further 2 weeks of control. The incidence of later epilepsy among infants who had neonatal seizures caused by HIE is 30% to 40%; this outcome is not influenced by continuing anticonvulsant therapy after the initial seizures have stopped (Hellström-Westas et al, 1995).

Trauma and Intracranial Hemorrhage

Neonatal head trauma occurs most often in large term newborns of primiparous mothers. Usually labor was prolonged and extraction was difficult because of fetal malposition or a precipitous delivery before the maternal cervix was suf-

ficiently dilated. Intracranial hemorrhage may be subarachnoid, subdural, or intraventricular. Intraventricular hemorrhage is discussed in Chapter 4.

Primary Subarachnoid Hemorrhage

CLINICAL FEATURES. Blood in the subarachnoid space probably originates from tearing of the superficial veins by shearing forces during a prolonged delivery with the head engaged. Mild HIE is often associated with subarachnoid hemorrhage, but the newborn is usually well when an unexpected seizure occurs on the first or second day of life. Lumbar puncture is performed because of suspected sepsis, and blood is found in the cerebrospinal fluid. Most newborns with subarachnoid hemorrhages will be neurologically normal later.

DIAGNOSIS. CT is useful to document the extent of hemorrhage. Blood is present in the interhemispheric fissure and the supratentorial and infratentorial recesses. Routine ultrasound does not reliably show blood in the subarachnoid space. Epileptiform activity may be seen on the EEG, but the background is not suppressed. This indicates that seizures are not caused by HIE and that the prognosis is more favorable. Clotting studies should be performed to exclude the possibility of a coagulopathy.

TREATMENT. Seizures usually respond to phenobarbital. Specific therapy is not available for the hemorrhage, and posthemorrhagic hydrocephalus is uncommon.

Subdural Hemorrhage

CLINICAL FEATURES. Subdural hemorrhage is usually the consequence of a tear in the tentorium near its junction with the falx. The tear is caused by excessive vertical molding of the head in vertex presentation, anteroposterior elongation of the head in face and brow presentations, or prolonged delivery of the aftercoming head in breech presentation. Blood collects in the posterior fossa and may produce brainstem compression. The initial features are those of mild to moderate HIE. Clinical evidence of brainstem compression is delayed for 12 hours or longer and is characterized by irregular respiration, abnormal cry, declining consciousness, hypotonia, seizures, and a tense fontanelle. Intracerebellar hemorrhage is sometimes present. Mortality is high, and neurologic impairment among survivors is common.

DIAGNOSIS. Subdural hemorrhage is readily visualized by CT and ultrasound.

TREATMENT. Small hemorrhages do not require treatment, but large collections should be evacuated surgically to relieve brainstem compression.

Idiopathic Cerebral Venous Thrombosis

Cerebral venous thrombosis in newborns may be caused by coagulopathies, polycythemia, sepsis, and asphyxia. Cerebral venous thrombosis, especially that involving the superior sagittal sinus, also occurs without known predisposing factors (Rivkin et al, 1992).

CLINICAL FEATURES. The initial symptom is focal seizures or lethargy beginning anytime during the first month. Intracranial pressure remains normal, lethargy slowly resolves, and seizures respond to phenobarbital. Long-term outcome is uncertain and probably depends upon the extent of hemorrhagic infarction of the hemisphere.

DIAGNOSIS. CT is satisfactory for diagnosis, but MRI provides a more comprehensive assessment of involved vessels and the extent of brain damage.

TREATMENT. Anticoagulation does not influence outcome and is not recommended.

Hypoglycemia

A transitory, asymptomatic hypoglycemia can be detected in 11% of newborns during the first hours after delivery and before oral feeding is initiated. Hypoglycemia is not associated with neurologic impairment later in life. Symptomatic hypoglycemia may result from cerebral stress or inborn errors of metabolism (Table 1–5).

CLINICAL FEATURES. The time of onset of symptoms depends upon the underlying disorder. Early onset is generally associated with perinatal asphyxia or intracranial hemorrhage, and late onset with inborn errors of metabolism. Hypoglycemia is rare and mild among newborns with classic maple syrup urine disease, ethylmalonic aciduria, and isolaveric acidemia, and invariably severe in 3-methylglutaconic aciduria, glutaric aciduria type 2, and disorders of fructose metabolism (Worthen et al, 1994).

The syndrome includes any of the following symptoms: apnea, cyanosis, tachypnea, jitteriness, high-pitched cry, poor feeding, vomiting, apathy, hypotonia, seizures, and coma. Symptomatic hypoglycemia is often associated with later neurologic impairment.

DIAGNOSIS. Neonatal hypoglycemia is defined as a whole-blood glucose concentration of less than 20 mg/dl (1 mmol/L) in premature and low–birth-weight newborns, less than 30 mg/dl (1.5 mmol/L) in term newborns during the first 72 hours, and less than 40 mg/dl (2 mmol/L) in full-term newborns after 72 hours.

TREATMENT. Normal blood glucose concentrations can be restored by intravenous administration of glucose, but the underlying cause must be determined before definitive treatment can be provided.

Hypocalcemia

Hypocalcemia is defined as a blood calcium concentration less than 7 mg/dl (1.75 mmol/L). The onset of hypocalcemia in the first 72 hours after delivery is associated with low birth weight, asphyxia, maternal diabetes, transient neonatal hypoparathyroidism, maternal hyperparathyroidism, and the DiGeorge syndrome. Later-onset hypocalcemia is seen in children fed evaporated cow's milk and other improper formulas, in maternal hyperparathyroidism, and in the DiGeorge syndrome

Hypoparathyroidism in the newborn may result from maternal hyperparathyroidism or be a transient phenomenon of unknown cause. Hypocalcemia occurs in less than 10% of stressed newborns and enhances their vulner-

■ TABLE 1–5
Causes of Neonatal Hypoglycemia

Primary Transitional Hypoglycemia
Complicated labor and delivery
Intrauterine malnutrition
Maternal diabetes
Prematurity
Secondary Transitional Hypoglycemia
Asphyxia
Central nervous system disorders
Cold injuries
Sepsis
Persistent Hypoglycemia
Aminoacidurias
    Maple syrup urine disease
    Methylmalonic acidemia
    Propionic acidemia
    Tyrosinosis
Congenital hypopituitarism
Defects in carbohydrate metabolism
    Fructose 1,6-diphosphatase deficiency
    Fructose intolerance
    Galactosemia
    Glycogen storage disease type 1
    Glycogen synthase deficiency
Hyperinsulinism
Organic acidurias
    Glutaric aciduria type 2
    3-methylglutaryl-CoA lyase deficiency

ability to seizures, but it is rarely the primary cause.

DiGeorge Syndrome

The DiGeorge syndrome is associated with microdeletions of chromosome 22q11 (Driscoll, 1994).

CLINICAL FEATURES. The DiGeorge syndrome is a congenital hypoplasia of organs derived from the third and fourth pharyngeal pouches (thymus, parathyroid gland, and great vessels). The main features are multiple minor facial anomalies, hypocalcemic seizures, lymphocytopenia, and congenital heart disease. The symptoms may be due to congenital heart disease, hypocalcemia, or both. Jitteriness and tetany usually begin in the first 48 hours after delivery. The peak onset of seizures is on the third day but may be delayed for 2 weeks. Many affected newborns die of cardiac causes during the first month; survivors fail to thrive and have frequent infections because of the failure of cell-mediated immunity.

DIAGNOSIS. In newborns who come to medical attention because of heart disease, hypocalcemia may be suspected when a prolonged Q-T interval is detected on the electrocardiogram (ECG). All newborns with symptoms of hypocalcemia should be examined for cardiac defects.

TREATMENT. Hypocalcemia generally responds to parathyroid hormone or to oral calcium and vitamin D.

Aminoacidopathies

Maple Syrup Urine Disease

The neonatal form of maple syrup urine disease (MSUD) is caused by an almost complete absence (less than 5% of normal) of branched-chain ketoacid dehydrogenase (BCKD). The BCKD complex is composed of four subunits and the gene for each subunit is on a different chromosome (19-6-1-7) (Pfeinemann and Danner, 1994).

The incidence of MSUD is 1:200,000 live births. Leucine, isoleucine, and valine cannot be decarboxylated, and they accumulate in blood, urine, and tissues (Figure 1-1). Later-onset forms are described in Chapters 5 and 10. The defect is transmitted by autosomal recessive inheritance.

CLINICAL FEATURES. Affected newborns appear healthy at birth, but lethargy, feeding difficulty, and hypotonia develop after ingestion of protein. Seizures begin in the second week and are associated with the development of cerebral edema (Riviello et al, 1991). Once seizures begin, they continue with increasing frequency and severity. Without therapy, cerebral edema becomes progressively worse and results in coma and death within 1 month.

DIAGNOSIS. Rapid screening of urine for MSUD can be accomplished by the addition of ferric chloride, which colors urine deep blue, or with 2,4-dinitrophenylhydrazine, which causes a cloudy, yellow precipitate. The diagnosis is established by showing increased plasma concentrations of the three branch-chained amino acids or enzyme deficiency in peripheral leukocytes. Heterozygotes can be detected by diminished levels of enzyme activity.

TREATMENT. Exchange transfusions or peritoneal dialysis transiently lowers the plasma concentration of branch-chained amino acids and ketoacids. Administration of glucose and insulin provides a more prolonged reduction by promoting the uptake of amino acids into skeletal muscle.

A special diet, low in branched-chain amino acids (MSUD formula, Mead-Johnson), may prevent further encephalopathy and should be started immediately by nasogastric tube. Thiamine supplementation, 10 to 20 mg/kg/day, should be tried as well. Early diagnosis and treatment can result in normal intellectual outcome (Kaplan et al, 1991).

Glycine Encephalopathy

Glycine encephalopathy (nonketotic hyperglycinemia) is caused by a defect in the glycine cleaving system. It is inherited as an autosomal recessive trait (Hamosh et al, 1995).

CLINICAL FEATURES. Affected newborns are normal at birth but become irritable and refuse feeding anytime from 6 hours to 8 days after delivery. The onset of symptoms is usually within 48 hours but may be delayed by a few weeks in milder allelic forms. Hiccupping is an early and continuous feature; some mothers relate that the child hiccupped in utero. Progressive lethargy, hypotonia, respiratory disturbances, and myoclonic seizures follow. Some newborns survive the acute illness, but their subsequent course is characterized by mental retardation, epilepsy, and spasticity.

DIAGNOSIS. During the acute encephalopathy the EEG demonstrates a burst-suppression pattern, which later evolves into hypsarrhythmia during infancy. MRI shows partial agenesis of the corpus callosum. The diagnosis is estab-

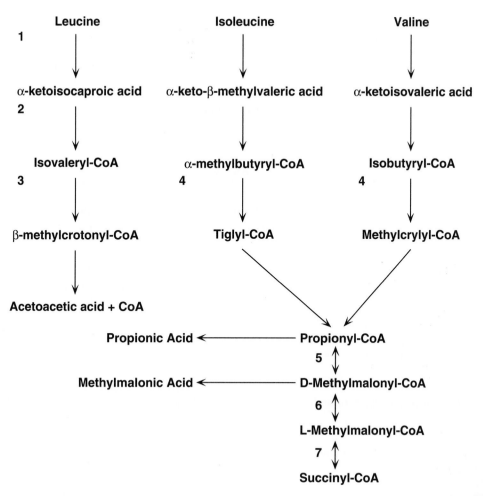

☐ F I G U R E 1 – 1 Branched-chain amino acid metabolism. 1, Transaminase system. 2, Branched-chain α-ketoacid dehydrogenase. 3, Isovaleryl-CoA dehydrogenase. 4, α-Methyl branched-chain acyl-CoA dehydrogenase. 5, Propionyl-CoA carboxylase (biotin cofactor). 6, Methylmalonyl-CoA racemase. 7, Methylmalonyl-CoA mutase (adenosylcobalamin cofactor).

lished by showing hyperglycinemia, and especially elevated concentrations of glycine in the cerebrospinal fluid, in the absence of hyperammonemia or organic acidemia.

TREATMENT. Exchange transfusion provides only temporary relief of the encephalopathy, and diet therapy has not proved successful in modifying the course. Diazepam, a competitor for glycine receptors, in combination with choline, folic acid, and sodium benzoate, may stop the seizures. Benzoate doses as high as 250 to 750 mg/kg are tolerated and should be tried (Hamosh et al, 1995).

Urea Cycle Disturbances

Carbamyl phosphate synthetase (CPS) *deficiency, ornithine transcarbamylase* (OTC) *de-ficiency, citrullinemia, argininosuccinic aci-demia,* and *argininemia* (arginase deficiency) are the disorders caused by defects in the enzyme systems responsible for urea synthesis (Figure 1–2). Arginase deficiency does not cause symptoms in the newborn. OTC deficiency is an X-linked trait; all others are transmitted by autosomal recessive inheritance. The prevalence of urea cycle enzyme deficiencies is estimated to be 1:30,000 live births.

CLINICAL FEATURES. The clinical features of urea cycle disorders are due to ammonia intoxication (Table 1–6). Progressive lethargy, vomiting, and hypotonia may develop on the first day after delivery, even before the initiation of protein feeding, and are followed by progressive loss of consciousness and seizures on subsequent days. Vomiting and lethargy correlate well

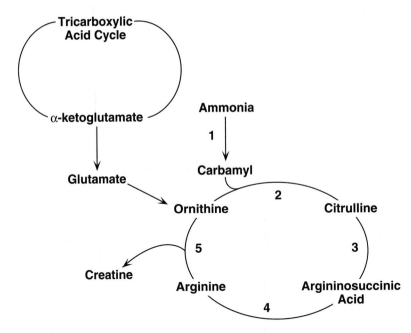

☐ F I G U R E   1 – 2 Ammonia metabolism. 1, Carbamyl phosphate sythetase (CPS). 2, Orithine transcarba-mylase (OTC). 3, Argininosuccinate sythetase (AS). 4, Argininosuccinate lyase (AL). 5, Arginase.

■ T A B L E   1 – 6
Causes of Neonatal Hyperammonemia

LIVER FAILURE

Primary Enzyme Defects in Urea Synthesis
Argininosuccinic acidemia
Carbamyl phosphate synthetase deficiency
Citrullinemia
Ornithine transcarbamylase deficiency
Other Disorders of Amino Acid Metabolism
Glycine encephalopathy
Isovaleric acidemia
Methylmalonic acidemia
Multiple carboxylase deficiency
Propionic acidemia
Transitory Hyperammonemia of Prematurity

with plasma ammonia concentrations greater than 200 µg/dl (120 µmol/L); coma with concentrations greater than 300 µg/dl (180 µmol/L); and seizures with those greater than 500 µg/dl (300 µmol/L). Death follows quickly in untreated newborns.

Newborns with partial deficiency of CPS and female carriers of OTC deficiency may become symptomatic after ingesting a large protein load.

DIAGNOSIS. The diagnosis of a urea cycle disturbance should be suspected in every newborn with a compatible clinical syndrome and hyperammonemia without organic acidemia. Hyperammonemia can be life-threatening, and rapid diagnosis, within 24 hours, is essential. Blood ammonia concentration should be analyzed immediately and plasma studied for acid-base status and concentrations of quantitative amino acids, creatinine, sodium, potassium, chloride, calcium, glucose, free and total carnitine, and lactate. A spot urine should be analyzed for quantitative amino acids, orotic acid, organic acids, and carnitine concentrations.

The diagnosis is established by identification of the specific enzyme defect in hepatic tissue or peripheral leukocytes.

TREATMENT. Treatment cannot await specific diagnosis in newborns with symptomatic hyperammonemia due to inborn errors of urea synthesis (Batshaw, 1994). Nitrogen intake is limited to 1.2 to 2.0 g/kg/day and a large percentage of the protein content should be essential amino acids. Arginine concentrations are low in all inborn errors of urea synthesis except for arginase deficiency and must be supplemented. Alternative pathways for nitrogen excretion must be provided. In addition to removal of ammonia by peritoneal dialysis or hemodialysis, waste nitrogen excretion through pathways other than urea synthesis can be promoted by sodium benzoate and phenylacetic acid. Nitrogen can be removed by peritoneal dialysis when blood ammonia concentrations become dangerously high.

Long-term management of disorders of urea synthesis requires a protein-restricted diet and arginine supplementation. Sodium benzoate and sodium phenylacetate (1.75 mmol/kg/day) should be continued as well. Even with optimal supervision, episodes of hyperammonemia may occur and may lead to coma and death. In such cases, intravenous administration of sodium benzoate, sodium phenylacetate, and arginine, coupled with nitrogen-free alimentation, is indicated. Peritoneal dialysis or hemodialysis is indicated if the patient does not respond to drug therapy.

Organic Acid Disorders

Organic acid disorders are characterized by the accumulation of compounds, usually ketones or lactic acid, that cause acidosis in biologic fluids (Ozand and Gascon, 1991). More than 50 organic acid disorders have been described. They can be caused by abnormalities in vitamin metabolism, lipid metabolism, glycolysis, the citric acid cycle, oxidative metabolism, glutathione metabolism, and 4-aminobutyric acid metabolism. The clinical presentations vary considerably and are described in several chapters.

Defects in the further metabolism of branched-chain amino acids are the organic acid disorders that most often cause neonatal seizures.

Isovaleric Acidemia

Isovaleric acid is a fatty acid derived from leucine. Its conversion to propionyl-coenzyme A (CoA) is metabolized by the enzyme isovaleryl-CoA dehydrogenase (Figure 1–1). Isovaleric acidemia is transmitted by autosomal recessive inheritance, and the heterozygote state can be detected in cultured fibroblasts.

CLINICAL FEATURES. Two phenotypes are associated with the same enzyme defect. One is an acute, overwhelming disorder of the newborn; the other is a chronic infantile form. Newborns are normal at birth but within a few days become lethargic, refuse to feed, and vomit. The clinical syndrome is similar to MSUD except that the urine is described as smelling like "sweaty feet" instead of maple syrup. Sixty percent of affected newborns die within 3 weeks. The survivors have a clinical syndrome identical to the chronic infantile phenotype.

DIAGNOSIS. Isovaleric acidosis is detected by the excretion of isovaleryl-lysine in the urine. Isovaleryl-CoA dehydrogenase activity can be assayed in cultured fibroblasts. The clinical phenotype correlates not with the percentage of residual enzyme activity, but with the ability to detoxify isovaleryl-CoA with glycine.

TREATMENT. Dietary restriction of protein, especially leucine, decreases the occurrence of later psychomotor retardation. L-Carnitine, 50 mg/kg/day, is a beneficial supplement to the diet of some children with isovaleric acidemia. In acutely ill newborns, oral glycine, 250 to 500 mg/day, in addition to protein restriction and carnitine, lowers mortality.

Propionic Acidemia

Propionyl-CoA is formed as a catabolite of methionine, threonine, and the branched-chain amino acids. Its further carboxylation to D-methylmalonyl-CoA requires the enzyme propionyl-CoA carboxylase and the coenzyme biotin (Figure 1–1). Isolated deficiency of propionyl-CoA carboxylase causes propionic acidemia (Hamilton et al, 1995). The defect is transmitted as an autosomal recessive trait.

CLINICAL FEATURES. Most affected children appear normal at birth; symptoms may begin as early as the first day after delivery but can be delayed for months or years. In newborns, the symptoms are nonspecific: feeding difficulty, lethargy, hypotonia, and dehydration. The subsequent course is characterized by recurrent attacks of profound metabolic acidosis often associated with hyperammonemia, which respond poorly to buffering. Untreated newborns rapidly become dehydrated, have generalized or myoclonic seizures, and become comatose.

Hepatomegaly caused by a fatty infiltration occurs in 28% of patients. Neutropenia, thrombocytopenia, and occasionally pancytopenia may be present. A bleeding diathesis accounts for massive intracranial hemorrhage in some newborns.

Children who survive beyond infancy develop infarctions in the basal ganglia.

DIAGNOSIS. Propionic acidemia should be considered in any newborn with ketoacidosis but must also be considered in newborns with hyperammonemia without ketoacidosis, since an erroneous diagnosis of carbamyl phosphate synthesis deficiency may be suggested. Propionic acidemia is the probable diagnosis when the plasma concentrations of glycine and propionate and the urinary concentrations of glycine, methylcitrate, and beta-hydroxypropionate are increased. While the urinary concentration of propionate may be normal, the plasma concentration is always elevated without a concurrent increase in the concentration of methylma-lonate.

The definitive diagnosis of propionic acidemia is established by showing a deficiency of enzyme activity in peripheral blood leukocytes or in skin fibroblasts. Prenatal diagnosis is accomplished by detecting methylcitrate, a unique metabolite of propionate, in the amniotic fluid, and by showing deficient enzyme activity in amniotic fluid cells.

TREATMENT. The newborn in ketoacidosis requires dialysis to remove toxic metabolites, parenteral fluids to prevent dehydration, and protein-free nutrition. The frequency and sever-ity of subsequent attacks are decreased by re-stricting protein intake to 0.5 to 1.5 g/kg/day. Oral administration of L-carnitine reduces the ke-togenic response to fasting and may be useful as a daily supplement. Biotin supplementation is often used, although its benefit has not been established.

Methylmalonic Acidemia

D-Methylmalonyl-CoA is racemized to L-methylmalonyl-CoA by the enzyme D-methyl-malonyl racemase and then isomerized to succinyl-CoA, which enters the tricarboxylic cycle (Rosenblatt, 1994). Isomerization is cata-lyzed by the enzyme D-methylmalonyl-CoA mu-tase, with the cobalamin (vitamin B_{12}) coen-zyme adenosylcobalamin required as a cofactor. Several defects in this pathway are known; all are transmitted by autosomal recessive inheritance (Ozand et al, 1994). Mutase deficiency is the most common abnormality. Propionyl-CoA, pro-pionic acid, and methylmalonic acid accumulate and cause hyperglycinemia and hyperammone-mia. Each of the enzyme defects responsible for methylmalonic acidemia is believed to be trans-mitted as an autosomal recessive trait.

CLINICAL FEATURES. Affected children ap-pear normal at birth. In 80% of those with complete mutase deficiency, the symptoms ap-pear during the first week after delivery; those with defects in the synthesis of adenosylcobal-amin generally show symptoms after 1 month. Symptoms include lethargy, failure to thrive, recurrent vomiting, dehydration, respiratory distress, and hypotonia after the initiation of protein feeding. Leukopenia, thrombocytope-nia, and anemia are present in more than one half of patients. Intracranial hemorrhage may result from a bleeding diathesis. The outcome for newborns with complete mutase deficiency is usually poor. Most die within 2 months of diagnosis; survivors have recurrent acidosis, growth retardation, and mental retardation.

DIAGNOSIS. The diagnosis should be sus-pected in any newborn with metabolic acidoses, especially if associated with ketosis, hyperam-monemia, and hyperglycinemia. The diagnosis is confirmed by the demonstration of increased concentration of methylmalonate in the plasma and urine. The specific enzyme defect can be determined in fibroblasts. Techniques for prena-tal detection are available.

TREATMENT. Treatment of newborns with mutase deficiency is confined to dietary therapy and management of metabolic disturbances as in propionic acidemia. Vitamin B_{12} supplementa-tion is useful in some defects of adenosylcobal-amin synthesis, and hydroxocobalamin, 1 mg, should be administered while the definitive diagnosis is awaited. Treatment is then main-tained with protein restriction (0.5 to 1.5 g/kg/day) and hydroxocobalamin, 1 mg, weekly. As in propionic acidemia, oral supplementation of L-carnitine reduces ketogenesis in response to fasting.

Herpes Simplex Encephalitis

Herpes genitalis (herpes simplex virus type 2, HSV-2) accounts for the majority of herpetic infections of the newborn (Overall, 1994). The newborn is most commonly infected during the second stage of labor by contact with maternal genital herpes, which is asymptomatic or unrec-ognized in 60% to 80% of women. Symptomatic infections occur in 8% of newborns whose mothers have a history of recurrent genital HSV infection. The risk of contamination at birth is greatest when the mother has primary genital herpes involving the cervix at delivery and the newborn is premature and delivered with instru-mentation, including scalp electrodes.

CLINICAL FEATURES. The clinical spectrum of perinatal HSV infection is wide. Among symptomatic newborns, two thirds have dis-seminated disease and one third have localized involvement of the brain, eyes, skin, or mouth. Whether disseminated or localized, approxi-mately half of infections involve the central nervous system. The overall mortality rate is 62%, and 50% of survivors have permanent neurologic impairment.

The onset of symptoms may be as early as the fifth day but is usually in the second week. A vesicular rash is present in 30%, usually on the scalp after vertex presentation and on the buttocks after breech presentation. Conjunctivitis, jaundice, and a bleeding diathesis may be present. The first symptoms of encephalitis are irritability and seizures. Seizures may be focal or generalized and are frequently refractory to therapy. Neurologic deterioration is progressive and characterized by coma and quadriparesis.

DIAGNOSIS. The EEG is always abnormal and shows a periodic pattern of slow waves or spike discharges. The cerebrospinal fluid examination demonstrates lymphocytic leukocytosis, red blood cells, and an elevated protein concentration. Diagnosis is established by culturing the virus or by viral identification in the cerebrospinal fluid using the polymerase chain reaction (Whitley and Lakeman, 1995).

TREATMENT. The best treatment is prevention. Recurrent genital herpes in adults can be suppressed by administration of acyclovir, 800 mg, as a single oral dose. All women with genital herpes at term whose membranes are intact or have been ruptured for less than 4 hours should be delivered by cesarean section. Acyclovir, 10 mg/kg every 8 hours for 10 to 14 days, is recommended for therapy in the newborn, but 10% with disseminated disease will relapse within 2 weeks after completion of the course. Mortality remains 50% or greater in newborns with disseminated disease.

Drug Withdrawal

Marijuana, alcohol, narcotic-analgesics, and hypnotic-sedatives are the drugs most commonly used during pregnancy. Marijuana and alcohol do not cause drug dependence in the fetus and are not associated with withdrawal symptoms. Hypnotic-sedatives, such as barbiturates, do not ordinarily produce withdrawal symptoms unless very large doses are ingested. Phenobarbital has a sufficiently long half-life in newborns that sudden withdrawal does not occur.

The prototype of narcotic withdrawal in the newborn is with heroin or methadone, but a similar syndrome occurs with codeine and propoxyphene.

CLINICAL FEATURES. Symptoms of opiate withdrawal are more severe and tend to occur earlier in full-term (first 24 hours) than in premature (24 to 48 hours) newborns (Doberczak et al, 1991). The initial feature is a coarse tremor, present only during the waking state, that can shake an entire limb. This is followed by irritability; a shrill, high-pitched cry; and hyperactivity. The newborn seems hungry but has difficulty feeding and vomits afterward. Diarrhea

and other symptoms of autonomic instability are common.

Myoclonic jerking is present in 10% to 25% of newborns undergoing withdrawal. Whether these movements are seizures or jitteriness is not clear. Definite seizures occur in fewer than 5%.

Maternal use of cocaine during pregnancy is associated with premature delivery, growth retardation, and microcephaly. Newborns exposed to cocaine in utero or after delivery through the breast milk often show features of cocaine intoxication including tachycardia, tachypnea, hypertension, irritability, and tremulousness.

DIAGNOSIS. Drug withdrawal should be suspected and anticipated in every newborn whose mother has a history of substance abuse. Even when such a history is not available, the combination of irritability, hyperactivity, and autonomic instability should provide a clue to diagnosis. Careful questioning of the mother concerning her use of prescription and nonprescription drugs is imperative. Specific drug identification is accomplished by blood and urine analyses.

TREATMENT. Symptoms remit spontaneously in 3 to 5 days, but appreciable mortality occurs among untreated newborns. Phenobarbital, 8 mg/kg/day, or chlorpromazine, 3 mg/kg/day, relieves symptoms and reduces mortality. Morphine, meperidine, opium, and methadone are not sufficiently secreted in breast milk to cause or relieve addiction in the newborn.

The occurrence of seizures does not in itself indicate a poor prognosis. Long-term outcome is closely related to the other risk factors associated with substance abuse in the mother.

Bilirubin Encephalopathy

Unconjugated bilirubin is bound to albumin in the blood. *Kernicterus,* a yellow discoloration of the brain especially severe in the basal ganglia and hippocampus, occurs when the serum unbound or free fraction becomes excessive. An excessive level of the free fraction in an otherwise healthy newborn is approximately 20 mg/100 ml (340 μmol/L). Kernicterus was an important complication of hemolytic disease from maternal-fetal blood group incompatibility, but this condition is now uncommon (Watchko and Claassen, 1994). Other causes of hyperbilirubinemia in full-term newborns are generally managed without difficulty. The group now at greatest risk are critically ill premature infants with respiratory distress syndrome, acidosis, and sepsis. In such newborns a serum unbound level of 10 mg/dl (170 μmol/L) may be sufficient to cause bilirubin encephalopathy, and even the albumin-bound fraction may pass the blood-brain barrier.

CLINICAL FEATURES. Three distinct clinical phases of bilirubin encephalopathy occur in full-term newborns with untreated hemolytic disease. Hypotonia, lethargy, and a poor sucking reflex are noted within 24 hours of delivery. Bilirubin staining of the brain is already evident in newborns who die during this first clinical phase. On the second or third day the newborn becomes febrile and shows increasing tone and opisthotonic posturing. Seizures are not a constant feature but may occur at this time. The third phase is characterized by apparent improvement with normalization of tone. This may cause second thoughts about the accuracy of the diagnosis, but the improvement is short lived. Evidence of neurologic dysfunction begins to appear toward the end of the second month and the symptoms become progressively worse throughout infancy.

In premature newborns, the clinical features are more subtle and may lack the phases of increased tone and opisthotonos. The majority of affected premature infants are believed to die in the newborn period.

The typical clinical syndrome after the first year includes extrapyramidal dysfunction, usually athetosis, which occurs in virtually every case (see Chapter 14); disturbances of vertical gaze, upward more often than downward, in 90%; high-frequency hearing loss in 60%; and mental retardation in 25%.

DIAGNOSIS. In newborns with hemolytic disease, a clinical diagnosis can be presumed on the basis of significant hyperbilirubinemia and a compatible evolution of symptoms. However, the diagnosis is difficult to establish in critically ill premature newborns, whose brain damage is more often caused by asphyxia and its consequences than by kernicterus.

The brainstem auditory evoked response (BAER) may be useful in assessing the severity of bilirubin encephalopathy and its response to treatment. The auditory nerve and pathways are especially susceptible to bilirubin encephalopathy. The generators of wave I and wave V of the BAER are the auditory nerve and the inferior colliculus. The latency of both waves increases in proportion to the concentration of free albumin and decreases after exchange transfusion.

TREATMENT. Kernicterus can be prevented by maintaining serum bilirubin concentrations below the toxic range either by phototherapy or exchange transfusion. Once kernicterus has occurred, further damage can be limited, but not reversed, by lowering serum bilirubin concentrations.

Pyridoxine Dependency

Pyridoxine dependency is a rare disorder, transmitted as an autosomal recessive trait. It may be caused by impaired glutamic decarboxylase activity. Neurotoxic concentrations of glutamate are measured in the cerebrospinal fluid (Baumeister et al, 1994).

CLINICAL FEATURES. Multifocal clonic seizures begin almost immediately after birth and progress rapidly to status epilepticus. However, a later onset, even after the first year, does not exclude the diagnosis. The seizures are refractory to standard anticonvulsants and respond only to pyridoxine. If pyridoxine supplementation is discontinued, seizures return within 3 weeks.

DIAGNOSIS. In most cases the diagnosis is suspected because a sibling was affected by the same syndrome and died. In the absence of a family history of the disorder, the diagnosis need be considered only in newborns with continuous seizures. The infantile-onset variety may be characterized by intermittent myoclonic seizures, focal clonic seizures, or generalized tonic-clonic seizures. The EEG is continuously abnormal because of generalized or multifocal spike discharges. An intravenous injection of pyridoxine, 100 mg, stops the clinical seizure activity and often converts the EEG to normal in less than 10 minutes.

Pyridoxine-responsive seizures also occur in newborns of mothers treated with isoniazid. The onset of seizures is in the third week after delivery.

TREATMENT. A life-long dietary supplement of pyridoxine, which varies from 10 to 30 mg/kg/day, prevents further seizures. The higher dose is used during infancy and the smaller dose in childhood. Subsequent psychomotor development is best when treatment is initiated early, but this does not ensure a normal outcome. The dose needed to prevent mental retardation may be higher than that needed to stop seizures.

Incontinentia Pigmenti (Bloch-Sulzberger Syndrome)

Incontinentia pigmenti is a rare neurocutaneous syndrome involving the skin, teeth, eyes, and central nervous system. It is transmitted as an X-linked trait (Xq28) lethal in the hemizygous male (Smahi et al, 1994).

CLINICAL FEATURES. The female-to-male ratio is 20:1. An erythematous and vesicular rash resembling epidermolysis bullosa is present on the flexor surfaces of the limbs and lateral aspect of the trunk at birth or soon thereafter. Neurologic disturbances occur in less than half of cases. In newborns, the prominent feature is the onset of seizures on the second or third day, often confined to one side of the body. The rash persists for the first few months and is replaced by a verrucous eruption that lasts weeks or months. Between 6 and 12 months of age, pigment is deposited in the previous area of rash in bizarre polymorphic arrangements. The pigmentation later regresses and may disappear.

Residual neurologic handicaps may include mental retardation, epilepsy, hemiparesis, and hydrocephalus. Two rare neurologic disturbances that may be associated with incontinenta pigmenti are degeneration of anterior horn cells, producing clinical features similar to those of infantile spinal muscular atrophy (see Chapter 6), and recurrent encephalomyelitis caused by transient loss of suppressor T cells.

DIAGNOSIS. Information about the character and evolution of the rash is essential for diagnosis.

TREATMENT. Neonatal seizures caused by incontinentia pigmenti usually respond to standard anticonvulsant drugs.

Benign Familial Neonatal Seizures

In some families several members have seizures in the first weeks of life but do not have epilepsy or other neurologic abnormalities later on. The trait is transmitted by autosomal dominant inheritance and the epileptic syndrome is considered one of the benign genetic epilepsies of childhood. The abnormal gene is localized to chromosome 20 in most families and on chromosome 8 in others (Berkovic et al, 1994, Steinlein et al, 1995).

CLINICAL FEATURES. Brief multifocal clonic seizures develop during the first week, sometimes associated with apnea. The onset may be delayed as long as 4 weeks. With or without treatment, the seizures usually stop spontaneously within 6 weeks. Febrile seizures occur in up to one third of children with chromosome 20-linked disease; some have febrile seizures without neonatal seizures. Epilepsy develops later in life in 10% to 15% of affected newborns.

DIAGNOSIS. The syndrome should be suspected when seizures develop without apparent cause in a healthy newborn. Laboratory tests, including the interictal EEG, show no abnormalities. During a seizure, the initial apnea and tonic activity is associated with flattening of the EEG; generalized spike-wave discharges occur during the clonic activity (Hirsch et al, 1993). A family history of neonatal seizures is critical to diagnosis but may not be discovered until grandparents are interviewed; parents are frequently unaware that they had neonatal seizures.

TREATMENT. Phenobarbital is usually effective to stop seizures. After 4 weeks of complete seizure control the drug can be tapered and discontinued. If seizures return, a longer trial should be initiated.

TREATMENT OF NEONATAL SEIZURES

Animal studies suggest that continuous seizure activity, even in the normoxemic brain, may cause brain damage by inhibiting protein synthesis and breaking down polyribosomes. In premature newborns, an additional concern is that the increased cerebral blood flow associated with seizures will increase the risk of intraventricular hemorrhage. Protein binding of anticonvulsant drugs may be impaired in premature newborns and the free fraction concentration may be toxic, whereas the measured protein-bound fraction appears therapeutic.

The initial steps in managing newborns with seizures are to maintain vital function, identify and correct the underlying cause (i.e., hypocalcemia) when possible, and rapidly provide a therapeutic blood concentration of an anticonvulsant drug when needed.

Phenobarbital

Intravenous phenobarbital is the treatment of choice for newborns with seizures. A unitary relationship usually exists between the intravenous dose of phenobarbital in milligrams per kilogram of body weight and the blood concentration in micrograms per milliliter measured 24 hours after the load (Gherpelli et al, 1993). A blood concentration of 20 µg/ml can be safely achieved with a single intravenous loading dose of 20 mg/kg injected at a rate of 5 mg/min. The usual maintenance dose is 4 mg/kg/day, but those who do not respond to the initial load should be given additional boluses of 10 mg/kg to a total of 40 mg/kg. Phenobarbital monotherapy is effective in 70% to 85% of newborns with seizures when blood levels of 40 µg/ml are achieved. In term newborns with intractable seizures from hypoxic-ischemic encephalopathy, additional boluses of phenobarbital can be used to achieve a blood concentration of 70 µg/ml, because such newborns are always being ventilated. If such concentrations of phenobarbital are ineffective, the addition of other drugs is unlikely to be helpful.

The half-life of phenobarbital in newborns varies from 50 to 200 hours, and additional doses should be administered only on the basis of current blood concentration information. After the tenth day the half-life shortens as the result of enzyme induction and a steady state is easier to achieve.

Phenytoin

Phenytoin can only be administered intravenously. Oral doses are poorly absorbed in newborns, and intramuscular doses are not absorbed at any age. A therapeutic blood concentration of 15 to 20 µg/ml (40 to 80 µmol/L) can be safely achieved by a single intravenous injection of 20 mg/kg at a rate of 0.5 mg/kg/min. The half-life is long during the first week, and further administration should be based on current knowledge of blood concentration. Most newborns require a maintenance dosage of 5 to 10 mg/kg/day.

Duration of Therapy

Seizures caused by an acute, self-limited encephalopathy, such as hypoxic-ischemic encephalopathy, do not ordinarily require prolonged maintenance therapy. In most newborns seizures stop when the acute encephalopathy is over. Therefore therapy should be discontinued after 2 weeks of complete seizure control. If seizures recur, anticonvulsant therapy can be reinitiated.

In contrast to newborns with seizures caused by acute encephalopathy, those with seizures caused by cerebral dysgenesis should be treated continuously. Eighty percent will be epileptic in childhood.

➡ Paroxysmal Disorders in Children Less Than 2 Years

The pathophysiology of paroxysmal disorders is more varied in infants than in newborns (Table 1-7). Seizures, especially febrile seizures, remain the major cause of paroxysmal disorders, but apnea and syncope (breathholding spells)

■ TABLE 1-7
Paroxysmal Disorders in Children Younger Than 2 Years

Apnea and Breathholding
Cyanotic
Pallid
Dystonia
Glutaric aciduria (see Chapter 14)
Transient paroxysmal dystonia of infancy
Migraine
Benign paroxysmal vertigo (see Chapter 10)
Cyclic vomiting
Paroxysmal torticollis (see Chapter 14)
Seizures
Febrile seizures
　Epilepsy triggered by fever
　Infection of the nervous system
　Simple febrile seizure
Nonfebrile seizures
　Generalized tonic-clonic seizures
　Partial seizures
　　Benign
　　Ictal laughter
Myoclonic seizures
　Infantile spasms
　Benign myoclonic epilepsy
　Severe myoclonic epilepsy
　Myoclonic status
　Lennox–Gastaut syndrome

are relatively common as well. Infants with paroxysmal disorders are frequently referred for neurologic consultation because of the suspicion of seizures. The determination of which "spells" are seizures is often difficult and relies more on obtaining a complete description of the spell than on laboratory tests. The parents should be asked to provide a sequential history. If more than one spell occurred, they should first describe the one that was best observed or most recent. The following questions should be included: What was the child doing before the spell? Did anything provoke the spell? Did the child's color change? If so, when and to what color? Did the eyes move in any direction? Was one part of the body affected more than another?

In addition to obtaining a home video of the spell, ambulatory EEG is useful in young infants to determine whether episodes of uncertain cause are seizures. It is almost impossible to keep an ambulatory EEG on a 1 to 2-year-old at home for very long. In some children, however, prolonged split-screen video-EEG monitoring is the only way to identify the nature of unusual spells.

APNEA AND SYNCOPE

Infant *apnea* is defined as cessation of breathing for 15 seconds or longer, or for less than 15 seconds if accompanied by bradycardia. Premature newborns with respiratory distress syndrome may continue to have apneic spells as infants, especially if they are neurologically abnormal.

Persistent apnea is often thought to be a seizure manifestation, but EEG monitoring in children with this condition rarely shows epileptiform activity in association with apneic spells or episodic tonic posturing.

Breathholding spells with loss of consciousness occur in almost 5% of infants (DiMario, 1992). They are a disturbance in central autonomic regulation probably transmitted by autosomal dominant inheritance with incomplete penetrance (DiMario and Burlson, 1993). Approximately 20% to 30% of parents of affected children have a history of the condition. The term "breathholding" is a misnomer because breathing always stops in expiration. Cyanotic and pallid varieties are described; cyanotic spells are 3 times more common than pallid spells. Most children experience only one or the other, but 20% have both.

The spells are involuntary responses to adverse stimuli. In approximately 80% of affected children the spells begin before 18 months of age, and in all cases start before 3 years of age. The last episode usually occurs by age 4 and no later than age 8.

Cyanotic Syncope

CLINICAL FEATURES. Cyanotic spells are usually provoked by anger, frustration, or fear. If the infant's sibling takes away a toy, the child cries and then stops breathing in expiration. Cyanosis develops rapidly, followed quickly by limpness and loss of consciousness. Occasional cyanotic episodes are provoked by pain, and these may not be preceded by crying.

If the attack lasts only a few seconds, the infant may resume crying on awakening. Most spells, especially the ones referred for neurologic evaluation, are longer and are associated with tonic posturing of the body and clonic movements of the hands or arms. The eyes may roll upward. These movements are regarded as seizures by even experienced observers, but they are probably a brainstem release phenomenon and concurrent EEG shows flattening of the record and not epileptiform activity.

After a short spell, the child rapidly recovers and seems normal immediately; after a prolonged spell the child first arouses and then goes to sleep. Once an infant begins having breathholding spells, the frequency increases for several months and then declines, and finally the spells cease.

DIAGNOSIS. The typical sequence of cyanosis, apnea, and loss of consciousness is critical for diagnosis. Cyanotic syncope is often misdiagnosed as epilepsy because of lack of attention to the precipitating event. It is not sufficient to ask, "Did the child hold his breath?" The question conjures up the image of breathholding during inspiration. Instead, questioning should be focused on precipitating events, absence of breathing, facial color, and family history. The family often has a history of breathholding spells.

Between attacks the EEG is normal. During an episode the EEG first shows diffuse slowing and then rhythmic slowing during the tonic-clonic activity.

TREATMENT. No treatment is available to prevent future breathholding spells or to stop a spell in progress. However, I believe that the spell is prolonged by picking up the child, which is the natural act of the mother or other observer. People who have lost consciousness because of decreased cerebral perfusion should not be placed in an upright position. You would not recommend that for a child who has fainted. I always caution parents to leave the child on the floor.

Most important is to identify the nature of the spell and explain that it is harmless. Children do not die during breathholding spells, and the episodes always cease spontaneously. Does anyone know an adult who has breathholding spells?

Pallid Syncope

CLINICAL FEATURES. Pallid syncope is usually provoked by a sudden, unexpected, painful event, such as a bump on the head. The child rarely cries but instead becomes white and limp and loses consciousness. These are truly terrifying to behold. Parents invariably believe the child is dead and begin mouth-to-mouth resuscitation. After the initial limpness the body may stiffen and clonic movements of the arms may occur. As in cyanotic syncope, these movements represent a brainstem release phenomenon and not seizure activity. The duration of the spell is difficult to determine because the observer is so frightened that seconds seem like hours. Afterward the child often falls asleep and is normal on awakening.

DIAGNOSIS. Pallid syncope is the result of reflex asystole. An attack sometimes can be provoked by pressure on the eyeballs to initiate a vagal reflex. I do not recommend provoking an attack as an office procedure. The diagnosis can be made by history alone.

TREATMENT. As with cyanotic spells, the major goal is to reassure the family that the child will not die during an attack. The physician must be very convincing.

FEBRILE SEIZURES

An infant's first seizure often occurs at the time of fever. Three explanations are possible: (1) an infection of the nervous system; (2) an underlying seizure disorder in which the initial seizure is triggered by the stress of fever, although subsequent seizures may be afebrile; and (3) a *simple febrile seizure,* a genetic age-limited epilepsy in which seizures only occur with fever. Infections of the nervous system are discussed in Chapters 2 and 4. The distinction between epilepsy and simple febrile seizures is sometimes difficult and may require time rather than laboratory tests.

CLINICAL FEATURES. Febrile seizures not caused by infection or other definable cause occur in approximately 4% of children. Only 2% of children whose first seizure is associated with fever will have nonfebrile seizures (epilepsy) by age 7. The most important predictor of subsequent epilepsy is an abnormal neurologic or developmental state. Complex seizures—defined as prolonged, focal, or multiple—slightly increase the probability of subsequent epilepsy.

A single, brief, generalized seizure occurring in association with fever is likely to be a simple febrile seizure. The seizure need not occur during the time when fever is rising (Berg, 1993). "Brief" and "fever" are difficult to define. Parents do not use a stop watch, and when a child is having a seizure, seconds seem like minutes. A prolonged seizure is one that is still in progress after the family has contacted the doctor or has left the house for the emergency room. Postictal sleep should not be counted as seizure time. Similarly, body temperature is not measured during a seizure and may be considerably different 30 minutes later.

Simple febrile seizures are familial and probably transmitted by autosomal dominant inheritance with incomplete penetrance. One third of infants who have a first simple febrile seizure will have a second at the time of a subsequent febrile illness, and half of these will have a third febrile seizure. The risk of recurrence is increased if the first febrile seizure occurs before 18 months of age or at a body temperature less than 40° C (Berg et al, 1992). More than three episodes of simple febrile seizures are unusual and suggest that the child may later have nonfebrile seizures.

DIAGNOSIS. Any child who is thought to have an infection of the nervous system should undergo a lumbar puncture for examination of the cerebrospinal fluid. Approximately one quarter of children with bacterial or viral meningitis have seizures (Green et al, 1993). Ninety percent are obtunded after the seizure and the other 10% have nuchal rigidity or complex seizures that suggest meningitis. In contrast, infants who have simple febrile seizures usually look normal after the seizure. Lumbar puncture is not needed following a brief, generalized seizure from which the child recovers rapidly and completely, especially if the fever subsides spontaneously or is otherwise explained.

Blood cell counts, measurements of glucose, calcium, electrolytes, urinalysis, and EEG on a routine basis are not cost effective and should not be performed. The decision for laboratory testing can be individualized to the circumstances of the case. EEG should be performed on every infant who is not neurologically normal or who has a family history of epilepsy. MRI is indicated in many infants with focal seizures or with focal deficits, even transitory, following a seizure.

TREATMENT. Because only one third of children with an initial febrile seizure have a second seizure, treating every affected child is unreasonable. The low-risk group with a single, brief, generalized seizure should not be treated. No evidence has shown that a second or third simple febrile seizure, even if prolonged, causes epilepsy or brain damage.

As a rule, I recommend anticonvulsant prophylaxis only if I believe the child has a condition other than simple febrile seizures, and I follow these guidelines:

1. Infants with an abnormal neurologic examination or developmental delay should be considered candidates for prophylactic anticonvulsant therapy.

2. When the initial febrile seizure is complex (multiple, prolonged, or focal) but the child recovers rapidly and completely, treatment is not indicated unless the family has a history of nonfebrile seizures.

3. A family history of simple febrile seizures is a relative contraindication to therapy in the situations just listed.

4. Children who have frequent and prolonged febrile seizures should be treated. The alternatives are prophylactic phenobarbital or oral administration of diazepam, 0.33 mg/kg, every 8 hours during a febrile illness (Rosman et al, 1993). The side effects of diazepam—ataxia, lethargy, and irritability—are transitory.

NONFEBRILE SEIZURES

Disorders that produce nonfebrile tonic-clonic or partial seizures in infancy are not substantially different from those that cause nonfebrile seizures in childhood (see the section that follows). Major risk factors for the development of epilepsy in infancy and childhood are congenital malformations, neonatal seizures, and a family history of epilepsy.

A complex partial seizure syndrome that has its onset during infancy, sometimes in the newborn period, is *ictal laughter* associated with hypothalamic hamartoma. The attacks are brief, occur several times each day, and may be characterized by pleasant laughter or giggling. At first the laughter is thought to be normal, but then facial flushing and pupillary dilatation are noted. With time the child begins to have drop attacks and generalized seizures, and undergoes personality change. Precocious puberty may be an associated condition.

A first partial motor seizure before the age of 2 is associated with a recurrence rate of 87%, whereas afterward the rate is 51%. The recurrence rate after a first nonfebrile, nonsymptomatic, generalized seizure is 60% to 70% at all ages. The younger the age at onset of a nonfebrile seizure of any type, the more likely that the seizure is symptomatic rather than idiopathic.

Approximately 25% of children who have recurrent seizures during the first year, excluding neonatal seizures and infantile spasms, are developmentally or neurologically abnormal at the time of the first seizure. The initial EEG has prognostic significance; normal EEG results are associated with a favorable neurologic outcome.

Intractable seizures in children less than 2 years of age are often associated with later mental retardation (Huttenlocher and Hapke, 1990). The following relationship exists between the seizure type and probability of mental retardation: myoclonic 94%, tonic-clonic 78%, complex partial 60%, and simple partial 61%.

A *benign familial epilepsy* transmitted by autosomal dominant inheritance occurs in infants, with onset as early as 3 months (Echenne et al, 1994). The seizures are characterized by motion arrest, decreased responsiveness, staring or blank eyes, and mild convulsive movements of the limbs. They are easily controlled with anticonvulsant drugs and stop spontaneously within 2 to 4 years.

MYOCLONUS AND MYOCLONIC SEIZURES

Infantile Spasms

Infantile spasms are age-dependent myoclonic seizures that occur with an incidence of 25 per 100,000 live births in the United States and Western Europe. An underlying cause can be determined in approximately 75% of patients; congenital malformations and perinatal asphyxia are common causes, and tuberous sclerosis accounts for 20% of cases in some series (Table 1–8). Despite considerable concern in the past, pertussis immunization is not a cause of infantile spasms (Institute of Medicine, 1991).

The combination of infantile spasms, agenesis of the corpus callosum (as well as other midline cerebral malformations), and retinal malformations is referred to as *Aicardi syndrome* (Menezes et al, 1994). All affected children are females and the disorder is believed to be transmitted as an X-linked dominant trait with hemizygous lethality in males.

CLINICAL FEATURES. The peak age at onset is between 4 and 7 months, and onset always occurs before 1 year of age. The spasm can be a flexor or an extensor movement; some children have both. Spasms generally occur in clusters, shortly after the infant awakens from sleep, and are not activated by stimulation. A rapid flexor spasm involving the neck, trunk, and limbs is followed by a tonic contraction sustained for 2 to 10 seconds. Less severe flexor spasms are characterized only by dropping of the head and abduction of the arms or by flexion at the waist resembling colic. Extensor spasms resemble the second component of the Moro reflex: the head moves backward and the arms are suddenly spread. Whether flexor or extensor, the movement is almost always symmetric and brief.

When the cause of spasms is identifiable (symptomatic spasms), the infant is usually abnormal neurologically or developmentally

■ TABLE 1-8
Neurocutaneous Disorders Causing Seizures in Infancy

Incontinentia Pigmenti

Seizure type
  Neonatal seizures
  Generalized tonic-clonic
Cutaneous manifestations
  Erythematous bullae (newborn)
  Pigmentary whorls (infancy)
  Depigmented areas (childhood)

Linear Nevus Sebaceous Syndrome

Seizure type
  Infantile spasms
  Lennox-Gastaut syndrome
  Generalized tonic-clonic
Cutaneous manifestation
  Linear facial sebaceous nevus

Neurofibromatosis

Seizure type
  Generalized tonic-clonic
  Partial complex
  Partial simple motor
Cutaneous manifestations
  Café au lait spots
  Axillary freckles
  Neural tumors

Sturge-Weber Syndrome

Seizure type
  Epilepsia partialis continuans
  Partial simple motor
  Status epilepticus
Cutaneous manifestation
  Hemifacial hemangioma

Tuberous Sclerosis

Seizure type
  Neonatal seizures
  Infantile spasms
  Lennox-Gastaut syndrome
  Generalized tonic-clonic
  Partial simple motor
  Partial complex
Cutaneous manifestations
  Abnormal hair pigmentation
  Adenoma sebaceum
  Café au lait spots
  Depigmented areas
  Shagren patch

---

when the spasms begin. Microcephaly is common in this group. Prognosis depends on the cause, but as a rule the symptomatic group does poorly: only 5% have normal development or only mild impairment.

Idiopathic spasms characteristically occur in children who had been developing normally at the onset of spasms and have no history of prenatal or perinatal disorders. Neurologic findings, including head circumference, are normal. Approximately 40% of children with idiopathic

spasms are neurologically normal or only mildly retarded subsequently.

DIAGNOSIS. The delay from spasm onset to diagnosis is often considerable. Infantile spasms are so unlike the usual perception of seizures that even experienced pediatricians may be slow to realize the significance of the movements. Colic is often considered and treated for several weeks before seizures are suspected.

Infantile spasms must be differentiated from benign myoclonus of early infancy, benign myoclonic epilepsy of infants, severe myoclonic epilepsy of infancy, and the Lennox-Gastaut syndrome (Table 1-9). However, there is some reason to believe that infantile spasms, severe myoclonic epilepsy, and the Lennox-Gastaut syndrome are a continuum of epileptic encephalopathies (Donat, 1992).

The EEG is the single most important test for diagnosis. However, EEG findings vary with duration of recording, sleep state, and underlying disorder. Hypsarrhythmia is the usual pattern recorded during the early stages of infantile spasms. It is characterized by a chaotic and continuously abnormal background of very high voltage and random slow waves and spikes. The spikes vary in location from moment to moment and at times become generalized, but they are never repetitive. Typical hypsarrhythmia is most often recorded during wakefulness or active sleep. During quiet sleep, greater interhemispheric synchrony occurs and the background may have a burst-suppression appearance.

The EEG may transiently become normal immediately upon arousal, but when spasms occur, either an abrupt attenuation of the background or high-voltage slow waves appears. Within a few weeks the original chaotic pattern of hypsarrhythmia is replaced by greater interhemispheric synchrony. The distribution of epileptiform discharges changes from multifocal to generalized, and the generalized discharges are followed by attenuation of the record.

TREATMENT. Hormonal therapy with adrenocorticotropic hormone (ACTH) or corticosteroids is effective in stopping infantile spasms, but it need not be used in every case. Hormonal therapy does not affect outcome in infants whose spasms are due to prenatal or perinatal brain abnormalities. In such infants clonazepam or nitrazepam should be tried first and usually proves effective, at least temporarily. Valproate monotherapy controls spasms in 70% of infants when doses of 100 to 300 mg/kg are used (Prats et al, 1991) but is not a first drug of choice

■ TABLE 1–9

Electroencephalographic (EEG) Appearance in Myoclonic Seizures in Infancy

SEIZURE TYPE	EEG APPEARANCE
Infantile spasms	Hypsarrhythmia
	Slow spike and wave
	Burst-suppression
Benign myoclonus	Normal
Benign myoclonic epilepsy	Spike and wave (3 cps)
	Polyspike and wave (3 cps)
Severe myoclonic epilepsy	Polyspike and wave (>3 cps)
Lennox-Gastaut syndrome	Spike and wave (2-2.5 cps)
	Polyspike and wave (2-2.5 cps)

because of an unacceptable rate of fatal hepatotoxicity in this age group.

If clonazepam fails, hormonal therapy should be initiated. However, clonazepam should be continued in neurologically abnormal infants; ACTH or prednisone usually provides only temporary respite from seizures, and long-term anticonvulsant therapy is needed. The ideal dose and duration of ACTH or prednisone have not been established. An initial ACTH dose of 20 to 30 IU/day for 2 to 6 weeks, tapered to zero during a 1-week period, is just as effective as an initial dose of 150 IU/day tapered over 10 weeks (Hrachovy et al, 1994). A 2-week course of oral prednisone, 2 mg/kg/day, and intramuscular ACTH gel, 20 IU/day, is equally effective.

The response to hormonal therapy is never graded; control is either complete or not at all. Even when the response is favorable, one third have relapses during or after the course of treatment. Failure to respond and relapse occur more often in symptomatic than idiopathic cases. A second course of treatment is effective in 75% of cases in which the first course was successful, albeit at the price of increased adverse reactions.

High-dose pyridoxine should be considered in the treatment of infantile spasms when ACTH fails initially or relapses occur. Some cases of infantile spasms or other seizures of infancy may be atypical presentations of pyridoxine-dependent seizures. However, in most cases the anticonvulsant properties of pyridoxine and ACTH are unrelated to their physiologic functions. The recommended dosage of pyridoxine is 30 to 40 mg/kg/day.

Some children with idiopathic infantile spasms who are refractory to medical therapy have an area of cortical abnormality demonstrable by some combination of positron emission tomography, closed-circuit television EEG,

and MRI (Shields et al, 1992). Surgical removal of the hypometabolic area, which usually proves to contain dysplastic tissue, often provides seizure control.

Benign Myoclonus of Infancy

CLINICAL FEATURES. Many series of patients with infantile spasms include a small number with normal EEG results. Such infants cannot be distinguished from others with infantile spasms by clinical features because the age at onset and the appearance of the movements are the same. The spasms occur in clusters, frequently at mealtime. Clusters increase in intensity and severity over a period of weeks or months and then abate spontaneously. After 3 months the spasms usually stop altogether, and although occasional episodes may recur, no spasms occur after 2 years of age. Affected infants are normal neurologically and developmentally and remain so afterward. The term *benign myoclonus* is used because the spasms are believed to be an involuntary movement and not a seizure.

DIAGNOSIS. A normal EEG result distinguishes this group from other types of myoclonus in infancy. The MRI findings are also normal.

TREATMENT. Infants who are neurologically normal and have normal EEGs should not be treated.

Benign Myoclonic Epilepsy

CLINICAL FEATURES. Benign myoclonic epilepsy is a rare disorder of uncertain cause. A genetic basis is presumed because one third of patients have family members with epilepsy. Onset is between 4 months and 2 years of age. Affected infants are neurologically normal at onset of seizures and remain so afterward. The seizures are characterized by brief myoclonic attacks, which may be restricted to head nodding or may be so severe as to throw the child to the floor. The head drops to the chest, eyes roll upward, arms are thrown upward and outward, and legs flex. Myoclonic seizures may be single or repetitive, but consciousness is not lost. No other seizure types are observed in infancy, but generalized tonic-clonic seizures may occur in adolescence.

DIAGNOSIS. During a seizure the EEG shows generalized 3 cycles/second (cps) spike-wave or polyspike-wave discharges. Sensory stimuli do not activate seizures. The pattern is consistent with primary, generalized epilepsy.

TREATMENT. Valproate produces complete seizure control. If left untreated, seizures may persist for years. The use of valproate is potentially dangerous in infants because of hepatotoxicity, but barbiturates and benzodiazepines are not effective.

Severe Myoclonic Epilepsy

Severe myoclonic epilepsy is an important, but poorly understood, syndrome. A seemingly healthy infant has a seizure and then undergoes progressive neurologic deterioration that ends in a chronic brain damage syndrome. Because its cause is unknown, the disorder is blamed on any and all preceding events. It is often, but improperly, blamed on immunization.

CLINICAL FEATURES. A family history of epilepsy is present in 25% of cases. The first seizures are frequently febrile, are usually prolonged, and can be generalized or focal clonic in type. Febrile and nonfebrile seizures recur, sometimes as status epilepticus. Generalized myoclonic seizures appear after 1 year of age. At first mild and difficult to recognize as a seizure manifestation, they later become frequent and repetitive and disturb function. Partial complex seizures with secondary generalization may also occur. Coincident with the onset of myoclonic seizures are the slowing of development and the gradual appearance of ataxia and hyperreflexia.

DIAGNOSIS. The initial differential diagnosis is the same as for febrile seizures. Because the febrile seizures are usually prolonged and sometimes focal, epilepsy should be suspected. A specific diagnosis is not possible until the appearance of myoclonic seizures in the second year.

Interictal EEG findings are normal at first. Paroxysmal abnormalities appear in the second year and are characterized by generalized spike-wave and polyspike-wave complexes with a frequency greater than 3 cps. Discharges are activated by photic stimulation, drowsiness, and quiet sleep.

TREATMENT. The seizures are resistant to therapy with anticonvulsant drugs. Valproate and benzodiazepines should be tried first. Carbamazepine may increase seizure frequency.

Biotinidase Deficiency

This relatively rare disorder of biotin metabolism is transmitted as an autosomal recessive trait. It was originally called *late-onset multiple (holo)carboxylase deficiency.*

CLINICAL FEATURES. Age at onset is usually between 1 and 6 months. Seizures and hypoto-

nia are the initial features. The seizures may be generalized tonic-clonic, myoclonic, or infantile spasms (Salbert et al, 1993). Other features that may be seen initially or develop later are ataxia, respiratory disturbances, dermatitis, and alopecia.

DIAGNOSIS. Ketoacidosis, hyperammonemia, and organic aciduria are present as in holocarboxylase deficiency. Biotinidase should be suspected when the onset of symptoms is after the newborn period. The diagnosis is established by showing biotinidase deficiency in serum.

TREATMENT. Treatment with biotin, 5 to 20 mg/day, successfully reverses most of the symptoms if started during early infancy, and may prevent mental retardation.

Lennox-Gastaut Syndrome

Lennox-Gastaut syndrome is characterized by the triad of seizures (atypical absence, atonic, and myoclonic), slow spike-wave complexes on EEG, and mental retardation. In most patients the seizures are secondary to underlying brain damage, but some are primary epilepsies. Some authorities reserve the term *myoclonic-astatic epilepsy* for Lennox-Gastaut syndrome that is due to primary epilepsy.

CLINICAL FEATURES. The peak age at onset is 3 to 5 years; less than half of cases begin before age 2. An underlying cause can be identified in approximately 60%: neurocutaneous disorders, perinatal disturbances, and postnatal brain injuries are most common. Twenty percent of children with the Lennox-Gastaut syndrome have a history of infantile spasms, sometimes with a seizure-free interval before development of the syndrome.

Although the syndrome can begin in a normal child, most children are identified as neurologically abnormal before its onset. The first seizures may be generalized tonic-clonic or focal clonic, but are usually tonic. Tonic seizures are characterized by stiffening of the body, upward deviation of the eyes, dilatation of the pupils, and alteration in the respiratory pattern. The seizures frequently occur during sleep, and enuresis may be an associated condition.

Atypical absence seizures occur in almost every patient. In addition to the stare, trembling of the eyelids and mouth occurs, followed by loss of facial tone so that the head leans forward and the mouth hangs open. Atonic seizures are characterized by sudden dropping of the head or body, at times throwing the child to the ground. More than 90%

of patients are mentally retarded by 5 years of age.

DIAGNOSIS. An EEG is essential for diagnosis. The characteristic feature during atypical absence or atonic seizures is a generalized burst of 2- to 2.5-cps spike-wave complexes. Tonic seizures are associated with 1-cps slow waves followed by generalized rapid discharges without postictal depression.

In addition to EEG, a thorough evaluation is needed to look for an underlying cause. Special attention should be given to skin manifestations suggesting a neurocutaneous syndrome (Table 1–8). MRI is useful for the diagnosis of congenital malformations, postnatal disorders, and neurocutaneous syndromes.

TREATMENT. Seizures are difficult to control. Valproate and clonazepam are the drugs most often effective. Felbamate, at increasing dosages to a maximum of 45 mg/kg/day, further reduces seizure frequency when added to other anticonvulsant drugs (Felbamate Study Group in Lennox-Gastaut Syndrome, 1993).

MIGRAINE

CLINICAL FEATURES. Migraine attacks are uncommon in infancy, but when they occur, the clinical features are often "paroxysmal" and suggest the possibility of seizures. Cyclic vomiting is probably the most common manifestation. Attacks of vertigo (see Chapter 10) or torticollis (see Chapter 14) may be especially perplexing, and some infants have attacks in which they rock back and forth and appear uncomfortable.

DIAGNOSIS. Benign paroxysmal vertigo is sufficiently stereotyped in presentation to be recognizable as a migraine variant. Other syndromes often remain undiagnosed until the episodes evolve into a typical migraine pattern. A history of migraine in one parent, usually the mother, is essential for diagnosis.

TREATMENT. Antimigraine drugs are generally not used in infants.

TRANSIENT PAROXYSMAL DYSTONIA OF INFANCY

CLINICAL FEATURES. Transient paroxysmal dystonia of infancy is a nonfamilial disorder characterized by episodes of opisthotonos and symmetric or asymmetric dystonia of limbs, without alteration in consciousness. Onset is between 6 and 22 months of age. The initial episodes usually last for several minutes but may last as long as 2 hours. Later, the episodes increase in duration (up to 7 days) and frequency and are characterized by torsion dystonia of the neck and trunk. Eventually the episodes decrease in frequency and disappear. Afterward the child is neurologically and developmentally normal.

DIAGNOSIS. The disorder must be differentiated from familial choreoathetosis, glutaric aciduria, and dopa-responsive dystonia (see Chapter 14). EEG findings during an episode are normal, as are levels of serum electrolytes and organic acids.

TREATMENT. Treatment is not needed to ensure a favorable outcome, but centrally acting muscle relaxants may be useful during prolonged episodes. A trial of dopa-carbidopa is warranted in every child with dystonia.

➡ Paroxysmal Disorders of Childhood

Like infants, children with paroxysmal disorders are generally thought to have seizures until proven otherwise. Seizures are the most common paroxysmal disorder requiring medical consultation. Syncope, especially presyncope, is considerably more common but is generally diagnosed and managed at home unless associated symptoms suggest a seizure.

Migraine is probably the most common causes of paroxysmal neurologic disorders in childhood; its incidence is 10 times greater than epilepsy. Migraine syndromes that may suggest epilepsy are described in Chapters 2, 3, 10, 11, 14, and 15.

Sleep disorders often have a paroxysmal quality and may be confused with complex partial seizures. Adding to the confusion is the fact that complex partial seizures are often activated by sleep.

SYNDROMES SIMULATING SEIZURES

Paroxysmal Dyskinesia

Two main forms of paroxysmal dyskinesia are recognized depending on whether the paroxysms are exertion-induced (Demirkiran and Jankovic, 1995): paroxysmal kinesigenic dyskinesia (PKD) and paroxysmal nonkinesigenic dyskinesia (PNKD). PNKD is transmitted as an autosomal dominant trait and is also known as *familial paroxysmal choreoathetosis*. Similar attacks are seen in children with episodic ataxia- type 1 (see Chapter 10), suggesting that PNKD is an ion-channel gene defect (Griggs and Nutt, 1995).

CLINICAL FEATURES. PKD usually begins in childhood. Most cases are sporadic. The paroxysms are precipitated by sudden movement or startle and usually last less than a minute. Several attacks occur each day. Each attack may include dystonia, choreoathetosis, or ballismus (see Chapter 14). One or both sides of the body can be affected. Some patients have an "aura" described as tightness or tingling of the face or limbs.

PNKD begins in childhood or adult life and is usually familial. Only a few attacks occur each year but they last for several hours or days. Consciousness is always preserved during attacks of paroxysmal dyskinesia, and life expectancy is not shortened.

DIAGNOSIS. Ictal and interictal EEGs are normal. Children with EEG evidence of epileptiform activity should be considered to have a seizure disorder and not a paroxysmal dyskinesia.

TREATMENT. Phenytoin in ordinary anticonvulsant dosages is effective in PKD but not in PNKD.

Hyperventilation Syndrome

Hyperventilation induces alkalosis by altering the proportion of blood gases. This is more readily accomplished in children than adults.

CLINICAL FEATURES. During times of emotional upset, respiratory rate and depth may increase insidiously, first appearing like sighing and then as obvious hyperventilation. The occurrence of tingling of the fingers disturbs the patient further and may induce greater hyperventilation. Headache is an associated symptom. If hyperventilation is allowed to continue, the patient may lose consciousness.

DIAGNOSIS. The observation of hyperventilation as a precipitating factor of syncope is essential to diagnosis. Often patients are unaware that they were hyperventilating and probing questions are needed to elicit the history in the absence of a witness.

TREATMENT. An attack in progress can be aborted by having the patient breathe into a paper bag.

Narcolepsy-Cataplexy

Narcolepsy-cataplexy is a sleep disorder characterized by an abnormally short latency from sleep onset to rapid eye movement (REM) sleep.

REM sleep is attained in less than 20 minutes instead of the usual 90 minutes. Normal REM sleep is characterized by dreaming and severe hypotonia. In narcolepsy-cataplexy these phenomena occur during wakefulness.

CLINICAL FEATURES. Onset may occur at any time from early childhood to middle adulthood, usually in the second or third decade and rarely before age 5 (Aldrich, 1992). The syndrome has four components:

1. *Narcolepsy* refers to short sleep attacks. Three or four attacks occur each day, most often during monotonous activity, and are difficult to resist. Half of patients are easy to arouse from a sleep attack, and 60% feel refreshed afterward. Narcolepsy is usually a life-long condition.

2. *Cataplexy* is a sudden loss of muscle tone induced by laughter, excitement, or startle. Almost all patients who have narcolepsy have cataplexy as well. The patient may collapse to the floor and then arise immediately. Partial paralysis, affecting just the face or hands, is more common than total paralysis. Two to four attacks occur daily, usually in the afternoon. They are embarrassing but do not cause physical harm.

3. *Sleep paralysis* occurs in the transition between sleep and wakefulness. The patient has generalized hypotonia and, although mentally awake, is unable to move any body part. Partial paralysis is less common. The attack may end spontaneously or when the patient is touched. Two thirds of patients with narcolepsy-cataplexy also experience sleep paralysis once or twice each week. Occasional episodes of sleep paralysis may occur in people who do not have narcolepsy-cataplexy.

4. *Hypnagogic hallucinations* are vivid, usually frightening, visual and auditory perceptions occurring at the transition between sleep and wakefulness: a sensation of dreaming while awake. They are reported as an associated event by half of patients with narcolepsy-cataplexy. Episodes occur less than once a week.

DIAGNOSIS. The syndrome should be recognizable by history. The symptoms are embarrassing or sound "crazy" to the patient, and considerable prompting is often needed to elicit a full history.

Narcolepsy can be difficult to distinguish from

other causes of excessive daytime sleepiness. The multiple sleep latency test is the standard for diagnosis. Patients with narcolepsy enter REM sleep within a few minutes of falling asleep.

TREATMENT. Symptoms of narcolepsy-cataplexy are distressing and often associated with emotional disturbances. The realization that narcolepsy is not a mental disorder is comforting.

Amphetamine or methylphenidate is usually prescribed for narcolepsy but should be given with some caution because of potential abuse (Aldrich, 1992). Small doses should be used on schooldays or workdays and no medicine, if possible, on weekends and holidays. When not taking medicine, patients should be encouraged to schedule short naps.

Selegiline, a monoamine oxidase inhibitor, is useful in reducing the frequency of sleep attacks and cataplexy (Hublin et al, 1994). Cataplexy also can be treated with fluoxetine, 20 mg a day (Frey and Darbonne, 1994), trihexyphenidyl, 2 mg three times a day, or imipramine, 50 mg three times a day.

Night Terrors

Night terrors are a partial arousal from non-rapid eye movement (nonREM) sleep.

CLINICAL FEATURES. The onset usually occurs by 4 years of age and almost always by age 6. Two hours after falling asleep the child awakens in a terrified state, does not recognize people, and is inconsolable. An episode usually lasts 5 to 15 minutes but can last an hour. During this time the child screams incoherently, may run if not restrained, and then goes back to sleep. Afterward, the child has no memory of the event.

Most children with night terrors experience an average of one or more episodes each week. Night terrors stop by 8 years of age in one half of affected children but continue into adolescence in a one third.

DIAGNOSIS. Half of children with night terrors are also sleepwalkers, and many have a family history of either sleepwalking or night terrors. The diagnosis should be based on the history alone. A sleep laboratory evaluation may be helpful in unusual circumstances when the possibility of seizures cannot be excluded.

TREATMENT. Treatment is not needed, and regular bedtime sedation should be avoided except when spells are very frequent and intolerable to the family. Clonidine, starting at 0.1 mg at bedtime and slowly increased, may be useful to treat night terrors and sleep walking.

Startle Disease

Startle disease, also called *hyperekplexia,* is a rare disorder transmitted as an autosomal dominant trait. The abnormal gene is a subunit of the glycine receptor on chromosome 5q (Tijssen et al, 1995).

CLINICAL FEATURES. The onset is at birth or during infancy. When the onset is at birth, the newborn may appear hypotonic during sleep and develop generalized stiffening on awakening. Apnea and an exaggerated startle response may be associated signs. Hypertonia in the newborn is unusual and has a limited differential diagnosis (see Table 8-5). Rigidity diminishes but does not disappear during sleep. Tendon reflexes are brisk and the response spreads to other muscles.

The stiffness resolves spontaneously during infancy and by 3 years of age the children are normal; however, episodes of stiffness may recur during adolescence or early adult life in response to startle, cold exposure, or pregnancy. Throughout life, affected individuals show a pathologically exaggerated startle response to visual, auditory, or tactile stimuli that would not startle normal individuals. In some, the startle is associated with a transitory, generalized stiffness of the body that causes falling without protective reflexes, often leading to injury. The stiffening response is often confused with the stiff-man syndrome (see Chapter 8).

DIAGNOSIS. A family history of startle disease is critical to the diagnosis but may be difficult to elicit because of partial expression or embarrassment. Epileptiform activity is not present on EEG.

TREATMENT. Valproate or clonazepam is useful in abolishing the falling attacks and reducing the startle. The natural history of the disease is variable; some patients improve spontaneously, but others get worse.

Syncope

Syncope is loss of consciousness because of a transitory decline in cerebral blood flow. This may be caused by an irregular cardiac rate or rhythm or by alterations of blood volume or distribution.

CLINICAL FEATURES. Syncope is a common event in otherwise healthy children, especially in the second decade. The mechanism is a vasovagal reflex by which an emotional experience produces peripheral pooling of blood. The reflex may also be stimulated by overextension or sudden decompression of viscera, by the

Valsalva maneuver, and by stretching with the neck hyperextended. Fainting in a hot, crowded church, when the worshiper rises to stand after prolonged kneeling, is especially common. Healthy children do not faint while lying down and rarely while seated. Fainting from anything but standing or arising suggests a cardiac arrhythmia and requires further investigation.

The child may first feel faint (described as "faint," "dizzy," or "lightheaded") or may lose consciousness without warning. Color drains from the face, and the skin becomes cold and clammy. With loss of consciousness the child falls to the floor. Consciousness may be regained rapidly, or stiffening of the body and clonic movements of the arms may occur. The latter is not a seizure. The stiffening and shaking is more common when the reduction of cerebral blood flow is exaggerated and prolonged because the child is prevented from falling. A short period of confusion may follow, but recovery is complete within minutes.

DIAGNOSIS. The criteria for differentiating syncope from seizures are the precipitating factors and the child's appearance. Seizures do not produce pallor and cold, clammy skin. I always enquire about the child's color during the "spell" in all children having an initial evaluation for seizures. Laboratory investigations are not cost-effective when syncope occurs in expected circumstances and the results of clinical examination are normal. Recurrent orthostatic syncope requires investigation of autonomic function, and any suspicion of cardiac abnormality deserves ECG monitoring. Always ask the child if irregular heart rate or beats are noted at the time of syncope or at other times.

TREATMENT. Infrequent syncopal episodes of obvious cause do not require treatment.

MIGRAINE AND EPILEPSY

Migraine and epilepsy are thought to be linked because (1) they are both familial, paroxysmal, and associated with transitory neurologic disturbances, (2) the incidence of epilepsy is increased in migraine sufferers and the incidence of migraine is increased in epileptics, (3) headache can be a seizure manifestation, and (4) abnormal EEGs are common in both disorders.

CLINICAL FEATURES. In children who have epilepsy and migraine, both disorders may share a common aura and one may provoke the other. Basilar migraine (see Chapter 10) and benign occipital epilepsy best exemplify the fine line between epilepsy and migraine. Both are characterized by seizures, headache, and epileptiform activity on EEG.

DIAGNOSIS. Asymptomatic central spikes are observed in 9% of children with migraine as compared with 2% of healthy children. Fourteen-and-six positive spikes, a normal adolescent pattern, is twice as common in children with migraine as in age-matched control subjects.

TREATMENT. Children who have both epilepsy and migraine must be treated for each condition separately.

STARING SPELLS

Daydreaming is a pleasant escape for people of all ages. Children feel the need for escape most acutely when in school and may stare vacantly out the window to the place they would rather be. Daydreams can be hard to break, and a child may not respond to verbal commands. Many dreamers are seen by neurologists, who may recommend EEG. Sometimes the EEG shows sleep-activated central spikes or another abnormality not related to staring, which may lead the physician to prescribe inappropriate anticonvulsant drug therapy.

Absence (petit mal) and complex partial seizures are both characterized by staring. They are usually distinguishable because absence is brief (5 to 15 seconds) and the child feels normal immediately afterward, while complex partial seizures usually last more than 1 minute and are followed by fatigue. The associated EEG patterns and response to treatment are quite different and precise diagnosis is needed before treatment is initiated.

Childhood Absence Epilepsy

Absence seizures occur in four epileptic syndromes: childhood absence epilepsy, juvenile absence epilepsy, juvenile myoclonic epilepsy, and myoclonic absence (Porter, 1993). Childhood absence epilepsy is a genetic disorder, transmitted as an autosomal dominant trait with age-dependent penetrance. The mother is more often the affected parent than the father (Doose, 1994). Juvenile absence epilepsy may be a continuum of the childhood form that begins near puberty, and has a higher frequency of generalized tonic-clonic seizures.

CLINICAL FEATURES. The peak age at onset is usually between 4 and 8 years, with a range between 3 and 12 years. Absence is not believed to begin after 20 years of age, but may persist

☐ FIGURE 1–3 Absence epilepsy. A generalized burst of 3-cps spike-wave complexes appears during hyperventilation.

from childhood into adult life. Affected children are otherwise healthy.

The reported incidence of epilepsy in families of children with absence varies from 15% to 40%. Concurrence in monozygotic twins is 75% for seizures and 85% for the characteristic EEG abnormality.

Typical attacks last 5 to 10 seconds and occur up to 100 times each day. The child stops ongoing activity, stares vacantly, sometimes with rhythmic movements of the eyelids, and then resumes activity. Aura and postictal confusion never occur. Longer seizures may last up to a minute and are indistinguishable by observation alone from complex partial seizures. Associated features may include myoclonus, increased or decreased postural tone, picking at clothes, turning of the head, and conjugate movements of the eyes. Occasional children and adults are brought to emergency departments in a confusional state caused by absence status (see Chapter 2).

Approximately 50% of children with absence have at least one generalized tonic-clonic seizure. Many are first brought for medical care because of a tonic-clonic seizure, even though absence attacks have occurred undiagnosed for months or years. The occurrence of a generalized tonic-clonic seizure does not change the diagnosis, prognosis, or treatment plan.

DIAGNOSIS. The EEG is pathognomonic. Bilaterally synchronous and symmetric paroxysms of 3-cps spike-wave complexes appear concurrent with the clinical seizure (Figure 1-3). The amplitude of discharge is greatest in the fronto-central regions. Although the discharge begins with a frequency of 3 cps, it may slow to 2 cps as it ends. Hyperventilation almost always activates the discharge. The interictal EEG is usually normal. When it is abnormal, the typical features are focal or multifocal spike discharges or diffuse slowing. Children with interictal abnormalities are more likely to have mental retardation or developmental delay.

Although the EEG pattern of discharge is stereotyped, variations on the theme in the form of multiple spike and wave discharges are also acceptable. During sleep, the discharges often lose their stereotypy and become polymorphic in form and frequency, but remain generalized.

Once a correlation between clinical and EEG findings is made, looking for an underlying disease is unnecessary. Absence epilepsy is distinguished from *myoclonic absence* and *juvenile myoclonic epilepsy* (see Myoclonic Seizures, later on) by the absence of myoclonic seizures.

TREATMENT. Ethosuximide and valproate are equally effective in the treatment of absence, with each providing complete relief of seizures in 80% of children. Ethosuximide is the treatment of choice because of its lower incidence of serious side effects. If neither drug alone provides seizure control, they can be used in combination at reduced dosages or lamotrigine can be substituted for one or both drugs (see Lamotrigene, later on, for precautions concerning the combination of valproate and lamotrigine). The EEG becomes normal if treatment is successful, and repeating the EEG is useful to confirm the seizure-free state.

Children with only 3-cps spike-wave complexes on EEG should first be treated with ethosuximide alone, even if a tonic-clonic seizure occurred before initiation of therapy. If tonic-clonic seizures recur after therapy is initiated, valproate should be substituted for ethosuximide. Clonazepam is sometimes useful in the treatment of refractory absence and carbamazepine may accentuate the seizures and cause absence status (Callahan and Noetzel, 1992).

Complex Partial Seizures

Complex partial seizures arise in the cortex, most often the temporal lobe, but can originate from the frontal or parietal lobes as well. Complex partial seizures are partial seizures that may be symptomatic of an underlying focal disorder (see "Partial Seizures," later on).

CLINICAL FEATURES. Complex partial seizures occur spontaneously or may be activated by sleep. Most last 1 to 2 minutes and rarely less than 30 seconds. An aura is reported in fewer than 30% of children. It is usually a nondescript unpleasant feeling, but might also be a stereotyped auditory hallucination or abdominal discomfort. The first feature of the seizure can be staring, automatic behavior, tonic extension of one or both arms, or loss of body tone. Staring is associated with a change in facial expression and is followed by automatic behavior. Automatisms vary from facial grimacing and fumbling movements of the fingers to walking, running, and resisting restraint. Automatic behavior in a given patient tends to be similar from seizure to seizure.

The seizure usually terminates with a period of postictal confusion, disorientation, or lethargy. Transitory aphasia is sometimes present. If the child is not treated, or if treatment is abruptly withdrawn, secondary generalization is likely to occur.

Partial complex status epilepticus is a rare

event characterized by impaired consciousness, staring alternating with wandering eye movements, and automatisms of the face and hands. Such children may arrive at the emergency department in a confused or delirious state (see Chapter 2).

DIAGNOSIS. The etiology of complex partial seizures is heterogeneous and a cause is often not determined. Brain tumor was thought to be an unusual cause in children, but contrast-enhanced MRI can show a low-grade glioma in many otherwise normal children with hard-to-control seizures, and should be performed in all such cases. Focal dysplastic lesions, especially migrational defects, are another important cause of partial seizures that are identified on MRI (Palmini et al, 1991).

An EEG should be recorded in both the waking and sleeping states. Hyperventilation and photic stimulation are not useful as provocative measures. Results of a single EEG may be normal in the interictal period, but repeated EEGs usually reveal either a spike or slow-wave focus in the frontal or temporal lobe or multifocal abnormalities. During the seizure, repetitive focal spike discharges occur in the involved area of cortex, which change to spike-slow wave complexes, and then slow waves with amplitude attenuation as the seizure ends.

TREATMENT. Carbamazepine, phenytoin, primidone, and valproate are effective for seizure control, and the choice should be based on cost, side effects, and dosage schedule.

Temporal lobectomy should be considered when seizures are refractory to anticonvulsant drugs (see Surgical Approaches to Childhood Epilepsy). The underlying pathology is often dysplastic tissue or a low-grade glioma.

MYOCLONIC SEIZURES

Myoclonus is a brief, involuntary muscle contraction (jerk) that may represent (1) a seizure manifestation, as in infantile spasms (2) a physiologic response to startle or to falling asleep, or (3) an involuntary movement either alone or in combination with tonic-clonic seizures (see Table 14-8). Myoclonic seizures are often difficult to distinguish from myoclonus (the movement disorder) on clinical grounds alone. Essential myoclonus and other disorders in which myoclonus is a movement disorder and not a seizure manifestation are discussed in Chapter 14.

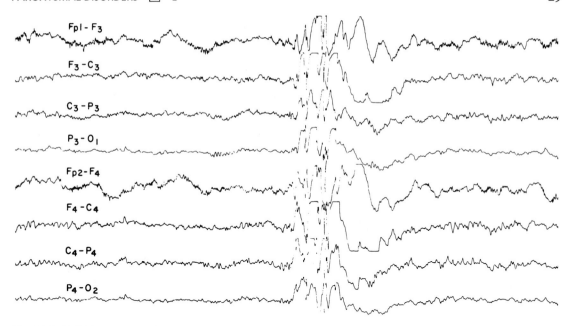

☐ F I G U R E 1 – 4 Juvenile myoclonic epilepsy. The interictal discharge is a 3.5- to 6-cps multispike-wave complex.

Juvenile Myoclonic Epilepsy (Janz)

Juvenile myoclonic epilepsy (Janz) is a hereditary disorder, probably inherited as an autosomal recessive trait. The responsible gene has been mapped to the short arm of chromosome 6.

CLINICAL FEATURES. Males and females are affected equally (Panayiotopoulos et al, 1994). Seizures in affected children and their affected relatives may be tonic-clonic, myoclonic, myoclonic absence, or simple absence. The usual age at onset of absence seizures is 7 to 13 years, of myoclonic jerks is 12 to 18 years, and of generalized tonic-clonic seizures is 13 to 20 years.

The myoclonic seizures are brief, bilateral but not always symmetric, flexor jerk of the arms, which may be repetitive. The jerk sometimes affects the legs, causing the patient to fall. Consciousness is usually retained so that the patient is aware of the jerking movement. Seizures are precipitated by sleep deprivation, alcohol ingestion, and awakening from nocturnal or daytime sleep.

Most patients also have generalized tonic-clonic seizures, and one third experience absence but are otherwise normal neurologically. The potential for seizures of one type or another continues throughout adult life.

DIAGNOSIS. The diagnosis is often missed, even by neurologists, because of unfamiliarity with the clinical syndrome. Seizures are accompanied by generalized polyspike discharges followed by a slow wave. The polyspike discharge is concurrent with the clinical seizure, and the slow wave occurs afterward. Seizures are sometimes precipitated by photic stimulation or eye closure. The interictal record may be normal or may show 3.5- to 6-cps multispike-wave complexes (Figure 1–4).

TREATMENT. Valproate is the treatment of choice and provides complete relief of seizures in 75% of cases. Other drugs, such as barbiturates and phenytoin, may be added in children whose seizures are refractory to valproate or who continue to experience generalized tonic-clonic seizures. Carbamazepine is not effective, and clonazepam monotherapy may precipitate generalized tonic-clonic seizures.

Myoclonic Absence

Myoclonic absence is a rare epilepsy, probably distinct from absence epilepsy, in which 85% of patients are boys. It is not a homogeneous entity but may be genetic in some cases and symptomatic of an underlying brain disorder in others.

CLINICAL FEATURES. Age at onset is between 2 and 12 years with the peak at 7 years. A family history of epilepsy is present in 25% of cases. Unlike absence epilepsy, 40% of affected children are mentally subnormal before the onset of seizures.

Seizures last 10 to 60 seconds and occur

several times each day. They are characterized by a combination of absence and intense rhythmic, bilateral myoclonus affecting the muscles of the shoulders, arms, and legs. The child does not lose consciousness and may be aware of and disturbed by the jerking. Other seizures types do not usually occur.

Myoclonic absence sometimes persists into adult life and other times ceases spontaneously. Some children, though intellectually normal before the onset of seizures, are retarded later.

DIAGNOSIS. Myoclonic absence is thought to be intermediary between primary and secondary epilepsy, but an underlying cause has not been determined. The EEG shows the same 3-cps spike-wave pattern associated with simple absence.

TREATMENT. The seizures are refractory to treatment. Occasional success may be achieved with a combination of valproate and ethosuximide.

Progressive Myoclonus Epilepsies

The term "progressive myoclonus epilepsies" is used to cover several progressive disorders of the nervous system characterized by (1) myoclonus; (2) seizures that may be tonic-clonic, tonic, or myoclonic; (3) progressive mental deterioration; and (4) cerebellar ataxia, involuntary movements, or both (Berkovic et al, 1993). Some of these disorders are due to specific lysosomal enzyme deficiencies, whereas others are probably mitochondrial disorders (Table 1–10).

Lafora Disease

Lafora disease is a rare hereditary disease probably transmitted by autosomal recessive inheritance.

CLINICAL FEATURES. Onset is between 11 and 18 years of age, with the mean at age 14. Tonic-clonic or myoclonic seizures are the initial feature in 80% of cases. Myoclonus becomes progressively worse, may be segmental or massive, and is increased by movement. Mental retardation begins early and is relentlessly progressive. Ataxia, spasticity, and involuntary movements occur late in the course. Death occurs 5 to 6 years from onset of symptoms.

DIAGNOSIS. The EEG is normal at first and later develops nonspecific generalized polyspike discharges that are not activated by sleep. The background becomes progressively disorganized and epileptiform activity more constant. Photosensitive discharges are a regular feature late in the course.

■ TABLE 1–10
Progressive Myoclonus Epilepsies

Ceroid lipofuscinosis juvenile form (see Chapter 5)
Glucosylceramide lipidosis (Gaucher type 3) (see Chapter 5)
Lafora disease
Myoclonus epilepsy and ragged-red fibers (see Chapter 5)
Ramsay-Hunt syndrome (see Chapter 10)
Sialidoses (see Chapter 5)
Unverricht-Lundborg syndrome

Antemortem diagnosis is sometimes accomplished by showing periodic acid-Schiff (PAS)-positive inclusion bodies consisting of aggregates of filaments composed of polyglucosans in biopsy specimens of liver or sweat gland, but may be absent even in late stages of the disease (Drury et al, 1993).

TREATMENT. The seizures become refractory to most anticonvulsant drugs, but the combination of valproate, clonazepam, and phenobarbital should be tried. Treatment of the underlying disease is not available.

Unverricht-Lundborg Syndrome

Unverricht-Lundborg syndrome is clinically similar to Lafora disease, except that inclusion bodies are not present. It is transmitted by autosomal recessive inheritance. The syndrome is most often reported in Finland and other Baltic countries, but has a worldwide distribution. Whether ethnic clusters are caused by distinct diseases is not known.

A combination of valproate, clonazepam, and phenobarbital is effective for seizure control.

Reading Epilepsy

Reading epilepsy may be a variant of juvenile myoclonic epilepsy; many children with reading epilepsy experience myoclonic jerks of the limbs shortly after arising in the morning (Radhakrishnan et al, 1995).

CLINICAL FEATURES. Age at onset is usually in the second decade. Myoclonic jerks involving orofacial and jaw muscles develop while reading. Reading time before seizure onset is variable. The initial seizure is almost always in the jaw and is described as "jaws locking or clicking." Other initial features are quivering of the lips, choking in the throat, or difficulty speaking. Myoclonic jerks of the limbs may follow and some children experience a generalized tonic clonic seizure if they continue reading. Generalized tonic-clonic seizures may also occur at other times.

DIAGNOSIS. The history of myoclonic jerks during reading and during other processes requiring higher cognitive function is critical to the diagnosis. The interictal EEG usually shows generalized discharges and brief spike-wave complexes can be provoked by reading that are simultaneous with jaw jerks.

TREATMENT. Some patients can control their seizures without the use of anticonvulsants drugs by quitting reading at the first sign of orofacial or jaw jerks. Most require anticonvulsant therapy. Phenytoin or carbamazepine is effective.

PARTIAL SEIZURES

This section discusses several different seizure types of focal cortical origin other than complex partial seizures. Such seizures may be purely motor or purely sensory or may affect higher cortical function. The most common cause of partial seizures in children are the *benign childhood partial epilepsies.* The most common benign childhood epilepsies are *benign centrotemporal (rolandic) epilepsy* and *benign occipital epilepsy.* The various benign partial epilepsy syndromes begin and cease at similar ages, have a similar course, and occur in the members of the same family. It seems likely that they are different phenotypic expressions of the same genetic defect.

Partial seizures are also secondary to underlying diseases, which can be focal, multifocal, or generalized. Intractable partial seizures are often caused by neuronal migrational disorders and gliomas. Cerebral cysticercosis is an important cause in Mexico and Central America. MRI is recommended for all children with intractable focal seizures. Many may be candidates for surgical therapy (Kuzniecky et al, 1993).

Any seizure that originates in the cortex may discharge into the brainstem, causing a generalized tonic-clonic seizure (secondary generalization). If the discharge remains focal for a few seconds, the patient experiences a focal seizure or an *aura* before losing consciousness. Often the secondary generalization occurs so rapidly that a tonic-clonic seizure is the initial symptom. In such cases, cortical origin of the seizure may be detectable on EEG. However, normal EEG findings are common during a simple partial seizure and do not exclude the diagnosis.

Acquired Epileptiform Aphasia

Acquired aphasia associated with epileptiform activity on EEG in children is called the *Landau-Kleffner syndrome* (Paquier et al, 1992). The syndrome appears to be a disorder of auditory processing. The cause is unknown except for occasional cases associated with temporal lobe tumors (Nass et al, 1993). Such diverse causes as cerebral arteritis, demyelinating encephalopathy, and genetic epilepsy have been considered.

CLINICAL FEATURES. Age at onset ranges from 2 to 11 years, with 75% beginning between 3 and 10 years. The first symptom may be aphasia or epilepsy. Aphasia is initially characterized by auditory verbal agnosia. The child has difficulty understanding what is said, spontaneous speech is reduced, and deafness or autism develops. Seizures, which may be partial or generalized, occur in 80% of children. Atypical absence is sometimes the initial feature and may be associated with continuous spike and slow waves during slow-wave sleep. Hyperactivity and personality change are noted in one half of affected children and may be caused by aphasia. Intelligence is not affected, and neurologic examination is otherwise normal.

Recovery of language is more likely to occur if the syndrome begins before 7 years of age. Seizures cease generally by age 10 and always by age 15.

DIAGNOSIS. Acquired epileptiform aphasia, as the name implies, can be differentiated from autism and hearing loss because the diagnosis requires that the child have normal language and cognitive development prior to onset of symptoms and normal hearing. The EEG shows multifocal cortical spike discharges with a predilection for the temporal and parietal lobes. Involvement is bilateral in 88% of cases. An intravenous injection of diazepam may normalize the EEG and improve speech transiently, but this should not suggest that aphasia is caused by epileptiform activity. Instead, both features reflect an underlying cerebral disorder.

MRI is needed in every case to exclude the rare possibility of a temporal lobe tumor.

TREATMENT. Standard anticonvulsant drugs such as carbamazepine and phenytoin usually control the seizures, but do not improve speech. Corticosteroid therapy, especially early in the course, may normalize the EEG and provide long-lasting remission of aphasia and seizures.

Autosomal Dominant Nocturnal Frontal Lobe Epilepsy

This epilepsy syndrome is characterized by bizarre behavior and motor features during sleep that are often misdiagnosed as a sleep or a psychiatric disorder (Scheffer et al, 1995). The abnormal gene is on chromosome 20q and may be allelic with one of the genes for benign neonatal familial epilepsy. It is transmitted as an autosomal dominant trait with a penetrance rate of approximately 70%.

CLINICAL FEATURES. Seizures begin in childhood and usually persist into adult life. Most attacks occur when dozing or first falling off to sleep. Clusters of 4 to 11 seizures, each lasting less than a minute, occur in one night. An aura, usually a gasp, grunt, or vocalization that awakens the individual, is common. Other auras include special sensory sensations, psychic phenomena (fear, malaise, etc.), shivering, and difficulty breathing. This is followed by thrashing or tonic stiffening with superimposed clonic jerks. The eyes are open and the individual is aware of what is happening. Many sit up and try to grab on to a bed part.

DIAGNOSIS. The family history is important to the diagnosis but many family members may not realize that their own attacks are seizures nor want others to know that they experience such bizarre symptoms. The interictal EEG is usually normal and concurrent video-EEG is often required to capture the event. During a seizure the discharge is generalized and distributed diffusely. The initial ictal EEG is often obscured by movement artefact.

TREATMENT. Carbamazepine is usually effective in preventing seizures.

Benign Occipital Epilepsy of Childhood

Benign occipital epilepsy of childhood is a genetic epilepsy, probably transmitted by autosomal dominant inheritance, that may be a phenotypic variation of benign rolandic epilepsy.

CLINICAL FEATURES. Age at onset is between 15 months and 17 years, generally between 4 and 8 years. One third of patients have a family history of epilepsy, frequently rolandic epilepsy. The initial seizure manifestation can consist of (1) visual hallucinations, usually flashing lights or spots; (2) blindness, hemianopia, or complete amaurosis; (3) visual illusions, such as micropsia, macropsia, or metamorphasia; or (4) loss of consciousness lasting up to 12 hours (Kivity and Lerman, 1992). More than one feature may occur simultaneously. The visual aura may be followed by unilateral clonic seizures, complex partial seizures, or generalized tonic-clonic seizures. Afterward, the child may have migraine-like headaches and nausea. Attacks occur when the child is awake or asleep, but the greatest frequency is at the transition from wake to sleep. Seizures may be induced by photic stimulation or by playing video games.

DIAGNOSIS. Results of neurologic examination, CT, and MRI are normal. The interictal EEG shows unilateral or bilateral, high-amplitude, occipital spike-wave discharges with a frequency of 1.5 to 2.5 cps. The discharges are inhibited by eye opening and enhanced by light sleep. A similar interictal pattern is seen in some children with absence epilepsy, suggesting a common genetic disorder among different benign genetic epilepsies (Talwar et al, 1992). During a seizure, rapid firing of spike discharges occurs in one or both occipital lobes.

Benign occipital epilepsy may be difficult to distinguish from basilar migraine (see Chapter 10). Reported cases of basilar migraine with occipital spikes are probably benign occipital epilepsy and not migraine. Such cases respond to anticonvulsant drugs and not antimigraine agents.

TREATMENT. Complete seizure control is usually accomplished with standard anticonvulsant drugs. Typical seizures never persist beyond 12 years. However, all children with occipital discharges do not have a benign epilepsy (Salanova et al, 1992). Persistent or hard to control seizures raise the question of a structural abnormality in the occipital lobe, and MRI is indicated.

Benign Rolandic Epilepsy of Childhood

Benign rolandic epilepsy of childhood is a genetic disorder thought to be transmitted as an autosomal dominant trait. Forty percent of close relatives have a history of febrile seizures or epilepsy. Absence and benign occipital epilepsy of childhood may be caused by the same genetic trait.

CLINICAL FEATURES. The age at onset is 18 months to 13 years, with the majority beginning between 5 and 10 years of age. Seizures almost always stop spontaneously by age 14. Even without drug therapy, 10% have only one seizure, 70% have infrequent seizures, and only 20% have frequent seizures. With drug therapy, 20% have isolated seizures and 6% have frequent seizures. Seventy percent of children have seizures only while asleep, 15% only when awake, and 15% both when awake and asleep.

The typical seizure wakes the child from sleep. Paresthesias occur on one side of the mouth, followed by ipsilateral twitching of the face, mouth, and pharynx, resulting in speech arrest and drooling. Consciousness is preserved. The seizure lasts for 1 or 2 minutes. Daytime seizures do not generalize, but nocturnal seizures in children younger than 5 years old often spread to the arm or evolve into a generalized tonic-clonic seizure.

DIAGNOSIS. Results of neurologic examination and brain imaging studies are normal. Interictal EEG shows unilateral or bilateral spike discharges in the central or centrotemporal region. The spikes are typically of high voltage and are activated by drowsiness and sleep. The frequency of spike discharge does not correlate with the subsequent course.

TREATMENT. Treatment is not needed if seizures are infrequent and only nocturnal. A single bedtime dose of phenobarbital is usually satisfactory for seizure control. After 2 years of treatment, medication can be withdrawn and 80% remain seizure free. Those who resume having seizures should be treated until age 14. All children eventually stop having seizures whether they are treated or not.

Epilepsia Partialis Continuans

Focal motor seizures that do not stop spontaneously are termed *epilepsia partialis continuans.* This is an ominous symptom and almost always indicates an underlying cerebral disorder. Possible causes include infarction, hemorrhage, tumor, and inflammation. Every effort should be made to stop the seizures with intravenous anticonvulsant drugs (see Treatment of Status Epilepticus, later on). The response to anticonvulsant drugs and the outcome depends on the underlying cause.

Hemiconvulsions-Hemiplegia Syndrome (Rasmussen Syndrome)

Rasmussen syndrome is a poorly understood disorder that was originally described as a focal viral encephalitis. However, an infectious etiology has never been established.

CLINICAL FEATURES. Focal jerking frequently begins in one body part, usually one side of the face or one hand, and then spreads to contiguous parts. Trunk muscles are rarely affected. The rate and intensity of the seizures vary at first, but then they become more regular and persist in

sleep. The affected limbs become progressively paretic and always remain so.

DIAGNOSIS. Affected children have focal motor seizures that defy treatment and progress to affect first both limbs on one side of the body and then the limbs on the other side. Progressive hemiplegia develops and remains after seizures have stopped.

EEG shows continuous spike discharges originating in one portion of the cortex, with spread to contiguous areas of the cortex and to a mirror focus on the other side. Secondary generalization may occur.

MRI should be performed in every case. The initial imaging studies are usually normal, but repeat studies after 6 months show atrophy of the hemisphere with dilation of the ipsilateral ventricle. Positron emission tomography (PET) shows widespread hypometabolism of the affected hemisphere at a time when the spike discharges are still localized.

The cerebrospinal fluid is usually normal, although a few monocytes may be present as a result of the prolonged seizure. In one patient the cerebrospinal fluid contained oligoclonal bands and an elevated IgG concentration (Andrews et al, 1990). Subsequent pathologic study of the affected hemisphere showed vasculitis and immune complex disease.

TREATMENT. The treatment of Rasmussen syndrome is especially difficult. Standard anticonvulsant therapy is not effective in stopping seizures and progressive hemiplegia is the rule. Medical treatment with high-dose steroids and intravenous immunoglobulin is worth trying (Hart et al, 1994), but early hemispherectomy may provide the best long-term results (Vining et al, 1993).

Subependymal Heterotopia

This may be a specific syndrome among the many migrational disorders associated with epilepsy (Raymond et al, 1994).

CLINICAL FEATURES. The onset of seizures may be anytime during childhood, with the median at 13 years. The female-to-male ratio is greater than 10:1. The heterotopic material is usually nodular, may be unilateral or bilateral, and is most often located in the occipital horn. Development and intelligence are normal before seizure onset and remain normal afterward. The seizures are usually focal motor or complex partial in type but may appear to be absence.

DIAGNOSIS. EEG may show generalized spike and wave discharges, suggesting a primary generalized epilepsy such as childhood absence. Diagnosis is only established by MRI.

TREATMENT. Seizures are reported as refractory to medical treatment, but this may reflect patient selection for MRI. Surgical resection of the heterotopic nodule can be curative.

GENERALIZED TONIC-CLONIC SEIZURES

Generalized tonic-clonic seizures are the most common seizures of childhood. They are dramatic and frightening events that invariably demand medical attention. Seizures that are prolonged or repeated without recovery are termed *status epilepticus.* The diagnostic considerations in a child who has had a generalized tonic-clonic seizure are summarized in Table 1–11.

CLINICAL FEATURES. The onset may occur anytime after the neonatal period, but the onset of primary generalized epilepsy without absence is usually during the second decade. With absence, age at onset shifts to the first decade.

The initial feature is sudden loss of consciousness. The child falls to the floor and the body stiffens (tonic phase). This is followed by repetitive jerking movements of the limbs (clonic phase); these movements at first are rapid and rhythmic and then become slower and more irregular as the seizure ends. The eyes roll backward in the orbits; breathing is rapid and deep, causing saliva to froth at the lips; and urinary and fecal incontinence may occur. Seizures are followed by a postictal sleep from which arousal is difficult. Afterward, the child appears normal but may have sore limb muscles and a painful tongue, bitten during the seizure.

DIAGNOSIS. A first, generalized tonic-clonic seizure requires laboratory evaluation. The extent of evaluation must be individualized. Important determining factors include neurologic

findings, family history, and known precipitating factors. An eyewitness report of focal features at the onset of the seizure, or the recollection of an aura, indicates a partial seizure with secondary generalization.

During the seizure the EEG shows generalized repetitive spikes in the tonic phase and then periodic bursts of spikes in the clonic phase. The clonic portion is usually obscured by movement artifact. As the seizure ends, the background rhythms are slow and the amplitude attenuated. Between seizures, brief generalized spike or spike-wave discharges that are polymorphic in appearance may occur. Discharge frequency is sometimes increased by drowsiness and light sleep. The presence of focal discharges indicates that the tonic-clonic seizure was secondarily generalized.

The cerebrospinal fluid is normal following a brief, tonic-clonic seizure due to primary epilepsy. However, prolonged or repeated seizures may cause leukocytosis (up to 80 cells/mm^3 with a polymorphonuclear predominance). Protein concentration can be mildly elevated, but glucose concentration is normal.

TREATMENT. I never start prophylactic anticonvulsant therapy in an otherwise normal child who has had a single, unexplained seizure. The recurrence rate is probably less than 50% after 1 year. Phenobarbital, phenytoin, and carbamazepine are equally effective in children with recurrent seizures that require treatment. Status epilepticus must be treated with intravenous drugs (see Treatment of Status Epilepticus).

Generalized Epilepsies of Adolescent Onset

Juvenile myoclonic epilepsy is probably the most common epileptic syndrome with adolescent onset. However, another epileptic syndrome has been identified that is not linked to the gene locus on chromosome 6 for juvenile myoclonic epilepsy (Greenberg et al, 1995). Seizures occur on awakening. Myoclonic jerks do not occur.

Pseudoseizures

"Hysterical" seizures are an effective method of seeking attention and secondary gain. They occur more often in adolescence than childhood and in females than males (3:1). A history of sexual abuse is common in women who experience pseudoseizures. People with pseudoseizures may also have true seizures; the pseudoseizures begin when true seizures come under

■ TABLE 1–11
Diagnostic Considerations for a First Nonfebrile Tonic-Clonic Seizure After 2 Years of Age

Acute encephalopathy or encephalitis (see Chapter 2)
Isolated unexplained seizure
Partial seizure of any cause with secondary generalization
Primary generalized epilepsy
Progressive disorder of the nervous system (see Chapter 5)

control and the secondary gain of epilepsy is lost.

CLINICAL FEATURES. Pseudoseizures rarely simulate true seizures but sometimes may be difficult to distinguish by observation alone (Lancman et al, 1994). The clinical features include a rich variety of motor and behavioral phenomena, but three broad patterns are often observed:

1. Unilateral or bilateral motor activity characterized by tonic posturing and tremulousness in which the patient's movements are thrashing or jerking rather than tonic-clonic; different movements may occur simultaneously.
2. Behavioral or emotional changes in which distress or discomfort is expressed, followed by semipurposeless, but not stereotyped, behaviors such as fumbling with objects or walking.
3. Periods of unresponsiveness.

Attacks may be precipitated and ended by suggestion. Patients usually do not hurt themselves and are not incontinent.

DIAGNOSIS. Pseudoseizures usually occur at home and are believed to be real. If the child has epilepsy, the seizures are reported by telephone to the physician and drug schedules are needlessly revised, often to the patient's detriment. The possibility of pseudoseizures must be considered when frequent seizures develop in children whose epilepsy has recently come under control.

Children who do not have epilepsy and in whom pseudoseizures develop are frequently brought to an emergency department and may be given anticonvulsant drugs before any investigation is initiated. It is then difficult to stop the medications and obtain a baseline EEG. Most pseudoseizures are diagnosed by observation alone. When doubt remains, video-EEG monitoring is the best method of diagnosis.

TREATMENT. The diagnosis of pseudoseizures should be presented in a positive and supportive manner. The diagnosis does not mean that the person is crazy or faking. The spells can be stopped, but not with anticonvulsant drugs. Psychiatric referral is not always necessary, but psychological counseling is often needed. Pseudoseizures are managed best by determining the secondary gain provided by seizures and offering alternative methods of satisfaction. In 78% of children with pseudoseizures the attacks stop once the diagnosis is established (Wyllie et al, 1990).

Video-Game Induced Seizures

Children who experience seizures while playing video games usually have a photosensitive seizure disorder than is demonstrable on EEG during intermittent photic stimulation (Ferrie et al, 1994). Two thirds have primary generalized epilepsy (generalized tonic-clonic, absence, and juvenile myoclonic epilepsy), and the remainder have partial epilepsies, usually benign occipital epilepsy.

 Anticonvulsant Drug Therapy

The goal of anticonvulsant therapy is to achieve the maximum normal function by balancing seizure control against drug toxicity.

INDICATIONS FOR STARTING THERAPY

Prophylactic therapy should be initiated whenever there is a reasonable expectation that seizures will recur. Approximately two thirds of otherwise normal children will have a second seizure within 1 year after a first unexplained and untreated tonic-clonic seizure. The risk of recurrence after a second untreated generalized tonic-clonic seizure is 90%. The recurrence rates in children with partial seizures is considerably lower because of the benign cortical epilepsies of childhood. Although most children who have a first nonfebrile seizure are expected to have more, a significant minority do not. Therefore, it is reasonable to withhold anticonvulsant therapy in an otherwise normal child until a second seizure occurs. Epileptiform activity on EEG, a family history of adult epilepsy, and an abnormal neurologic or developmental examination are factors that support initiating therapy after a single seizure.

In contrast to nonfebrile seizures, the risk of recurrence after a first febrile seizure is relatively small (see Febrile Seizures).

DISCONTINUING THERAPY

Children who have seizures during an acute encephalopathy (e.g., anoxia, head trauma, encephalitis) should be treated with anticonvulsant drugs. When the acute encephalopathy is over and seizures have stopped, anticonvulsant therapy should be discontinued. Only a minority of children later have epilepsy, and they can be treated when seizures recur. It is not established that later epilepsy can be prevented by the continuous use of anticonvulsant drugs after an acute encephalopathy.

It is generally true that anticonvulsant therapy can be successfully discontinued in most children whose seizures have been controlled for 2 years. I suspect that many otherwise normal children who were started on anticonvulsant medication after a first seizure and then remain seizure free for 2 years should not have been started in the first place. The decision to stop therapy should be individualized to the child and the cause of the epilepsy (Shinnar et al, 1994). Children who are neurologically abnormal (remote symptomatic epilepsy) and those with specific epileptic syndromes that are known to persist into adult life (juvenile myoclonic epilepsy) are likely to have recurrences, while those with benign epilepsies of childhood are likely to remain seizure free. Three fourths of relapses occur during the withdrawal phase and in the 2 years thereafter. Contrary to popular belief, seizures are not caused by the rapid withdrawal of anticonvulsant drugs in a person who does not need them (Marks et al, 1991; Tennison et al, 1994). Seizures occur in people with epilepsy when the blood concentration is no longer therapeutic, without regard to the rate of decline.

As a general rule, I try to stop anticonvulsant therapy 1 year before driving age in children who are seizure free and neurologically normal.

PRINCIPLES OF THERAPY

Therapy should be started with a single drug. In approximately 75% of children with epilepsy the seizures can be fully controlled with monotherapy. Even patients whose seizures are never controlled are likely to do better on monotherapy than polytherapy. Polytherapy poses several problems: (1) drugs compete with each other for protein binding sites, (2) one drug can increase the rate and pathway of catabolism of a second drug, (3) drugs have cumulative toxicity, and (4) compliance is more difficult.

When more than one drug is needed, drugs that have different spectrums of activity or mechanisms of action should be chosen. Only one drug should be changed at a time. If several changes are made simultaneously, it is impossible to determine which drug is responsible for a beneficial or an adverse effect.

Anticonvulsant drugs should not be administered more often than three times each day. With many drugs an acceptable steady state can be attained using a twice-a-day regimen and some can be administered once a day. Compliance usually falls when drugs are taken more than twice each day. Children often have difficulty taking medicine at school.

BLOOD CONCENTRATIONS

The development of techniques to measure blood concentrations of anticonvulsant drugs was an important advance in the treatment of epilepsy. Measuring total drug concentrations, protein-bound and free fractions, is customary even though the free fraction is responsible for efficacy and toxicity. While the ratio of free to bound fractions is relatively constant, some drugs, such as valproate, have a greater affinity for binding protein than other drugs and will displace them when used together. The free fraction of the displaced drug is then increased and causes toxicity even though the measured total drug concentration is "therapeutic."

Reference values of drug concentrations are guidelines. Some patients are seizure free with concentrations that are below the reference value, and others are unaffected by apparent toxic concentrations.

Most anticonvulsants follow first-order kinetics; that is, blood levels increase proportionately with increases in oral dose. The major exception is phenytoin, whose metabolism changes from first-order to zero-order kinetics when the enzyme system responsible for its catabolism is saturated. Then a small increment in oral dose produces large increments in blood concentration. The half-lives of anticonvulsants listed in Table 1–12 are at steady state. Half-lives are generally longer when a patient is first exposed to a drug. Steady state is usually achieved after five half-lives. Similarly, five half-lives are required to eliminate a drug after administration has been discontinued. Drug half-lives vary from individual to individual and may be shortened or increased by the concurrent use of other anticonvulsants, antibiotics, and antipyretics. This is one reason that children with epilepsy may have a toxic response to drug or increased seizures at the time of a febrile illness.

Some anticonvulsants are metabolized to active metabolites that have anticonvulsant and toxic properties. With the exception of phenobarbital derived from primidone, these metabolites are not usually measured. Active metabolites may provide seizure control or have

■ TABLE 1-12

Anticonvulsant Drugs for Children

DRUG	INITIAL DOSAGE (MG/KG/DAY)	MAINTENANCE DOSAGE (MG/KG/DAY)	BLOOD CONCENTRATION (µG/ML)	HALF-LIFE (H)
Carbamazepine	5	15–20	4–12	14–27
Clonazepam	0.025	0.1–0.15	0.2–0.7*	20–40
Clorazepate	0.3	0.3–1	>1.2*	20–60
Ethosuximide	20	20–40	40–100	30–60
Felbamate	15	45	40–80	14–20
Gabapentin	4–13	10–50	2–20	5–7
Lamotrigine	1–2†	5–10	1–3	12–48
Methsuximide	20	20–40	*	*
Nitrazepam	0.2	0.5–1		18–30
Phenacemide	20	40–50	50–75	24
Phenobarbital	3–5	3–5	10–40	37–73
Phenytoin	5–7	5–7	10–20	5–14
Primidone	2–5	10–15	8–12	5–11
Trimethadione	20	30–60	*	16
Valproate	20	30–60	50–100	6–15
Vigabatrin			*	Days

*Not clinically useful.
†Dosage depends on concomitant therapy with other drugs (see text).

toxic effects when the blood concentration of the parent compound is low.

ADVERSE REACTIONS

Many anticonvulsant drugs irritate the gastric mucosa and cause nausea and vomiting. When this occurs, symptoms may be relieved by taking smaller doses at more frequent intervals, using enteric coated preparations, and administering the drug after meals.

Toxic adverse reactions are dose related. All anticonvulsant drugs cause sedation when blood concentrations are excessive. Subtle cognitive and behavioral disturbances, which are recognized only by the patient or family, often occur at low blood concentrations. The patient's observation of a toxic effect should not be discounted because the blood concentration is within the therapeutic range. As doses are increased, attention span, memory, and interpersonal relations may become seriously impaired. This is especially common with barbiturates, but can occur with any drug.

Idiosyncratic reactions are not entirely dose related. They may occur on the basis of hypersensitivity (usually manifest as rash, fever, and lymphadenopathy) but may also be caused by the production of toxic metabolites. Idiosyncratic reactions are not always predictable, and the patient's observation should be respected, even when the reaction was not previously reported.

SELECTION OF AN ANTICONVULSANT DRUG

The use of generic drugs is difficult to avoid in managed care health programs. Unfortunately, several different manufacturers provide generic versions of each drug; the bioavailability and half-life of these products vary considerably and maintaining a predictable blood concentration is difficult. The most common reasons for loss of seizure control in children who were previously seizure free are noncompliance and changing from the brand name to a generic drug, or from one generic to another. I tell patients to ask their pharmacist to tell them when their source of generic drug is going to change.

The drugs most often selected for the treatment of tonic-clonic and partial seizures are carbamazepine, phenobarbital, and phenytoin. Clonazepam, felbamate, gabapentin, primidone, and valproate are used in refractory cases. Valproate has become very popular as a primary drug of choice because it is effective against so many different seizure types. However, it is considerably more expensive and toxic than several other drugs and should not be chosen first when other drugs are equally effective.

The initial drugs used to treat absence and myoclonic seizures are ethosuximide and valproate. Secondary drugs are benzodiazepines (clonazepam, clorazepate, and nitrazepam) and lamotrigene. The ketogenic diet is an alternative to drug therapy.

ACTH, prednisone, and pyridoxine provide

transitory relief of intractable seizures in infants (see "Infantile Spasms"), but are not ordinarily used in older children. Intravenous immunoglobulin has been used to treat children with intractable seizures, especially those with Rasmussen syndrome. Controlled studies are not reported and its efficacy is not established (van Engelen et al, 1994).

Carbamazepine (Tegretol, Geigy)

INDICATIONS. Tonic-clonic and partial seizures. Atypical absence and myoclonic seizures may be exacerbated to the point of status (Callahan and Noetzel, 1992).

ADMINISTRATION. Absorption from the gastrointestinal tract is slow and variable. The rectal route may be used for maintenance if the dose is increased by one third. Approximately 85% of the drug is protein bound. Carbamazepine induces its own metabolism, and the initial dose should be 25% of the maintenance dose to prevent toxicity. The usual maintenance dosage is 15 to 20 mg/kg/day to provide a blood concentration of 4 to 12 µg/ml (17 to 51 µmol/L). However, 30 mg/kg/day is often required in infants. Half-life at steady state is 5 to 27 hours, and children usually require doses three times a day.

Concurrent use of erythromycin, propoxyphene, verapamil, and cimetidine interferes with carbamazepine metabolism and has a toxic effect.

ADVERSE EFFECTS. A depression of peripheral leukocytes is expected, but rarely sufficient (absolute neutrophil count less than 1,000) to warrant discontinuation of therapy. It is reasonable to measure the white blood cell count 6 weeks after therapy is started. Repeat white blood cell counts each time the patient returns for a routine follow-up visit is not cost-effective and does not allow the prediction of life-threatening events (Pellock and Willmore, 1991). The most informative time to repeat the white blood cell count is concurrent with a febrile illness.

Cognitive disturbances occur within the therapeutic range. Sedation, ataxia, and nystagmus occur at toxic blood concentrations. Nonepileptic myoclonus is an allergic reaction.

Clonazepam (Klonopin, Roche)

INDICATIONS. Infantile spasms, myoclonic seizures, absence, and partial seizures. Tolerance to clonazepam often develops in children with severe myoclonic epilepsy, such as those with infantile spasms and the Lennox-Gastaut syndrome (Specht et al, 1989). Once tolerance is established, discontinuation of the drug may actually improve seizure control.

ADMINISTRATION. The initial dosage is 0.025 mg/kg/day in two divided doses. Increments of 0.025 mg/kg are recommended every 3 to 5 days as needed and tolerated. The usual maintenance dosage is 0.1 mg/kg/day in three divided doses. Most children cannot tolerate dosages more than 0.15 mg/kg/day. Therapeutic blood concentrations are 0.02 to 0.07 µg/ml; 47% is protein bound and the half-life is 20 to 40 hours. The rectal route may be used for maintenance.

ADVERSE EFFECTS. Toxic effects with doses within the therapeutic range include sedation, cognitive impairment, hyperactivity, and excessive salivation. Idiosyncratic reactions are unusual.

Clorazepate (Tranxene, Abbott)

INDICATIONS. Adjunct therapy for refractory myoclonic and partial seizures. Clorazepate should not be used as a primary anticonvulsant.

ADMINISTRATION. The smallest capsule, 3.75 mg, is given once each day and increased by one capsule every 3 days as needed and tolerated. Maintenance dosage is 1 to 3 mg/kg/day in three divided doses. The total dosage is limited by toxicity, and blood concentration measurements are not useful.

ADVERSE EFFECTS. Sedation occurs within the therapeutic range and limits usefulness. Higher doses cause ataxia, diplopia, and impairment of cognitive function.

Ethosuximide (Zarontin, Parke-Davis)

INDICATIONS. Treatment of absence; also useful for myoclonic absence.

ADMINISTRATION. The drug is absorbed rapidly, and peak blood concentrations appear within 4 hours. It is not bound to plasma proteins. The half-life is 30 hours in children and up to 60 hours in adults. The initial dosage is 20 mg/kg/day in three divided doses after meals to avoid gastric irritation. Increments of 10 mg/kg/day are administered as needed and tolerated to provide a blood concentration above 40 µg/ml (280 µmol/L).

ADVERSE EFFECTS. Ethosuximide does not interact with other anticonvulsants because it is not protein bound. Idiosyncratic reactions include dystonia and a lupus-like syndrome. Aplastic anemia is a rare complication. Common toxic reactions include nausea, abdominal pain, headache, and sedation. Gastrointestinal symptoms occur within the therapeutic range and limit usefulness.

Felbamate (Felbatol, Wallace Laboratories)

INDICATIONS. Felbamate has a wide spectrum of antiepileptic activity. Its primary use is in the Lennox-Gastaut syndrome, juvenile myoclonic epilepsy, absence, and atonic seizures, but it is quite effective also in children with refractory partial and generalized seizures.

ADMINISTRATION. Felbamate is rapidly absorbed after oral intake and is not affected by food or antacids. Maximal plasma concentrations occur in 2 to 6 hours. The initial dosage is 15 mg/kg/day in three divided doses. Nighttime doses should be avoided if the drug causes insomnia. Increments of 15 mg/kg are made weekly to a maintenance dose of approximately 45 mg/kg/day. The therapeutic serum concentration is between 30 and 80 μg/ml.

ADVERSE EFFECTS. Initially, adverse effects of felbamate were thought to be mild (nausea, anorexia, insomnia, weight loss) except when used in combination with other anticonvulsants. The addition of felbamate increases the plasma concentrations of phenytoin and valproate as much as 30%. Carbamazepine serum concentrations fall but the concentration of its active epoxide metabolite increases almost 50%.

However, post-marketing experience showed that felbamate caused fatal liver damage and aplastic anemia. Its use is now limited to patients who do not respond to any other drug, and regular monitoring of blood counts and liver function are required. However, a complete profile of the conditions that were conducive to serious side adverse events was not established. More information is needed, as this is too valuable a drug to be discarded.

Gabapentin (Neurontin, Parke-Davis)

INDICATIONS. Mainly used as adjunct therapy with carbamazepine or phenytoin, especially for refractory partial onset seizures and secondarily generalized seizures (Ramsay, 1994).

ADMINISTRATION. Gabapentin is rapidly absorbed and not metabolized. It is not protein bound, does not induce hepatic enzymes, does not interact with other drugs, and is excreted unchanged in the urine. The original recommendation was to achieve blood concentrations of 2 to 3 μg/ml by administering 20 to 40 mg/kg/day in three divided doses. More recent evidence indicates that dosages that are three times greater may be needed.

ADVERSE EFFECTS. These are usually mild and mainly consist of somnolence, dizziness, and ataxia.

Lamotrigine (Lamictal, Burroughs Wellcome)

INDICATIONS. Adjunctive therapy in absence epilepsy, atonic seizures, and the Lennox-Gastaut syndrome (Schlumberger et al, 1994).

ADMINISTRATION. The therapeutic plasma concentration of 2 to 3 μg/ml is usually achieved with an oral dosage of 5 mg/kg/day in two divided doses. The concomitant use of lamotrigine and other anticonvulsants shortens the half-life of lamotrigine but does not lower the blood concentration of the other drugs. In contrast, the concomitant use of valproate markedly extends the half-life of lamotrigine (Pellock, 1994). The initial dose and the incremental doses of lamotrigine must be reduced by 50% when administered to children who are taking valproate.

ADVERSE EFFECTS. The incidence of adverse effects is low and consists mainly of dizziness, ataxia, diplopia, and headache.

Methsuximide (Celontin, Parke-Davis)

INDICATIONS. A secondary drug for absence and myoclonic seizures if ethosuximide and valproate cannot be used. It may also be useful as a secondary drug for partial seizures.

ADMINISTRATION. Methsuximide is rapidly absorbed and reaches peak blood concentrations within 2 hours. However, active metabolites rather than the parent compound are probably responsible for efficacy and toxicity. Some of these accumulate for 30 to 40 hours. The initial dosage is 20 mg/kg/day in three divided doses. Increments of 10 mg/kg/day are administered as needed and tolerated. Measuring the blood concentration of the parent compound is not helpful.

ADVERSE EFFECTS. Drowsiness is the most common side effect, but gastric irritation and personality change may occur as well.

Nitrazepam (Mogadon, Roche)

INDICATIONS. Infantile spasms and myoclonic seizures.

ADMINISTRATION. Nitazepam is not approved for use in the United States. The half-life is 18 to 30 hours. Initial dosage is 0.2 mg/kg/day in two divided doses. Biweekly increments of 0.3 mg/kg are administered as needed until a maintenance dosage of 0.5 to 1 mg/kg/day is achieved.

ADVERSE EFFECTS. Drowsiness, hypotonia, and increased secretions are the usual side effects.

Phenytoin (Dilantin, Parke-Davis)

INDICATIONS. Tonic-clonic seizures, partial seizures, status epilepticus.

ADMINISTRATION. Oral absorption is slow and unpredictable in newborns, erratic in infants, and probably not reliable until 3 to 5 years of age. Even in adults there is considerable individual variability. Once absorbed, phenytoin is 70% to 95% protein bound. A typical maintenance dosage is 7 mg/kg/day in newborns and 5 mg/kg/day in children. The half-life is up to 60 hours in term newborns, up to 140 hours in premature infants, 5 to 14 hours in children, and 10 to 34 hours in adults. Capsules are usually taken in two divided doses, but tablets are more rapidly absorbed and may require three divided doses a day.

Rapid loading of phenytoin can be performed by giving three times the maintenance dosage by either the oral or intravenous route (see "Treatment of Status Epilepticus"). Intramuscular injections are not absorbed and should not be used.

Blood concentrations less than 10 μg/ml (40 μmol/L) are metabolized by first-order kinetics, but higher concentrations are metabolized by zero-order kinetics. The usual therapeutic range is 10 to 20 μg/ml (40 to 80 μmol/L), and once within that range, dosage increments must be small.

ADVERSE EFFECTS. The major adverse reactions are hypersensitivity, gum hypertrophy, and hirsutism. Hypersensitivity reactions usually occur with 6 weeks of the initiation of therapy and are characterized by rash, fever, and lymphadenopathy. Once such a reaction has occurred, the drug should be discontinued. Concurrent use of antihistamines is not appropriate management. Continued use of the drug may produce a Stevens-Johnson syndrome or a lupus-like disorder.

Gum hypertrophy is caused by a combination of phenytoin metabolites and plaque on the teeth. Persons with good oral hygiene are unlikely to have gum hypertrophy. The importance of good oral hygiene should be discussed at the onset of therapy. Hirsutism is rarely a

problem, and then only for girls. When it occurs the drug can be discontinued without permanent harm.

Memory impairment, decreased attention span, and personality change may occur at therapeutic concentrations, but they occur less often and less severe than with phenobarbital.

Phenobarbital

INDICATIONS. Tonic-clonic and simple partial seizures.

ADMINISTRATION. Oral absorption is slow, and daily doses are better given with the evening meal than at bedtime if seizures are hypnagogic. Since intramuscular absorption requires 1 to 2 hours, the intramuscular route should not be used for rapid loading (see Treatment of Status Epilepticus); 50% is protein bound, and 50% is free.

Initial and maintenance dosages are 3 to 5 mg/kg/day. The half-life is 46 to 136 hours in adults, 37 to 73 hours in children, and 61 to 173 hours in term newborns. Because of the very long half-life at all ages, once-a-day doses are usually satisfactory, and steady-state blood concentrations should be measured after 2 weeks of therapy. Therapeutic blood concentrations are 10 to 40 μg/ml (40 to 160 μmol/L).

ADVERSE EFFECTS. Hyperactivity is the most common and limiting side effect in children. Adverse behavioral changes occur in one half of children between ages 2 and 10. Parents should be warned of this possibility at the onset of therapy. Behavioral changes are dose related, and other barbiturates that are converted to phenobarbital produce the same adverse effects at equivalent phenobarbital blood concentrations.

Drowsiness and cognitive dysfunction, rather than hyperactivity, are the usual adverse effects after 10 years of age. Infants tolerate phenobarbital well, and it remains a drug of choice for oral use in newborns and infants. Idiosyncratic reactions are unusual.

Primidone (Mysoline, Ayerst)

INDICATIONS. Tonic-clonic and partial seizures.

ADMINISTRATION. Primidone is metabolized to at least two active metabolites, phenobarbital and phenyl-ethyl-malonamide (PEMA). Primidone half-life is 6 to 12 hours and PEMA half-life is 20 hours. The usual maintenance dosage is 10 to 15 mg/kg/day, but the initial dosage should be 25% of maintenance or intolerable sedation occurs. A therapeutic blood concentration of primidone is 8 to 12 µg/ml (36 to 52 µmol/L). The blood concentration of phenobarbital derived from primidone is generally four times greater, but this ratio is altered when other anticonvulsant drugs are administered concurrently.

ADVERSE EFFECTS. The adverse effects are the same as for phenobarbital, except that the risk of intolerable sedation from the first tablet is great.

Valproate (Depakene, Abbott)

INDICATIONS. Myoclonic seizures, simple absence, myoclonic absence, myoclonus, and tonic-clonic seizures. Valproate is especially useful for mixed seizure disorders.

ADMINISTRATION. Oral absorption is rapid, and half-life is 6 to 15 hours. Doses three times a day are needed to achieve constant blood concentrations. An enteric-coated capsule (Depakote) slows absorption and allows twice-a-day doses in many children.

The initial dosage is 20 mg/kg/day. Increments of 10 mg/kg/day are administered to provide a blood concentration of 50 to 100 µg/ml (350 to 700 µmol/L). Blood concentrations of 80 to 120 µg/ml (560 to 840 µmol/L) are often required to achieve seizure control. Protein binding is 95% at blood concentrations of 50 µg/ml and 80% at 100 µg/ml. Therefore doubling the blood concentration increases the free fraction eightfold. Valproate has a strong affinity for plasma proteins and displaces other anticonvulsant drugs.

Valproate is absorbed when given rectally and can be administered by this route when oral administration is not possible. A peak concentration is attained 3 hours after rectal administration, and the serum concentration is approximately 75% of the oral dose.

ADVERSE EFFECTS. Valproate has dose-related and idiosyncratic hepatotoxicity. Dose-related hepatotoxicity is harmless and characterized by increased serum concentrations of transaminases. Important dose-related effects are a reduction in the platelet count, pancreatitis, and hyperammonemia. Thrombocytopenia may result in serious bleeding after trivial injury, whereas pancreatitis and hepatitis are both associated with nausea and vomiting. Hyperammonemia, caused by interference with the urea cycle, causes cognitive disturbances and nausea. These adverse reactions are reversible when the daily dose is reduced.

Plasma carnitine concentrations are reduced in children taking valproate, and some believe that carnitine supplementation helps relieve cognitive impairment.

The major idiosyncratic reaction is fatal liver necrosis attributed to the production of an aberrant and toxic metabolite. The major risk (1:800) is in children younger than 2 years of age receiving polytherapy. Many such cases may not be caused by valproate, or valproate alone, but by an underlying disorder that causes both hepatic and cerebral degeneration (Bicknese et al, 1992). Fatal hepatotoxicity has not been reported in children over 10 years of age treated with valproate alone.

The clinical manifestations of idiosyncratic hepatotoxicity are similar to those of Reye syndrome (see Chapter 2). It may begin after 1 day of therapy or not appear for 6 months. No reliable way exists to monitor patients for idiosyncratic hepatotoxicity or to predict its occurrence.

Vigabatrin

INDICATIONS. Adjunctive therapy in partial seizures and infantile spasms (Appleton, 1993). A better response is seen in children with symptomatic than cryptogenic infantile spasms.

ADMINISTRATION. Vigabatrin is a very long-acting drug and needs only single-day dosing but twice-daily dosing is preferable to reduce adverse effects. The maintenance dosage in children is 50 to 100/mg/kg/day. Vigabatrin and lamotrigine have complementary modes of action and may be more effective when given in combination (Stolarek et al, 1994).

ADVERSE EFFECTS. Behavioral problems, fatigue, confusion, and gastrointestinal upset are usually mild and dose related.

TREATMENT OF STATUS EPILEPTICUS

Status epilepticus is defined as a prolonged single seizure (longer than 20 minutes) or repeated seizures without interictal recovery. Generalized tonic-clonic status is life threatening and is the most common emergency in pediatric neurology. Status may be caused by a new acute illness such as encephalitis, a progressive neurologic disease, loss of seizure control in a known epileptic, or a febrile seizure in an otherwise normal child (Shinnar et al, 1992). The outcome is mainly determined by the cause. Recurrence of status epilepticus is most likely in children who are neurologically abnormal and is rare in children with febrile seizures.

Absence status and complex partial status are often difficult to identify as status epilepticus. The child may appear to be in a confusional state.

Immediate Management

Prolonged seizures or clusters of seizures in children with known epilepsy can sometimes be managed at home with rectal diazepam to prevent or abort status epilepticus (Kriel et al, 1991). A rectal preparation of diazepam is not commercially available in the United States, but the intravenous preparation can be given rectally (0.4 mg/kg) through a lubricated syringe. Pharmacists can make up suppositories for home use. If the rectal dose fails to stop the seizures, the child should be brought to an emergency service.

Status epilepticus is a medical emergency requiring prompt attention. Initial assessment should be rapid and includes cardiorespiratory function, history leading up to the seizure, and neurologic examination. A controlled airway must be established immediately and mechanical ventilation made available. Venous access is established next. Blood is withdrawn for measurement of glucose, electrolytes, and anticonvulsant concentrations when applicable. Other tests (i.e., toxic screen) are performed as indicated. After blood is withdrawn, an intravenous infusion of saline solution is started for the administration of anticonvulsant drugs. An intravenous bolus of a 50% glucose solution, 1 mg/kg, is then administered.

Drug Treatment

The ideal drug for treating status epilepticus is one that acts rapidly, has a long duration of action, and does not produce sedation. Diazepam is used widely for this purpose but is inadequate because the duration of action is brief. In addition, children who are given intravenous diazepam after a prior load of barbiturate often have respiratory depression. If diazepam is chosen as a first drug, the dose is 0.2 mg/kg, not to exceed 10 mg at a rate of 1 mg/min. Lorazepam may be preferable to diazepam because of its longer action (Labar et al, 1994). The usual dose in children 12 years or younger is 0.1 mg/kg. After age 12 it is 0.07 mg/kg.

My preference is intravenous phenytoin because of its very long duration of action. A dose of 20 mg/kg is injected at a rate not to exceed 0.5 mg/kg/min. Infants generally require 30 mg/kg. The slow rate of administration is necessary to avoid causing cardiac arrhythmias.

Phenytoin is usually effective unless status epilepticus is caused by severe, acute encephalopathy. EEG should be done after clinical signs of status have stopped to be certain that electrical status is terminated. This is especially important in children who fail to wake up at an expected time.

When phenytoin fails, several alternatives are available; my preference is pentobarbital coma. The patient should have been transferred from the emergency department to an intensive care unit, intubated, and mechanically ventilated. After an arterial line is placed, the patient's blood pressure, cardiac rhythm, body temperature, and blood oxygen saturation are monitored

With an EEG monitor recording continuously, 10-mg/kg boluses of pentobarbital are infused until a burst-suppression pattern appears on the EEG (Figure 1-5); a minimum of 30 mg/kg is generally required. Hypotension is the most serious complication and requires treatment with vasopressors. It is generally not observed until 40 to 60 mg/kg is administered. Barbiturates tend to accumulate and the usual dosage needed to maintain pentobarbital coma is 3 mg/kg/h. The coma can be maintained safely for several days. The EEG should be checked several times each day for the burst-suppression pattern. During barbiturate coma, the patient has gastroparesis and medications given through a nasogastric tube are not adequately absorbed but may remain in the stomach and then be rapidly absorbed when coma is lifted. The coma can be lifted every 24 to 48 hours to see whether the seizures have stopped.

 ## Surgical Approaches to Childhood Epilepsy

Surgery is sometimes recommended for children with epilepsy that is intractable to optimal anticonvulsant therapy. Surgery is never a substitute for good medical therapy and anticonvulsant drugs are often needed after surgery is performed. Three procedures are used: hemispherectomy, interhemispheric commissurotomy, and temporal lobectomy. None of these procedures is new, and all have gone through phases of greater or lesser popularity since being introduced.

HEMISPHERECTOMY

Hemispherectomy, or more correctly hemidecortication, has been used exclusively for

☐ FIGURE 1 – 5 Burst-suppression pattern in pentobarbital coma. Long intervals of amplitude suppression are interrupted by bursts of mixed frequencies.

children with intractable epilepsy and hemiplegia. The original procedure consisted of removing the cortex of one hemisphere along with a variable portion of the underlying basal ganglia. The extent of surgery depended partly upon the underlying disease. The resulting cavity communicated with the third ventricle and became lined with a subdural membrane. The immediate results were good. Seizures were relieved in about 80% of children, and behavior and spasticity was improved without deterioration of intellectual function.

However, late complications of hemorrhage, hydrocephalus, and hemosiderosis occurred in up to 35% of children and were sometimes fatal. It is believed that the subdural membrane repeatedly tears, bleeding into the ventricular system and staining the ependymal lining and the pia arachnoid with iron.

Because of these complications, less radical alternatives are generally preferred. These alternatives are the Montreal-type hemispherectomy and interhemispheric commissurotomy. The Montreal-type hemispherectomy is a modified procedure in which most of the damaged hemisphere is removed but portions of the frontal and occipital lobes are left in place, disconnected from the other hemisphere and brainstem. The best results are obtained when presurgical evaluation with single photon emmission computed tomography (SPECT) or PET shows that only one hemisphere is abnormal and the source of seizures (Carmant et al, 1994).

INTERHEMISPHERIC COMMISSUROTOMY

Disconnecting the hemispheres from each other and from the brainstem is an alternative to hemispherectomy in children with intractable epilepsy and hemiplegia. This operation is also used to decrease the occurrence of secondary generalized tonic-clonic seizures from partial or minor generalized seizures. The efficacy of commissurotomy and hemispherectomy in children with infantile hemiplegia is probably comparable, but the efficacy of commissurotomy in other forms of epilepsy has not been established.

Complete and partial commissurotomies have been recommended. Complete commissurotomy entails division of the entire corpus callosum, anterior commissure, one fornix, and the hippocampal commissure. Complete commissurotomies may be performed in one stage or two. Partial commissurotomies vary from division of the corpus callosum and hippocampal commissure to division of only the anterior portion of the corpus callosum.

Two immediate, but transitory, postoperative complications may follow interhemispheric commissurotomy: (1) a syndrome of mutism, left arm and leg apraxia, and urinary incontinence and (2) hemiparesis. They are both more common after one-stage, complete commissurotomy than after two-stage procedures or partial commissurotomy and are probably caused by prolonged retraction of one hemisphere during surgery. Long-term complications may include stuttering and poorly coordinated movements of the hands.

TEMPORAL LOBECTOMY

The results of temporal lobectomy depends upon the selection criteria and the skill of the epileptology team. Complete seizure relief should be attainable in more than 50% children with intractable partial complex seizures of temporal lobe origin. Only children who have a unilateral temporal focus are candidates for surgery. PET is proving valuable for identifying the epileptic focus. The surgical procedure is a subpial resection of the superior temporal gyrus, hippocampus, and amygdala. The extent of resection is determined by intraoperative EEG. Benign tumors, gliomas and ganglioneuromas, are found in 12% of the specimens.

The most common complication is superior quadrantanopsia (40%) and the most serious complication is aphasia (10%), which is usually transitory.

REFERENCES

Aldrich MS. Narcolepsy. Neurology 1992;42(suppl):34-43.

Andrews JM, Thompson JA, Pysher TJ, et al. Chronic encephalitis, epilepsy, and cerebrovascular immune complex deposits. Ann Neurol 1990;28:88-90.

Appleton RE. The role of vigabatrin in the management of infantile epileptic syndromes. Neurology 1993;43(suppl 5):S21-S23.

Batshaw ML. Inborn errors of urea synthesis. Ann Neurol 1994;35:133-141.

Baumeister FA, Gsell W, Shin YS, et al. Glutamate in pyridoxine-dependent epilepsy: Neurotoxic glutamate concentration in the cerebrospinal fluid and its normalization by pyridoxine. Pediatrics 1994;94:318-321.

Berg AT. Are febrile seizures provoked by a rapid rise in temperature? Am J Dis Child 1993;147:1101-1103.

Berg AT, Shinnar S, Hauser WA, et al. A prospective study of recurrent febrile seizures. N Engl J Med 1992;327:122-127.

Berkovic SF, Cocius J, Andermann E, et al. Progressive myoclonus epilepsies: Clinical and genetic issues. Epilepsia 1993;34(suppl 3):S19-S30.

Berkovic SF, Kennerson ML, Howell RA, et al. Phenotypic expression of benign familial neonatal convulsions linked to chromosome 20. Arch Neurol 1994;51:1125-1128.

Bicknese AR, May W, Hickey WF, et al. Early childhood hepatocerebral degeneration misdiagnosed as valproate hepatotoxicity. Ann Neurol 1992;32:767-775.

Callahan DJ, Noetzel MJ. Prolonged absence status associated with carbamazepine therapy, increased intracranial pressure, and transient MRI abnormalities. Neurology 1992;42:2198-2201.

Carmant L, O'Tuama LA, Roach PJ, et al. Technetium-99m HmPAO brain SPECT and outcome of hemispherectomy for intractable seizures. Pediatr Neurol 1994;11:203-207.

Daoust-Roy J, Seshia SS. Benign neonatal sleep myoclonus. A

differential diagnosis of neonatal seizures. Am J Dis Child 1992;146:1236-1241.

DiMario FJ Jr. Breath-holding spells in children. Am J Dis Child 1992;146:125-131.

DiMario FJ Jr, Burleson JA. Autonomic nervous system function in severe breath-holding spells. Pediatr Neurol 1993;9:268-274.

Doberczak TM, Kandall SR, Wilets I. Neonatal opiate abstinence syndrome in term and preterm infants. J Pediatr 1991;118:933-937.

Donat J. The age-dependent epileptic encephaliecs. J Child Neurol 1992;7:7.

Doose H. Absence epilepsy of early childhood—genetic aspects. Eur J Pediatr 1994;153:372-377.

Driscoll DA. Genetic basis of DiGeorge syndrome and velocardial syndromes. Curr Opin Pediatr 1994;6:702-706.

Drury I, Blaivas M, Abou-Khalil BW, et al. Biopsy results in a kindred with Lafora disease. Arch Neurol 1993;50:102-105.

Echenne B, Humbertclaude V, Rivier F, et al. Benign infantile epilepsy with autosomal dominant inheritance. Brain Dev 1994;16:108-111.

Felbamate Study Group in Lennox-Gastaut Syndrome. Efficacy of felbamate in childhood epileptic encephalopathy (Lennox-Gastaut syndrome). N Engl J Med 1993;328:29-33.

Ferrie CD, De Marco P, Grünewald RA, et al. Video game induced seizures. J Neurol Neurosurg Psychiatry 1994;57:925-931.

Frey J, Darbonne C. Fluoxetine suppresses human cataplexy: A pilot study. Neurology 1994;44:707-709.

Gherpelli JLD, Cruz AM, Tsanaclis LM, et al. Phenobarbital in newborns with neonatal seizures: A study of plasma levels after intravenous administration. Brain Dev 1993;15:258-262.

Green SM, Rothrock SG, Clem KJ, et al. Can seizures be the sole manifestation of meningitis in febrile children? Pediatrics 1993;92:527-534.

Greenberg DA, Durner M, Resor S, et al. The genetics of idiopathic generalized epilepsies of adolescent onset: Differences between juvenile myoclonic epilepsy and epilepsy with random grand mal and with awakening grand mal. Neurology 1995;45:942-946.

Griggs RC, Nutt JG. Episodic ataxias as channelopathies. Ann Neurol 1995;37:285-287.

Hamilton RL, Haas RH, Nyhan WL, et al. Neuropathology of propionic acidemia: A report of two patients with basal ganglia lesions. J Child Neurol 1995;10:25-30.

Hamosh A, Johnston MV, Valle D. Nonketotic hyperglycinemia. In Scriver CR, Beaudet AL, Sly WS, et al, eds. The Metabolic and Molecular Basis of Inherited Disease, 7th edition. McGraw-Hill, New York, 1995;1337-1348.

Hart YM, Cortez M, Andermann F, et al. The medical treatment of Rasmussen syndrome (chronic encephalitis and epilepsy): Effect of high dose steroids and/or immunoglobulin in 19 patients. Neurology 1994;44:1030-1036.

Hellström-Westas L, Blennow G, Lindroth M, et al. Low risk of seizure recurrence after early withdrawal of antiepileptic treatment in the neonatal period. Arch Dis Child 1995;72:F97-F101.

Hirsch E, Velez A, Sellal F, et al. Electroclinical signs of benign neonatal familial seizures. Ann Neurol 1993;34:835-841.

Holmes GB, Rosenfeld WE, Graves NM, et al. Absorption of valproate suppositories in human volunteers. Arch Neurol 1989;46:906-909.

Hrachovy RA, Frost JD Jr, Glaze D. High-dose, long-duration versus low-dose, short-duration corticotropin therapy for infantile spasms. J Pediatr 1994;124:803-806.

Hublin C, Partinen M, Heinonen EH, et al. Selegiline in the treatment of narcolepsy. Neurology 1994;44:2095-2101.

Huttenlocher PR, Hapke RJ. A follow-up study of intractable seizures in childhood. Ann Neurol 1990;28:699-705.

Institute of Medicine. Adverse Effects of Pertussis and Rubella Vaccines. National Academy Press, Washington, DC, 1991.

Kaplan P, Mazur A, Field M, et al. Intellectual outcome in children with maple syrup urine disease. J Pediatr 1991; 119:46-50.

Kivity S, Lerman P. Stormy onset with prolonged loss of consciousness in benign childhood epilepsy with occipital paroxysms. J Neurol Neurosurg Psychiatry 1992;55:45-48.

Kriel RL, Cloyd JC, Hadsall RS, et al. Home use of rectal diazepam for cluster and prolonged seizures: Efficacy, adverse reactions, quality of life, and cost analysis. Pediatr Neurol 1991;7:13-17.

Kuzniecky R, Murro A, King D, et al. Magnetic resonance imaging in childhood intractable partial epilepsies: Pathologic correlations. Neurology 1993;43:681-687.

Labar DR, Ali A, Root J. High-dose intravenous lorazepam for the treatment of refractory status epilepticus. Neurology 1994;44:1400-1403.

Lancman ME, Asconapé GJ, Graves S, et al. Psychogenic seizures in children: Long-term analysis of 43 cases. J Child Neurol 1994;9:404-407.

Marks DA, Katz A, Scheyer R, et al. Clinical and electrographic effects of acute anticonvulsant withdrawal in epileptic patients. Neurology 1991;41:508-512.

Menezes AV, MacGregor DL, Buncic JR. Aicardi syndrome: Natural history and possible predictors of severity. Pediatr Neurol 1994;11:313-318.

Nass R, Heier L, Walker R. Landau-Kleffner syndrome: Temporal lobe tumor resection results in good outcome. Pediatr Neurol 1993;9:303-305.

Overall JC Jr. Herpes simplex virus infection of the fetus and newborn. Pediatr Ann 1994;23:131-136.

Ozand PT, Gascon GG. Organic acidurias: A review. Part 1. J Child Neurol 1991;6:196-219.

Ozand PT, Nyhan WL, al Aqeel A, et al. Malonic aciduria. Brain Dev 1994;16:7-11

Palmer C, Vannucci RC. Potential new therapies for perinatal cerebral hypoxia-ischemia. Clin Perinatol 1993;20:411-432.

Palmini A, Andermann F, Olivier A, et al. Focal neuronal migration disorders and intractable partial epilepsy: A study of 30 patients. Ann Neurol 1991;30:741-749.

Panayiotopoulos CP, Obeid T, Tahan AR. Juvenile myoclonic epilepsy: A 5-year prospective study. Epilepsia 1994;35:285-296.

Paquier PF, Dongen HRV, Loonen CB. The Landau-Kleffner syndrome or "acquired aphasia with convulsive disorder": Long-term follow-up of six children and a review of the recent literature. Arch Neurol 1992;49:354-359.

Pellock JM. The clinical efficacy of lamotrigine as an epileptic drug. Neurology 1994;44(suppl 8):S29-S35.

Pellock JM, Willmore LJ. A rational guide to routine blood monitoring in patients receiving antiepileptic drugs. Neurology 1991;41:961-964.

Pfeinemann F, Danner DJ. Maple syrup urine disease 1954 to 1993. J Inherited Metab Dis 1994;17:3-15.

Porter RJ. The absence epilepsies. Epilepsia 1993;34(suppl 3):S42-S48.

Prats JM, Garaizar C, Rua MJ, et al. Infantile spasms treated with high doses of sodium valproate: Initial response and follow-up. Dev Med Child Neurol 1991;33:617-625.

Radhakrishnan K, Silbert PL, Klass DW. Reading epilepsy: An appraisal of 20 patients diagnosed at the Mayo Clinic,

Rochester, Minnesota, between 1949 and 1989, and delineation of the syndrome. Brain 1995;118:75-89.

Ramsay RE. Clinical efficacy and safety of gabapentin. Neurology 1994;44(suppl 5):S23-S30.

Raymond AA, Fish DR, Stevens JM, et al. Subependymal heterotopia: A distinct neuronal migration disorder associated with epilepsy. J Neurol Neurosurg Psychiatry 1994; 57:1195-1202.

Riviello JJ Jr, Rezvani I, DiGeorge AM, et al. Cerebral edema causing death in children with maple syrup urine disease. J Pediatr 1991;119:42-45.

Rivkin MJ, Anderson ML, Kaye EM. Neonatal idiopathic cerebral venous thrombosis: An unrecognized cause of transient seizures or lethargy. Ann Neurol 1992;32:51-56.

Rosenblatt DS. Inborn errors of vitamin B_{12} metabolism: Clinical and genetic heterogeneity. Int Pediatr 1994;9: 209-213.

Rosman NP, Colton T, Labazzo J, et al. A controlled trial of diazepam administered during febrile illnesses to prevent recurrence of febrile seizures. N Engl J Med 1993;329: 79-84.

Salanova V, Andermann F, Olivier A, et al. Occipital lobe epilepsy: Electrocortical manifestations, electrocorticography, cortical stimulation and outcome in 42 patients treated between 1930 and 1991. Surgery of occipital lobe epilepsy. Brain 1992;115:1655-1680.

Salbert BA, Pellock JM, Wolf B. Characterization of seizures associated with biotinidase deficiency. Neurology 1993;43: 1351-1355.

Scheffer IE, Bhatia KP, Lopes-Cendes I, et al. Autosomal dominant nocturnal frontal lobe epilepsy: A distinctive clinical disorder. Brain 1995;118:61-73.

Scher MS, Kosaburo A, Beggarly ME, et al. Electrographic seizures in preterm and full-term neonates: clinical correlates, associated brain lesions, and risk for neurologic sequelae. Pediatrics 1993;91:128-134.

Schlumberger E, Chavez F, Palacios L, et al. Lamotrigine in treatment of 120 children with epilepsy. Epilepsia 1994; 35:359-367.

Shields WD, Shewmon DA, Chugani HT, et al. Treatment of infantile spasms: Medical or surgical? Epilepsia 1992;33 (suppl 4):S26-S31.

Shinnar S, Berg AT, Moshé SL, et al. Discontinuing antiepileptic drugs in children with epilepsy: A prospective study. Ann Neurol 1994;35:534-545.

Shinnar S, Maytal J, Krasnoff L, et al. Recurrent status epilepticus in children. Ann Neurol 1992;31:598-604.

Smahi A, Hyden-Granskog C, Peterlin B, et al. The gene for the familial form of incontinentia pigmenti (IP) maps to the distal part of Xq28. Hum Mol Genet 1994;3:273-278.

Specht U, Boenigk HE, Wolf P. Discontinuation of clonazepam after long-term treatment. Epilepsia 1989;30: 458-463.

Steinlein O, Schuster V, Fischer C, et al. Benign familial neonatal convulsions: Confirmation of genetic heterogeneity and further evidence for a second locus on chromosome 8q. Hum Genet 1995;95:411-415.

Stolarek I, Blacklaw J, Forrest G, et al. Vigabatrin and lamotrigine in refractory epilepsy. J Neurol Neurosurg Psychiatry 1994;57:921-924.

Talwar D, Rask CA, Torres F. Clinical manifestations in children with occipital spike-wave paroxysms. Epilepsia 1992;33:667-674.

Tennison M, Greenwood R, Lewis D, et al. Discontinuing antiepileptic drugs in children with epilepsy. A comparison of a six-week and a nine-month period. N Engl J Med 1994;330:1407-1410.

Tijssen MAJ, Shiang R, Deutekom Jv, et al. Molecular genetic reevaluation of the Dutch hyperekplexia family. Arch Neurol 1995;52:578-582.

van Engelen BGM, Renier WO, Weemaes CMR, et al. Immunoglobulin treatment in epilepsy, a review of the literature. Epilepsy Res 1994;19:181-190.

Vining EPG, Freeman JM, Brandt J, et al. Progressive unilateral encephalopathy of childhood (Rasmussen's syndrome): A reappraisal. Epilepsia 1993;34:639-650.

Watchko JF, Claassen D. Kernicterus in premature infants: Current prevalence and relationship to NICHD Phototherapy Study exchange criteria. Pediatrics 1994;93: 996-999.

Whitley R, Lakeman F. Herpes simplex virus infections of the nervous system: Therapeutic and diagnostic considerations. Clin Infect Dis 1995;20:414-420.

Worthen HG, Ashwal A, Ozand PT, et al. Comparative frequency and severity of hypoglycemia in selected organic acidemias, branched chain amino acidemia, and disorders of fructose metabolism. Brain Dev 1994;16(suppl 1): S81-S85.

Wyllie E, Friedman D, Rothner AD, et al. Psychogenic seizures in children and adolescents: Outcome after diagnosis by ictal video and electroencephalographic recording. Pediatrics 1990;85:480-484.

2
Altered States of Consciousness

The terms used in this text to describe states of decreased consciousness are provided in Table 2-1. With the exception of *coma,* these definitions are not standard. However, they are more precise and therefore more useful than such terms as *semicomatose* and *semistuporous.* The term *encephalopathy* is used to describe a diffuse disorder of the brain in which at least two of the following symptoms are present: (1) altered states of consciousness, (2) altered cognition or personality, and (3) seizures. *Encephalitis* is an encephalopathy accompanied by cerebrospinal fluid pleocytosis.

Lack of responsiveness is not always caused by lack of consciousness. For example, infants with botulism (see Chapter 6) may have such severe hypotonia and ptosis that they cannot move their limbs or eyelids in response to stimulation. They appear to be in coma or stupor but are actually alert. The locked-in syndrome (a brainstem disorder in which the individual can process information, but cannot respond) and catatonia are other examples of diminished responsiveness in the alert state.

Progression from consciousness to coma may be characterized by increased or decreased neuronal excitability. Patients with increased neuronal excitability (the *high road*) become restless, then confused; next tremor, hallucinations, and delirium (an agitated confusional state) develop. Myoclonic jerks may occur. Seizures herald the end of delirium and are followed by stupor or coma. Table 2-2 summarizes the differential diagnosis of the high road to coma.

Tumors and other mass lesions are not expected causes. Instead, the diagnosis is weighted in favor of metabolic, toxic, and inflammatory disorders.

Decreased neuronal excitability (the *low road*) lacks an agitated stage. Instead, awareness progressively deteriorates from lethargy to obtundation, to stupor, and to coma. The differential diagnosis is considerably larger than that with the "high road" and includes mass lesions and other causes of increased intracranial pressure (Table 2-3). Conditions that cause recurrent encephalopathies are listed in Table 2-4. A comparison of Tables 2-2 and 2-3 shows a considerable overlap between conditions whose initial features are agitation and confusion and those that begin with lethargy and coma; therefore the disorders responsible for each are described together in the text to prevent repetition.

Diagnostic Approach to Delirium

Any child with the acute behavioral changes of delirium (agitation, confusion, delusions, or hallucinations) should be assumed to have an organic encephalopathy until proven otherwise. Delirium is usually caused by a toxic or metabolic disorder diffusely affecting both cerebral hemispheres. Schizophrenia should not be a consideration in a prepubertal child with acute delirium. *Delusions* are fixed beliefs that cannot be altered by reason. The paranoid delusions of

States of Decreased Consciousness

TERM	DEFINITION
Lethargic	Difficulty in maintaining in the aroused state
Obtunded	Responsive to stimulation other than pain*
Stuporous	Responsive only to pain*
Comatose	Unresponsive to pain

*Responsive indicates cerebral alerting and not just reflex withdrawal.

schizophrenia are logical to the patient and frequently part of an elaborate system of irrational thinking in which the patient feels menaced. Delusions associated with organic encephalopathy are less logical, are not systematized, and tend to be stereotyped.

A *hallucination* is the perception of sensory stimuli that are not present. Visual hallucinations are almost always caused by organic encephalopathy, and auditory hallucinations, especially if accusatory, usually indicate psychiatric illness. Stereotyped auditory hallucinations that represent a recurring memory are an exception and suggest temporal lobe seizures.

HISTORY AND PHYSICAL EXAMINATION

Delirious children, even with stable vital function, must be assessed rapidly because the potential for deterioration to a state of diminished consciousness is always present. Careful history must be obtained of (1) the events leading to the behavioral change, (2) drug or toxic exposure (prescription drugs are more often at fault than substances of abuse, and a medicine cabinet inspection should be ordered in every home the child has visited), (3) personal or family history of migraine or epilepsy, (4) recent or concurrent fever, infectious disease, or systemic illness, and (5) previous personal or family history of encephalopathy.

Examination of the eyes, in addition to determining the presence or absence of papilledema, provides other etiologic clues. Drug or toxic exposure is suggested by small or large pupils that respond poorly to light, nystagmus, or impaired eye movements. Fixed deviation of the eyes in one lateral direction may indicate that (1) the encephalopathy has focal features, (2) seizures are a cause of the confusional state, or (3) seizures are part of the encephalopathy.

Causes of Agitation and Confusion

Epileptic
Absence status (see Chapter 1)
Complex partial seizure (see Chapter 1)
Infectious Disorders
Bacterial infections
  Cat scratch disease
  Meningitis (see Chapter 4)
Rickettsial infections
  Lyme disease
  Rocky Mountain spotted fever
Viral infections
  Aseptic meningitis
  Arboviruses
  Herpes simplex encephalitis
  Measles encephalitis
  Postinfectious encephalomyelitis
  Reye syndrome
Metabolic and Systemic Disorders
Disorders of osmolality
  Hypoglycemia
  Hyponatremia
Endocrine disorders
  Adrenal insufficiency
  Hypoparathyroidism
  Thyroid disorders
Hepatic encephalopathy
Inborn errors of metabolism
  Disorders of pyruvate metabolism (see Chapter 5)
  Medium-chain acyl-CoA dehydrogenase (MCAD) deficiency
  Respiratory chain disorders (see Chapters 5, 6, 8, 10)
  Urea cycle disorder, heterozygote (see Chapter 1)
Renal disease
  Hypertensive encephalopathy
  Uremic encephalopathy
Migraine
Acute confusional
Aphasic
Transient global amnesia
Psychological
Panic disorder
Schizophrenia
Toxic
Immunosuppressive drugs
Prescription drugs
Substance abuse
Toxins
Vascular
Congestive heart failure
Embolism
Hypertensive encephalopathy
Lupus erythematosus
Subarachnoid hemorrhage
Vasculitis

The general and neurologic examinations should specifically include a search for evidence of trauma, needle marks on the limbs, meningismus, and cardiac disease.

■ T A B L E 2 – 3
Causes of Lethargy and Coma

Epilepsy

Postictal state (see Chapter 1)
Status epilepticus (see Chapter 1)

Hypoxia-Ischemia

Cardiac arrest
Cardiac arrhythmia
Congestive heart failure
Hypotension
   Autonomic dysfunction
   Dehydration
   Hemorrhage
   Pulmonary embolism
Near drowning
Neonatal (see Chapter 1)

Increased Intracranial Pressure

Cerebral abscess (see Chapter 4)
Cerebral edema (see Chapter 4)
Cerebral tumor (see Chapters 4 and 10)
Herniation syndromes (see Chapter 4)
Hydrocephalus (see Chapters 4 and 18)
Intracranial hemorrhage
   Spontaneous (see Chapter 4)
   Traumatic

Infectious Disorders

Bacterial infections
   Cat scratch disease
   Gram negative sepsis
   Hemorrhagic shock and encephalopathy
    syndrome
   Meningitis (see Chapter 4)
   Toxic shock syndrome
Rickettsial infections
   Lyme disease
   Rocky Mountain spotted fever
Viral infections
   Aseptic meningitis
   Arboviruses
   Herpes simplex encephalitis
   Measles encephalitis
   Postinfectious encephalomyelitis
   Reye syndrome

Metabolic and Systemic Disorders

Disorders of osmolality
   Diabetic ketoacidosis (hyperglycemia)
   Hypoglycemia
   Hypernatremia
   Hyponatremia

Endocrine disorders
   Adrenal insufficiency
   Hypoparathyroidism
   Thyroid disorders
Hepatic encephalopathy
Inborn errors of metabolism
   Disorders of pyruvate metabolism (see Chapter 5)
   Glycogen storage disorders (see Chapter 1)
   Medium-chain acyl-CoA dehydrogenase (MCAD)
    deficiency
   Respiratory chain disorders (see Chapters 5, 6, 8, 10)
   Urea cycle disorder, heterozygote (see Chapter 1)
Renal disorders
   Acute uremic encephalopathy
   Chronic uremic encephalopathy
   Dialysis encephalopathy
   Hypertensive encephalopathy
Other metabolic disorders
   Burn encephalopathy
   Hypomagnesemia
   Parenteral hyperalimentation
   Vitamin B complex deficiency

Migraine Coma

Toxic

Immunosuppressive drugs
Prescription drugs
Substance abuse
Toxins

Trauma

Concussion
Contusion
Intracranial hemorrhage
   Epidural hematoma
   Subdural hematoma
   Intracerebral hemorrhage
Neonatal (see Chapter 1)

Vascular

Hypertensive encephalopathy
Intracranial hemorrhage, nontraumatic (see Chapter 4)
Lupus erythematosus (see Chapter 11)
Neonatal idiopathic cerebral venous thrombosis
  (see Chapter 1)
Vasculitis (see Chapter 11)

LABORATORY INVESTIGATIONS

Laboratory evaluation should be individualized; not every test is essential for each clinical situation. The first step is to obtain blood and urine. Studies of potential interest include culture; complete blood count; sedimentation rate; toxicity screen; blood concentrations of glucose, electrolytes, calcium, and phosphorus, urea nitrogen, ammonia, and thyroid-stimulating hormone; and liver function tests. If possible, computed tomography (CT) of the head should be obtained while these results are pending. If sedation is required to perform the study, a short-acting benzodiazepine is preferred. Nondiagnostic blood studies and normal CT results are an indication for lumbar puncture to look for infection, hemorrhage, and increased intracra-

■ TABLE 2-4
Causes of Recurrent Encephalopathy

Burn encephalopathy
Epilepsy
Hashimoto thyroiditis
Hypoglycemia
Increased intracranial pressure (recurrent)
Medium-chain acyl-CoA dehydrogenase (MCAD)
  deficiency
Mental disorders
Migraine
Mitochondrial disorders
Pyruvate metabolism disorders
Substance abuse
Urea cycle disorder

nial pressure. A manometer should always be available to measure cerebrospinal fluid pressure.

An electroencephalogram (EEG) can be useful in the evaluation of delirious patients and should be obtained at an opportune time. Findings are almost always abnormal in acute organic encephalopathies and normal in psychiatric illnesses. The minimal EEG finding in encephalopathy is slowing of the posterior rhythm; more severe encephalopathies are characterized by diffuse theta and delta activity, absence of faster frequencies, and intermittent rhythmic delta activity. Specific abnormalities may include epileptiform activity consistent with absence or complex partial status; triphasic waves, indicating hepatic or uremic encephalopathy; and periodic lateralizing epileptiform discharges in one temporal lobe, suggesting herpes encephalitis.

 Diagnostic Approach to Lethargy and Coma

The diagnostic approach to states of diminished consciousness in children is similar to that suggested for delirium, except for greater urgency. Progressive decline in state of consciousness can be caused by diffuse or multifocal disturbances of the cerebral hemispheres or by focal injury to the brainstem. The anatomic site of abnormality can often be determined by physical examination.

HISTORY AND PHYSICAL EXAMINATION

The historical data to be obtained are the same as for delirium, except that mass lesions are an important consideration. Further inquiry must be made concerning trauma or preceding symptoms of increasing intracranial pressure.

Physical examination is directed at determining both the anatomic site of disturbed cerebral function and its cause. The important variables in locating the site of abnormality are state of consciousness, pattern of breathing, pupillary size and reactivity, eye movements, and motor responses. Lethargy and obtundation are generally caused by mild depression of hemispheric function. Stupor and coma are characteristic of much more extensive disturbance of hemispheric function or involvement of the diencephalon and upper brainstem. Derangements of the dominant hemisphere may have a greater effect on consciousness than derangements of the nondominant hemisphere.

Cheyne-Stokes respiration, in which periods of hyperpnea alternate with periods of apnea, is usually caused by bilateral hemispheric or diencephalic injuries, but can result from bilateral damage anywhere along the descending pathway between the forebrain and upper pons. Alertness, pupillary size, and heart rhythm may vary during Cheyne-Stokes respiration. Alertness is greater during the waxing portion of breathing. Lesions just ventral to the aqueduct or fourth ventricle cause a sustained, rapid, deep hyperventilation (*central neurogenic hyperventilation*). Abnormalities within the medulla and pons affect the respiratory centers and cause several different patterns of respiratory control: (1) *apneustic breathing,* a pause at full inspiration; (2) *ataxic breathing,* haphazard breaths and pauses without a predictable pattern; and (3) *Ondine's curse,* failure of automatic breathing when asleep.

The pupillary light reflex is usually retained in metabolic disturbances, and its absence in a comatose patient indicates a structural abnormality. The major exception is drugs: fixed dilation of the pupils in an alert patient is caused by topical administration of mydriatics. In comatose patients, hypothalamic damage causes unilateral pupillary constriction and a Horner syndrome; midbrain lesions cause midposition fixed pupils; pontine lesions cause small but reactive pupils; and lateral medullary lesions cause a Horner syndrome.

Tonic lateral deviation of both eyes indicates a seizure originating in the hemisphere opposite the direction of gaze or a destructive lesion in the hemisphere in the direction of gaze. Ocular motility in comatose patients can be assessed by instilling ice water sequentially 15 minutes apart in each ear to chill the tympanic membrane. Ice water in the right ear causes both eyes to deviate rapidly to the right and then slowly return to the midline. The rapid movement to the right is a brainstem reflex, and its presence indicates that much of the brainstem is intact. Abduction of the right eye with failure of left eye adduction indicates a lesion in the medial longitudinal fasciculus (see Chapter 15). The slow movement that returns the eyes to the left requires a corticopontine pathway originating in the right hemisphere and terminating in the left pontine lateral gaze center. Its presence indicates unilateral hemispheric function.

Trunk and limb position at rest, spontaneous movements, and response to noxious stimuli must be carefully observed. Spontaneous movement of all limbs generally indicates a mild depression of hemispheric function without structural disturbance. Monoplegia or hemiplegia, except in the postictal state, suggests a structural disturbance of the contralateral hemisphere. An extensor response of the trunk and limbs to a noxious stimulus is termed *decerebrate rigidity.* The most severe form is called *opisthotonos:* the neck is hyperextended and the teeth are clenched; the arms adducted, hyperextended, and hyperpronated; and the legs extended with the feet plantar flexed. Decerebrate rigidity indicates brainstem compression and should be considered an ominous sign whether present at rest or in response to noxious stimuli. Flexion of the arms and extension of the legs is termed *decorticate rigidity.* It is uncommon in children except following head injury and indicates hemispheric dysfunction with brainstem integrity.

LABORATORY INVESTIGATIONS

Laboratory investigations are similar to those described for the evaluation of delirium. Head CT with contrast enhancement should be performed promptly in order to exclude the possibility of a mass lesion and herniation. It is a great error to send a child whose condition is uncertain for CT without someone in attendance who knows how to monitor deterioration and intervene appropriately.

 Hypoxia and Ischemia

Hypoxia and ischemia usually occur together. Prolonged hypoxia causes personality change first and then loss of consciousness; acute anoxia results in immediate loss of consciousness.

PROLONGED HYPOXIA

CLINICAL FEATURES. Prolonged hypoxia can result from severe anemia (oxygen-carrying capacity reduced by at least half), congestive heart failure, chronic lung disease, and neuromuscular disorders.

The best-studied model of prolonged, mild hypoxia is ascent to high altitudes. Mild hypoxia causes impaired memory and judgment, confusion, and decreased motor performance. Greater degrees of hypoxia result in obtundation, multifocal myoclonus, and sometimes focal neurologic signs such as monoplegia and hemiplegia. Children with chronic cardiopulmonary disease may have an insidious alteration in behavioral state as arterial oxygen concentration slowly declines.

Neuromuscular disorders that weaken respiratory muscles, such as muscular dystrophy, often produce nocturnal hypoventilation as a first symptom of respiratory insufficiency. This is characterized by frequent awakenings and fear of sleeping (see Chapter 7).

DIAGNOSIS. Chronic hypoxia should be considered in children with chronic cardiopulmonary disorders who become depressed or undergo personality change. Arterial oxygen pressure (Pao_2) values below 40 mm Hg are regularly associated with obvious neurologic disturbances, but minor mental disturbances may occur at Pao_2 concentrations of 60 mm Hg, especially when hypoxia is chronic.

TREATMENT. Encephalopathy usually reverses when PaO_2 is increased, but persistent cerebral dysfunction may occur in mountain climbers after returning to sea level, and permanent cerebral dysfunction may develop in children with chronic hypoxia. As a group, children with chronic hypoxia from congenital heart disease have a lower IQ than nonhypoxic children. The severity of mental decline is related to the duration of hypoxia.

Children with neuromuscular disorders who have symptoms during sleep can be treated overnight with intermittent positive-pressure ventilation applied by mouth (see Chapter 7).

ACUTE ANOXIA AND ISCHEMIA

The usual circumstance in which acute anoxia and ischemia occur is cardiac arrest or sudden hypotension. Anoxia without ischemia occurs with suffocation (near-drowning, choking). Prolonged anoxia leads to bradycardia and cardiac arrest. In adults, hippocampal and Purkinje cells begin to die after 4 minutes of total anoxia and ischemia and the outside limit of brain viability is believed to be 10 minutes. Exact timing may be difficult in clinical situations when ill-defined intervals of anoxia and hypoxia occur. Remarkable survivals are sometimes associated with near-drowning in water cold enough to lower cerebral temperature and metabolism. The pattern of hypoxic-ischemic brain injury in newborns is different and depends largely on brain maturity (see Chapter 1).

CLINICAL FEATURES. Consciousness is lost within 8 seconds of cerebral circulatory failure, but the loss may take longer when anoxia occurs without ischemia. Presyncopal symptoms of lightheadedness and visual disturbances sometimes precede loss of consciousness. Seizures and extensor rigidity follow.

Considerable effort has been made to identify predictors of outcome after hypoxic-ischemic events. Only 13% of adults who have had a cardiac arrest regain independent function in the first year after arrest. Outcome in children is somewhat better because the incidence of pre-existing cardiopulmonary disease is lower. Absence of pupillary responses on initial examination is an ominous sign; such patients do not recover independent function. Twenty-four hours after arrest, patients with poor prognoses are identified by lack of motor responses in the limbs and eyes. In contrast, a favorable outcome can be predicted for patients who rapidly recover roving or conjugate eye movements and limb withdrawal from pain. Children who are unconscious for longer than 60 days will not regain language skills or the ability to walk (Kriel et al, 1994).

Two delayed syndromes of neurologic deterioration follow anoxia. The first is *delayed postanoxic encephalopathy*, the appearance of apathy or confusion 1 to 2 weeks after apparent recovery. This is followed by motor symptoms, usually rigidity or spasticity, and may progress to coma or death. Demyelination is the suggested mechanism. The other syndrome is *postanoxic action myoclonus*. This usually follows a severe episode of anoxia and ischemia caused by cardiac arrest. All voluntary activity initiates disabling myoclonus (see Chapter 14). Symptoms of cerebellar dysfunction are also present.

DIAGNOSIS. Cerebral edema is prominent during the first 72 hours after severe hypoxia.

CT during that time shows decreased density with loss of the differentiation between gray and white matter. Severe, generalized loss of density on CT correlates with a poor outcome.

An EEG that shows a burst-suppression pattern or absence of activity is associated with poor neurologic outcome or death; lesser abnormalities are not useful in predicting prognosis.

TREATMENT. The principles of treating patients who have sustained hypoxic-ischemic encephalopathy do not differ substantially from the principles of caring for other comatose patients. Oxygenation, circulation, and blood glucose concentration must be maintained. Intracranial pressure must be lowered sufficiently to allow satisfactory cerebral perfusion (see Chapter 4). Seizures are managed with anticonvulsant drugs (see Chapter 1). Anoxia is invariably associated with lactic acidosis, and acid-base balance must be restored.

Barbiturate coma is frequently used to slow cerebral metabolism, but neither clinical nor experimental evidence indicates a beneficial effect following cardiac arrest or near-drowning. Hypothermia prevents brain damage during the time of hypoxia and ischemia, but has questionable value after the event. Corticosteroids do not improve neurologic recovery in patients with global ischemia following cardiac arrest (Jastremski et al, 1989).

Postanoxic action myoclonus can be treated with valproate.

PERSISTENT VEGETATIVE STATE

The term *persistent vegetative state* (PVS) is used to describe patients who, after recovery from coma, return to a state of wakefulness without cognition. PVS is a form of eyes-open permanent unconsciousness with loss of cognitive function and awareness of the environment but preservation of sleep-wake cycles and vegetative function. Survival is indefinite with good nursing care. The usual causes, in order of frequency, are anoxia and ischemia, metabolic or encephalitic coma, and head trauma. Anoxia-ischemia has the worst prognosis. Children who remain in a persistent vegetative state for 3 months do not regain functional skills (Kriel et al, 1993).

The American Academy of Neurology (1989) has adopted the policy that all medical treatment, including the provision of nutrition and hydration, may be ethically discontinued when a patient's condition has been diagnosed as PVS, it

■ TABLE 2–5
Diagnostic Criteria for the Clinical Diagnosis of Brain Death

Prerequisites
Cessation of all brain function
Proximate cause of brain death is known
Condition is irreversible
Cardinal Features
Coma
Absent brainstem reflexes
   Pupillary light reflex
   Corneal reflex
   Oculocephalic reflex
   Oculovestibular reflex
   Oropharyngeal reflex
Apnea (established by formal apnea test)
Confirmatory Tests (optional)
Cerebral angiography
Electroencephalography
Radioisotope cerebral blood flow study
Transcranial doppler ultrasonography

is clear that the patient would not want to be maintained in this state, and the family agrees to discontinue therapy.

BRAIN DEATH

Various standards for the diagnosis of brain death have been proposed, but the guidelines suggested by The American Academy of Neurology (1995) are generally accepted. The important features of the report are summarized in Table 2-5. The Commission urged caution in applying the criteria to children younger than 5 years, but subsequent experience supports the validity of the standards in the newborn and through childhood (Ashwal and Schneider, 1989). Absence of cerebral blood flow is the earliest and most definitive proof of brain death. EEG activity may still be present 24 hours after cessation of cerebral blood flow but subsequently becomes isoelectric.

▶ Infectious Disorders
BACTERIAL INFECTIONS

Cat Scratch Disease

Cat scratch disease is caused by *Rochalimaea henselae* a gram-negative bacillus that is transmitted by a cat scratch and perhaps by cat fleas (Zangwill et al, 1993). Three thousand cases were diagnosed in the United States between 1959 and 1987. Most cases are probably undi-

agnosed. The age range is 1 to 65 years, and males and females are equally affected. Eighty-two percent of cases occur in children less than 12 years of age (Carithers and Margileth, 1991).

CLINICAL FEATURES. The major feature is lymphadenopathy proximal to the site of scratch. Fever is present in only 60% of cases. The disease is usually benign and self-limited. Unusual systemic manifestations are oculoglandular disease, erythema nodosum, osteolytic lesions, and thrombocytopenic purpura. The most common neurologic manifestation is encephalopathy. Rare cases of transverse myelitis, cerebral arteritis, and neuroretinitis are reported.

Encephalitis occurs in less than 1% of patients with cat scratch disease. The mechanism is unknown, but it may be caused by direct infection or vasculitis. The male-to-female ratio is 2:1. Only 17% occur in children less than 12 years, and 15% in children 12 to 18 years. The frequency of fever and the site of scratch are no different in patients with cat scratch disease encephalitis as compared to those who had the disease without encephalitis. The initial and most prominent feature is a decreased state of consciousness ranging from lethargy to coma. Seizures occur in 46%, and combative behavior in 40%. Focal findings are rare.

DIAGNOSIS. The diagnosis requires local lymphadenopathy, contact with a cat, and an identifiable site of inoculation. An indirect fluorescent antibody test for the detection of an antibody response to *R. henselae* has been developed that appears to be sensitive (88%) and specific (94%). The cerebrospinal fluid is normal in 70% of cases. Lymphocytosis in the cerebrospinal fluid, when present, does not exceed 30 cells/mm^3. EEG is diffusely slow, and cranial magnetic resonance imaging (MRI) or CT is normal.

TREATMENT. All affected children recover completely, 50% within 4 weeks. Intravenous gentamicin (5 to 7/mg/kg/day) or oral trimethoprim (10 mg/kg/twice daily) and sulfamethoxazole (100 mg/kg/twice daily) may speed recovery in children with severe encephalopathy (Collio, 1992).

Gram-Negative Sepsis

CLINICAL FEATURES. The onset of symptoms in gram-negative sepsis may be explosive and is characterized by fever or hypothermia, chills, hyperventilation, hemodynamic instability, and mental changes (irritability, delirium, or coma).

Neurologic features may also include asterixis, tremor, and multifocal myoclonus. Multiple organ failure follows (1) renal shutdown caused by hypotension, (2) hypoprothrombinemia caused by vitamin K deficiency, (3) thrombocytopenia caused by nonspecific binding of immunoglobulin, (4) disseminated intravascular coagulation with infarction or hemorrhage in several organs, and (5) progressive respiratory failure (Bolton et al, 1993).

DIAGNOSIS. Sepsis should always be considered in the differential diagnosis of shock, and blood cultures must be obtained. When shock is the initial feature, gram-negative sepsis is likely. In *Staphylococcus aureus* infections, shock is more likely to occur during the course of the infection and not as an initial feature. The cerebrospinal fluid is usually normal or may have an elevated concentration of protein. MRI or CT of the brain is normal early in the course and shows edema later on.

TREATMENT. Septic shock is a medical emergency. Antibiotic therapy should be initiated promptly at maximal doses (see Chapter 4). Hypotension must be treated by restoration of intravascular volume, and each factor contributing to coagulopathy must be addressed. Mortality is high even with optimal treatment.

Hemorrhagic Shock Encephalopathy Syndrome

The hemorrhagic shock and encephalopathy syndrome is presumed to be caused by bacterial sepsis, but this has not been proven (Bonham et al, 1992).

CLINICAL FEATURES. Most affected children are younger than 1 year of age, but cases are described up to 26 months. One half of children have mild prodromal symptoms of a viral gastroenteritis or respiratory illness. In the rest the onset is explosive; a previously well child is found unresponsive and having seizures. Fever of 38° C or higher is a constant feature. Marked hypotension with poor peripheral perfusion is followed by profuse watery or bloody diarrhea with metabolic acidosis and compensatory respiratory alkalosis. Disseminated intravascular coagulopathy develops, and bleeding occurs from every venipuncture site.

The mortality rate is 50%; the survivors have mental and motor impairment.

DIAGNOSIS. The syndrome resembles toxic shock syndrome, gram-negative sepsis, heatstroke, and Reye syndrome. Abnormal renal

function occurs in every case, but serum ammonia concentrations remains normal, hypoglycemia is unusual, and blood cultures yield no growth.

Cerebrospinal fluid is normal except for increased pressure. CT shows small ventricles and loss of sulcal marking caused by cerebral edema. The initial EEG background is diffusely slow or may be isoelectric. A striking pattern called "electric storm" evolves over the first hours or days. The pattern is characterized by runs of spikes, sharp waves, or rhythmic slow waves that fluctuate in frequency, amplitude, and location (Harden et al, 1991).

TREATMENT. Affected children require intensive care with ventilatory support, volume replacement, correction of acid-base and coagulation disturbances, anticonvulsant therapy, and control of cerebral edema.

Toxic Shock Syndrome

Toxic shock syndrome is a potentially lethal illness caused by infection or colonization with some strains of *S. aureus.*

CLINICAL FEATURES. The onset is abrupt and characterized by high fever, hypotension, vomiting, diarrhea, myalgia, headache, and a desquamating rash. Multiple organ failure may occur during desquamation. Serious complications include cardiac arrhythmia, pulmonary edema, and oliguric renal failure. Initial encephalopathic features are agitation and confusion. These may be followed by lethargy, obtundation, and generalized tonic-clonic seizures.

Most pediatric cases have occurred in menstruating girls who use tampons, but may also occur in children with occlusive dressings after burns or surgery (Bacha et al, 1994), and as a complication of influenza-like illness in children with staphylococcal colonization of the respiratory tract.

DIAGNOSIS. No diagnostic laboratory test is available. The diagnosis is based on the typical clinical and laboratory findings. Over half of patients have sterile pyuria, immature granulocytic leukocytes, coagulation abnormalities, hypocalcemia, low serum albumin and total protein concentrations, and elevated concentrations of blood urea nitrogen, transaminase, bilirubin, and creatine kinase. Cultures of specimens from infected areas yield *S. aureus.*

TREATMENT. Hypotension usually responds to volume restoration with physiologic saline solutions. Some patients require vasopressors or fresh-frozen plasma. Antibiotic therapy should be initiated promptly with an agent effective against *S. aureus.*

RICKETTSIAL INFECTIONS

Lyme Disease

Lyme disease, caused by a spirochete *(Borrelia burgdorferi)* and transmitted by tick bite, is now the most common vector-borne infection in the United States. Six northeastern states account for 80% of cases.

CLINICAL FEATURES. Three stages of disease are described, but this sequence is variable. The first symptom (stage 1) in 60% to 80% of patients is a skin lesion of the thigh, groin, or axilla (erythema chronicum migrans), which may be associated with fever, regional lymphadenopathy, and arthralgia. The rash begins as a red macule at the site of the tick bite and then spreads to form a red annular lesion with partial clearing, sometimes appearing as alternating rings of rash and clearing.

Neurologic involvement (neuroborreliosis) develops weeks or months later when the infection becomes disseminated (stage 2). Most children have only headache, which clears completely within 6 weeks; this may be caused by mild aseptic meningitis or encephalitis (Belman et al, 1993). Fever may not occur. Other neurologic symptoms in children are facial palsy, sleep disturbances, and papilledema. Polyneuropathies are uncommon in children. Transitory cardiac involvement (myopericarditis and atrioventricular block) may occur in stage 2.

A year or more of continual migratory arthritis begins weeks to years after the onset of neurologic features (stage 3). Only one joint, often the knee, or a few large joints are affected. During stage 3 the patient feels ill. Fatigue may be the most prominent symptom, but chronic encephalopathy and polyneuropathy also occur.

DIAGNOSIS. The spirochete can be grown on cultures from the skin rash during stage 1 of the disease. At the time of meningitis the cerebrospinal fluid may be normal at first but then shows a lymphocytic pleocytosis (about 100 cells/mm^3), an elevated protein concentration, and a normal glucose concentration.

A two-test approach is recommended to establish the diagnosis of neuroborreliosis (Garcia-Monco and Benach, 1995). The first step is to show the production of specific IgG and IgM antibodies in cerebrospinal fluid. Antibody production begins 2 weeks after infection and IgG is always detectable at 6 weeks. The second step, to be used when the first is inconclusive, is the polymerase chain reaction (PCR) to detect the organism.

TREATMENT. Intravenous therapy for 2 weeks with either ceftriaxone, 2 g/day as a single dose, or penicillin G, 20 million U/day in six divided doses, is used for children with neurologic manifestations; however, oral amoxicillin, 250 mg three times a day, or tetracycline, 250 mg three times a day, can be used if Bell's palsy is the only feature.

Rocky Mountain Spotted Fever

Rocky Mountain spotted fever is an acute, tick-borne disorder caused by *Rickettsia rickettsii* (Kirk et al, 1990). Its geographic name is a misnomer; the disease occurs in much of the United States, with a special predilection for southwestern and southeastern states.

CLINICAL FEATURES. Fever, myalgia, and rash are constant symptoms. The rash appears within 14 days of onset (average 4 days), and may be maculopapular, petechial, or both. Headache is present in 66% of patients, meningismus in 33%, focal neurologic signs in 14%, and seizures in 6%.

DIAGNOSIS. The diagnosis is confirmed by a fourfold rise in the Weil-Felix agglutination reaction, or the presence of complement fixing or immunofluorescent antibody. The cerebrospinal fluid shows a mild pleocytosis.

VIRAL INFECTIONS

Because encephalitis usually affects the meninges as well as the brain, the term *meningoencephalitis* may be more accurate. However, distinguishing encephalitis from aseptic meningitis is useful for viral diagnosis, because most viruses cause primarily one or the other, but not both. An annual incidence of 7.4:100,000 for encephalitis and 10.9:100,000 for aseptic meningitis remained relatively constant in one Minnesota county over a 32-year period. Both conditions are more common in the summer, in childhood, and in males.

Routine childhood immunization has reduced the number of pathogenic viruses circulating in the community. Enteroviruses and herpes simplex are now the most common viral causes of meningitis and encephalitis in children. However, specific viral identification is established in only 15% to 20% of cases.

The classification of viruses undergoes frequent change, but a constant first step is the separation of viruses with a DNA nucleic acid core from those with an RNA core. The only DNA viruses that cause acute, postnatal encephalitis in immunocompetent hosts are herpes viruses. RNA viruses causing encephalitis are myxoviruses (influenza and measles encephalitis), arboviruses (St. Louis encephalitis, eastern equine encephalitis, western equine encephalitis, and LaCrosse-California encephalitis), retroviruses (acquired immune deficiency syndrome encephalitis), and rhabdoviruses (rabies). RNA viruses (especially enteroviruses and mumps) are responsible for aseptic meningitis.

Some viruses, such as herpes simplex, are highly neurotropic (almost always infect the nervous system) but rarely neurovirulent (rarely cause encephalitis), whereas others, such as measles, are rarely neurotropic but are highly neurovirulent. In addition to viruses that directly infect the brain and meninges, encephalopathies may also follow systemic viral infections. These are thought to result from demyelination caused by immune-mediated responses of the brain to infection.

Aseptic Meningitis

The term *aseptic meningitis* is used to define a syndrome of meningismus and cerebrospinal fluid leukocytosis without bacterial or fungal infection. It is generally caused by drugs and viral infections. Viral meningitis is a benign, self-limited disease from which 95% of children recover completely.

CLINICAL FEATURES. Twenty percent of children have a history of antecedent respiratory infection or gastrointestinal illness. The onset of symptoms is abrupt and characterized by fever, headache, and stiff neck, except in infants who do not have meningismus (Rorabaugh et al, 1993). Irritability, lethargy, and vomiting are also common. "Encephalitic" symptoms are not part of the syndrome in children, but seizures and coma may occur in infants. Systemic illness is uncommon, but its presence may suggest specific viral disorders (parotitis suggestive of mumps, myalgia of coxsackie viral infection, rash of echovirus infection and Lyme disease, diarrhea of enterovirus infection).

The acute illness usually lasts less than 1 week, but malaise and headache may continue for several weeks. Communicating hydrocephalus is an unusual long-term sequela.

DIAGNOSIS. In most cases of aseptic meningitis the cerebrospinal fluid contains 10 to 200 leukocytes/mm^3, but cell counts of 1,000 cells/mm^3 or greater may occur with lymphocytic choriomeningitis. The response is primarily lymphocytic, but polymorphonuclear leukocytes may predominate early in the course. Protein concentration is generally between 50 and 100 mg/dl (0.5 and 1 g/L) and glucose concentration is normal, although it may be slightly reduced in mumps and lymphocytic choriomeningitis.

Aseptic meningitis usually occurs in the spring or summer, and enteroviruses are responsible for most cases in children. The mumps and poliomyelitis viruses remain important causative agents in countries where immunization is not mandatory. Nonviral causes of aseptic meningitis are rare but must be considered; these include Lyme disease, Kawasaki disease, leukemia, systemic lupus erythematosus, migraine, and irritation of the meninges from blood, drugs, and contrast materials.

Patients with a personal or family history of migraine may have attacks of severe headache associated with stiff neck and focal neurologic disturbances, such as hemiparesis and aphasia. Cerebrospinal fluid examination shows a pleocytosis of 5 to 300 cells/mm^3 that is mainly lymphocytes and a protein concentration of 50 to 100 mg/dl (0.5 to 1 g/L). Whether the attacks are migraine provoked by intercurrent aseptic meningitis or represent a "meningitic" form of migraine is not known. The recurrence of attacks in some patients suggests that the mechanism is wholly migrainous.

Bacterial meningitis is the major concern when a child has meningismus. Although cerebrospinal fluid examination provides several clues that differentiate bacterial from viral meningitis, antibiotic therapy should be initiated for every child with a clinical syndrome of aseptic meningitis until cerebrospinal fluid culture is negative for bacteria (see Chapter 4). This is especially true for children who received antibiotic therapy before examination of the cerebrospinal fluid.

TREATMENT. Children with viral meningitis or encephalitis are now routinely treated for herpes encephalitis until that diagnosis can be excluded; treatment with acyclovir is harmless. Treatment of viral aseptic meningitis is directed at the symptoms. Bed rest in a quiet environment and mild analgesics provide satisfactory relief of symptoms in most children.

Arboviral (Arthropod-Borne) Encephalitis

Arboviruses are classified on the basis of ecology rather than structure. Ticks and mosquitos are the usual vectors, and epidemics occur in the spring and summer. Each encephalitis has a defined geographic area. Arboviruses account for 10% of encephalitis cases reported in the United States.

California-LaCrosse Encephalitis

LaCrosse virus is the most common cause of encephalitis by California serogroup viruses in the United States.

CLINICAL FEATURES. Before 1984 most cases were reported from Wisconsin and Minnesota. Later epidemics occurred in Indiana and sporadic cases are reported throughout the Midwest and western New York. Small woodland mammals serve as a reservoir, and mosquitos as the vector.

Most cases of encephalitis occur in children, and asymptomatic infection is common in adults. The initial feature is a flulike syndrome that lasts for 2 or 3 days. Encephalitis is heralded by headache followed by seizures and rapid progression to coma. Focal neurologic disturbances are present in 20% of cases. Symptoms begin to resolve 3 to 5 days after onset, and most children recover without neurologic sequelae. Death is uncommon and occurs mainly in infants.

DIAGNOSIS. Examination of cerebrospinal fluid shows a mixed pleocytosis with lymphocytes predominating. The count is usually 50 to 200 cells/mm^3, but may range from 0 to 600. The virus is difficult to culture and diagnosis depends on showing a fourfold or greater increase in hemagglutination inhibition and neutralizing antibody titers between acute and convalescent sera.

TREATMENT. Treatment is supportive. No effective antiviral agent is available.

Eastern Equine Encephalitis

CLINICAL FEATURES. Eastern equine encephalitis is a perennial infection of horses from New York to Florida. Human cases do not exceed five each year, and they follow epidemics in horses (Centers for Disease Control, 1991a). The mortality rate is 30%. Wild birds serve as a reservoir, and mosquitoes as a vector. Consequently, almost all cases occur during the summer months.

Onset is usually abrupt and characterized by high fever, headache, and vomiting, followed by drowsiness, coma, and seizures. The longer the duration of non-neurologic prodromal symptoms, the better the outcome. In infants, seizures and coma are often the first manifestation. Signs of meningismus are usually present in older children. Children usually survive the acute encephalitis, but mental impairment, seizures, and disturbed motor function can be expected in survivors.

DIAGNOSIS. The cerebrospinal fluid pressure is usually elevated, and examination reveals 200 to 2,000 leukocytes/mm^3, of which half are polymorphonuclear leukocytes. Diagnosis relies on the showing a fourfold or greater rise in complement fixation and neutralizing antibody titers between acute and convalescent sera.

TREATMENT. Treatment is supportive. No effective antiviral agent is available.

Japanese B Encephalitis

Japanese B encephalitis is a major form of encephalitis in Asia and is an important health hazard to nonimmunized travelers during summer months.

CLINICAL FEATURES. The initial features are malaise, fever, and headache or irritability lasting 2 to 3 days. These are followed by meningismus, confusion, and delirium. During the second or third week, photophobia and generalized hypotonia develop. Seizures may occur at any time. Finally, rigidity, a masklike facies, and brainstem dysfunction ensue. Mortality rates are very high among indigenous populations and lower among Western travelers, probably because of a difference in the age of the exposed populations.

DIAGNOSIS. Examination of the cerebrospinal fluid shows pleocytosis (20 to 500 cells/mm^3). The cells are initially mixed, but later lymphocytes predominate. Protein concentration is usually between 50 and 100 mg/dl (0.5 and 1 mg/L), and glucose concentration is normal. Diagnosis depends on demonstrating a fourfold or greater elevation in the level of complement-fixing antibodies between acute and convalescent sera.

TREATMENT. Treatment is supportive. No effective antiviral agent is available, but immunization with an inactivated vaccine protects against encephalitis in more than 90% of individuals.

St. Louis Encephalitis

CLINICAL FEATURES. St. Louis encephalitis is endemic in the western United States and epidemic in the Mississippi valley and Atlantic states. It is the most common cause of epidemic viral encephalitis in the United States (Centers for Disease Control; 1991b). The vector is a mosquito, and birds are the major reservoir.

Most infections are asymptomatic. The spectrum of neurologic illness varies from aseptic meningitis to severe encephalitis leading to death within days. The mortality rate is low. Headache, vomiting, and states of decreased consciousness are typical features. Stiff neck and seizures are less common, and focal neurologic disturbances are rare. The usual duration of illness is 1 to 2 weeks. Children usually recover completely, but adults may be left with mental or motor impairment.

DIAGNOSIS. Cerebrospinal fluid examination reveals a lymphocytic pleocytosis (50 to 500 cells/mm^3) and a protein concentration between 50 and 100 mg/dl (0.5 and 1 g/L). Glucose concentration is normal.

The virus is difficult to grow on culture and diagnosis requires a fourfold or greater increase in complement fixation and hemagglutination inhibition antibody titers between acute and convalescent sera.

TREATMENT. Treatment is supportive. No effective antiviral agent is available.

Western Equine Encephalitis

CLINICAL FEATURES. Western equine encephalitis is a rare disorder. Wild birds serve as the reservoir and mosquitoes as the vector. All recent cases have been reported from North Dakota, South Dakota, and Canada. Between 20% and 30% of cases occur in infants.

In infants the infection is characterized by irritability, fever, meningismus, bulging of the fontanelles, seizures, and coma. Older children may have a flulike syndrome before symptoms of meningoencephalitis develop. The initial symptom is usually behavioral change, including delirium, which is followed by drowsiness and coma. The EEG shows focal abnormalities lateralizing to one temporal lobe that suggest herpes encephalitis.

Symptoms last for 1 to 2 weeks, and although the overall mortality rate is 10%, most fatalities are infants. Fifty percent of surviving infants have permanent mental impairment and seizures.

DIAGNOSIS. Cerebrospinal fluid pleocytosis is first a mixture of polymorphonuclear leukocytes and lymphocytes and then lymphocytes alone. Protein concentration is between 50 and 100 mg/dl (0.5 and 1 g/L). Diagnosis relies on showing a fourfold or greater rise in complement-fixing or neutralizing antibodies between acute and convalescent sera.

Western equine encephalitis may be difficult to distinguish from herpes encephalitis without brain biopsy.

TREATMENT. Treatment is supportive. The child should be treated for herpes encephalitis until a definitive diagnosis is made. No effective antiviral agent is available for western equine encephalitis.

Herpes Simplex Encephalitis

Two similar strains of herpes simplex virus (HSV) are pathogenic to humans. HSV-1 is associated with orofacial infections and HSV-2 with genital infections. Both are worldwide in distribution. Forty percent of children have antibodies to HSV-1, but antibodies to HSV-2 are not routinely detected until puberty. HSV-1 is the important causative agent of acute herpes simplex encephalitis after the newborn period, and HSV-2 of encephalitis in the newborn (see Chapter 1).

Initial orofacial infection with HSV-1 may be asymptomatic. The virus replicates in the skin, infecting nerve fiber endings and then the trigeminal ganglia. Further replication occurs within the ganglia before the virus enters a latent stage during which it cannot be recovered from the ganglia. Reactivation occurs during time of stress, especially intercurrent febrile illness. The reactivated virus ordinarily retraces its neural migration to the facial skin, but occasionally spreads proximally to the brain, causing encephalitis. The hosts immunocompetence maintains the virus in a latent state. An immunocompromised state results in frequent reactivation and severe, widespread infection.

Herpes simplex is the single most common cause of nonepidemic encephalitis and accounts for 10% to 20% of cases. The annual incidence is estimated at 2.3 cases per million population. Thirty-one percent of cases occur in children.

CLINICAL FEATURES. Primary infection is often the cause of encephalitis in children. Only 22% of patients give a history of recurrent labial herpes infection. Typically the patient has an acute onset of fever, headache, lethargy, nausea, and vomiting. Eighty percent of patients show focal neurologic disturbances (hemiparesis, cranial nerve deficits, visual field loss, aphasia, and focal seizures), and the remainder show behavioral changes or generalized seizures without clinical evidence of focal neurologic deficits. However, both groups have focal abnormalities on neuroradiographic studies or EEG. The acute stage of encephalitis lasts approximately a week. Recovery takes several weeks and is often incomplete.

Herpes meningitis is usually associated with genital lesions and caused by HSV-2. The clinical features are similar to those of aseptic meningitis caused by other viruses.

DIAGNOSIS. Prompt diagnosis of herpes simplex encephalitis is important because treatment is available. Cerebrospinal fluid pleocytosis is present in 97% of cases. The median count is 130 leukocytes/mm^3 (range 0 to 1,000). Up to 500 red blood cells/mm^3 may be present as well. Median protein concentration is 80 mg/dl (0.8 g/L), but 20% of patients have normal protein concentrations and 40% have concentrations exceeding 100 mg/dl (1 g/L). The glucose concentration in the cerebrospinal fluid is usually normal, but in 7% of cases it is less than half of the blood glucose concentration.

In the past the demonstration of periodic lateralizing epileptiform discharges on EEG was considered presumptive evidence of herpes encephalitis. However, MRI has proved to be a more sensitive early indicator of herpes encephalitis. T$_2$-weighted studies show increased signal intensity in one or both temporal lobes (Figure 2–1).

The identification of the organism in the cerebrospinal fluid by polymerase chain reaction has obviated the need for brain biopsy to establish the diagnosis.

TREATMENT. Most physicians begin acyclovir treatment in every child with a compatible clinical history. The dosage is 10 mg/kg every 8 hours, infused in 100 ml of standard intravenous fluid over a 1-hour period. The mortality rate is 28% and is highest in patients who are already in coma when treatment is initiated. In 38% of patients function returns to normal. The prognosis is best for noncomatose children younger than 10 years of age.

Measles (Rubeola) Encephalitis

Compulsory immunization had almost eliminated natural measles infection in the United States, but the incidence began climbing again in 1990 because of reduced immunization rates. The risk of encephalitis from natural disease is 1:1,000. During the first 20 years of the measles vaccine program, an estimated 52 million cases of measles, 5,200 deaths, and 17,400 cases of

☐ FIGURE 2–1 MRI scan of herpes encephalitis. T$_2$-weighted images show increased signal intensity in both temporal lobes.

mental retardation were prevented. The mechanism of measles encephalitis has been contested, but evidence for both direct viral infection and allergic demyelination has been presented. A chronic form of measles encephalitis (subacute sclerosing panencephalitis) is described in Chapter 5.

CLINICAL FEATURES. Measles is a neurotropic virus, and EEG abnormalities are often present even without clinical symptoms of encephalopathy. Symptoms of encephalitis usually begin 1 to 8 days after the appearance of rash, but can be delayed for 3 weeks. The onset is usually abrupt and is characterized by lethargy or obtundation that may rapidly progress to coma. Generalized seizures occur in half of patients. The spectrum of neurologic disturbances includes hemiplegia, ataxia, and involuntary movement disorders. Acute transverse myelitis may occur as well (see Chapter 12). The incidence of neurologic morbidity (mental retardation, epilepsy, and paralysis) is high but does not correlate with the severity of acute encephalitis.

Measles immunization does not cause an acute encephalopathy or any chronic brain damage syndrome (Institute of Medicine, 1993). Generalized seizures may occur during the second week following immunization; these are mainly febrile seizures and recovery is complete.

DIAGNOSIS. Examination of cerebrospinal fluid shows a lymphocytic pleocytosis. The number of lymphocytes is usually highest in the first few days but rarely exceeds 100 cells/mm^3. Protein concentrations are generally between 50 and 100 mg/dl (0.5 and 1 g/L), and the glucose concentration is normal.

TREATMENT. Treatment is supportive. Anticonvulsant drugs usually provide satisfactory seizure control.

Postinfectious Encephalomyelitis

Demyelinating disorders that occur during or after systemic viral illnesses are called postinfectious and are presumed to be immune mediated. The nervous system is not thought to be infected. Either central or peripheral myelin may be affected, but whether both can be affected simultaneously has not been determined. Examples of postinfectious disorders appear in several chapters of the text and include the Guillain-Barré syndrome (see Chapter 7), acute cerebellar ataxia (see Chapter 10), transverse myelitis (see Chapter 12), brachial neuritis (see Chapter 13), optic neuritis (see Chapter 16), and Bell's palsy (see Chapter 17). The incidence of some postinfectious disorders is increased in immunocompromised populations, which provides further support for the immune hypothesis.

The cause-and-effect relationship between viral infection and many of these syndromes is virtually impossible to establish if 30 days is used as the latency period between viral infection and onset of neurologic dysfunction. The average school-aged child has four to six "viral illnesses" each year, so that 33% to 50% of children will report a viral illness 30 days before the onset of any life event. A greater than 50% incidence of viral illness, 30 days before onset, is not reported for any syndrome listed previously.

CLINICAL FEATURES. MRI has expanded the spectrum of clinical features associated with postinfectious encephalopathy by allowing the demonstration of small demyelinating lesions. Lethargy and weakness are at one end of the spectrum, and coma is at the other.

The encephalopathy is often preceded by lethargy, headache, and vomiting. Whether these "systemic features" are symptoms of a viral illness or of early encephalopathy is not clear. The onset of neurologic symptoms is abrupt and characterized by declining consciousness and seizures. In some cases the generalized encephalopathy is preceded by optic neuritis, trans-

verse myelitis, or both (see Chapter 12). Some children never have focal neurologic signs, whereas in others the initial features suggest a focal mass lesions (Kepes, 1993).

Mortality is highest in the first week. Although recovery among survivors is variable, the degree of recovery may be astonishing.

DIAGNOSIS. Diagnosis is based on T$_2$-weighted MRI scan that show a marked increase in signal intensity throughout the white matter (Figure 2–2). The lesions resolve in the weeks that follow, and no new lesions are expected (Kesselring et al, 1990). Adrenoleukodystrophy must be excluded in boys.

The cerebrospinal fluid is frequently normal. Occasional abnormalities are a mild lymphocyte pleocytosis and elevation of protein concentration.

TREATMENT. Most children with severe demyelinating encephalopathies are treated with corticosteroids, despite the absence of conclusive evidence that such treatment is beneficial.

Reye Syndrome

Reye syndrome is a systemic disorder of mitochondrial function that occurs during or following viral infection. The disorder occurs more often when salicylates are administered during viral illness for relief of symptoms. Recognition of this relationship has led to decreased use of salicylates in children and a marked decline in the incidence of Reye syndrome.

CLINICAL FEATURES. In the United States sporadic cases are generally associated with varicella (chickenpox) or nonspecific respiratory infections; small epidemics are associated with influenza B infection. When varicella is the precipitating infection, the initial stage of Reye syndrome occurs 3 to 6 days after the appearance of rash.

The clinical course is relatively predictable and has been divided into five stages:

Stage 0	Vomiting, but no symptoms of brain dysfunction
Stage I	Vomiting, confusion, and lethargy
Stage II	Agitation, delirium, decorticate posturing, and hyperventilation
Stage III	Coma and decerebrate posturing
Stage IV	Flaccidity, apnea, and dilated fixed pupils

The progression from stage I to stage IV may be explosive, evolving in less than 24 hours. More commonly, the period of recurrent vomit-

□ F I G U R E 2 – 2 Postinfectious demyelination of the cerebral hemispheres. Areas of increased signal intensity are seen in both hemispheres (arrows).

ing and lethargy lasts for a day or longer. In most children with vomiting and laboratory evidence of hepatic dysfunction following varicella or respiratory infection, liver biopsy shows the features of Reye syndrome, despite normal cerebral function. This has been designated as Reye stage 0. Stages I and II represent increasing degrees of encephalopathy with metabolic dysfunction and edema. Stages III and IV indicate generalized increased intracranial pressure and herniation.

Focal neurologic disturbances and meningismus are not part of the syndrome. Fever is not a prominent feature, and hepatomegaly occurs in one half of patients late in the course.

Outcome is variable, but as a rule, infants do worse than older children. Progression to stages III and IV at all ages is associated with a high death rate and with impaired neurologic function in survivors.

DIAGNOSIS. Typical blood abnormalities are hypoglycemia, hyperammonemia, and increased concentration of hepatic enzymes. Serum bilirubin concentrations remain normal and jaundice does not occur. Acute pancreatitis sometimes develops and can be identified by increased concentrations of serum amylase.

The cerebrospinal fluid is normal except for increased pressure. The EEG shows abnormalities consistent with a diffuse encephalopathy.

Liver biopsy is definitive. Light microscopy shows panlobular accumulation of small intracellular lipid droplets and depletion of succinic acid dehydrogenase in the absence of other abnormalities. Electron microscopic changes include characteristic mitochondrial abnormalities, peroxisomal proliferation and swelling, proliferation of smooth endoplasmic reticulum, and glycogen depletion.

Conditions that mimic Reye syndrome are disorders of fatty acid oxidation, ornithine transcarbamylase deficiency, and valproate hepatotoxicity (Coates, 1994). Inborn errors of metabolism should be assumed and sought for in any child with recurrent Reye syndrome (Table 2–4) or a family history of similar illness. Metabolic products of valproate are mitochondrial poisons that have been used to produce an experimental model of Reye syndrome.

TREATMENT. Children with stage I or II disease should be watched closely in a pediatric intensive care unit and treated with intravenous hypertonic (10% to 15%) glucose solution at normal maintenance volumes. Stages III and IV require treatment of increased intracranial pressure (see Chapter 4), by elevation of the head, controlled mechanical ventilation, and mannitol. Corticosteroids are of limited benefit and should not be used routinely. Some authorities continue to advocate intracranial pressure monitors and pentobarbital coma, although they have never been shown to affect outcome. Fortunately, this once common and deadly disease has almost disappeared with discontinuation of salicylate therapy for children.

POSTIMMUNIZATION ENCEPHALOPATHY

Three types of vaccines are in general use in the United States: live-attenuated viruses, whole- or fractionated-killed organisms, and toxoids.

Live-attenuated virus vaccines (measles, mumps, rubella, varicella, and oral poliomyelitis) are intended to produce a mild and harmless infection with subsequent immunity. However, even under ideal circumstances of vaccine preparation and host resistance, symptoms of the natural disease and its known neurologic complications may develop in vaccine recipients.

Whole-killed organisms (pertussis, influenza, rabies, and inactivated poliomyelitis) do not reproduce their natural disease, but are alleged to injure the nervous system by a toxic or an allergic mechanism. Whole-cell pertussis vaccine causes seizures, and while it is not established that it causes chronic brain damage, The Institute of Medicine has conceded the possibility based on The National Childhood Encephalopathy Study (Institute of Medicine, 1994). Rabies vaccine had been an important cause of encephalomyelitis in the past, but the newer vaccine, prepared from virus grown on human diploid cells, has been only rarely implicated as a cause of polyneuropathy. The older vaccine (Semple), still in use in some parts of the world, contains myelin-basic protein and is known to cause encephalomyelitis. None of the other whole-killed organism vaccines causes encephalopathy.

Toxoids are produced by the inactivation of toxins produced by bacteria. Diphtheria and tetanus toxoids are the only such vaccines now in use. Tetanus toxoid is associated with the Guillain-Barré syndrome and brachial plexitis; neither is associated with encephalopathy.

 ## Metabolic and Systemic Disorders

DISORDERS OF OSMOLALITY

The osmolality of a solution is determined by the number of particles in the solution. Sodium salts, glucose, and urea are the primary osmoles of the extracellular space, potassium salts of the intracellular space, and plasma proteins of the intravascular space. Because cell membranes are permeable to water and osmotic equilibrium must be maintained, the volume of intracellular fluid is determined by the osmolality of the extracellular space.

Hypernatremia and hyperglycemia are the major causes of serum hyperosmolality, and hyponatremia is the main cause of serum hypoosmolality.

Diabetic Ketoacidosis

The major cause of symptomatic hyperglycemia in children is diabetic ketoacidosis. Nonketotic, hyperglycemic coma, associated with mild or non-insulin-requiring diabetes, is unusual in children.

CLINICAL FEATURES. Diabetic ketoacidosis develops rapidly in children who have neglected to take prescribed doses of insulin or who have a superimposed infection. Initial features are polydipsia, polyuria, and fatigue. The child

hyperventilates to compensate for metabolic acidosis. Lethargy rapidly progresses to coma. Ketoacidosis is the leading cause of death in children with diabetes, and mortality rates are still as high as 10%.

Cerebral edema is an early and almost constant feature of diabetic ketoacidosis. The mechanism is not established. The severity of cerebral edema correlates with changes in level of consciousness. Edema may contribute to death in some cases. Other, less common, neurologic complications of diabetic ketoacidosis are venous sinus thrombosis and intracerebral hemorrhage. Both are associated with focal or generalized seizures.

DIAGNOSIS. The diagnosis is based on the combination of a blood glucose level greater than 400 mg/dl (22 mmol/L), the presence of serum and urinary ketones, an arterial pH less than 7.25, and a serum bicarbonate concentration less than 15 mmol/L.

TREATMENT. In children with moderate to severe diabetic ketoacidosis, the rapid administration of hypotonic fluids at a time of high serum osmolality should be avoided. Fluid deficits should be replaced evenly over 48 hours. The sodium deficit should be reduced by half in the first 12 hours, and the remainder eliminated over the next 36 hours. Bicarbonate ion should be given in physiologic proportions.

Hypoglycemia

Symptomatic hypoglycemia after the neonatal period is usually associated with insulin use in the treatment of diabetes mellitus. Sepsis and inborn errors of metabolism account for only a minority of cases.

CLINICAL FEATURES. Clinical features are not precisely predictable from blood glucose concentration. Hypoglycemia does not usually become symptomatic until blood concentrations are less than 50 mg/dl (2.8 mmol/L). The rate of fall may be important in determining the clinical features. Dizziness and tremor may occur at blood concentrations below 60 mg/dl (3.1 mmol/L) and serve as a warning of insulin overdose. Greater declines in blood glucose concentration result in confusion, delirium, and loss of consciousness. Sudden hemiplegia, usually transitory and sometimes shifting between the two sides, is a rare feature of hypoglycemia. The mechanism is unknown, and CT shows no evidence of infarction.

DIAGNOSIS. Hypoglycemia should always be suspected in diabetic children with an altered mental status or decreased consciousness. Blood glucose concentration should be measured promptly.

TREATMENT. Diabetic children should be encouraged to carry a source of sugar for use at the first symptom of hypoglycemia. Children who are comatose from hypoglycemia should receive immediate intravenous glucose replacement. Complete recovery is the rule.

Hypernatremia

Hypernatremia is usually caused by dehydration in which water loss exceeds sodium loss, and by overhydration with hypertonic saline solutions. It is a medical emergency and, if not corrected promptly, may lead to permanent brain damage and death.

CLINICAL FEATURES. Hypernatremic dehydration may be a consequence of vomiting or diarrhea, especially if water intake is restricted. Iatrogenic hypernatremia is usually caused by overzealous correction of hyponatremia. Rapid alterations in sodium concentration are much more likely to cause encephalopathy than are equivalent concentrations attained slowly. The symptoms of hypernatremia are all referable to the nervous system and include irritability, lethargy progressing to coma, and seizures. The presence of focal neurologic deficits suggests cerebral venous sinus thrombosis.

DIAGNOSIS. Symptomatic hypernatremia develops at sodium concentrations greater than 160 mEq/L (160 mmol/L). EEG shows the nonspecific slowing associated with metabolic encephalopathies. Focal slowing on the EEG or focal abnormalities on examination warrant CT to look for venous sinus thrombosis.

Chronic or recurrent episodes of hypernatremia may result from hypodipsia (lack of thirst), a rare condition encountered in children with congenital or acquired brain disorders. The syndrome is usually associated with a defect in secretion of antidiuretic hormone.

TREATMENT. Rapid water replacement can lead to cerebral edema. The recommended approach is to correct abnormalities of intravascular volume before correcting the water deficit.

Hyponatremia

Hyponatremia may result from water retention, sodium loss, or both. Water retention is often caused by the syndrome of inappropriate antidiuretic hormone secretion (SIADH), and sodium loss results from renal disease, vomiting, and diarrhea. Permanent brain damage from hyponatremia is uncommon, but may occur in otherwise healthy children if the serum sodium concentration is allowed to remain less than 115 mEq/L for several hours (Arieff et al, 1992).

Syndrome of Inappropriate Antidiuretic Hormone Secretion

SIADH occurs in association with several neurologic disorders, including head trauma, infections, and intracranial hemorrhage.

CLINICAL FEATURES. Most patients with SIADH have a pre-existing loss of consciousness from their underlying neurologic disorder. In such patients hyponatremia is the only feature of SIADH. In those who are alert, lethargy develops from the hyponatremia but rarely progresses to coma or seizures.

DIAGNOSIS. Those who provide care for children with acute intracranial disorders must be vigilant for SIADH; repeated determinations of serum sodium concentration are required. Once hyponatremia is documented, urinary sodium concentration must be measured. The urinary sodium concentration is usually greater than 20 mEq/L (20 mmol/L) and parallels intake. The diagnosis is established by showing inappropriately high plasma concentrations of arginine vasopressin in the presence of hyponatremia.

TREATMENT. All signs of SIADH respond to fluid restriction. An intake of 50% to 75% of daily water maintenance is generally satisfactory.

Sodium Loss

CLINICAL FEATURES. Hyponatremic encephalopathy is caused by the movement of water into the brain. Nausea, vomiting, muscular twitching, and lethargy appear when the serum sodium concentration falls below 125 mEq/L (125 mmol/L). A further decline to less than 115 mEq/L (115 mmol/L) is associated with seizures and coma.

DIAGNOSIS. Hyponatremia should be recognized as a potential problem in children with vomiting or diarrhea or with renal disease. Serum and urinary sodium concentrations are both decreased.

TREATMENT. Hypertonic sodium chloride (514 mEq/L) is infused with the goal of increasing the serum sodium concentration to 125 to 130 mEq/L (125 to 130 mmol/L) but by no more than 25 mEq/L (25 mmol/L) in the first 48 hours (Arieff et al, 1992). More rapid corrections are associated with seizures, hypernatremic encephalopathy, and the possibility of central pontine myelinolysis.

ENDOCRINE DISORDERS

Adrenal Disorders

Adrenal hypersecretion causes agitation or depression but does not produce coma. Adrenal failure may result from sepsis, abrupt withdrawal of corticosteroid therapy, or adrenal hemorrhage. Initial symptoms are nausea, vomiting, abdominal pain, and fever. Lethargy progresses to coma and is associated with hypovolemic shock. Prompt intravenous infusion of fluids, glucose, and corticosteroids is life-saving.

Parathyroid Disorders

The neurologic features of hyperparathyroidism are all related to hypercalcemia. Weakness and myopathy are relatively common. Alterations in mental status occur in 50% of patients and include apathy, delirium, paranoia, and dementia. Apathy and delirium occur at serum calcium concentrations greater than 11 mg/dl (2.75 mmol/L), and psychosis and dementia develop at concentrations of 16 mg/dl (4.0 mmol/L) or greater.

Seizures are the main feature of hypoparathyroidism and hypocalcemia. They may be generalized or focal and are often preceded by tetany. Hypocalcemic seizures do not respond to anticonvulsant drugs and must be treated with calcium replacement.

Thyroid Disorders

Hyperthyroidism causes exhilaration bordering on mania and may be associated with seizures and chorea (see Chapter 14). Thyroid storm (crisis) is a life-threatening event characterized by restlessness, cardiac arrhythmia, vomiting, and diarrhea. Delirium is an early feature and may progress to coma.

Acquired hypothyroidism affects both the central and the peripheral nervous system. Peripheral effects include neuropathy and myopathy. Central effects are cranial nerve abnormalities, ataxia, psychoses, dementia, seizures, and coma. Delusions and hallucinations occur in more than half of patients with long-standing disease. Myxedema coma, a rare manifestation of long-standing hypothyroidism in adults, is even more uncommon in children. It is characterized by profound hypothermia without shivering.

Hashimoto's Encephalopathy

Hashimoto's thyroiditis is an immune-mediated disease associated with high titers of antithyroid antibodies (Shaw et al, 1991).

CLINICAL FEATURES. The progression of symptoms is variable but usually begins with headache and confusion that progress to stupor. Focal or generalized seizures and transitory neurologic deficits (strokelike episodes) may be an initial or a late feature. Tremulousness and myoclonus commonly occur during some stage in the illness. The encephalopathy lasts several days and then gradually disappears. Recurrent episodes are the rule and lead to permanent neurologic sequelae.

DIAGNOSIS. Hashimoto thyroiditis should be suspected in every case of recurrent encephalopathy. The cerebrospinal fluid protein concentration is elevated, sometimes above 100 mg/dl (1 g/L), but the pressure and cell count are normal. Affected individuals are usually euthyroid. The diagnosis depends on the presence of antithyroid antibodies. Antibodies against thyroglobulin and the microsomal fraction are most common, but antibodies against other thyroid elements and other organs may be present as well.

TREATMENT. Corticosteroids and other immunosuppressive agents are beneficial in ending an attack and preventing further episodes.

HEPATIC ENCEPHALOPATHY

Fulminant hepatic failure in children is caused by viral hepatitis, drugs, toxins, and Reye syndrome. The encephalopathy that accompanies hepatic failure cannot be explained by abnormalities of any single factor, such as the ammonia concentration, but is due to multifactorial metabolic derangements. Severe viral hepatitis with marked elevation of the unconjugated bilirubin concentration may even lead to kernicterus in older children.

In children with chronic choleastatic liver disease, demyelination of the posterior columns and peripheral nerves may develop as a result of vitamin E deficiency. The major features are ataxia, areflexia, and gaze paresis, without evidence of encephalopathy (see Chapter 10).

CLINICAL FEATURES. Malaise and fatigue are early symptoms that accompany the features of hepatic failure: jaundice, dark urine, and abnormal results of liver function tests. Nausea and vomiting occur when hepatic failure is fulminant. The onset of coma may be spontaneous or induced by gastrointestinal bleeding, infection, high-protein intake, and excessive use of tranquilizers or diuretics. The first features are disturbed sleep and a change in affect. These are followed by drowsiness, hyperventilation, and asterixis, a flapping tremor at the wrist when the arms are extended and the wrists flexed. Hallucinations sometimes occur during early stages, but a continuous progression to coma is more common. Seizures and decerebrate rigidity develop as the patient becomes comatose.

DIAGNOSIS. In hepatic coma, the EEG pattern is not specific but is always abnormal and suggests a metabolic encephalopathy: loss of posterior rhythm, generalized slowing of background, and frontal triphasic waves.

Biochemical markers of liver failure include a sharp rise in transaminase activity (serum glutamic oxaloacetic transaminase [SGOT] and serum glutamic pyruvate transaminase [SGPT]), increased prothrombin time, mixed hyperbilirubinemia, and a decline in serum albumin concentration.

TREATMENT. The goal of treatment is to maintain cerebral, renal, and cardiopulmonary function until liver regeneration or transplantation can occur. Cerebral function is impaired, not only by abnormal concentrations of metabolites but also by cerebral edema.

INBORN ERRORS OF METABOLISM

The inborn errors of metabolism that cause states of decreased consciousness are usually associated with hyperammonemia, hypoglycemia, or organic aciduria. Neonatal seizures are an early feature in most of these conditions (see Chapter 1), but some may not cause symptoms until infancy or childhood. Inborn errors with a delayed onset of encephalopathy include disorders of pyruvate metabolism and respiratory chain disorders (see Chapters 5, 6, 8, and 10); hemizygotes for ornithine carbamylase deficiency and heterozygotes for carbamyl phosphate synthetase deficiency (see Chapter 1); glycogen storage diseases (see Chapter 1); and primary carnitine deficiency.

Medium-Chain Acyl-Coenzyme A Dehydrogenase Deficiency

Medium-Chain Acyl-Coenzyme A (CoA) dehydrogenase (MCAD) deficiency is a disorder of beta-oxidation of fatty acids. The trait is transmitted by autosomal recessive inheritance (Iafolla et al, 1994). It is the main cause of what had been described as *primary carnitine deficiency* (Table 2–6). L-Carnitine is essential for (1) the transfer of long-chain fatty acids across the inner mitochondrial membrane, (2) the facilitation of branched chain alpha-ketoacid oxidation, (3) the shuttle of acyl-CoA products of peroxi-

■ TABLE 2–6

Differential Diagnosis of Carnitine Deficiency

Inborn Errors of Metabolism

Aminoacidurias
  Glutaric aciduria
  Isovaleric acidemia
  Methylmalonic acidemia
  Propionic acidemia
Disorders of pyruvate metabolism
  Multiple carboxylase deficiency
  Pyruvate carboxylase deficiency
  Pyruvate dehydrogenase deficiency
Disorders of the respiratory chain
Medium-chain acyl-CoA dehydrogenase (MCAD)
  deficiency
Phosphoglucomutase deficiency

Acquired Conditions

Hemodialysis
Malnutrition
Pregnancy
Reye syndrome
Total parenteral nutrition
Valproate hepatotoxicity

somal beta-oxidation to the mitochondrial matrix in the liver, (4) the modulation of the acyl-CoA/CoA ratio, and (5) the esterification of potentially toxic acyl-CoA metabolites. The transfer of fatty acids across the mitochondrial membrane requires the conversion of acyl-CoA to acylcarnitine. If the carnitine concentration is deficient, toxic levels of acyl-CoA accumulate and impair the citric acid cycle, gluconeogenesis, the urea cycle, and fatty acid oxidation (De Vivo and Tein, 1990).

CLINICAL FEATURES. Affected children are normal at birth. Recurrent attacks of nonketotic hypoglycemia, vomiting, confusion, lethargy, and coma are provoked by intercurrent illness or fasting during infancy and early childhood. Cardiorespiratory arrest and sudden infant death may occur, but MCAD is not considered an important cause of the sudden infant death syndrome (SIDS). Between attacks the child may appear normal. In some families the deficiency causes cardiomyopathy, whereas in others it causes only mild to moderate proximal weakness (see Chapters 6 and 7). Similar clinical phenotypes are caused by deficiencies of long-chain and short-chain acyl-CoA dehydrogenase (Tein et al, 1991).

DIAGNOSIS. All affected children have low or absent urinary ketones during episodes of hypoglycemia and elevated serum concentrations of aspartate aminotransferase and lactate dehydrogenase. Blood carnitine concentrations are less than 20 μmol/mg noncollagen protein. The diagnosis is established by showing the enzyme deficiency or the genetic mutation.

TREATMENT. All affected children must avoid fasting. Dietary supplementation with L-carnitine is recommended. The initial dosage is 50 mg/kg/day, which is increased as tolerated (up to 800 mg/kg/day) until the desired blood concentration is attained. Adverse effects of carnitine include nausea, vomiting, diarrhea, and abdominal cramps. Dietary supplementation with riboflavin and glycine is also recommended but their efficacy is less well established.

During an acute attack, a diet rich in medium-chain triglycerides and low in long-chain triglycerides should be provided in addition to carnitine. General supportive care is required for hypoglycemia and hypoprothrombinemia.

RENAL DISORDERS

Children with chronic renal failure are at risk for acute or chronic uremic encephalopathy, dialysis encephalopathy, hypertensive encephalopathy, and neurologic complications of the immunocompromised state.

Acute Uremic Encephalopathy

CLINICAL FEATURES. In children with acute renal failure, symptoms of cerebral dysfunction develop over several days. Asterixis is often the initial feature. This is followed by periods of confusion and headache, sometimes progressing to delirium and then to lethargy. Weakness, tremulousness, and muscle cramps develop. Myoclonic jerks and tetany may be present. If uremia continues, decreasing consciousness and seizures follow.

Transitory or permanent hemiparesis may occur in children with *hemolytic-uremic syndrome*. Encephalopathy is the usual initial feature, but hemiparesis and aphasia caused by thrombotic stroke can occur in the absence of seizures or altered states of consciousness.

DIAGNOSIS. The mechanism is multifactorial and does not correlate with concentrations of blood urea nitrogen alone. Hyperammonemia and disturbed equilibrium of ions between the intracellular and extracellular spaces are probably important factors.

Late in the course, acute uremic encephalopathy may be confused with hypertensive encephalopathy. A distinguishing feature is that increased intracranial pressure is an early feature of hypertensive encephalopathy but not of acute uremic encephalopathy. Early in the course the

EEG shows slowing of the background rhythms and periodic triphasic waves.

TREATMENT. Hemodialysis reverses the encephalopathy and should be performed as quickly as possible after diagnosis.

Chronic Uremic Encephalopathy

CLINICAL FEATURES. Chronic uremic encephalopathy is usually caused by congenital renal hypoplasia. Renal failure begins during the first year, and encephalopathy occurs between 1 and 9 years of age. Growth failure precedes the onset of encephalopathy. Three stages are described.

Stage 1 consists of delayed motor development, dysmetria and tremor, or ataxia. Examination during this stage shows hyperreflexia, mild hypotonia, and extensor plantar responses. Within 6 to 12 months the disease progresses to stage 2.

Stage 2 is characterized by myoclonus of the face and limbs, partial motor seizures, dementia, and then generalized seizures. Facial myoclonus and lingual apraxia make speech and feeding difficult, and limb myoclonus interferes with ambulation. The duration of stage 2 is variable and may be months to years.

Stage 3 consists of progressive bulbar failure, a vegetative state, and death.

DIAGNOSIS. The diagnosis is based on clinical findings. Serial EEG shows progressive slowing and then superimposed epileptiform activity, and serial CT shows progressive cerebral atrophy. The disorder may be difficult to distinguish from dialysis encephalopathy; they may be the same disease.

Hyperparathyroidism with hypercalcemia occurs in some children with chronic uremic encephalopathy, but parathyroidectomy does not reverse the process. A suggested cause is aluminum toxicity from antacids administered as phosphate binders. Plasma concentrations of aluminum should be determined during stage 1 and, if they are elevated, aluminum ingestion discontinued.

TREATMENT. Hemodialysis and renal transplantation have not altered the course in most patients.

Dialysis Encephalopathy

Long-term dialysis may be associated with acute, transitory neurologic disturbances attributed to the rapid shift of fluids and electrolytes between intracellular and extracellular spaces. Most common are vascular headaches and seizures. Seizures usually occur toward the end of dialysis or up to 24 hours later and may be preceded by lethargy and delirium.

In contrast, progressive encephalopathies associated with dialysis are often fatal. Two important causes exist: (1) opportunistic infections in the immunodeficient host, usually caused by cytomegalovirus and mycoses in children, and (2) the dialysis dementia syndrome.

Dialysis Dementia Syndrome

CLINICAL FEATURES. The mean interval between commencement of dialysis and onset of symptoms is 4 years (range 1 to 7 years), and subsequent progression of symptoms varies from weeks to years. Patients have a characteristic speech disturbance either as an initial feature or later in the course. It begins as intermittent hesitancy of speech (stuttering and slurring) and may progress to aphasia. Agraphia and apraxia may be present as well. Subtle personality changes suggestive of depression occur early in the course. A phase of hallucinations and agitation may occur, and progressive dementia develops.

Myoclonic jerking of the limbs is often present before the onset of dementia. First noted during dialysis, it soon becomes continuous and interferes with normal activity. Generalized tonic-clonic seizures develop in most patients and become more frequent and severe as the encephalopathy progresses. Complex partial seizures may be observed, but focal motor seizures are unusual.

Neurologic examination reveals the triad of speech arrest, myoclonus, and dementia. In addition, many patients show symmetric proximal weakness (myopathy) or distal weakness and sensory loss (neuropathy) with loss of tendon reflexes.

DIAGNOSIS. EEG changes correlate with disease progress. A characteristic early feature is the appearance of paroxysmal high-amplitude delta activity in the frontal areas, despite a normal posterior rhythm. Eventually the background becomes generally slow and frontal triphasic waves are noted. Epileptiform activity develops in all patients with dialysis dementia and is the EEG feature that differentiates dialysis dementia from uremic encephalopathy. The activity consists of sharp, spike, or polyspike discharges that may have a periodic quality.

TREATMENT. Aluminum toxicity is an important contributory cause, but no single factor has been established as causative. Excessive aluminum may be derived from orally administered aluminum gels or from the dialysate. Removal of aluminum from dialysate prevents the appearance of new cases and progression in some established cases, even if oral gels are still administered.

Renal transplantation prevents development of the syndrome but does not always provide relief in established cases. Benzodiazepines are useful in treating myoclonus and seizures, and may improve the speech disturbance.

Hypertensive Encephalopathy

Hypertensive encephalopathy occurs when increases in systemic blood pressure exceed the limits of cerebral autoregulation. The result is damage to small arterioles, which leads to patchy areas of ischemia and edema. Therefore, focal neurologic deficits are relatively common.

CLINICAL FEATURES. The initial features are transitory attacks of cerebral ischemia and headache. Such symptoms may be dismissed as part of uremic encephalopathy, despite the warning signs of focal neurologic deficits. Headache persists and is accompanied by visual disturbances and vomiting. Seizures and diminished consciousness follow. The seizures are frequently focal at onset and then generalized. Examination reveals papilledema and retinal hemorrhages.

DIAGNOSIS. Because the syndrome occurs in children receiving long-term renal dialysis while awaiting transplantation, the differential diagnosis includes disorders of osmolality, uremic encephalopathy, and dialysis encephalopathy. The EEG shows nonspecific abnormalities, including generalized slowing of the background rhythms and sometimes paroxysmal discharges and periodic complexes.

Hypertensive encephalopathy can be distinguished from other encephalopathies associated with renal disease by the greater elevation of blood pressure and the presence of focal neurologic disturbances.

TREATMENT. Hypertensive encephalopathy is a medical emergency. Treatment consists of anticonvulsant therapy and aggressive efforts to reduce hypertension. Measures to reduce cerebral edema are required in some patients.

OTHER METABOLIC ENCEPHALOPATHIES

Several less common causes of metabolic encephalopathy are listed in Table 2–3. Some are attributable to derangements of a single substance, but most are multifactorial.

In 5% of children with burns covering 30% of the body surface, an encephalopathy that may be intermittent develops *(burn encephalopathy)*. The onset may be days to weeks after the burn. Altered mental states (delirium or coma) and seizures (generalized or focal) are the major features. Multiple metabolic alterations are present, and the encephalopathy usually cannot be attributed to a single factor.

Encephalopathies that occur during total parenteral hyperalimentation are generally due to hyperammonemia caused by excessive loads of amino acids.

Hypomagnesemia in infancy may be caused by prematurity, maternal deficiency, maternal or infant hypoparathyroidism, high-phosphorus diets, exchange transfusion, intestinal disorders, and specific defects in magnesium absorption. These conditions are often associated with hypocalcemia. Excessive use of diuretics causes hypomagnesemia in older children. Symptoms develop when plasma magnesium concentrations are less than 1.2 mg/dl (0.5 mmol/L), and include jitteriness, hyperirritability, and seizures. Further decline in serum magnesium concentrations leads to obtundation and coma.

Deficiency of one or more B vitamins may be associated with lethargy or delirium, but only thiamine deficiency causes coma. Thiamine deficiency is relatively common in alcoholic adults and produces Wernicke encephalopathy but is uncommon in children. Subacute necrotizing encephalopathy (Leigh disease) is a thiamine deficiency-like state in children (see Chapters 5 and 10).

⮕ Migraine

Migraine causes several neurologic syndromes and is discussed in many chapters. Among its less common syndromes are a confusional state, coma, and an amnestic state.

ACUTE CONFUSIONAL MIGRAINE

CLINICAL FEATURES. A confused and agitated state resembling toxic-metabolic psychosis occurs as a migraine variant in children between the ages of 5 and 16 (Sheth et al, 1995). Most affected children are 10 years or older. The symptoms develop rapidly. The child becomes delirious and appears to be in pain but does not complain of headache. Impaired awareness of environment, retarded responses to painful stimuli, hyperactivity, restlessness, and combat-ive behavior are evident. The duration of an attack is usually 3 to 5 hours but may be as long as 20 hours. The child eventually falls into a deep sleep, appears normal on awakening, and has no memory of the episode. Confusional attacks tend to recur over days or months and then evolve into typical migraine episodes.

DIAGNOSIS. Migraine is always a clinical diagnosis and should be arrived at only after other possibilities are excluded. The diagnosis relies heavily on a family history of migraine, but not necessarily of confusional migraine. During or shortly after a confusional attack the EEG shows unilateral temporal or occipital slowing.

TREATMENT. The acute attack can be treated with intramuscular chlorpromazine, 1 mg/kg. Propranolol provides prophylaxis (see Chapter 3).

MIGRAINE COMA

Migraine coma is a rare but extreme form of migraine that can be fatal.

CLINICAL FEATURES. The major features of migraine coma are (1) recurrent episodes of coma precipitated by trivial head injury and (2) apparent meningitis associated with life-threatening cerebral edema. Migraine coma has been reported in a kindred with *familial hemiplegic migraine* (see Chapter 11), but a similar syndrome may occur in sporadic cases as well. Coma develops following trivial head injury and is associated with fever. Intracranial pressure is increased because of cerebral edema, which can be localized to one hemisphere and cause sufficient midline shift to produce herniation. States of decreased consciousness may last several days. Recovery is then complete.

DIAGNOSIS. Coma following even trivial head injury causes concern for intracranial hemorrhage. The initial CT scan may be normal, especially if obtained early in the course. Scans obtained between 24 and 72 hours show generalized or focal edema.

Examination of the cerebrospinal fluid reveals increased pressure and pleocytosis (up to 100 cells/mm^3. The combination of fever, coma, and cerebrospinal fluid pleocytosis suggests viral encephalitis, and herpes is a possibility if edema is localized to one temporal lobe.

TREATMENT. Patients who have experienced migraine coma should be treated afterward with a prophylactic agent to prevent further attacks (see Chapter 3). The major treatment goal during the acute attack is to decrease intracranial pressure by reducing cerebral edema (see Chapter 4).

TRANSIENT GLOBAL AMNESIA

Transient global amnesia usually occurs in adults and is characterized by sudden inability to form new memories and repetitive questioning about events, without other neurologic symptoms or signs. Migraine is the probable cause when such attacks occur in children or in more than one family member (Sheth et al, 1995).

CLINICAL FEATURES. Attacks last from 20 minutes to several hours, and retrograde amnesia is present on recovery. Many adults with transient global amnesia have a history of migraine, and a similar syndrome may be seen in children with migraine following trivial head injury. The attacks are similar to acute confusional migraine except that the patient has less delirium and greater isolated memory deficiency.

DIAGNOSIS. A personal or family history of migraine is essential for diagnosis. The CT scan shows no abnormalities, but the EEG may show slowing of the background rhythm in one temporal lobe.

TREATMENT. Management is the same as for migraine with aura (see Chapter 3).

 Psychological Disorders

Panic disorders and schizophrenia may have an acute onset of symptoms suggesting delirium or confusion and must be distinguished from acute organic encephalopathies.

PANIC DISORDER

CLINICAL FEATURES. Panic attacks were thought to be confined to adults but now are recognized to occur in adolescents and school-aged children. A panic attack is an agitated state caused by anxiety. Principal features are paroxysmal dizziness, headache, and dyspnea. Hyperventilation often occurs and results in further dizziness, paresthesias, and lightheadedness. Attacks may be provoked by phobias, such as fear of going to school. They can last for minutes to hours and recur daily.

DIAGNOSIS. Panic attacks simulate cardiac or neurologic disease, and many children undergo extensive and unnecessary medical evaluation before the correct diagnosis is reached. Panic disorder should be suspected in children with recurrent attacks of hyperventilation, dizziness, or dyspnea.

TREATMENT. Antidepressant drugs have varying degrees of efficacy. Imipramine has the best success rate. Initial dosages are less than those used for depression (0.25 mg/kg/day), but higher dosages may be needed if concurrent depression must be treated.

SCHIZOPHRENIA

CLINICAL FEATURES. Schizophrenia is a disorder of adolescence or early adult life and should not be suspected in prepubertal children. Schizophrenic individuals do not have an antecedent history of an affective disorder. An initial feature is often declining work performance simulating dementia. Intermittent depersonalization (not knowing where or who one is) may occur early in the course and suggests complex partial seizures.

Thoughts move with loose association from one idea to another until they become incoherent. Delusions and hallucinations are common and usually have paranoid features. Motor activity can be either lacking, with the patient remaining stationary, or excessive and purposeless. This combination of symptoms in an adolescent may be difficult to distinguish clinically from drug encephalopathy.

DIAGNOSIS. The diagnosis is established by careful evaluation of mental status. The family may have a history of schizophrenia. Neurologic and laboratory findings are normal. A normal EEG in an awake child with the clinical symptoms of an acute encephalopathy points to a psychologic disturbance, including schizophrenia.

TREATMENT. Schizophrenia is generally considered a chemical disorder of the brain. It is incurable, but many of the symptoms are alleviated by antipsychotic drugs. Phenothiazines and haloperidol are most often used.

 Toxic Encephalopathies

Accidental poisoning with drugs and chemicals left carelessly within reach are relatively common in children from ages 1 to 4. Between ages 4 and 10 there is a trough in the frequency of poisoning, which is followed by increasing frequency of intentional poisoning with substances of abuse and prescription drugs.

IMMUNOSUPPRESSIVE DRUGS

Immunosuppressive drugs are used widely in children undergoing organ transplant (Patchell, 1994). Encephalopathy in children who are immunosuppressed may be caused by the drugs themselves, by secondary metabolic disturbances, or by cerebral infection. Three children being treated with amphotericin B to treat aspergillosis after bone marrow transplant for leukemia developed a severe encephalopathy with parkinsonian features (Mott et al, 1995).

Corticosteroid Psychosis

Daily use of corticosteroids at doses lower than 1 mg/kg may cause hyperactivity, insomnia, and anxiety. The higher dosages used for immunosuppression, generally >2mg/kg/day, may precipitate a psychosis similar to schizophrenia or delirium. Stopping the drug reverses the symptoms.

Cyclosporine Encephalopathy

Cyclosporine, the drug most commonly used to prevent organ rejection, causes encephalopathy in 5% of recipients. The blood concentration of drug does not correlate simply with any neurologic complication. The more common syndrome consists of lethargy, confusion, cortical blindness, and visual hallucinations without any motor disturbances. A second syndrome is a combination of motor symptoms (ataxia, tremor, paralysis) and altered states of consciousness and cognition.

MRI shows widespread edema and leukoencephalopathy. In children with the syndrome of visual disturbances and encephalopathy, the most intense disturbances are in the occipital lobes. The encephalopathy clears completely when the drug is stopped. Sometimes, the drug can be restarted at a lower dose without causing encephalopathy.

OKT3 Meningoencephalitis

OKT3 is an anti-T-cell monoclonal antibody used to initiate immunosuppression and to treat rejection. Up to 14% of patients develop fever, and a sterile meningitis 24 to 72 hours after the first injection, and up to 10% develop encephalopathy within 4 days. The encephalopathy slowly resolves over the next 2 weeks whether or not the drug is stopped.

PRESCRIPTION DRUGS OVERDOSES

Most intentional overdoses are with prescription drugs, because they are readily available. Delirium or coma may be due to toxic effects of psychoactive drugs (anticonvulsants, antidepressants, antipsychotics, and tranquilizers), hypoglycemia (insulin and oral hypoglycemia agents), and acid-base disturbances (salicylates).

The encephalopathies that occur when drugs cause disorders of osmolality or organ failure are described in the section on metabolic encephalopathies.

CLINICAL FEATURES. Psychoactive drugs are present in many households and are a frequent cause of poisoning. As a rule, toxic doses produce lethargy, nystagmus, or ophthalmoplegia, and loss of coordination. Higher concentrations cause coma and seizures. Involuntary movements may occur as an idiosyncratic or dose-related effect.

Diazepam is remarkably safe and overdose does not cause coma or death when taken alone. Other benzodiazepines are also reasonably safe.

Tricyclic antidepressants are among the most widely prescribed drugs in the United States and account for 25% of serious overdoses. The major features of overdosage are coma, hypotension, and anticholinergic effects (flushing, dry skin, dilated pupils, tachycardia, decreased gastrointestinal motility, and urinary retention). Seizures and myocardial depression may be present as well.

The onset of symptoms following phenothiazine or haloperidol ingestion may be delayed for 6 to 24 hours, and symptoms may be intermittent. Extrapyramidal disturbances (see Chapter 14), and symptoms of anticholinergic poisoning are prominent features. Fatalities are uncommon and probably caused by cardiac arrhythmia.

DIAGNOSIS. Most drugs can be identified in the laboratory within 2 hours. A drug screen of the urine should be performed in all cases of unidentified coma or delirium. If an unidentifiable product is found in the urine, further identification may be possible in the plasma. Blood concentration should be determined when the identity of a drug is known.

TREATMENT. The specificities and degree of supportive care needed depend on the drug and the severity of the poisoning. Most children need an intravenous line and careful monitoring of cardiorespiratory status. A continuous electrocardiogram (ECG) is often required because of concern for arrhythmia. Unabsorbed drug must be removed from the stomach by lavage and repeated doses of activated charcoal (30 mg every 6 hours) administered to prevent absorption and increase drug clearance. Extrapyramidal symptoms are treated with intravenous diphenhydramine, 2 mg/kg.

POISONING

Most accidental poisonings occur in small children who ingest common household products. The ingestion is usually discovered quickly because the child becomes sick and vomits. Insecticides, herbicides, and products containing hydrocarbons or alcohol are frequently implicated. Clinical features vary depending on the agent ingested. Optimal management requires identification of constituent poisons, estimation of amount ingested, interval since exposure, cleansing of the gastrointestinal tract, specific antidotes when available, and supportive measures.

SUBSTANCE ABUSE

Alcohol remains the most common substance of abuse in the United States. More than 90% of high school seniors have used alcohol one or more times, and 6% are daily drinkers. Approximately 6% of high school seniors use marijuana daily, but less than 0.1% are regular users of hallucinogens or opiates. The use of cocaine, stimulants, and sedatives has been increasing in recent years. Daily use of stimulants is reported by up to 1% of high school seniors.

CLINICAL FEATURES. The American Psychiatric Association defines the diagnostic criteria for substance abuse as (1) a pattern of pathologic use with inability to stop or reduce use; (2) impairment of social or occupational functioning, which includes school performance in children; and (3) persistence of the problem for 1 month or longer.

The clinical features of acute intoxication vary with the substance used. Almost all disturb judgment, intellectual function, and coordination. Alcohol and sedatives lead to drowsiness, sleep, and obtundation. In contrast, hallucinogens cause bizarre behavior, which includes hallucinations, delusions, and muscle rigidity. Such drugs as phencyclidine (angel dust) and lysergic acid diethylamide (LSD) produce a clinical picture that simulates schizophrenia.

The usual symptoms of marijuana intoxication are euphoria and a sense of relaxation at low doses and a dreamlike state with slow response time at higher doses. Very high blood concentrations produce depersonalization, disorientation, and sensory disturbances. Hallucinations and delusions are unusual with marijuana and suggest mixed drug use.

Amphetamine abuse should be considered when an agitated state is coupled with peripheral evidence of adrenergic toxicity: mydriasis, flushing, diaphoresis, and reflex bradycardia caused by peripheral vasoconstriction.

Cocaine affects the brain and heart. Early symptoms include euphoria, mydriasis, headache, and tachycardia. Higher doses produce emotional lability, nausea and vomiting, flushing, and a syndrome that simulates paranoid schizophrenia. Life-threatening complications are hyperthermia, seizures, cardiac arrhythmia, and stroke. Associated stroke syndromes include transient ischemic attacks in the distribution of the middle cerebral artery, lateral medullary infarction, and anterior spinal artery infarction.

DIAGNOSIS. The major challenge is to differentiate acute substance intoxication from schizophrenia. Important clues are a history of substance abuse obtained from family or friends, associated autonomic and cardiac disturbances, and alterations in vital signs. Urinary and plasma screening generally detects the substance or its metabolites.

TREATMENT. Management of acute substance abuse depends on the substance used and the amount ingested. Physicians must be alert to the possibility of multiple drug or substance exposure. An attempt should be made to empty the gastrointestinal tract of substances taken orally. Support of cardiorespiratory function and correction of metabolic disturbances are generally required. Intravenous diazepam reduces the hallucinations and seizures produced by stimulants and hallucinogens. Standard cardiac drugs are used to combat arrhythmias.

The most vexing problem with substance abuse is generally not the acute management of intoxication, but rather breaking the habit. This requires the patient's motivation and long-term inpatient and outpatient treatment.

 Trauma

Trivial head injuries, without loss of consciousness, are commonplace in children and are an almost constant occurrence in toddlers. Migraine should be suspected whenever transitory neurologic disturbances (e.g., amnesia, ataxia, blindness, coma, confusion, hemiplegia) follow trivial head injuries. Important causes of significant head injuries are child abuse in infants, sports and play injuries in children, and motor vehicle accidents in adolescents.

Neonatal head injuries generally cause seizures (see Chapter 1). Loss of consciousness is the major feature of head injuries beyond the neonatal period. Mild head injuries are characterized by temporary loss of consciousness without evidence of focal neurologic disturbances. Such events are usually termed *concussion*. Severe head injuries are characterized by prolonged intervals of coma associated with brain swelling and intracranial hemorrhage.

MILD AND MODERATE HEAD INJURIES

CLINICAL FEATURES. A mild closed head injury is characterized by no more than brief loss of consciousness and the absence of localizing neurologic signs *(concussion)*. The child may be stunned without definite loss of consciousness. A moderate head injury is one in which the child is obtunded for several hours but is not in coma. Once consciousness is restored, the child is invariably tired and sleeps long and soundly if left undisturbed. As a rule recovery is complete, but the child may not remember the event or the period before and after it. The length of the amnestic interval correlates with the severity of injury.

Many children complain of headache and dizziness for several days or weeks following concussion. They may be irritable and have memory disturbances. The severity and duration of these symptoms usually correlate with the severity of injury but sometimes seem disproportionate (Klonoff et al, 1993).

Focal or generalized seizures, and sometimes status epilepticus, may occur 1 or 2 hours following mild head injury. Seizures may even occur in children who did not lose consciousness. Such seizures rarely portend later epilepsy.

DIAGNOSIS. A CT scan of the head (without contrast and with windows adjusted for bone and soft tissue) should be obtained whenever loss of consciousness, no matter how brief, follows a head injury. This is probably cost-effective because it reduces the number of hospital admissions. MRI in children with moderate head injury may show foci of hypointensity in the white matter that indicate axonal injury as the mechanism of lost consciousness (Mittl et al, 1994).

EEG should be performed if there is any suspicion that the head injury occurred during a seizure or if neurologic disturbances are disproportionate to the severity of injury.

TREATMENT. Mild head injuries do not require treatment, and a child whose neurologic examination and CT scan findings are normal does not require hospitalization (Ghajar and

Hariri, 1992). If the child does not need hospitalization, asking the parents to awaken the child at regular intervals and assess neurologic status is unreasonable. Normal children are difficult to arouse from sleep, and a child who has had a head injury and spent several hours in an emergency department will sleep all the sounder. A child who does not need hospital observation does not need home observation.

SEVERE HEAD INJURIES

The outcome following severe head injuries is usually better for children than for adults, but children less than 1 year of age have double the mortality of those between 1 and 6, and three times the mortality of those between 6 and 12 (Ghajar and Hariri, 1992). CT evidence of diffuse brain swelling on the day of injury is associated with a 53% mortality rate (Aldrich et al, 1992).

Shaking Injuries

CLINICAL FEATURES. Shaking is a common method of child abuse in infants. An unconscious infant is brought to the emergency department with bulging fontanelles. Seizures may have precipitated the hospital visit. The history is fragmentary and inconsistent among informants. Typically the child has been left in the care of a babysitter or the mother's boyfriend.

The child shows no external evidence of head injury, but ophthalmoscopic examination shows retinal and optic nerve sheath hemorrhages. Retinal hemorrhages are more common after inflicted than accidental injuries and may be due to rotational forces (Duhaime et al, 1992). Many of the hemorrhages may be old, suggesting repeated shaking injuries. On the thorax or back the examiner may note bruises that conform to the shape of a hand where the child was held during the shaking. Healing fractures of the posterior rib cage indicate child abuse.

Death may result from uncontrollable increased intracranial pressure or contusion of the cervicomedullary junction (Hadley et al, 1989).

DIAGNOSIS. The CT scan shows a swollen brain but may not show subdural collections of blood if bleeding is recent. A subdural tap is both diagnostic and therapeutic.

TREATMENT. Bilateral subdural taps are needed to remove large collections of blood. The intention is to remove as much blood as possible. The amount available for drainage through a subdural tap is only a small percentage of the total volume in the subdural space. The goal of the subdural tap is not to remove all subdural blood, but rather to remove a sufficient quantity to relieve increased intracranial pressure and to aid reabsorptive mechanisms. Taps are repeated daily until the removable volume begins to decline; then an every-other-day schedule of subdural taps allows continued reduction of the accumulated fluid. A subdural-peritoneal shunt may be required if permanent effusion develops. Transfusion may be needed if the peripheral hematocrit is low and falling.

Protective service must be sought to prevent further injuries. Overall, the neurologic and visual outcome among victims of shaking is poor. Most are left with considerable handicap.

Closed Head Injuries

Supratentorial subdural hematomas are venous in origin, are frequently bilateral, and usually occur without associated skull fracture. Supratentorial epidural hematomas are usually associated with skull fracture and are described in the section on open head injuries. Epidural and subdural hematomas are almost impossible to distinguish on clinical grounds alone. Progressive loss of consciousness is a feature of both types, and both may be associated with a lucid interval between time of injury and neurologic deterioration.

Posterior fossa epidural and subdural hemorrhages occur most often in newborns (see Chapter 1) and older children with posterior skull fractures.

CLINICAL FEATURES. Loss of consciousness is not always immediate; a lucid period of several minutes may intervene between injury and onset of neurologic deterioration. The Glasgow Coma Scale is used widely to quantify the degree of responsiveness following head injuries (Table 2-7). Scores of 8 or less correlate well with severe injury.

Acute brain swelling and intracranial hemorrhage account for the clinical features. Increased intracranial pressure is always present and may lead to herniation if uncontrolled. Focal neurologic deficits suggest intracerebral hemorrhage.

Mortality rates in children with severe head injury are usually between 10% and 15% and have not changed substantially in the past decade (Kalff et al, 1989). Low mortality rates are sometimes associated with higher percentages of survivors in chronic vegetative states. Duration of coma is the best guide to long-term

TABLE 2-7
Glasgow Coma Scale*

Eye Opening (E)	
Spontaneously	4
To speech	3
To pain	2
None	1
Best Motor Response (M)	
Obeys	6
Localizes	5
Withdraws	4
Abnormal flexion	3
Abnormal extension	2
None	1
Verbal Response (V)	
Oriented	5
Confused conversation	4
Inappropriate words	3
Incomprehensible sounds	2
None	1

*Coma score = E + M + V.

morbidity. Permanent neurologic impairment is expected when coma persists for 1 month or longer.

DIAGNOSIS. Cranial CT should be performed as rapidly as possible after closed head injuries. Brain swelling and subarachnoid hemorrhage with blood collecting along the falx are typical findings. Intracranial hemorrhage may also be detected. Immediately after injury some subdural hematomas are briefly isodense and may not be observed. Later the hematoma appears as a region of increased density, convex toward the skull and concave toward the brain. With time the density decreases.

Intracerebral hemorrhage is usually superficial but may extend deep into the brain. Frontal or temporal lobe contusion is common. Discrete deep hemorrhages without a superficial extension are not usually caused by trauma.

Children with head injuries must be kept with the neck immobilized until radiographic examination for fracture-dislocation of the cervical spine is done, because the force of a blow to the skull is frequently propagated to the neck. The child must be examined for limb and organ injury when head injury occurs in a motor vehicle accident.

TREATMENT. Severe head injuries should be managed in an intensive care unit. Essential support includes controlled ventilation, prevention of hypotension, and sufficient reduction in brain swelling to maintain cerebral perfusion. Methods to reduce cerebral edema are reviewed

74

2 □ ALTERED STATES OF CONSCIOUSNESS

in Chapter 4. Barbiturate coma does not affect outcome.

Acute expanding intracranial hematomas warrant immediate surgery. Small subdural collections that do not produce a mass effect can be left in place until the patient's condition is stabilized and the options are considered.

Phenytoin is routinely administered intravenously to prevent post-traumatic epilepsy. It decreases seizure frequency during the first week but is ineffective in preventing subsequent epilepsy (Temkin et al, 1990).

Open Head Injuries

The clinical features, diagnosis, and management of open head injuries are much the same as described for closed injuries. The major differences are the greater risk of epidural hematoma and infection and the possibility of damage to the brain surface from depression of the bone.

Supratentorial epidural hematomas are usually temporal or temporoparietal in location. The origin of the blood may be arterial (tearing of the middle meningeal artery), venous, or both. Skull fracture is present in 80% of cases (Ersahin et al, 1993). Increased intracranial pressure accounts for the clinical features of vomiting and decreased states of consciousness. Epidural hematoma has a characteristic lens-shaped appearance (Figure 2–3).

Infratentorial epidural hematoma is venous in origin and associated with occipital fracture. The clinical features are headache, vomiting, and ataxia (Ciurea et al, 1993). Skull fractures, other than linear fractures, are associated with an increased risk of infection. A fracture is referred to as *depressed* if the inner table fragment is displaced by at least the thickness of the skull. Depressed fractures are termed *compound* if the scalp is lacerated and penetrating if the dura is torn. Most skull fractures heal spontaneously. Skull fractures that do not heal are usually associated with a dural tear and feel pulsatile (Johnson and Helman, 1995). In infants, serial radiographs of the skull may suggest that the fracture is enlarging because the rapid growth of the brain causes the fracture line to spread further in order to accommodate the increasing intracranial volume. The fracture line is not being held open by a leptomeningeal cyst and surgery is not needed.

Depressed fractures of the skull vault may injure the underlying brain and tear venous sinuses. The result is hemorrhage into the brain and subdural space. Treatment includes eleva-

□ FIGURE 2–3 Epidural hematoma. The hematoma appears as a lens-shaped density just below the skull.

tion of depressed fragments, debridement and closure of the scalp laceration, and systemic penicillin.

Basilar skull fractures with dural tear may result in leakage of cerebrospinal fluid from nose or ear and meningitis. Such leaks usually develop within 3 days of injury. The timing and need for dural repair are somewhat controversial, but the need for intravenous antibiotic coverage is established.

Post-traumatic Epilepsy

Post-traumatic epilepsy develops in about 50% of patients with penetrating head injuries. Half continue to have seizures as long as 15 years after injury. Two thirds have seizure onset during the first year after the injury, and 90% by 5 years, but onset is delayed by 10 to 15 years in 7%. The cause-an-effect relationship between trauma and epilepsy becomes harder to establish when the interval between the two is longer than one year. Patients with focal neurologic deficits and large cerebral lesions immediately after injury have the greatest risk for post-traumatic epilepsy. Initial seizures are generalized in 70 to 80% of cases.

Post-traumatic epilepsy is much less common with closed head injuries. The 5-year incidence is 11.5% after severe head trauma (brain contusion, intracranial hemorrhage, or 24 hours of unconsciousness or amnesia) and 1.6% after less severe head trauma (skull fracture or 30 minutes to 24 hours of unconsciousness or amnesia). Mild head injuries (less than 30 minutes of unconsciousness or amnesia) are not associated with an increased incidence of post-traumatic epilepsy.

 ## Vascular Disorders

SYSTEMIC LUPUS ERYTHEMATOSUS

Although systemic lupus erythematosus (SLE) is classified here as a "vascular" disorder, the pathophysiology of its neurologic manifestations may be secondary to immune complex deposition in the brain rather than by "vasculitis." The clinical features are consistent with a diffuse encephalopathy rather than stroke.

CLINICAL FEATURES. The symptoms of cerebral involvement in SLE ranges from mild cognitive disturbances to severe encephalopathy (West, 1994). Most common are seizures and psychosis. Some degree of cognitive dysfunction can be measured in most patients but dementia is uncommon. Depression and anxiety are relatively common and it is uncertain whether this is caused by the disease or a reaction to chronic illness. Corticosteroids, which are a mainstay of treatment, may also contribute to the anxiety. Frank psychosis as defined by impaired reality testing and hallucinations occur in less than 15% of patients.

DIAGNOSIS. The diagnosis of SLE is usually established by other criteria before the development of encephalopathy. Patients with encephalopathy usually have high serum titers of anti-DNA and lymphocytotoxic antibodies, and high cerebrospinal fluid titers of antineural antibodies. This further supports the concept that the encephalopathy is immune mediated.

TREATMENT. Some features of the encephalopathy can be treated symptomatically, but immunosuppressive therapy directed at the underlying disorder is the main therapeutic modality.

R E F E R E N C E S

Aldrich EF, Eisenberg HM, Saydjari C, et al. Diffuse brain swelling in severely head-injured children: A report from the NIH traumatic coma data bank. J Neurosurg 1992;76: 450-454.

American Academy of Neurology. Position of the American Academy of Neurology on certain aspects of the care and management of the persistent vegetative state patient. Neurology 1989;39:125-126.

American Academy of Neurology. Practice parameters for determining brain death in adults (summary statement). Neurology 1995;45:1012-1014.

Arieff AI, Ayus JC, Fraser CL. Hyponatremia and death or permanent brain damage in healthy children. Br Med J 1992;304:1218-1222.

Ashwal S, Schneider S. Brain death in the newborn. Pediatrics 1989;84:429-437.

Bacha EA, Sheridan RL, Donohue GA, et al. Staphylococcal toxic shock syndrome in a paediatric burn unit. Burn 1994;20:499-502.

Belman AL, Iyer M, Coyle PK, et al. Neurologic manifestations in children with North American Lyme disease. Neurology 1993;43:2609-2614.

Bolton CF, Young GB, Zochodne DW. The neurological complications of sepsis. Ann Neurol 1993;33:94-100.

Bonham JR, Meeks A, Levin M, et al. Complete recovery from hemorrhagic shock and encephalopathy. J Pediatr 1992:120:440-443.

Carithers HA, Margileth AM. Cat-scratch disease: Acute encephalopathy and other neurologic manifestations. Am J Dis Child 1991;145;98-101.

Centers For Disease Control. Eastern equine encephalitis— Florida, Eastern United States. MMWR 1991a;40:533-555.

Centers For Disease Control. St. Louis encephalitis outbreak—Arkansas, 1991. MMWR 1991b;40:605-607.

Ciurea AV, Nuteanu L, Simionescu N, et al. Posterior fossa extradural hematomas in children: Report of nine cases. Child Nerv Syst 1993;9:224-228.

Coates PM. New developments in the diagnosis and investigation of mitochondrial fatty acid oxidation disorders. Eur J Pediatr 1994;153(Suppl 1):S49-S56.

Collio PJ. Cat-scratch disease: Therapy with trimethoprim-sulfamethoxazole. Am J Dis Child 1992;146:397-399.

DeVivo DC, Tein I. Primary and secondary disorders of carnitine metabolism. Int Pediatr 1990;5:134.

Duhaime AC, Alario AJ, Lewander WJ, et al. Head injury to very young children: mechanisms, injury types, and ophthalmologic findings in 100 hospitalized patients younger than 2 years of age. Pediatrics 1992;90:179-185.

Ersahin Y, Mutluer S, Güzelbag E. Extradural hematoma: Analysis of 146 cases. Child Nerv Syst 1993;9:96-99.

Garcia-Monco JC, Benach JL. Lyme neuroborreliosis. Ann Neurol 1995;37:691-702.

Ghajar J, Hariri RJ. Management of pediatric head injuries. Pediatr Clin North Am 1992;39:1093-1125.

Hadley MN, Sonntag VKH, Rekate HL, et al. The infant whiplash-shake injury syndrome: A clinical and pathological study. Neurosurgery 1989;24:536-540.

Harden A, Boyd SG, Cole G, et al. EEG features and their evolution in the acute phase of haemorrhagic shock and encephalopathy syndrome. Neuropediatrics 1991;22: 194-197.

Iafolla AK, Thompson RJ Jr, Roe CP. Medium-chain acyl-coenzyme A dehydrogenase deficiency: Clinical course in 120 affected children. J Pediatr 1994;124:409-415.

Institute of Medicine. Adverse Events Associated with Childhood Vaccines. National Academy Press, Washington, DC, 1993.

Institute of Medicine. DPT Vaccine and Chronic Nervous System Dysfunction: A new analysis. National Academy Press, Washington, DC, 1994.

Jastremski M, Sutton-Tyrrell K, Vaagenes P, et al. Glucocorticoid treatment does not improve neurological recovery following cardiac arrest. JAMA 1989;262:3427-3430.

Johnson DL, Helman T. Enlarging skull fractures in children. Child Nerv Syst 1995;11:265-268.

Kalff R, Kocks W, Pospiech J, et al. Clinical outcome after head injury in children. Child Nerv Syst 1989;5: 156-159.

Kepes JJ. Large focal tumor-like demyelinating lesions of the brain: Intermediate entity between multiple sclerosis and acute disseminated encephalomyelitis? A study of 31 patients. Ann Neurol 1993;33:18-27.

Kesselring J, Miller DH, Robb SA, et al. Acute disseminated encephalomyelitis. MRI findings and the distinction from multiple sclerosis. Brain 1990;113:291-302.

Kirk JL, Fine DP, Sexron DJ, et al. Rocky Mountain spotted fever. A clinical review based on 48 confirmed cases, 1943-1986. Medicine 1990;69:35-45.

Klonoff H, Clark C, Klonnoff PS. Long-term outcome of head injuries: A 23 year follow up study of children with head injuries. J Neurol Neurosurg Psychiatry 1993;56:410-415.

Kriel RL, Krach LE, Jones-Saete C. Outcome of children with prolonged unconsciousness and vegetative states. Pediatr Neurol 1993;9:362-368.

Kriel RL, Krach LE, Luxemberg MG, et al. Outcome of severe anoxic/ischemic brain injury in children. Pediatr Neurol 1994;10:207-212.

Mittl RL, Grossman RI, Hiehle JF, et al. Prevalence of MR evidence of diffuse axonal injury in patients with mild head injury and normal head CT findings. Am J Neurol Radiol 1994;15:1583-1589.

Mott SH, Packer RJ, Vezina LG, et al. Encephalopathy with Parkinsonian features in children following bone marrow transplantations and high-dose amphotericin B. Ann Neurol 1995;37:810-814.

Patchell RA. Neurological complications of organ transplant. Ann Neurol 1994;36:688-703.

Rorabaugh ML, Berlin LE, Heldrich F, et al. Aseptic meningitis in infants younger than 2 years of age: Acute illness and neurologic complications. Pediatrics 1993;92:206-211.

Shaw PJ, Walls TJ, Newman MB, et al. Hashimoto's encephalopathy: A steroid-responsive disorder associated with high anti-thyroid antibody titers-report of 5 cases. Neurology 1991;41:228-233.

Sheth RD, Riggs JE, Bodensteiner JB. Acute confusional migraine: A variant of transient global amnesia. Pediatr Neurol 1995;12:129-131.

Tein I, De Vivo DC, Hale DE, et al. Short-chain L-3-hydroxyacyl-CoA dehydrogenase deficiency in muscle: A new cause for recurrent myoglobinuria and encephalopathy. Ann Neurol 1991;30:415-419.

Temkin NR, Dikmen SS, Wilensky AJ, et al. A randomized double-blind study of phenytoin for the prevention of post-traumatic seizures. N Engl J Med 1990;323:497-502.

West SG. Neuropsychiatric lupus. Rheum Dis Clin North Am 1994;20:129-151.

Zangwill KM, Hamilton DH, Perkins BA, et al. Cat scratch disease in Connecticut: Epidemiology, risk factors, and evaluation of a new diagnostic test. N Engl J Med 1993;329:8-13.

3 Headache

Approach to Headache

Ten percent of children ages 5 to 15 years have migraine and 1% have chronic tension headaches (Abu-Arefeh and Russell, 1994). Children with migraine average twice as many days lost from school as those without migraine. Among American adolescents, 12% miss a day of school each month because of headache, and 13% of males and 20% of females have consulted a physician because of headache.

Parents seek medical attention for a child with headache not so much looking for relief of pain as seeking assurance that the headache is not a sign of intracranial disease such as a brain tumor. If this is the understood purpose for consultation, identifying the cause of headache may not be necessary in all cases. The paramount goal is to provide assurance that headache is not a sign of serious illness. In some circumstances, this assurance is the only possible achievement. Not every headache can be explained, and the term *psychogenic* should not be used as a synonym for idiopathic. It is usually possible, often by history and physical examination alone but sometimes with the aid of diagnostic studies, to distinguish headaches that are only painful from those that are harmful. This distinction is usually made by identifying the structure or structures that are generating pain and is almost always ensured by imaging the brain.

SOURCES OF PAIN

Pain-sensitive structures of the head and neck are summarized in Table 3–1. The major pain-sensitive structures inside the skull are blood vessels. Mechanisms that stimulate pain from blood vessels are vasodilation, inflammation, and traction-displacement. Increased intracranial pressure causes pain mainly by the traction and displacement of intracranial arteries (see Chapter 4). The brain parenchyma, its ependymal lining, and the meninges are insensitive to pain.

The innervation of pain from supratentorial intracranial vessels is transmitted by the trigeminal nerve, whereas pain from infratentorial intracranial vessels is transmitted by the first three cervical nerves. Arteries in the superficial portion of the dura are innervated by the ophthalmic division of the trigeminal nerve and refer pain to the eye and forehead. The middle meningeal artery is innervated by the second and third divisions of the trigeminal nerve and refers pain to the temple. Cerebral arteries are innervated by all three divisions of the trigeminal nerve and refer pain to the eye, forehead, and temple. In contrast, pain from all structures in the posterior fossa is referred to the occiput and neck.

Several extracranial structures are pain sensitive. Major scalp arteries are present around the eye, forehead, and temple and produce pain when dilated or stretched. Cranial bones are insensitive, but periosteum, especially in the sinuses and near the teeth, is painful when inflamed. The inflamed periosteum is usually tender to palpation or to other forms of physical stimulation. Muscles attached to the skull are a possible source of pain. The largest groups of such muscles are the neck extensors, which attach to the occipital ridge, the masseter

■ TABLE 3-1
Sources of Headache Pain

Intracranial
Cerebral and dural arteries
Large veins and venous sinuses
Extracranial
Cervical roots
Cranial nerves
Extracranial arteries
Muscles attached to skull
Periosteum/sinuses

---

muscles, and the frontalis muscle. The mechanism of muscle pain is not fully understood but probably involves prolonged contraction. The extraocular muscles are a source of muscle contraction pain in patients with heterophoria. When an imbalance exists, especially in convergence, long periods of close work cause difficulty in maintaining conjugate gaze and pain is felt in the orbit.

Pain from the cervical roots and cranial nerves is generally due to mechanical traction from injury or malformation. Pain follows this nerve distribution: the neck and back of the head up to the vertex for the cervical roots, and the face for the cranial nerves.

DESCRIPTIONS OF PAIN

History is everything when attempting to diagnose the cause of headache. Most children, especially very young ones, are incapable of describing pain. A child asked to describe the quality of pain usually responds with sullen silence. This is rarely important information, even in older children. "Throbbing" and "splitting" are more often used to describe intensity than character.

Asking a child younger than 10 years of age how often headaches occur or how long they last is rarely productive. Young children have no sense of time (Are we almost there?), but parents are usually quite helpful in this regard. The exception is the parent who replies, either through conviction or to impress the physician with the severity of the situation, that the child who is sitting comfortably in the examining room has had a headache every day for the past 6 months or 1 year. Four questions should be asked in response:

1. "How many days of school have been missed?" The answer tells a great deal about frequency, severity, and disability.

2. "What is the longest period of time that you have been headache free?" This identifies a common headache pattern in which the child has a flurry of headaches over a period of a week or two, then after a prolonged headache-free interval experiences another flurry of daily headaches.

3. "How many different kinds of headache do you have?" A common response is that the child has two kinds of headache: one headache is severe and causes the child to look sick (migraine), and the other is a mild headache that is almost constant but is not disabling (analgesic rebound headache).

4. "What analgesics have you used, and how often?" This helps establish what does and does not work and may also establish the diagnosis of analgesic rebound headache as a contributing factor.

Helpful responses to traditional questions concerning the history of headache can be obtained from children aged 10 years or older. Several typical headache patterns, when present, allow recognition of either the source or the mechanism of pain. Temporal pain is usually vascular in origin. Steady, tight pain, especially in the occipital region or in a band around the head, is likely to be muscular in origin. Periosteal pain, especially inflammation of the sinuses, is localized and tender to palpation. Cervical root and cranial nerve pain has a radiating or shooting quality. Confusion arises when several mechanisms of pain are experienced concurrently. Individuals with migraine often have other headaches as well.

Sinusitis is overdiagnosed as a cause of headache. Computed tomography (CT) evidence of sinusitis is commonplace in children being evaluated for other reasons. In my experience, "sinusitis" is the most frequent radiographic finding in children evaluated for dementia. The physician should no sooner conclude that CT evidence of sinusitis is causally related to headache than that it is related to dementia.

A continuous, low-intensity, chronic headache, in the absence of associated symptoms or signs, is not likely to indicate a serious intracranial disease. The most common cause is analgesic rebound headache. Intermittent headaches, especially those that make the child look and feel sick, from which the child recovers completely and is normal between attacks, are likely to be migraine. A severe headache of recent onset, unlike anything previously experienced, from which the child never returns to a normal baseline is probably due to significant intracranial disease.

Most bilateral or generalized headaches are not caused by serious intracranial disease. Unilateral headache suggests migraine or intracranial mass lesions that are displacing local vessels without producing generalized increased intracranial pressure. Time of onset may indicate a stressful period for a child, such as attending school or visitation by a separated parent.

EVALUATION

Children referred to a pediatric neurologist for headache commonly arrive with a cranial CT scan or at least a report of a normal study. The only question asked by the primary physician was, "Does this child have a brain tumor?" Unfortunately, the normal CT scan neither explained nor cured the headache. A routine brain imaging study on every child with chronic headache is not a substitute for an adequate history and physical examination. As a rule, neuroimaging is not indicated in people with headache who have a normal neurologic examination, especially when the headache is of the migraine type (Frishberg, 1994; Nevo et al, 1994).

 ## Migraine

Migraine accounts for 75% of headaches in young children referred for neurologic consultation (Chu and Shinnar, 1992). It is a hereditary disorder transmitted by autosomal dominant inheritance. A history of migraine in at least one parent is reported in 90% of cases if both parents are interviewed and in 80% if only one parent is interviewed. The prevalence of migraine is 2.5% under the age of 7 (both sexes equally affected), 5% from age 7 to puberty (female-to-male ratio of 3:2), 5% in postpubertal boys, and 10% in postpubertal girls. The prevalence in preschool children is probably higher than the recorded figure, because migraine symptoms in preschool children tend to be atypical and may not be identified as migraine at the time. The higher incidence of migraine in pubertal girls than in boys is probably related to the triggering effect of the menstrual cycle on migraine attacks.

TRIGGERING FACTORS

Among persons with a predisposition to migraine, individual attacks are usually provoked by an idiosyncratic triggering factor. Common triggering factors are stress, exercise, head trauma, and the premenstrual decline in circulating estrogen. An allergic basis for migraine has been considered but never established.

Stress and Exercise

Migraine symptoms may first occur during stress or exercise or, more often, during a time of relaxation following a period of stress. When stress is the triggering factor, attacks are most likely to occur during school or just after returning home. Attacks rarely occur upon awakening. Children with migraine do not have a specific personality type. Migraine is just as likely in a "slug" as in an overachiever.

Head Trauma

The mechanism by which blows to the head and whiplash head movements provoke migraine attacks is unknown. Trivial blows to the head during competitive sports are significant triggering factors because they occur against a background of vigorous exercise and stress. A severe migraine attack—headache, vomiting, and transitory neurologic deficits—following a head injury suggests the possibility of intracranial hemorrhage. The number of diagnostic tests can be reduced if the cause-and-effect relationship between head trauma and migraine is appreciated and the diagnosis of migraine established.

Transitory cerebral blindness, as well as other transitory neurologic deficits, sometimes occurs after head trauma in children with migraine (see Chapter 16).

Menstrual Cycle

The higher rate of migraine among postpubertal girls as compared either with prepubertal children of both sexes or with postpubertal boys supports the observation that hormonal changes in the normal female cycle trigger attacks of migraine. The widespread use of oral contraceptives has provided some insight into the relationship between the female hormonal cycle and migraine. Oral contraceptives increase the frequency and intensity of migraine attacks in many women with a history of migraine and may precipitate the initial attack in genetically predisposed women who have previously been migraine free. Among women taking oral contraceptives, the greatest increase in frequency of migraine occurs at midcycle. The decline in concentration of circulating estrogens is probably the critical factor in precipitating an attack (Silberstein and Merriam, 1991).

CLINICAL SYNDROMES

Migraine in children can be divided into three groups: migraine with aura (classic migraine), migraine without aura (common migraine), and migraine equivalent syndromes. Migraine without aura is more than twice as common as migraine with aura in school-age children. Migraine with and without aura are probably variable expressions of the same genetic defect; different members of a family may or may not have an aura with attacks. The main feature of migraine equivalent syndromes is a transitory disturbance in neurologic function. Headache is a minor feature or not present. These syndromes are discussed in several other chapters (Table 3-2).

Migraine With Aura

Migraine with aura is a biphasic event. In the initial phase, a wave of excitation followed by depression of cortical function spreads over both hemispheres from back to front. This is associated with decreased regional cerebral blood flow and transitory neurologic disturbances. These disturbances are caused primarily by neuronal depression rather than ischemia. The second phase is usually associated with increased blood flow in both the internal and external carotid circulation. Headache, nausea, and sometimes vomiting occur in the second phase. The mechanism of headache and nausea remains uncertain but is not explained by increased cerebral blood flow.

During an attack the main clinical features may be related only to the first phase (aura), only to the second phase, or to both. The usual features of the aura are visual aberrations: the perception of sparkling lights or colored lines, blind spots,

■ TABLE 3–2
Migraine Equivalents

Acute confusional migraine (see Chapter 2)
Basilar migraine (see Chapter 10)
Benign paroxysmal vertigo (see Chapter 10)
Cyclic vomiting
Hemiplegic migraine (see Chapter 11)
Ophthalmoplegic migraine (see Chapter 15)
Paroxysmal torticollis (see Chapter 14)
Transient global amnesia (see Chapter 2)

blurred vision, hemianopia, transitory blindness, micropsia, and visual hallucinations. Visual symptoms are identified in about a third of children when specific questions are asked. They tend to be stereotyped for each child and may be perceived in one eye, in one field, or without localization.

Visual hallucinations and other visual distortions may be associated with impairment of time sense and body image. This symptom complex in migraine is called the *Alice-in-Wonderland syndrome.* More extreme disturbances in mental state—amnesia, confusion, and psychosis—are discussed in the sections on confusional migraine and transient global amnesia (see Chapter 2).

Dysesthesias of the limbs and perioral region are the next most common sensory features. Other possible features of the aura are focal motor deficits, usually hemiplegia or ophthalmoplegia, and aphasia. Such deficits, although alarming, are transitory; normal function usually returns within 24 hours and always within 72 hours.

A migraine attack may terminate at the end of the initial phase without headache. Alternatively, the initial phase may be brief or asymptomatic and headache the major symptom. The pain is usually dull at first and then becomes throbbing, pulsating, or pounding. Severe headache that is maximal at onset is not migraine! Pain is unilateral in approximately two thirds of patients and bilateral in the rest. It is most intense in the region of the eye, forehead, and temple. Eventually the pain becomes constant and diffuse. Most headaches lasts 2 to 6 hours, and are associated with nausea and sometimes vomiting. Anorexia and photophobia are concomitant symptoms. The child looks sick and wants to lie down; I always ask the parent, "Does the child look sick?" With migraine, the answer is always "yes." Vomiting frequently heralds the end of the attack and the fatigued child falls into a deep sleep. Normal function resumes when the child awakens.

Most children average one attack per month but may have long intervals without attacks and other intervals when attacks occur weekly. The intervals with frequent headaches are probably times of stress.

Migraine Without Aura

The attacks of migraine without aura are monophasic. Headache and vomiting are the only features and attacks are less readily identified as migrainous. The typical initial symptoms are personality change, malaise, and nausea. Recurrent vomiting may be the only feature of the attack in preschool children.

The headache may be unilateral and pounding but more often the child has difficulty in localizing the pain and describing its quality. When the headache is prolonged, the pain is not of uniform intensity; instead, intermittent severe headaches are superimposed on a background of chronic discomfort in the neck and other pericranial muscles. The pain is aggravated by physical activity (Dalessio, 1994). Migraine without an aura may be difficult to separate from other headache syndromes or from intercurrent illness. The important clue is that the child appears sick, wants to lie down, and is sensitive to light and sound. Nausea and vomiting may occur repeatedly, need not herald the termination of the attack, and can be more prominent than the headache.

DIAGNOSIS

The diagnosis of migraine is based on the clinical features; migraine is one of the few remaining neurologic disorders in which the physician cannot stumble on the diagnosis by imaging the brain. Salient features are a family history of migraine and some combination of recurrent headache, nausea, or neurologic disturbances, especially if the symptoms are relieved by sleep. The physician should be reluctant to make the diagnosis if questioning of both parents does not elicit a family history of migraine. A history of motion sickness is obtained in almost half of children with migraine. The significance of this association is uncertain; the incidence of motion sickness in the general population approaches 100% depending on the amount of motion.

Diagnostic tests are unnecessary when the diagnosis of migraine can be clearly established on the basis of the family history and clinical features. Brain imaging is only indicated when there is uncertainty.

The most common electroencephalographic (EEG) abnormality during a classic migraine attack is a slow-wave focus in the temporal lobe of one hemisphere. An increased incidence of asymptomatic central spikes and 14-and-6 positive spikes is reported but both are of uncertain significance. The only reason to obtain an EEG in children with migraine-like headaches is to exclude the possibility of benign occipital epilepsy (see Chapter 1).

TREATMENT

The essential caveat for the treatment of migraine is that irrespective of treatment, about half of children have more than a 50% reduction in headache frequency in the 6 months following the initial visit to a neurologist. This is consistent with the experience of most blind controlled trials of drug therapy, in which the placebo success rate is usually 50%. Once the child's parents are convinced that headache is due to migraine and not a brain tumor, they are less anxious, the child is more relaxed, and headaches either decrease in frequency or are discussed less often. The therapeutic efficacy of neurologic consultation has the dual effect of making drug evaluation difficult and at the same time reinforcing the neurologist's belief that the drug regimen selected is useful.

The two approaches to migraine therapy are treatment of the acute attack and prophylaxis. Whichever approach is selected, the patient and family must be told that the migraine will not go away and that they will need to learn "how to live with migraine." After all, migraine is not a temporary condition, it is often life long.

1. Instruct the patient and parents to avoid, when possible, activities that are known to trigger attacks.

2. When an attack occurs, it must be managed by one technique or another; life can not go on as before.

3. Do not use narcotics or other addictive drugs to treat severe attacks.

4. Sleep ends the attack. Any medication that puts the child to sleep will end the attack.

Treating the Acute Attack

Over-the-counter analgesics and nonsteroidal anti-inflammatory drugs such as naproxen may relieve headache pain but not other symptoms of migraine (Welch, 1993). Ergotamine is the drug most often prescribed for the acute treatment of migraine. The response is variable and this drug should never be used for the purpose of diagnosis. Oral ergotamine is not more effective than placebo in double-blind controlled studies.

The best treatment for migraine is to have the child go to sleep. I generally prescribe oral promethazine, 25 mg (generally 1 mg/kg). It relieves nausea and causes drowsiness. Intramuscular chlorpromazine, 1 mg/kg, is a safe and effective alternative for severe attacks.

Sumatriptan, a selective agonist of 5-hydroxytryptamine-like receptors, is an effective but expensive treatment for acute attacks. A subcutaneous injection of 6 mg decreases the severity of the attack within 60 minutes in 72% of adults. Adverse effects include tiredness, tingling of the head and arms, and a sensation of pressure or stiffness in the neck, throat, and chest (Dahlöf et al, 1994). The 6-mg dose has been used successfully and safely in most school-age children (MacDonald, 1994). A half-dose (3 mg) is recommended for children of smaller size. An oral compound (sumatriptan succinate) is now available that will probably replace the injectable form, especially for children. The dosing schedule is not established, but 25 mg of the oral preparation may be equivalent to 6 mg of the injectable form.

Migraine Prophylaxis

An extraordinary number of agents with diverse pharmacologic properties have been administered daily to prevent migraine attacks (Baumel, 1994). I only suggest prophylactic agents for children who miss school more than once each month. The most commonly used are propranolol, calcium channel blocking agents, cyproheptadine, and amitriptyline. Cyproheptadine is commonly used by pediatricians but has never been proven more effective than placebo in controlled clinical trials. Propranolol is the only agent that has consistently shown greater efficacy than placebo in controlled clinical trials and should be considered the drug of choice in migraine prophylaxis. Calcium channel blocking agents are widely used but have not been studied rigorously in large controlled trials, and valproate, a relatively toxic drug in children, was shown more effective than placebo in migraine prophylaxis in one study (Mathew et al, 1995).

Propranolol

Propranolol is a beta-adrenergic blocking agent that was serendipitously found useful in preventing migraine attacks in patients being treated for cardiovascular disease. It decreases headache frequency by at least half in 80% of patients. The mechanism of action is probably central and not beta-adrenergic blockade. Propranolol must have central action because it causes depression. Other beta-adrenergic blocking agents have not been studied in migraine and should not be used.

The dosage in children is 2 mg/kg in three divided doses. Because depression is a dose-related adverse reaction and because lower doses may be effective, treatment should be started at 1 mg/kg/day. Depression is the most common reason to discontinue therapy, and parents should be warned of this reaction when the drug is started. The drug should not be used in children with asthma because it may provoke an attack. Hypotension and pulse rate reduction do not occur in children with normal cardiovascular systems. Once a maintenance dose is established, the sustained-release tablet can be used by increasing the daily dose by one third. Plasma levels of propranolol are not useful in determining the effective dose for migraine.

Patients who respond to propranolol do not develop tolerance. However, if the drug is abruptly stopped after 6 to 12 months of therapy, some patients will have rebound headaches of increased frequency. Others will continue to show the benefits achieved during therapy.

Calcium Channel Blocking Agents

Calcium channel blocking agents are vasodilators that prevent the influx of calcium into vascular smooth muscle. They have been used extensively for coronary artery disease and are effective dilators of the cerebral vasculature. Specific agents that have been tested in migraine are listed in Table 3–3. Flunarizine is considered the most promising agent for migraine prophylaxis, but an oral form is not available in the United States. Nifedipine is of questionable value and may cause headache. Nimodipine, flunarizine, and verapamil have not been tested in children with migraine, and the dosages provided in Table 3–3 are for adults. Calcium channel blocking agents as a group have little or no toxicity in children with normal cardiovascular systems.

In general, the efficacy of this class of drugs remains uncertain. Clinical trials have involved small numbers of patients and the results have not always been consistent. They may decrease the frequency of attacks but not their severity (Welch, 1993).

■ TABLE 3–3
Calcium Channel Blocking Agents

DRUG	DOSAGE
Cyproheptadine	0.2–0.4 mg/kg
Flunarizine	5 mg bid
Nifedipine	1 mg/kg
Nimodipine	40 mg tid
Verapamil	40–80 mg tid

➡ Headaches That Cluster

The three syndromes of paroxysmal hemicrania are cluster headache, chronic paroxysmal hemicrania, and hemicrania continua. All three are uncommon in children. Another syndrome, called *episodic paroxysmal hemicrania,* is so similar to chronic paroxysmal hemicrania that I (along with most neurologists) cannot tell them apart, and have lumped them together. Chronic paroxysmal hemicrania must be distinguished from cluster headache because the treatments are different.

CLUSTER HEADACHE

Cluster headache occurs mainly in boys and rarely affects other family members (Russell et al, 1995).

CLINICAL FEATURES. The onset is almost exclusively after age 10. Clusters of headaches recur over periods of weeks or months separated by intervals of 1 to 2 years. A cluster of daily attacks lasting 4 to 8 weeks may occur once or twice a year, often in the autumn or spring. Headaches do not occur in the interim.

Headache is the initial feature, often beginning during sleep. The pain occurs in bursts lasting 30 to 90 minutes, that repeats two to six times each day (Dalessio, 1994). It is always unilateral and affects the same side of the head in each attack. It begins behind and around one eye, then spreads to the entire hemicranium. During an attack the affected individual cannot lie still but typically walks the floor in anguish; this feature is important in distinguishing cluster headache from migraine, in which the child wants to go to bed. Pain is intense and may be described as throbbing or constant. The scalp may seem edematous and tender. One third of individuals with cluster headache experience sudden intense jabs of pain suggesting tic douloureux. Nausea and vomiting do not occur, but symptoms of hemicranial autonomic dysfunction—injection of the conjunctiva, tearing of the eye, Horner syndrome, sweating, flushing of the face, and stuffiness of the nose—develop ipsilateral to the headache.

DIAGNOSIS. The diagnosis of cluster headache is established on the clinical features alone and is not aided by laboratory studies.

TREATMENT. The management of cluster headache is to suppress recurrences of a bout in progress and to relieve acute pain. Suppression of bouts can be done with methysergide or corticosteroids. Methysergide maleate, a serotonin agonist, was once popular as a prophylactic agent for migraine and for cluster headache. Unfortunately, retroperitoneal fibrosis, as well as other fibrotic syndromes, occurs in patients taking the medication regularly for periods greater than 1 year. Methysergide maleate can be used safely for periods of less than 6 months and is useful for short-term therapy in 70% of patients with cluster. The dosage in adults is 2 mg three times a day after meals to avoid gastric upset. A dosage in milligrams per kilogram has not been established for children.

Prednisone suppresses bouts of cluster headache in three fourths of patients who are unresponsive to methysergide. An initial dose of 1 mg/kg is administered for the first 5 days and then tapered over the following 2 weeks. If headaches reappear during the tapering process, the dose is increased and maintained at a level sufficient to keep the patient headache free. If the bout of cluster headache is prolonged, the prednisone dosage should be tapered before the appearance of adverse side effects.

The acute attacks can be treated with sumatriptan (Sumatriptan Cluster Headache Study Group, 1991), by oxygen inhalation, or a combination of the two. Sumatriptan is given as a 6-mg injection in adults; the dosage in children is not established. Inhalation of 100% oxygen at a rate of 8 to 10 L/min relieves an acute attack in most patients. Lithium is useful for patients with a chronic form of cluster headache in which headache never ceases. Increasing doses are used to achieve a blood concentration of 1.2 mEq/L (1.2 mmol/L). Most patients have at least a partial response to lithium, but only 50% are relieved completely. The beneficial effect of lithium is enhanced by the addition of daily oral ergotamine.

CHRONIC PAROXYSMAL HEMICRANIA

CLINICAL FEATURES. Like cluster headache, the main features of chronic paroxysmal hemicrania are unilateral, throbbing pain associated with ipsilateral autonomic features. However, the painful attack is briefer in duration but more frequent than in cluster headaches (Newman et al, 1992). Attacks last for weeks to months and are separated by remissions that last months to years. The pain is located in the frontal and retro-orbital region and is accompanied by conjunctival injection and tearing.

DIAGNOSIS. The diagnosis is based on the clinical features and is not aided by laboratory studies.

TREATMENT. Chronic paroxysmal hemicrania responds to indomethacin. The typical adult dosage is 75 mg/day. Larger dosages may be needed in successive attacks. Acetazolamide may prove successful when indomethacin fails (Warner et al, 1994).

HEMICRANIA CONTINUA

CLINICAL FEATURES. Hemicrania continua is a continuous unilateral headache of moderate severity (Newman et al, 1994). Autonomic symptoms may be associated but are not prominent. Some patients have continuous headaches lasting from weeks to months separated by pain-free intervals; others never experience remissions. The episodic form may later become continuous.

DIAGNOSIS. The diagnosis is established by the clinical features. Other causes of chronic headache, such as increased intracranial pressure and chronic use of analgesics must be excluded.

TREATMENT. The headaches usually respond to indomethacin at dosages of 25 to 250 mg/day.

 Tension Headaches

The term *tension headache* is time honored and suggests that the headache is caused by stress. This is usually true with regard to episodic tension headaches, but the mechanism of chronic tension headache is less well established and is probably multifactorial.

EPISODIC TENSION HEADACHE

CLINICAL FEATURES. Episodic tension headache is common in people of all ages and both sexes. It is generally brought on by fatigue, exertion, and temporary life stress. The mechanism is probably prolonged contraction of muscles attached to the skull. The pain is described as constant, aching, and tight. It is localized mainly to the back of the head and neck, sometimes become diffuse, and may be described as a constricting band around the head. Nausea, vomiting, photophobia, and phonophobia are not present.

Headaches usually last from 30 minutes to all day. One episode may last for several days with some waxing and waning, but not for a week.

DIAGNOSIS. Episodic tension headache should be differentiated from chronic tension, which has similar clinical features but persists for weeks, months, and years. Most episodic tension headaches are self-diagnosed, and the individual rarely seeks medical attention.

TREATMENT. Pain is relieved by rest or relaxation and also responds to aspirin or acetaminophen.

CHRONIC TENSION HEADACHE

It is not always clear that a child with chronic tension headache is experiencing stress. When a stressful situation is identified (e.g., divorce of the parents, unsuitable school placement, physical or sexual abuse) the headache cannot be managed without resolution of the stress. A family history of chronic tension headache is often obtained, and about half of adults with chronic tension headache date the onset to childhood.

CLINICAL FEATURES. People with chronic headache of any cause may be depressed and anxious. Pain is almost always bilateral and diffuse, and the site of most intense pain may shift during the course of the day. Much of the time, headache is dull and aching; sometimes it is more intense. Headache is generally present upon awakening and may continue all day but is not aggravated by routine physical activity. Most children describe an undulating course characterized by long periods in which headache occurs almost every day and shorter intervals when they are headache free.

Nausea, vomiting, photophobia, phonophobia, and transitory neurologic disturbances are not associated. When these features are present, they usually occur only a few times a month and suggest intermittent migraine against a background of chronic tension headache. Neurologic examination is normal.

DIAGNOSIS. The diagnosis of chronic tension headache is to some extent a diagnosis of exclusion. Common causes of chronic headache in children that must be distinguished are migraine and analgesic withdrawal. Both may coexist with chronic tension headache. Increased intracranial pressure must also be considered and excluded by brain imaging in appropriate cases. The management of chronic tension headache is often easier when the specter of brain tumor has been laid to rest. EEG is indicated when the intermittent nature of the headache or associated features suggest the possibility of epilepsy.

TREATMENT. Chronic tension headache is by definition difficult to treat or it would not be a chronic headache. Most children have tried and received no benefit from several over-the-counter analgesics before coming to a physician, and analgesic rebound headache is often complicating management. The use of more powerful analgesics or analgesic-muscle relaxant combinations has limited value and generally adds upset stomach to the child's distress.

Amitriptyline is probably the most useful drug for chronic tension headache. It has analgesic properties beyond its effect as an antidepressant. I always start with a small dose (approximately 10 to 25 mg) at bedtime and rarely need to increase the dose.

Many children with chronic tension headache benefit from relaxation exercises or biofeedback. I routinely refer children for such therapy when the response to amitriptyline is unsatisfactory.

➡ Headaches Associated with Drugs and Foods

Many psychotropic drugs, analgesics, and cardiovascular agents have vasodilating properties. Cocaine use produces a migraine-like headache in individuals who do not have migraine at other times (Dhuna et al, 1991). Drug-induced headache should be suspected in a child who has headache following the administration of any drug.

Many other drugs and substances cause vasoconstriction. Withdrawal after acute excessive use or chronic use causes rebound vasodilation and headache.

ANALGESIC REBOUND HEADACHE

CLINICAL FEATURES. *Analgesic rebound* is one of the more common causes of chronic headache in people of all ages (Cantwell-Simmons et al, 1993). Individuals with migraine are especially predisposed to analgesic rebound headaches *(extended migraine)*. The term refers to the vicious cycle of headache–analgesic use–headache when the analgesic effect wears off–more analgesic use. The pain is generalized, of low intensity, and dull. It interferes with, but

does not prevent, routine activities, and is not aggravated by activity.

DIAGNOSIS. Any child who is taking analgesics every day, or even most days, should be assumed to have analgesic rebound headache.

TREATMENT. All analgesic use must be stopped; caffeine should be avoided as well. Bedtime amitriptyline often helps the transition to the analgesic-free state. The first few days may be difficult, but a positive effect is noted within days and reinforces the recommended management.

CAFFEINE WITHDRAWAL

CLINICAL FEATURES. Many children, especially adolescents, drink large volumes of carbonated beverages containing caffeine each day. The amount of caffeine in some beverages is sufficient to require a prescription were it to be used therapeutically. Caffeine has vasoconstricting properties and does not in itself cause headache. However, rebound vasodilation occurs when blood caffeine concentrations fall. Individuals who regularly drink large amounts of caffeine-containing beverages often notice a dull frontotemporal headache an hour or more after last use. More caffeine is taken to relieve the headache, and caffeine addiction is initiated. Withdrawal symptoms eventually become severe and include throbbing headache, anxiety, and malaise.

DIAGNOSIS. Most people associate caffeine with coffee and are unaware of the caffeine content of soft drinks. Adolescent girls frequently use diet colas as a substitute for food and become caffeine dependent.

TREATMENT. Caffeine addiction, like other addictions, is often hard to break. Some patients can be weaned from caffeine, but most require abrupt cessation and experience withdrawal symptoms. Hospitalization and sedation are sometimes necessary to help patients through withdrawal.

FOOD ADDITIVES

CLINICAL FEATURES. Chemicals are added to food as preservatives and to enhance its appearance. Ordinarily the concentration is low and adverse effects occur only in individuals who are genetically sensitive. Nitrites are powerful vasodilators used to enhance the appearance of cured meats such as hot dogs, salami, bacon, and ham. Diffuse, throbbing headaches may occur just after ingestion.

Monosodium glutamate (MSG) is used primarily in Chinese cooking and may cause generalized vasodilation. Sensitive individuals develop a throbbing bitemporal headache and a band headache, sometimes associated with pressure and tightness of the face and a burning sensation over the body. Symptoms occur 20 minutes after MSG ingestion.

DIAGNOSIS. The association between ingestion of a specific food and headache is quickly evident to the patient.

TREATMENT. Headache can be prevented only by avoidance of the offending chemical. This is not easy; prepared foods often do not list all additives.

MARIJUANA

Marijuana is a peripheral vasodilator and causes a sensation of warmth, injection of the conjunctivae, and sometimes frontal headache. The headache is mild and ordinarily experienced only during marijuana use. However, marijuana metabolites remain in the blood for several days, and chronic headaches occur in children who are regular users.

 ## Vasculitis

Headaches caused by vasculitis, especially temporal arteritis, are important in the differential diagnosis of vascular headaches in adults. Cerebral vasculitis is uncommon in children and usually occurs as part of a collagen vascular disease, as a result of hypersensitivity, or as part of an infection of the nervous system.

CONNECTIVE TISSUE DISORDERS

Headache is a relatively common feature of systemic lupus erythematosus and mixed connective tissue disease. In patients with connective tissue disease, it is not clear that neurologic symptoms, including headache, are caused by vasculitis of the cerebral arteries.

CLINICAL FEATURES. Headache is not an early symptom of lupus in children. The usual initial features are fever, arthritis, and skin rash. Symptoms referable to the nervous system—seizures and mental changes—are an initial feature in less than 5% of affected children. Hepatosplenomegaly and lymphadenopathy oc-

cur in 70% of children, twice the rate in adults.

Mixed connective disease is a syndrome with features of lupus erythematosus, scleroderma, and polymyositis. Its course is usually less severe than that of lupus. Thirty-five percent of patients with mixed connective disease report vascular headaches. The headaches are moderate and generally do not interfere with activities of daily living. Headaches may be unilateral or bilateral, but are generally throbbing. More than half of patients report a visual aura, and some have nausea and vomiting. Some of these children may be experiencing migraine aggravated by the underlying vasculitis; in others, the headache may be caused by the vasculitis itself.

DIAGNOSIS. The diagnosis of connective tissue disease depends on the combination of a compatible clinical syndrome and the demonstration of antinuclear antibodies in the blood. The presence of antinuclear antibodies in a child with headache who has no systemic symptoms of connective tissue disease should suggest the possibility of a hypersensitivity reaction.

TREATMENT. Children with connective tissue disease are ordinarily treated with corticosteroids. In many cases headaches develop while the child is already taking corticosteroids, and this is not an indication to increase the dose. Headache is not a disabling symptom, it does not indicate a generalized encephalopathy, and it should be treated with analgesics.

HYPERSENSITIVITY VASCULITIS

The important causes of hypersensitivity vasculitis in children are serum sickness, Henoch-Schonlein purpura (see Chapter 11), amphetamine abuse, and cocaine abuse. Children with serum sickness or Henoch-Schonlein purpura have systemic symptoms that precede the headache. Persistent headache and behavioral changes are often the only neurologic consequences of Henoch-Schonlein purpura (Ostergaard and Storm, 1991). In contrast, substance abuse can cause a cerebral vasculitis in the absence of systemic symptoms. The features are headache, encephalopathy, focal neurologic deficits, and subarachnoid hemorrhage.

 ## Other Causes of Headache
BENIGN EXERTIONAL HEADACHE

Exertion, especially during competitive sports, is a known trigger for migraine in predisposed individuals (see Migraine, earlier in this chapter). Aerobic (effort) and anerobic (exertion) exercises may cause headache in people who do not have migraine. Others, who do not have migraine, may also experience headaches during exercise (Williams and Nukada, 1994). Headache during sexual intercourse is probably a form of exertional headache, and affected individuals often experience the same headache during exercise (Silbert et al, 1991).

CLINICAL FEATURES. Effort headaches tend to be acute and severe, starting early in the course of exercise, while exertion headaches tend to start later and last longer. Both may be throbbing and bitemporal. Headache may occur during prolonged sexual arousal as well as during sexual intercourse.

More than one kind of headache is associated with sexual intercourse (Lance, 1993). A dull headache, primarily occipital but also in a band distribution, may be experienced as sexual excitement increases. This is probably caused by excessive contraction of head and neck muscles. It is not incapacitating and does not disrupt sexual activity. A more severe and dangerous headache is one that occurs just before and at the moment of orgasm. This headache, caused by sudden increase in blood pressure, is similar to the headache associated with pheochromocytoma. Blood pressure elevation during orgasm is considerable and can be associated with subarachnoid hemorrhage in adolescents with arteriovenous malformations.

DIAGNOSIS. The association between exertion and headache is easily recognized. Medical consultation is seldom requested unless the patient is a competitive athlete whose performance is impaired.

TREATMENT. Exertional headache can sometimes be prevented by taking indomethacin before activities known to induce benign exertional headache. The prophylactic use of indomethacin, 25 mg three times a day, or propranolol, 1 to 2/mg/kg/day, also reduces the incidence of attacks.

HYPERTENSION

A sudden rise in systemic blood pressure causes the explosive throbbing headache associated with orgasm and pheochromocytoma. Children with chronic hypertension may have low-grade occipital headache on awakening that diminishes as they get up and begin activity, or frontal throbbing heading during the day (Lieberman, 1994). However, most children with chronic hypertension are asymptomatic. The development of chronic headache in children with renal disease should not be ascribed to hypertension (see Chapter 2). Instead, alternative causes must be pursued. Headaches are common in patients undergoing dialysis and may be due to psychological tension, the precipitation of migraine attacks, and dialysis itself. *Dialysis headache* begins a few hours after the procedure is terminated and is characterized by mild bifrontal throbbing headache, which may be associated with nausea and vomiting.

POST-TRAUMATIC HEADACHE

Several different kinds of headache are associated with head trauma. Vascular headache is experienced by 40% of patients in the first day or two after head injury. It is a diffuse pounding headache made worse by movement of the head or by coughing and straining. Dizziness may be associated. Post-traumatic vascular headaches subside spontaneously. Prolonged post-traumatic headaches are not fully understood (see Chapter 2); some are analgesic rebound headache.

 Pain From Other Cranial Structures

EYESTRAIN

CLINICAL FEATURES. Prolonged ocular near fixation in a child with a latent disturbance in convergence may cause dull aching pain behind the eyes that is quickly relieved when the eyes are closed. The pain is of muscular origin and caused by the continuous effort to maintain conjugate gaze. If work is continued despite ocular pain, episodic tension headache may develop.

DIAGNOSIS. Children who complain of eyestrain are often thought to have refractive errors, and eyeglasses are fitted. However, refractive errors do not cause eyestrain in children as presbyopia does in adults.

TREATMENT. Eyestrain is relieved by resting the eyes.

SINUSITIS

When questioned about migraine symptoms, most parents identify their own episodic headache, preceded by scintillating scotoma and followed by nausea and vomiting, as sinusitis. This diagnosis is favored by physicians and patients to describe chronic or episodic headaches and is usually wrong.

CLINICAL FEATURES. Children with sinusitis are usually sick. They are febrile, feel stuffy, and have difficulty maintaining a clear airway. Localized tenderness is present over the infected frontal or maxillary sinuses, and inflammation of the ethmoidal or sphenoidal sinuses causes deep midline pain behind the nose. Pain is exaggerated by blowing the nose or by quick movements of the head, especially bending forward. Concurrent vascular headache caused by fever is common.

DIAGNOSIS. Radiographs reveal clouding of the sinuses and sometimes a fluid level. CT of the skull is exceptionally accurate in identifying sinusitis but is usually an unnecessary expense. It is impressive how often CT of the head, performed for reasons other than headache, shows radiographic evidence of asymptomatic sinusitis. Clearly, radiographic evidence of sinusitis does not necessarily explain a patient's headache.

TREATMENT. The primary objective of treatment is to allow the sinus to drain. This is usually accomplished with decongestants, but sometimes surgery is required. Antibiotics have limited usefulness if drainage is not established.

TEMPOROMANDIBULAR JOINT SYNDROME

Any discussion of temporomandibular joint (TMJ) syndrome must begin with the caveat that the association between TMJ disease and headache is not clearly understood.

CLINICAL FEATURES. TMJ syndrome is not generally recognized as a disease of childhood but occurs in children as young as 8 years. The duration of symptoms before diagnosis may be as long as 5 years and averages 2 years. The primary disturbance is an arthritis of the temporomandibular joint that causes localized pain in the lower face and crepitus in the joint. Because of pain on one side, chewing is performed on the opposite side. Unfortunately, this has the unwanted effect of overuse of the affected side. The overused masseter muscle becomes tender; a muscle contraction headache ensues and is felt on the side of the face and at the vertex. The cause of arthritis is generally attributed to dental malocclusion, but a prior injury of the jaw accounts for one third of TMJ syndromes in children.

DIAGNOSIS. Radiographs of the TMJ usually show some internal derangement of the joint and may show degenerative arthritis. Magnetic resonance imaging (MRI) using surface coils is considered the most effective technique to show disturbed joint architecture.

TREATMENT. Treatment for TMJ syndrome has not been established based on controlled experiments. Placebos provide considerable benefit and extensive oral surgery is not indicated. Nonsteroidal anti-inflammatory agents, application of heat to the tense muscles, and dental splints may prove useful.

WHIPLASH AND OTHER NECK INJURIES

Whiplash and other neck injuries cause pain by rupture of cervical disks, damage to soft tissue, injury to occipital nerves, and excessive muscle contraction. The muscles contract in an effort to splint the area of injury and thereby reduce further tissue damage.

CLINICAL FEATURES. Constant contraction of the neck extensors causes a dull aching pain not only in the neck but also in the shoulders and upper arms. This may persist for months after the injury. The head is generally kept in a fixed position. Nausea and vomiting are not associated symptoms.

DIAGNOSIS. Following any neck or head injury, radiographs of the cervical spine are needed to determine the presence of fracture or dislocation. Shooting pains that radiate either to the occiput or down the arm and into the fingers suggest the possibility of disk herniation and require further study with MRI or CT.

TREATMENT. Warn the patient and family at the onset that prolonged head and neck pain are expected after injury and do not indicate a serious condition. The pain is relieved in part by lying or sitting with the head supported, by superficial application of heat to the painful muscles, by muscle relaxants, and by use of non-narcotic analgesics.

➡ Seizure Headache

Diffuse headache caused by vasodilation of cerebral arteries is a frequent occurrence following a generalized tonic-clonic convulsion. In patients who have both epilepsy and migraine, one can trigger the other, and frequently headache and seizure occur concurrently. Approximately 1% of epileptic patients report headache as a seizure manifestation *(seizure headache).* Most patients with seizure headaches are known epileptics, but in some children, headache is the only feature of their seizure disorder. This is very uncommon!

CLINICAL FEATURES. Headache is part of several epilepsy syndromes, the most common in children being benign occipital epilepsy (see Chapter 1). The sequence of events suggests migraine.

I have seen one eloquent adolescent who complained of paroxysmal "head pain that is not like other headaches" that was associated with EEG evidence of generalized epileptiform activity. The head pain was relieved by anticonvulsants.

Headache may also occur as a seizure manifestation in patients known to have a seizure disorder. Such individuals usually have a long history of partial or generalized seizures before headache becomes part of the syndrome. Associated ictal events depend on the site of the cortical focus and may include auditory hallucinations, visual disturbances, vertigo, déja vu, and focal motor seizures. Headache may be the initial feature of the seizure or can follow other partial seizure manifestations, such as déja vu and vertigo. The headache may be described as throbbing, sharp, or without an identified quality. Complex partial seizures, simple partial seizures, or generalized tonic-clonic seizures follow the headache phase. Spike foci in patients with seizure headaches are usually temporal in location.

Two children with seizure headaches were studied with depth electrodes before surgery. Both had seizure activity confined to the right hippocampus and amygdala during seizure headaches. In one, pain was localized to the vertex and was associated with shortness of breath and lightheadedness. At times the seizure progressed to aphasia but consciousness was preserved. The other child had frequent attacks of dizziness and tinnitus associated with the sudden onset of pain in the temporal region. The pain lasted for 30 to 60 seconds. Temporal lobe surgery provided complete relief of seizure activity in both patients.

DIAGNOSIS. Most seizure headaches in children are diagnosed by showing interictal spike discharges on the EEG. However, some interictal discharges, especially rolandic spikes, do not necessarily indicate that the headaches are a seizure manifestation. A child who has a clinical syndrome and a family history of migraine, and who has never had a clinical seizure, probably has migraine and not epilepsy despite the presence of interictal spike discharges.

EEG is indicated for children with chronic paroxysmal headache who do not have a family history of migraine. If interictal spike discharges are seen, an effort should be made to record a seizure headache with an ambulatory EEG monitor. The observation of continuous epileptiform activity during a headache provides reassurance that headache is a seizure manifestation and that anticonvulsant drugs are indicated. However, the site of the seizure focus does not necessarily match the location of the headache.

TREATMENT. The response to anticonvulsant therapy is usually considered diagnostic as well as therapeutic. Because the seizure focus is usually cortical and most often in the temporal lobe, carbamazepine or phenytoin is recommended.

REFERENCES

Abu-Arefeh I, Russell G. Prevalence of headache and migraine in schoolage children. Br Med J 1994;309:765-769.

Baumel B. Migraine: A pharmacologic review with newer options and modalities. Neurology 1994;44(suppl 3): S13-S17.

Cantwell-Simmons E, Duckro PN, Richardson WD. A review of studies on the relationship of chronic analgesic use and chronic headaches. Headache Q 1993;4:28-35.

Chu ML, Shinnar S. Headaches in children younger than 7 years of age. Arch Neurol 1992;49:79-82.

Dahlöf C, Ekbom K, Persson L. Clinical experiences from Sweden on the use of subcutaneously administered sumatriptan in migraine and cluster headache. Arch Neurol 1994;51:1256-1261.

Dalessio DJ. Diagnosing the severe headache. Neurology 1994;44(suppl 3):S6-S12.

Dhuna A, Pascuel-Leone A, Belgrade M. Cocaine-related vascular headaches. J Neurol Neurosurg Psychiatry 1991; 54:803-806.

Frishberg BM. The utility of neuroimaging in the evaluation of headache in patients with normal neurological examinations. Neurology 1994;44:1191-1197.

Lance JW. Mechanism and Management of Headache. 5th edition. Butterworth-Heinemann, Oxford, 1993;194-197.

Lieberman E. Pediatric hypertension: Clinical perspective. Mayo Clin Proc 1994;69:1098-1107.

MacDonald JT. Treatment of juvenile migraine with subcutaneous sumatriptan. Headache 1994;34:581-582.

Mathew NT, Saper JR, Silberstein SD, et al. Migraine prophylaxis with divalproex. Arch Neurol 1995;52:281-286.

Nevo Y, Kramer U, Rieder-Groswasser I, et al. Clinical categorization of 312 children with chronic headache. Brain Dev 1994;16:441-444.

Newman LC, Gordon ML, Lipton RB, et al. Episodic paroxysmal hemicrania: Two new cases and a literature review. Neurology 1992;42:964-966.

Newman LC, Lipton RB, Solomon S. Hemicrania continua: Ten new cases and a review of the literature. Neurology 1994;44:2111-2114.

Ostergaard JR, Storm K. Neurologic manifestations of Schonlein-Henoch purpura. Acta Pediatr Scand 1991;80: 339-342.

Russell MB, Andersson PG, Thomsen LL. Familial occurrence of cluster headache. J Neurol Neurosurg Psychiatry 1995; 58:341-343.

Silberstein SD, Merriam GR. Estrogens, progestins, and headache. Neurology 1991;41:786-793.

Silbert PL, Edis RH, Stewart-Wynne EG, Gubbay SS. Benign vascular sexual headache and exertional headache: Interrelationships and long term prognosis. J Neurol Neurosurg Psychiatry 1991;54:417-421.

Sumatriptan Cluster Headache Study Group. Treatment of acute cluster headache with sumatriptan. N Engl J Med 1991;325:322-326.

Warner JS, Wamil AW, McLean MJ. Case report: Acetazolamide for the treatment of chronic paroxysmal hemicrania. Headache 1994;34:597-599.

Williams SJ, Nukada H. Sport and exercise headache: Part 2 Br J Sports Med 1994;28:96-100.

4
Increased Intracranial Pressure

atients do not come to a physician complaining of increased intracranial pressure (Table 4-1). Most often it is brought to attention because of headache, vomiting, personality change, and alterations in states of consciousness. Less frequently, the initial complaint is diplopia or the observation that one or both eyes are turning in. Some children are referred for neurologic consultation because a primary physician believes the child has papilledema. Conditions causing increased intracranial pressure are described elsewhere in the book, especially in chapters on altered states of consciousness, headache, ataxia, and disorders of ocular motility. This chapter is restricted to conditions in which symptoms of increased intracranial pressure are initial and prominent features.

Pathophysiology

Once the cranial bones fuse during childhood, the contents of the skull are enveloped by a rigid box. Intracranial pressure is then the sum of the individual pressures exerted by the brain, blood, and cerebrospinal fluid. An increase in the volume of any of these three components must be accommodated by an equivalent decrease in size of one or both of the other components, if intracranial pressure is to remain constant. Because cerebral blood flow must be kept relatively constant to provide oxygen and nutrients, the major adaptive mechanisms available to relieve pressure are the compressibility of the brain and the rapid reabsorption of cerebrospinal fluid by arachnoid villi. Infants and young children, in whom the cranial bones are still unfused, have the additional adaptive mechanism of spreading the cranial bones apart to increase cranial volume.

THE CEREBROSPINAL FLUID

The choroid plexus accounts for at least 70% of cerebrospinal fluid production, and the transependymal movement of fluid from the brain to the ventricular system accounts for the remainder. The average volumes of cerebrospinal fluid are 90 ml in children from 4 to 13 years of age and 150 ml in adults. The rate of formation is approximately 0.35 ml/min, or 500 ml/day. Therefore approximately 14% of total volume turns over every hour. The rate at which cerebrospinal fluid is formed remains relatively constant and declines only slightly as cerebrospinal fluid pressure increases. In contrast, the rate of absorption increases linearly as cerebrospinal fluid pressure exceeds 70 mm H_2O. At a pressure of 200 mm H_2O, the rate of absorption is three times the rate of formation.

Impaired absorption, not increased formation, is the usual mechanism of progressive

■ TABLE 4-1
Features of Increased Intracranial Pressure

In Infants
Bulging fontanelles
Failure to thrive
Large head (see Chapter 18)
Impaired upward gaze (setting sun sign)
Shrill cry
In Children
Diplopia (see Chapter 15)
Headache (see Chapter 3)
Mental changes
Nausea and vomiting
Papilledema

hydrocephalus. Choroid plexus papilloma is the only pathologic process in which formation can sometimes overwhelm absorption. When absorption is impaired, efforts to decrease the formation of cerebrospinal fluid are not likely to have a significant effect on volume.

CEREBRAL BLOOD FLOW

Systemic arterial pressure is the primary determinant of cerebral blood flow. Normal cerebral blood flow remains remarkably constant from birth to adult life and is generally 50 to 60 ml/min/100 g brain weight. Blood vessels on the surface and at the base of the brain are more richly innervated by autonomic nerve fibers than are vessels of any other organ. These nerve fibers allow the autoregulation of cerebral blood flow. *Autoregulation* refers to a buffering effect by which cerebral blood flow remains constant despite changes in systemic arterial perfusion pressure. Alterations in the arterial blood concentration of carbon dioxide have an important effect on total cerebral blood flow. Hypercarbia dilates cerebral blood vessels and increases blood flow, whereas hypocarbia constricts cerebral blood vessels and decreases flow. Alterations in blood oxygen content have the reverse effect, but are less potent stimuli for vasoconstriction or vasodilation than are alterations in blood carbon dioxide concentration.

Cerebral perfusion pressure is the difference between mean systemic arterial pressure and intracranial pressure. It can be reduced to dangerous levels either by reducing systemic arterial pressure or by increasing intracranial pressure. The autoregulation of the cerebral vessels is lost when cerebral perfusion pressure

falls below 50 cm H_2O or severe acidosis is present. Increased intracranial blood volume can be caused by arterial vasodilation or by obstruction of cerebral veins and venous sinuses. Increased intracranial blood volume, like increased cerebrospinal fluid volume, results in increased intracranial pressure.

CEREBRAL EDEMA

Cerebral edema is an increase in the brain's volume caused by an increase in its water and sodium content. Edema may be localized or generalized; when generalized, it increases intracranial pressure. Cerebral edema is generally categorized as *vasogenic, cytotoxic,* or *interstitial.*

Vasogenic edema is caused by increased capillary permeability and is encountered with brain tumor, abscess, trauma, and hemorrhage. The fluid is located primarily in the white matter and responds to treatment with corticosteroids. Osmotic agents have no effect on vasogenic edema, but they can decrease the volume of normal brain tissue and in that way reduce total intracranial pressure.

Cytotoxic edema is caused by swelling of neurons, glia, and endothelial cells. It is usually caused by hypoxia, ischemia, or infection of the nervous system. Increased fluid is located in both gray and white matter. Corticosteroids do not decrease edema, but osmotic agents may relieve intracranial pressure by reducing brain volume.

Interstitial edema is caused by transependymal movement of fluid from the ventricular system to the brain. This occurs when cerebrospinal fluid absorption is blocked and the ventricles are enlarged. The fluid collects chiefly in the periventricular white matter. Agents intended to reduce cerebrospinal fluid production, such as acetazolamide and furosemide, may be useful. Corticosteroids and osmotic agents are not effective.

MASS LESIONS

Mass lesions (e.g., tumor, abscess, hematoma, arteriovenous malformation) increase intracranial pressure by occupying space at the expense of other intracranial compartments, provoking cerebral edema, blocking the circulation and absorption of cerebrospinal fluid, increasing blood flow, and obstructing venous return.

Symptoms and Signs

The clinical features of increased intracranial pressure depend on the child's age and the rate at which pressure increases. Newborns and infants present a special case because increased pressure can be partially vented by expanding the volume of the skull. The rate of intracranial pressure increase is important at all ages. Intracranial structures accommodate slowly increasing pressure remarkably well, but sudden changes are intolerable and result in some combination of headache, personality change, and states of decreasing consciousness.

INCREASED INTRACRANIAL PRESSURE IN INFANCY

Measurement of head circumference and palpation of the anterior fontanelle are readily available methods of assessing intracranial volume and pressure rapidly. Head circumference is measured by determining its greatest anteroposterior circumference. Normal standards are different for premature and full-term newborns. Normal head growth in the term newborn is 2 cm/month for the first 3 months, 1 cm/month for the second 3 months, and 0.5 cm/month for the next 6 months. Excessive head growth is a major feature of increased intracranial pressure throughout the first year and even up to 3 years of age. However, normal head growth does not preclude the presence of increased intracranial pressure. In posthemorrhagic hydrocephalus, considerable ventricular dilatation precedes any measurable change in head circumference by compressing the brain parenchyma.

The palpable tension of the anterior fontanelle is an excellent measure of intracranial pressure. In a quiet child a fontanelle that bulges above the level of the bone edges and is sufficiently tense to cause difficulty in determining where bone ends and fontanelle begins is abnormal and indicates increased intracranial pressure. A full fontanelle, which is clearly distinguishable from the surrounding bone edges, may indicate increased intracranial pressure but can also be caused by crying, edema of the scalp, subgaleal hemorrhage, and extravasation of intravenous fluids. The normal fontanelle is clearly demarcated from bone edges, falls below the surface, and pulsates under the examining finger.

Although the size of the anterior fontanelle and its rate of closure are variable, increased intracranial pressure should be suspected when the metopic and coronal sutures are sufficiently separated to admit a fingertip.

When the separation of cranial sutures is no longer sufficient to decompress increased intracranial pressure, the infant experiences lethargy and vomiting and fails to thrive. Palsies of the sixth cranial nerve, impaired upward gaze (setting sun sign), and disturbances of blood pressure and pulse may ensue. Papilledema is uncommon.

INCREASED INTRACRANIAL PRESSURE IN CHILDREN

Headache

Headache is one of the more common symptoms of increased intracranial pressure at all ages. Traction and displacement of intracranial arteries are the major cause of headache from increased intracranial pressure (see Chapter 3). As a rule, pain fibers from supratentorial intracranial vessels are innervated by the trigeminal nerve and pain is referred to the eye, forehead, and temple. In contrast, infratentorial intracranial vessels are innervated by cervical nerves and pain is referred to the occiput and neck.

When increased intracranial pressure is generalized, as may occur from cerebral edema or obstruction of the ventricular system, headache is generalized and more often prominent in the morning on awakening and rising to a standing position. Pain is constant, but may vary in intensity. Coughing, sneezing, straining, and other maneuvers that transiently increase intracranial pressure exaggerate the headache. The quality of pain is often difficult to describe. Vomiting in the absence of nausea, especially on arising in the morning, is often a concurrent feature.

In the absence of generalized increased intracranial pressure, localized, or at least unilateral, headache can occur if a mass causes traction on contiguous vessels.

In children younger than 10 years, symptoms of increased intracranial pressure can be temporarily relieved by the separation of sutures. Such children may have a symptom-free interval of several weeks following weeks or months of chronic headache and vomiting. The relief of pressure is temporary, and symptoms return with their prior intensity. An intermittent course of symptoms should not direct attention away from the possibility of increased intracranial pressure.

Any individual who was previously well and then experiences an acute, intense headache described as "the worst headache I ever had in my life" has surely suffered a subarachnoid hemorrhage. A small hemorrhage may not cause loss of consciousness but still produces sufficient meningeal irritation to cause intense headache and some stiffness of the neck. Fever may be present.

Diplopia and Strabismus

Paralysis of one or both abducens nerves is a relatively common feature of generalized increased intracranial pressure and may be a more prominent feature than headache in children with pseudotumor cerebri (see Chapter 15).

Papilledema

Papilledema is passive swelling of the optic disk caused by increased intracranial pressure (Table 4–2). The mechanism of swelling is uncertain, but generally is believed to be the obstruction of venous return from the retina and nerve head. The edema is usually bilateral and, when unilateral, suggests a mass lesion behind the affected eye. Early papilledema is asymptomatic, and only when it is advanced does the patient experience transitory obscuration of vision. Preservation of visual acuity differentiates papilledema from primary optic nerve disturbances such as optic neuritis, in which visual acuity is always profoundly impaired early in the course (see Chapter 16).

The observation of papilledema in a child with headache or diplopia confirms the diagnosis of increased intracranial pressure. However, the diagnosis of papilledema is not always easy, and congenital variations of disk appearance may confuse the issue. The earliest sign of papilledema is loss of spontaneous venous pulsations in the vessels around the disk margin. Spontaneous venous pulsations are said to occur in approximately 80% of normal eyes, but this is closer to 100% in children. Spontaneous venous pulsa-

tions cease when intracranial pressure exceeds 200 mm H_2O. Therefore, papilledema is not present if spontaneous venous pulsations are present, no matter how obscure the disk margin may appear. Conversely, when spontaneous venous pulsations are lacking in children, papilledema should be suspected even though the disk margin is flat and well visualized.

As edema progresses, the disk swells and is raised above the plane of the retina, causing obscuration of the disk margin and tortuosity of the veins (Figure 4–1). Associated features include small flame-shaped hemorrhages and nerve fiber infarcts known as "cotton-wool" (Figure 4–2). If the process continues, the retina surrounding the disk becomes edematous so that the disk appears greatly enlarged and retinal exudates radiate from the fovea. Eventually, the hemorrhages and exudates clear, but optic atrophy ensues and blindness may be permanent. Even if increased intracranial pressure is relieved during the early stages of disk edema, 4 to 6 weeks is required before the retina appears normal again.

Congenitally elevated disks that give the false impression of papilledema are usually caused by hyaline bodies (drusen) within the nerve head. The actual drusen are not observable during the first decade, and therefore only the elevated nerve head is apparent. Drusen continue to grow and can be seen in older children and in their parents (Figure 4–3). Drusen are inherited

■ TABLE 4–2
Differential Diagnosis of a Swollen Disk

Congenital disk elevation
Increased intracranial pressure
Ischemic neuropathy
Juvenile diabetes
Optic glioma
Papillitis
Retinitis
Retrobulbar mass
Uveitis

□ F I G U R E   4 – 1   Acute papilledema. The optic disk is swollen and peripapillary nerve fiber layer hemorrhages are evident.

□ FIGURE 4-2 Established papilledema. The optic disk is elevated and opacification of the nerve fiber layer can be seen around the disk margin and retinal folds (Paton lines) temporally.

□ FIGURE 4-3 Drusen. The disk margin is indistinct, the physiologic cup is absent, and yellowish, globular bodies are present on the surface.

as an autosomal dominant trait and occur more often in whites than other racial groups. Anomalous nerve head elevations can be easily distinguished from papilledema because spontaneous venous pulsations are present.

■ TABLE 4-3
Herniation Syndromes

Unilateral (Uncal) Transtentorial Herniation
Declining consciousness
Respiratory irregularity
Dilated and fixed pupil
Homonymous hemianopia
Increased blood pressure, slow pulse
Decerebrate rigidity
Bilateral (Central) Transtentorial Herniation
Declining consciousness
Pupillary constriction or dilation
Impaired upward gaze
Irregular respiration
Decerebrate or decorticate rigidity
Cerebellar (Downward) Herniation
Neck stiffness or head tilt
Declining consciousness
Impaired upward gaze
Irregular respirations
Lower cranial nerve palsies

HERNIATION SYNDROMES

Increased intracranial pressure may cause portions of the brain to shift from their normal location into other compartments, compressing structures already occupying that space. Such shifts may occur under the falx cerebri, through the tentorial notch, and through the foramen magnum (Table 4-3).

Lumbar puncture is generally contraindicated in patients with increased intracranial pressure because of the fear that a change in fluid dynamics will cause herniation. It is especially hazardous when pressure between cranial compartments is unequal. This prohibition is relative, and early lumbar puncture is the rule in infants and children with suspected infections of the nervous system despite the presence of increased intracranial pressure. In other situations lumbar puncture is rarely essential for diagnosis, but it is usually accomplished safely in the absence of papilledema. Patients at increased risk for herniation following lumbar puncture can be defined by the following computed tomography (CT) criteria: lateral shift of midline structures, loss of the suprachiasmatic and basilar cisterns, obliteration of the fourth ventricle, and obliteration of the superior cerebellar and quadrigeminal plate cisterns.

Falx Herniation

Herniation of one cingulate gyrus under the falx cerebri is common when one hemisphere is enlarged. The major feature is compression of the internal cerebral vein and the anterior cerebral artery, resulting in still greater increased intracranial pressure because of reduced venous outflow and arterial infarction.

Unilateral (Uncal) Transtentorial Herniation

The tentorial notch allows structures to pass from the posterior to the middle fossa. Normally it is filled with the brainstem, the posterior cerebral artery, and the third nerve. Unilateral transtentorial herniation characteristically occurs when enlargement of one temporal lobe causes the uncus or hippocampus to bulge into the tentorial notch. Falx herniation is usually an associated feature. Because intracranial pressure must be considerable to cause such a shift, consciousness is decreased even before the actual herniation and continues to decline as the brainstem is compressed. Direct pressure on the oculomotor nerve causes ipsilateral dilatation of the pupil; sometimes the contralateral pupil is dilated because the displaced brainstem compresses the opposite oculomotor nerve against the incisura of the tentorium. Contralateral homonymous hemianopia occurs (but is impossible to test in an unconscious patient) because of compression of the ipsilateral posterior cerebral artery. With further pressure on the midbrain, both pupils become dilated and fixed, respirations become irregular, decerebrate posturing is noted, and death results from cardiorespiratory collapse.

Bilateral (Central) Transtentorial Herniation

Central herniation is usually associated with generalized cerebral edema. Both hemispheres are displaced downward, and the diencephalon and midbrain are pushed caudad through the tentorial notch. The diencephalon becomes edematous, and the pituitary stalk may be avulsed. The clinical features are states of decreasing consciousness, pupillary constriction and then dilatation, impaired upward gaze, irregular respiration, disturbed control of body temperature, decerebrate or decorticate posturing, and death.

Cerebellar Herniation

Increased pressure in the posterior fossa may cause upward herniation of the cerebellum through the tentorial notch or downward displacement of one or both cerebellar tonsils through the tentorial notch. Upward displacement causes compression of the midbrain, resulting in impairment of upward gaze, dilated or fixed pupils, and respiratory irregularity. Downward cerebellar herniation causes compression of the medulla, resulting in states of decreasing consciousness, impaired upward gaze, and lower cranial nerve palsies. One of the earliest features of cerebellar herniation into the foramen magnum is neck stiffness or head tilt as an effort is made to relieve the pressure by enlarging the surface area of the foramen magnum.

 Medical Treatment

Several measures to lower increased intracranial pressure are available, even in circumstances where surgical intervention is required (Table 4-4).

MONITORING INTRACRANIAL PRESSURE

The enthusiasm for continuous monitoring of intracranial pressure in children is declining. Despite advances in technology, the effect of pressure monitoring on outcome is questionable. It has no value in children with hypoxic-ischemic encephalopathies and has marginal value in children with other kinds of encephalopathies (Le Roux et al, 1991). The symptoms and prognosis of increased intracranial pressure depend more on its cause than on the level of pressure attained.

HEAD ELEVATION

Elevating the head of the bed 30 to 45 degrees above horizontal decreases intracranial pressure by improving jugular venous drainage. Systemic blood pressure is not affected, so that the overall result is increased cerebral perfusion. A continuous wave doppler technique has been used to measure the effect of head elevation on intracranial pressure in normal and in asphyxiated newborns. Pressure is higher in the dependent position and lower in the elevated position in both groups, but the effect is greater in asphyxiated newborns.

HYPERVENTILATION

Intracranial pressure is reduced within seconds of the initiation of hyperventilation. The

■ T A B L E 4 – 4

Medical Measures to Decrease Intracranial Pressure

Elevation of head
Hyperventilation
Osmotic diuretics
Mannitol
Glycerol
Corticosteroids
Hypothermia
Pentobarbital coma

mechanism is vasoconstriction resulting from hypercarbia. The goal is to lower the arterial pressure of carbon dioxide to 25 cm H_2O from 40 cm H_2O. Further reduction may cause ischemia and is contraindicated. Vasoconstriction is not maintained so long as hyperventilation is continued. However, as the vessels redilate and blood flow returns to normal, "rebound," in which blood flow increases above baseline, does not occur.

OSMOTIC DIURETICS

Mannitol and glycerol are the two osmotic diuretics most widely used in the United States. Mannitol, 0.25 g/kg, is given intravenously as a 20% solution. Much larger doses were previously recommended, but the lower dose is equally effective and produces less rebound. Mannitol does not cross the blood-brain barrier. It remains in the plasma and creates an osmotic gradient that draws water from the brain into capillaries. Onset of action is within 30 minutes, and the peak effect is generally 1 to 2 hours after administration. The effect is short lasting, and infusions must be given 3 to 6 times each day to keep serum osmolality below 320 mOsm/L (320 nmol/L). Because repeated infusions of mannitol produce dehydration, as well as fluid and electrolyte imbalance, it is generally used for only 2 or 3 days. Rebound may occur when mannitol is discontinued.

Glycerol, 1 g/kg, is given intravenously as a 10% solution three or four times a day. The onset of action is within 30 minutes, and the effect usually lasts 24 hours or longer. As with mannitol, dehydration and electrolyte disturbances may follow repeated administration. Rebound is less prominent than with mannitol.

CORTICOSTEROIDS

Corticosteroids such as dexamethasone are effective in the treatment of vasogenic edema.

The intravenous dosage is 0.1 to 0.2 mg/kg every 6 hours. Onset of action is 12 to 24 hours, and peak action may be delayed even longer. The mechanism is uncertain. Cerebral blood flow is not affected. Corticosteroids are most useful for reducing edema surrounding mass lesions.

HYPOTHERMIA

Hypothermia decreases cerebral blood flow and is frequently used concurrently with pentobarbital coma. Body temperature is generally kept between 27° and 31° C. It is not clear how much is gained by hypothermia in addition to other measures that decrease cerebral blood flow, such as head elevation, hyperventilation, and pentobarbital coma.

PENTOBARBITAL COMA

Barbiturates reduce cerebral blood flow, decrease edema formation, and lower the brain's metabolic rate. These effects do not occur at anticonvulsant plasma concentrations but require brain concentrations sufficient to produce a burst-suppression pattern on the electroencephalogram (EEG). Barbiturate coma is particularly useful in patients with increased intracranial pressure resulting from disorders of mitochondrial function such as Reye syndrome. Pentobarbital is preferred to phenobarbital (see Chapter 1).

 Hydrocephalus

Hydrocephalus is a condition marked by an excessive volume of intracranial cerebrospinal fluid. It is termed *communicating* or *noncommunicating,* depending on whether or not the cerebrospinal fluid communicates between the ventricular system and subarachnoid space. Congenital hydrocephalus occurs in approximately one birth per thousand. It is generally associated with other congenital malformations and may be caused by genetic disturbances or intrauterine disorders such as infection and hemorrhage. Often, no cause can be determined. Congenital hydrocephalus is discussed in Chapter 18 because its initial feature is almost always macrocephaly.

Acquired hydrocephalus may be caused by brain tumor, intracranial hemorrhage, or infection. Solid brain tumors generally produce hydrocephalus by obstructing the ventricular system, whereas nonsolid tumors such as leukemia impair the reabsorptive mechanism in the subarachnoid space.

Intracranial hemorrhage and infection may produce communicating and noncommunicating hydrocephalus and also may increase intracranial pressure through the mechanisms of cerebral edema and impaired venous return. Because several factors contribute to increased intracranial pressure, the discussion of acquired hydrocephalus is categorized by cause in the sections that follow.

 Brain Tumors

Primary tumors of the posterior fossa and middle fossa are discussed in Chapters 10, 15, and 16 (Table 4–5). This section deals with tumors of the cerebral hemispheres. Supratentorial tumors comprise approximately half of brain tumors in children (Pollack, 1994). They occur more commonly in children less than 2 years, and again in adolescents.

■ TABLE 4–5
Brain Tumors in Children

Hemispheric Tumors
Choroid plexus papilloma
Glial tumors
  Astrocytoma
  Ependymoma
  Oligodendroglioma
  Primitive neuroectodermal tumors
Pineal region tumors
  Pineal-parenchymal tumors
    Pineoblastoma
    Pineocytoma
  Germ cell tumors
    Embryonal cell carcinoma
    Germinoma
    Teratoma
  Glial tumors
    Astrocytoma
    Ganglioglioma
Other tumors
  Angiomas
  Dysplasia
  Meningioma
  Metastatic tumors
Middle Fossa Tumors
Optic glioma (see Chapter 16)
Sellar and parasellar tumors (see Chapter 16)
Posterior Fossa Tumors
Astrocytoma (see Chapter 10)
Brainstem glioma (see Chapter 15)
Ependymoma (see Chapter 10)
Hemangioblastoma (see Chapter 10)
Medulloblastoma (see Chapter 10)

CHOROID PLEXUS PAPILLOMA

Choroid plexus papilloma is an unusual tumor, representing less than 2% of childhood brain tumors. It generally occurs during infancy and may be present at birth.

CLINICAL FEATURES. Choroid plexus tumors are usually located in one lateral ventricle (Ellenbogen et al, 1989). The main features are those of increased intracranial pressure from hydrocephalus. Communicating hydrocephalus is sometimes caused by excessive production of cerebrospinal fluid by the tumor, but noncommunicating hydrocephalus caused by obstruction of the ventricular foramen is the rule. If the tumor is pedunculated, its movement may cause intermittent ventricular obstruction by a ball-valve mechanism. The usual course is one of rapid progression with only a few weeks from first symptoms to diagnosis.

Infants with choroid plexus tumors usually have macrocephaly and are thought to have congenital hydrocephalus. Older children have nausea, vomiting, diplopia, headaches, and weakness. Papilledema is the rule.

DIAGNOSIS. Because affected children show clear evidence of increased intracranial pressure, CT is usually the first test performed. The tumor is visualized within one ventricle as a mass of increased density with marked contrast enhancement. Hydrocephalus of one or both lateral ventricles is visualized as well. Because choroid plexus papillomas are highly vascular, angiography should be considered before surgery. Many tumors bleed spontaneously, and the spinal fluid may be xanthochromic or grossly bloody. The concentration of protein in the cerebrospinal fluid is usually elevated.

TREATMENT. Complete surgical extirpation is the treatment of choice. The 5-year survival rate is 50% with most deaths occurring within 7 months of surgery. Operative mortality may be high because the tumor has a tendency to hemorrhage. If the tumor is removed completely, hydrocephalus is relieved without the need of a shunt and recurrences are unusual.

GLIAL TUMORS

Tumors of glial origin comprise approximately 40% of supratentorial tumors in infants and children. The common glial tumors of childhood in order of frequency are astrocytoma, ependymoma, and oligodendroglioma. A mixture of two or more cell types is the rule. Oligodendroglioma occurs exclusively in the cerebral hemispheres, whereas astrocytoma and ependymoma may be found in either a supratentorial or infratentorial location.

Oligodendroglioma is generally not encountered until adolescence. These tumors grow slowly and tend to calcify. The initial symptom is usually a seizure rather than increased intracranial pressure.

Astrocytoma

Hemispheric astrocytomas are graded by histologic appearance into three classes: low-grade, anaplastic, and glioblastoma multiforme. Anaplastic tumors and glioblastoma multiforme are referred to as high-grade tumors. Glioblastoma multiforme accounts for fewer than 10% of childhood supratentorial astrocytomas and is more likely to occur in adolescence than in infancy. High-grade tumors may evolve from low-grade tumors

CLINICAL FEATURES. The initial features of glial tumors in children depend on location and may include seizures, hemiparesis, and movement disorders affecting one side of the body. Seizures are the most common initial feature of low-grade gliomas. Tumors infiltrating the basal ganglia and internal capsule are less likely to cause seizures than those closer to cortical structures. A mass effect may not be present early in the course because slow-growing, infiltrating tumors can be accommodated by surrounding neural structures. Such tumors may cause only seizures for several years before causing weakness of the contralateral limbs.

Headache is a relatively common complaint and may be focal if the tumor is producing localized displacement of vessels without increasing intracranial pressure. A persistent focal headache usually correlates well with tumor location.

Symptoms of increased intracranial pressure—generalized headache, nausea, and vomiting—are an initial feature of hemispheric astrocytoma in only a third of children, but are common at the time of diagnosis. Intracranial pressure is likely to increase when rapidly growing tumors provoke edema of the hemisphere. A mass effect is produced that causes collapse of one ventricle, shift of midline structures, and pressure on the aqueduct. When herniation occurs, or when the lateral ventricles are dilated because of pressure on the aqueduct, the early features of headache, nausea, vomiting, and diplopia are followed by generalized weakness

or fatigability, lethargy, and declining consciousness.

Papilledema occurs in children with generalized increased intracranial pressure; those under 2 years of age, however, macrocephaly may develop instead. When papilledema is present, abducens palsy is usually associated. Other neurologic findings depend on the site of the tumor and may include hemiparesis, hemisensory loss, or homonymous hemianopia.

DIAGNOSIS. High-grade hemispheric astrocytomas are readily identified by contrast-enhanced CT, but low-grade tumors are much better visualized with magnetic resonance imaging (MRI). MRI is always preferable to CT when tumor is suspected as the cause of seizures. Low-grade gliomas appear as low-density or cystic areas that are enhanced when contrast material is injected (Figure 4–4). Cerebral edema is identified as a low-density area surrounding the tumor that does not demonstrate contrast enhancement.

High-grade gliomas have patchy areas of low and high density, sometimes evidence of hemorrhage, and cystic degeneration. Marked contrast enhancement is noted, often in a ring pattern. When a mass effect is present, MRI shows a shift of midline structures, deformity of the ipsilateral ventricle, and swelling of the affected hemisphere with obliteration of sulcal markings (Figure 4–5). A mass effect is identified in half of low-grade astrocytomas and in almost all high-grade tumors.

TREATMENT. All children with increased intracranial pressure caused by hemispheric astrocytoma should be treated with dexamethasone to reduce vasogenic cerebral edema. Headache and nausea are frequently relieved within 24 hours, and neurologic deficits are often improved as well. Surgical resection of the tumor is the next step in treatment. Complete removal is rarely possible, except with cystic cerebral astrocytoma, which resembles cerebellar astrocytomas in having a mural nodule within the cyst. In these tumors, the 5-year survival rate following surgery alone is 90%.

Children with low-grade astrocytomas of the cerebral hemisphere have a 20-year survival rate of 85% after surgical resection alone (Pollack et al, 1995). Postoperative radiotherapy impairs cognition without increasing survival. Postoperative radiation is recommended for anaplastic astrocytomas. Children with anaplastic astrocytomas have less than a 30% 5-year survival rate even with radiotherapy, and those with glioblas-

□ F I G U R E 4 – 4 Low-grade glioma. MRI *(left)* reveals an area of increased signal intensity in the right temporal lobe, which appears as a cystic lesion on CT *(right)*.

□ F I G U R E 4 – 5 Malignant glioma. MRI shows a malignant astrocytoma invading the corpus callosum.

toma multiforme have less than a 3% 5-year survival.

Because the 5-year survival rate is poor with high-grade astrocytomas, several chemotherapy protocols have been tried. Children treated with a combination of lomustine, vincristine, and prednisone following radiotherapy have a 5-year, event-free survival rate of 46% (Sposto et al, 1989).

Ependymoma

Ependymomas are tumors derived from cells that line the ventricular system, and they may be found in either a supratentorial or an infratentorial location. Infratentorial ependymoma is discussed in Chapter 10 because the initial symptom is often ataxia. However, symptoms of increased intracranial pressure are the first feature in 90% of children with posterior fossa ependymoma, and papilledema is present in 75% at the time of initial examination. Approximately 60% of children with ependymoma are younger than 5 years old at the time of diagnosis and only 4% are older than 15 years. As a rule, children with infratentorial ependymoma are younger than children with supratentorial ependymoma.

The expected location of supratentorial ependymoma is in relation to the third and lateral ventricles. However, ependymal tumors may arise within the hemispheres at a site distant from the ventricular system. Such tumors are thought to be derived from ependymal cell rests.

CLINICAL FEATURES. Symptoms of increased intracranial pressure are less prominent with supratentorial tumors than with infratentorial tumors. Common manifestations are focal weakness, seizures, and visual disturbances. Papilledema is a common physical finding in all patients with ependymoma. Hemiparesis, hyperreflexia, and hemianopia are typical features, but some children show only ataxia. The duration of symptoms before diagnosis averages only 7 months but can be as little as 1 month for malignant tumors and as long as several years for low-grade tumors.

DIAGNOSIS. Tumor density on CT is usually greater than brain density, and contrast enhancement is present. Small cysts within the tumor are relatively common. Approximately one third of supratentorial ependymomas contain calcium.

Tumors within the third ventricle cause marked dilatation of the lateral ventricles with edema of the hemispheres and obliteration of sulcal markings. High-grade tumors are likely to seed the subarachnoid space, producing metastases in the spinal cord and throughout the ventricular system. In such cases, tumor cells may line the lateral ventricles and produce a "cast" of contrast enhancement around the ventricles.

TREATMENT. Complete surgical resection is possible in only 30% of cases. Even after complete resection, the 5-year rate of progression-free survival is between 60% and 80% (Vanuytsel et al, 1992). The relation between histologic grading and prognosis is not established.

Whole-brain and craniospinal radiation is not proven to provide a better outcome than limited-field radiotherapy to the tumor bed and its margins. Most incompletely resected tumors will progress despite radiotherapy. No chemotherapy protocol has proven useful.

PRIMITIVE NEUROECTODERMAL TUMORS

Primitive neuroectodermal tumors (PNET) are tumors of childhood consisting of small, undifferentiated, darkly staining cells that have neuronal, glial, and mesenchymal elements. Medulloblastoma is now classified as an infratentorial PNET. This section deals with supratentorial PNET tumors. Medulloblastoma is dealt with in Chapter 10.

CLINICAL FEATURES. Age at onset may be anytime during childhood, but is usually the first decade. Males and females are affected equally. Because these tumors are highly malignant, the progression of symptoms is rapid and time to diagnosis is usually less than 3 months. Approximately half of children show features of increased intracranial pressure. Other manifestations are determined by tumor site. Two thirds of tumors are located in the frontal or parietal lobe. Seizures, monoparesis, hemiplegia, and ophthalmoplegia are initial features in approximately 10% of patients. Hydrocephalus or head enlargement is unusual early in the course.

DIAGNOSIS. CT and MRI are effective techniques for determining tumor location and size. On CT, PNET appear as poorly defined, infiltrating and lobular masses, sometimes containing multiple cysts and hemorrhage. The tumor mass is surrounded by cerebral edema, and midline structures are frequently shifted under the falx.

TREATMENT. Cerebral edema may be relieved by the use of dexamethasone. Complete tumor resection is attempted but rarely accomplished. Postoperative craniospinal irradiation is believed to prolong survival. Several chemotherapeutic trials are ongoing.

Unfortunately, the mean survival of all patients is only 26 months. The best results are attributed to complete surgical resection, postoperative radiation therapy, and aggressive chemotherapy (Tomita et al, 1988). However, the tumor metastasizes throughout the subarachnoid space of brain and spinal cord so recurrence is possible even when the primary tumor is believed to be fully resected.

PINEAL REGION TUMORS

Tumors in the pineal region may be derived from several histologic types. Germ cell tumors are the most common, then tumors of the pineal parenchyma, and finally other histologic types. The incidence of pineal region tumors is 10 times higher in Japan than in the United States or Western Europe. Pineal region tumors are more common in boys than girls and generally become symptomatic during the second decade.

CLINICAL FEATURES. Because pineal region tumors are in a midline location, where they can invade or compress the third ventricle or aqueduct, symptoms of increased intracranial pressure are common. The first symptoms may be acute and accompanied by midbrain dysfunction. Midbrain dysfunction resulting from pressure by pineal region tumors on the periaqueductal gray is usually referred to as *Parinaud syndrome:* loss of pupillary light reflex, supranuclear palsy of upward gaze with preservation of downward gaze, and retraction-convergence nystagmus when upward gaze is attempted. Eventually, paralysis of both upward and downward gaze and loss of accommodation may occur.

Tumors growing into or compressing the anterior hypothalamus produce loss of vision, diabetes insipidus, precocious puberty, and emaciation. Precocious puberty occurs almost exclusively in males. Extension of tumor into the posterior fossa produces multiple cranial neuropathies and ataxia, and lateral extension causes hemiparesis.

DIAGNOSIS. CT or MRI accurately image tumor location and the presence of secondary hydrocephalus but cannot distinguish histologic types. As a rule, germinomas are isodense and noncalcified and have irregular margins. Contrast enhancement is not homogeneous. Teratomas appear lobulated and have both hyperdense and multicystic areas. Calcification may be present, and contrast enhancement is not uniform. Tumors that spread into the ventricular system and have intense contrast enhancement are likely to be malignant. Tumors that contain abundant amounts of calcium are likely to be benign.

Asymptomatic non-neoplastic pineal cysts are sometimes identified by CT or MRI in children who are being imaged for other reasons. These are developmental variants of the pineal gland that may contain calcium. Only rarely do they grow to sufficient size to obstruct the aqueduct or cause a Parinaud syndrome.

TREATMENT. Stereotactic biopsy is essential to establish histologic type and plan therapy. Ventricular drainage may be needed to relieve hydrocephalus. Germinomas are highly radiosensitive, and 5-year survival rates of 50% to 80% are reported. Other tumors of the pineal region are less radiosensitive. Complete surgical removal of pineal region tumors has been discouraged in the past because mortality and morbidity rates have been prohibitive. Improved surgical techniques are now allowing successful removal in many cases.

OTHER TUMORS

Cerebral metastatic disease is unusual in childhood. Tumors with the highest frequency of producing cerebral metastases are osteogenic sarcoma and rhabdomyosarcoma in patients younger than 15 years and testicular germ cell tumors after age 15. The cerebral hemispheres are affected more often than posterior fossa structures. Pulmonary involvement always precedes cerebral metastasis. Brain metastasis is rarely present at the time of initial cancer diagnosis.

Meningioma is uncommon in children. The initial features are usually focal neurologic signs and seizures and not increased intracranial pressure (Germano et al, 1994).

Intracranial Arachnoid Cysts

Primary arachnoid cysts are cavities that are within the arachnoid and are filled with cerebrospinal fluid. The cause of cyst formation is uncertain, but cysts are generally considered a minor disturbance in arachnoid formation and not a pathologic process. Arachnoid cysts are identifed in 0.5% of postmortem examinations.

CLINICAL FEATURES. Most cysts are asymptomatic structures identified by CT or MRI. Deciding whether the cyst is the cause of the symptom for which the imaging study was ordered is sometimes a problem. Subarachnoid cysts are usually present from infancy, but may develop, or at least enlarge enough to be detected, during adolescence.

Large cysts can produce symptoms by compressing adjacent structures or by increasing intracranial pressure. Focal neurologic disturbances vary with location but are most often hemiparesis or seizures when the cyst is supratentorial and ataxia when infratentorial. Compression of the parietal lobe from early infancy may result in undergrowth of contralateral limbs.

Increased intracranial pressure can be caused by mass effect or hydrocephalus and is associated with cysts in all locations. Manifestations include macrocephaly, headache, and behavioral change.

DIAGNOSIS. It has become commonplace for children with headache, learning or behavioral disorders, and suspected seizures to undergo imaging studies of the brain. Many have incidental arachnoid cysts. A cause-and-effect relationship should be considered only if the cyst is large and if it clearly explains the symptoms. Positron emission tomography (PET) may be useful in deciding whether an arachnoid cyst is having a pressure effect on the brain (De Volder et al, 1994). Brain compression sufficient to disturb function is characterized by hypometabolism in the surrounding brain.

TREATMENT. Simple drainage of the cyst often results in reaccumulation of fluid and recurrence of symptoms. Superficial cysts can be excised and deeply located cysts shunted into the peritoneal space (Oberbauer et al, 1992).

Intracranial Hemorrhage

HEAD TRAUMA

Head trauma is a major cause of intracranial hemorrhage from the newborn period through childhood and adolescence. It is associated with intracerebral hemorrhage, subarachnoid hemorrhage, subdural hematoma, and epidural hematoma. Increased intracranial pressure is a constant feature of intracranial hemorrhage and also occurs from cerebral edema following concussion without hemorrhage. Intracranial hemorrhage from head trauma is discussed in Chapter 2.

INTRAVENTRICULAR HEMORRHAGE IN THE NEWBORN

Intraventricular hemorrhage is primarily a disorder of live-born premature newborns with respiratory distress syndrome. The autoregulation of cerebral blood flow, which meets local tissue needs by altering cerebrovascular resistance, is impaired in premature newborns with respiratory distress syndrome. During episodes of systemic hypotension, cerebral blood flow is decreased and the potential for cerebral infarction exists. Such infarctions usually occur symmetrically in the white matter adjacent to the lateral ventricles and are termed *periventricular leukomalacia.*

During episodes of systemic hypertension, cerebral blood flow increases. Hemorrhage occurs first in the subependymal germinal matrix and then bursts through the ependymal lining into the lateral ventricle. Such hemorrhages are called *periventricular-intraventricular hemorrhages.* The predilection of the germinal matrix for hemorrhage during episodes of increased cerebral blood flow has not been fully explained. The likely explanation is prior ischemic injury that weakens the capillary walls and their supporting structures, making them vulnerable to rupture during episodes of increased cerebral blood flow.

Intraventricular hemorrhage also occurs in full-term newborns, but the mechanism of hemorrhage at term is different from that before term.

Periventricular-Intraventricular Hemorrhage in Premature Newborns

The incidence of periventricular-intraventricular hemorrhage (PIVH) in premature newborns whose birth weight is less than 2000 g has fallen in recent years from 40% to 25% (Philip et al, 1989). The reason for the decline is not fully explained. PIVH is still identified in 62% of very small premature newborns, with birth weights between 500 and 700 g, and is associated with

a high mortality rate. In newborns weighing less than 1500 g the incidence is approximately 40%. A grading system has been developed to quantify the severity of hemorrhage:

I. Isolated subependymal hemorrhage
II. Intraventricular hemorrhage without ventricular dilatation
III. Intraventricular hemorrhage with ventricular dilatation
IV. Intraventricular hemorrhage with ventricular dilatation and hemorrhage into the parenchyma of the brain.

Hemorrhage into the parenchyma of the brain (grade IV) is a coexistent process caused by hemorrhagic infarction (*periventricular hemorrhagic infarction*) and is not an extension of the first three grades of intraventricular hemorrhage.

CLINICAL FEATURES. Routine ultrasound examinations are now the standard of care for all newborns whose birth weight is 1,800 g or less. Ultrasound often shows PIVH in newborns for whom there was no clinical suspicion of hemorrhage. Among this group some have blood in the cerebrospinal fluid and others have clear cerebrospinal fluid. Only newborns with grade III or IV hemorrhage have predictable clinical features.

In some premature newborns, PIVH produces rapid neurologic deterioration characterized by decreasing states of consciousness, severe hypotonia, and respiratory insufficiency. Within minutes to hours the infants shows obvious evidence of increased intracranial pressure: bulging fontanelle, decerebrate posturing, loss of pupillary reflexes, and respiratory arrest. Hypothermia, bradycardia, hypotension, and a 10% fall in the hematocrit may be associated features.

More commonly the hemorrhage is manifested by stepwise progression of symptoms over a period of hours or even days. The initial symptoms are subtle and include a change in behavior, diminished spontaneous movement, and either an increase or a decrease in appendicular tone. The fontanelles remain soft, and vital signs are stable. These first symptoms may correspond to grade I hemorrhage. Some newborns then become stabile and have no further difficulty. Others undergo clinical deterioration characterized by hypotonia and declining consciousness. This deterioration probably corresponds to the presence of blood in the ventricles. The child becomes lethargic or obtunded and then may stabilize. If continued bleeding causes acute ventricular dilatation, apnea and coma follow. Seizures occur when blood dissects into the cerebral parenchyma.

Newborns with intraventricular hemorrhage are at risk for progressive hydrocephalus. The likelihood is much greater among children with grade III or IV hemorrhage. Initial ventricular dilatation is probably due to plugging of the arachnoid villi and impaired reabsorption of cerebrospinal fluid. The ventricles can enlarge by compressing the brain without causing a measurable change in head circumference. Therefore, weekly ultrasound studies are imperative to follow the progression of hydrocephalus.

A progressive hydrocephalus develops in 10% to 15% of premature newborns with PIVH (Dykes et al, 1989). The hydrocephalus ultimately arrests or regresses in two thirds of children, and progresses to severe hydrocephalus in the remainder.

DIAGNOSIS. Ultrasound is the standard for the diagnosis of intraventricular hemorrhage in the newborn. Ultrasound is preferred over other brain imaging techniques because it can be performed in the intensive care nursery, study time is briefer, and no radiation is involved. MRI during infancy or childhood is useful to show the extent of brain damage from the combination of periventriculat leukomalacia and PIVH.

PREVENTION. Prevention is the best treatment for PIVH. This could be accomplished, to a great extent, by preventing prematurity and by delivering premature newborns at specialized perinatal centers. A premature newborn transported to an intensive care nursery has a far greater chance of hemorrhage than a fetus transported to the delivery room in utero. Normal tension of carbon dioxide and oxygen, normal osmolality and viscosity, normal perfusion pressure without episodic hypertension from undue stimulation, and good ventilatory control in the early hours postpartum can best be maintained in a specialized neonatal unit (Volpe, 1989).

Several promising medical interventions for preventing PIVH have been introduced (Table 4-6); none of the drug treatments has gained wide acceptance (Vannucci, 1990). Even more vexing is the management of progressive posthemorrhagic hydrocephalus.

TREATMENT. Once intraventricular hemorrhage has occurred, treatment is directed at preventing or stabilizing progressive posthemorrhagic hydrocephalus. The efficacy of treatment for posthemorrhagic hydrocephalus is difficult to assess because the role of ventricular dilation in causing chronic neurologic impairment is not

■ T A B L E   4 – 6
Prevention of Periventricular-Intraventricular Hemorrhage

Antenatal
Prevention of prematurity
Delivery in specialized center
Treatment of mothers with
  Phenobarbital
  Vitamin K supplementation
Postnatal
Avoidance of rapid volume expansion
Maintenance of stable systemic blood pressure
Muscle paralysis of ventilated premature
Correction of coagulation abnormalities
Potential pharmacologic agents
  Ethamsylate
  Indomethacin
  Phenobarbital
  Vitamin E

established. Newborns with progressive posthemorrhagic hydrocephalus have also experienced asphyxial encephalopathy, germinal matrix hemorrhage, and periventricular leukomalacia. Neurologic morbidity correlates better with the degree of parenchymal damage than with ventricular size (Dykes et al, 1989).

Children with progressive posthemorrhagic hydrocephalus require a ventriculoperitoneal shunt. However, early shunt placement, while the ventricles still contain blood, has a high incidence of shunt failure and infection. Several methods of preventing posthemorrhagic hydrocephalus have been tried to either delay the time of shunt surgery or obviate the need for it.

The procedure that has undergone the greatest scrutiny is serial lumbar punctures. The main problem is the technical difficulty of performing repeated lumbar punctures on a small premature newborn. Different groups have reported contradictory results on the efficacy of serial lumbar punctures. Although its value is not established, the method is recommended for at least temporary amelioration of posthemorrhagic hydrocephalus if, in response to the procedure, a decrease in ventricular size is shown by ultrasound.

Alternatives to serial lumbar punctures are (1) external ventricular reservoir drainage, which is technically easier than serial lumbar punctures but may cause ventriculitis (Marro et al, 1991); (2) intraventricular instillation of urokinase (10,000 IU), a thrombolytic agent, instilled twice each day into the ventricles, which obviated the need for surgical shunt in one small series (Hudgins et al, 1994), and (3) the use of acetazolamide and furosemide, which are presumed to reduce the production of spinal fluid. Acetazolamide is started at a dosage of 25 mg/kg/day for 1 day and then increased by 25 mg/kg/day each day to a maximum of 100 mg/kg/day. Metabolic acidosis may occur at the maintenance dosage of 100 mg/kg/day. Base replacement with a systemic alkalizing agent must be initiated simultaneously to maintain a serum bicarbonate level greater than 18 mEq/l (18 mmol/L). Furosemide is started at a dosage of 1 mg/kg/day in three divided doses and may be increased to 3 mg/kg/day. The results with this protocol are encouraging, but the number of treated infants reported is not large enough to support a definite conclusion.

The neurologic outcome for newborns following PIVH is linked to the grade of hemorrhage. Following grade II hemorrhage, up to 75% of children may have normal intellectual and motor development, whereas virtually all children with grade IV hemorrhage have some neurologic morbidity. However, some newborns who have only grade I hemorrhage may be neurologically impaired, whereas others with grade III hemorrhage are normal. Neurologic outcome is determined by multiple factors of which asphyxia and periventricular infarction probably play an important role.

Intraventricular Hemorrhage at Term

Unlike intraventricular hemorrhage in the premature newborn, which originates almost exclusively from the germinal matrix, intraventricular hemorrhage at term may originate from the veins of the choroid plexus, from the germinal matrix, or both.

CLINICAL FEATURES. Full-term newborns with intraventricular hemorrhage may be divided into two groups. More than half are delivered with difficulty, frequently in the breech position, and have suffered some degree of intrauterine asphyxia. These newborns are usually bruised and require resuscitation. At first they appear to be improving, and then multifocal seizures occur on the second day postpartum. The fontanelle is tense, and the cerebrospinal fluid is bloody. The other half have experienced neither trauma nor asphyxia and appear normal at birth. During the first hours postpartum, however, apnea, cyanosis, and a tense fontanelle develop. The mechanism of hemorrhage is not understood. Posthemorrhagic hydrocephalus is common in both groups, and 35% require shunt placement.

DIAGNOSIS. Ultrasound is as useful for diagnosis of intraventricular hemorrhage in full-term newborns as in the premature newborns.

TREATMENT. Full-term newborns with intraventricular hemorrhage are treated in the same manner as premature newborns with intraventricular hemorrhage.

ARTERIAL ANEURYSMS

Arterial aneurysms are vestiges of the embryonic circulation and are present in a rudimentary form before birth. Only rarely do they rupture during childhood (Ito et al, 1992). Symptomatic arterial aneurysms in childhood may be associated with coarctation of the aorta or polycystic kidney disease. Aneurysms tend to be located at the bifurcation of major arteries at the base of the brain.

CLINICAL FEATURES. Subarachnoid hemorrhage is usually the first feature of a ruptured aneurysm. The initial symptoms may be catastrophic: sudden loss of consciousness, tachycardia, hypotension, and evidence of increased intracranial pressure, but in most patients the first bleeding is a "warning leak" that may go unrecognized. The warning leak is characterized by severe headache, stiff neck, and low-grade fever. Occasionally aneurysms produce neurologic signs by exerting pressure on adjacent cranial nerves. The oculomotor nerve is most frequently affected, resulting in disturbances of gaze and pupillary function.

Physical activity is not related to time of rupture. Aneurysmal size is the only predictor of rupture; those smaller than 1 cm in diameter have a low probability of rupture.

The patient's state of consciousness is the most important predictor of survival. Approximately 50% of patients die during the first hospitalization, some from the initial hemorrhage during the first 14 days. Untreated, another 30% die from recurrent hemorrhage in the next 10 years.

Unruptured aneurysms may cause acute severe headache without nuchal rigidity (Raps et al, 1993). The mechanism of headache may be aneurysmal thrombosis or localized meningeal inflammation.

DIAGNOSIS. On the day of aneurysmal rupture, CT shows intracranial hemorrhage in all patients, but the blood is rapidly reabsorbed and can be demonstrated in only two thirds on the fifth day. Most aneurysms can be visualized by standard MRI or by using MRI angiography.

Lumbar puncture is often performed because the stiff neck, headache, and fever suggest bacterial meningitis. The fluid is usually grossly bloody and therefore indicative of subarachnoid hemorrhage. Unfortunately, blood in the cerebrospinal fluid is often attributed to a traumatic tap when time is not taken to centrifuge the fluid and examine it for xanthochromia. Once a diagnosis of subarachnoid hemorrhage is established, either by imaging studies or by lumbar puncture, four-vessel cerebral arteriography is essential. All vessels must be visualized in order to determine the aneurysmal site and the presence of multiple aneurysms.

TREATMENT. The initial goals of therapy are to prevent early rebleeding and cerebral ischemia from arterial spasm. Nimodipine, a calcium channel blocking agent, reduces the incidence of spasm and should be administered as quickly as possible. The definitive treatment is surgical clipping and excision of the aneurysm. Early surgery is recommended in conscious patients to prevent rebleeding. The 6-month survival rate in patients who are conscious at time of admission is approximately 86%. In contrast, only 20% of patients who are comatose on admission are alive 6 months later.

ARTERIOVENOUS MALFORMATIONS

Arteriovenous malformations account for almost 9% of subarachnoid hemorrhage at all ages, but comprise a considerably larger share of subarachnoid hemorrhage in childhood. Approximately 0.1% to 0.2% of the population has an arteriovenous malformation. No familial occurrence has been documented. Two types of malformations are described. The first arises early in gestation from an abnormal communication between primitive choroidal arteries and veins. Such malformations are in the midline and give rise to the vein of Galen malformation, malformations involving the choroid plexus, and shunts between cerebellar arteries and the straight sinus. The other type arises later in gestation or even after birth between superficial arteries and veins and results in an arteriovenous malformation within the parenchyma of the cerebral hemisphere. The vessels of the scalp, skull, and dura are interconnected, causing anastomotic channels between the extracranial and intracranial circulations to remain patent (Lasjaunias et al, 1995). Approximately 90% of arteriovenous malformations are supratentorial and 10% are infratentorial.

Deep Midline Malformations

Large deep midline malformations, especially those involving the great vein of Galen, produce hydrocephalus and cardiac failure during infancy. They do not bleed. These are discussed in Chapter 18.

CLINICAL FEATURES. Small, deep midline malformations are rarely symptomatic in childhood. The initial feature is often caused by bleeding into the parenchyma of the brain or the subarachnoid space. Bleeding occurs when secondary venous changes reroute the drainage to the pial veins. Because the bleeding is from the venous rather than the arterial side of the malformation, the initial symptoms are not as catastrophic as with arterial aneurysms. Symptoms may evolve over several hours and no characteristic clinical syndrome has been established. Most patients describe sudden severe headache, neck stiffness, and vomiting. Fever is frequently an associated symptom. The presence of focal neurologic deficits depends on the location of the malformation and may include hemiparesis, sensory disturbances, and oculomotor palsies. Many patients recover completely from the first hemorrhage; the risk of recurrent hemorrhage is small.

DIAGNOSIS. Most arteriovenous malformations are easily visualized on MRI or CT with contrast enhancement. The degree of ventricular enlargement is shown by either study. However, the development of a therapeutic plan requires four-vessel arteriography to demonstrate fully all arterial and venous channels.

TREATMENT. Deep midline malformations are usually managed by venous embolization. The results vary with the size and location of the malformation.

Supratentorial Malformations

CLINICAL FEATURES. Among children with arteriovenous malformations in and around the cerebral hemispheres, the initial feature is intracranial hemorrhage in half and seizures in the other half. Recurrent vascular headache may precede the onset of hemorrhage and seizures or may develop concurrently. Headaches are usually unilateral but may not occur consistently on the same side. In some patients the headaches have a migraine quality: scintillating scotoma and unilateral throbbing pain. The incidence of such migraine-like headaches in patients with arteriovenous malformations does not appear to be greater than in the population at large. The malformation probably provokes a migraine attack in people who are genetically predisposed.

Most patients who have seizures have at least one focal seizure, but among seizures associated with arteriovenous malformations half are focal and half are generalized. No specific location of the malformation is associated with a higher incidence of seizures. However, small superficial malformations, especially in the centroparietal region, are associated with the highest incidence of hemorrhage. Hemorrhage may be only subarachnoid or may dissect into the brain parenchyma.

DIAGNOSIS. MRI and contrast-enhanced CT provide excellent visualization of the malformation in most children. Four-vessel arteriography is required to define all arterial and venous channels, but may be replaced by magnetic resonance angiography (MRA) as the technology improves.

TREATMENT. The photon knife is becoming the standard of treatment for small malformations. Other options for management include surgical excision and embolization. Superficial malformations are more accessible for direct surgical excision than those deep in the midline. In considering treatment modes the physician must balance the decision to do something against the decision to do nothing based on the likelihood of further bleeding and the morbidity of intervention.

COCAINE ABUSE

Intracranial hemorrhage has been associated with use of cocaine abuse, especially crack, in young adults (Mangiardi et al, 1988). The hemorrhages may be subarachnoid or intracerebral in location and are thought to be caused by sudden transitory increases in systemic blood pressure.

 Infectious Disorders

Infections of the brain and meninges produce increased intracranial pressure by causing cerebral edema, by obstructing the flow and reabsorption of cerebrospinal fluid, and by impairing venous outflow. Symptoms of increased intracranial pressure are frequently the initial features of bacterial and fungal infections and may also be the initial feature of viral encephalitis. However, viral infections are more likely to cause seizures, personality change, or decreased consciousness and therefore are discussed in Chapter 2.

BACTERIAL MENINGITIS

The offending organism and the clinical features of bacterial meningitis vary with age (Table 4–7). Therefore, it is useful to discuss the syndromes of bacterial meningitis by age group: newborn, infants and young children (28 days to 5 years), and school-age children.

Meningitis in the Newborn

Meningitis occurs in 1 live birth per 2,500 and accounts for up to 4% of all neonatal deaths. It is a consequence of septicemia, and organs other than the brain are infected. The two risk factors that correlate best with sepsis and meningitis are low birth weight and maternal infection. An early-onset (first 5 days) and a late-onset (after 5 days) pattern of meningitis have been identified in newborns. In early-onset meningitis the infection is acquired at the time of delivery and the responsible organisms are almost always *Escherichia coli* or group B *Streptococcus.* The child becomes symptomatic during the first week, and the mortality rate is 20% to 50%. In late-onset meningitis the infection is acquired postnatally and symptoms may begin as early as the fourth day postpartum but usually begin after the first week. Newborns requiring intensive care are specifically at risk for late-onset meningitis because infection is introduced by instrumentation. The responsible organisms are not only *E. coli* and group B *Streptococcus,* but also enterococci, gram-negative enteric bacilli (*Pseudomonas* and *Klebsiella*), and *Listeria monocytogenes.* The mortality rate is 10% to 20%.

■ T A B L E 4 – 7
Organisms Most Commonly Responsible for Bacterial Meningitis

Newborn
Group B *Streptococcus*
Escherichia coli
Listeria monocytogenes
Other Enterobacteriaceae
Infancy and Preschool
Haemophilus influenzae
Mycobacterium tuberculosis
Neisseria meningitidis
Streptococcus pneumoniae
School Age
Mycobacterium tuberculosis
Neisseria meningitidis
Streptococcus pneumoniae

CLINICAL FEATURES. Newborns infected in utero or during delivery may experience respiratory distress and shock within 24 hours of birth. Other features that may be associated with septicemia include hyperthermia, hypothermia, jaundice, hepatomegaly, lethargy, anorexia, and vomiting.

In meningitis of late onset the clinical manifestations are variable. Initial symptoms are usually nonspecific and include lethargy, disturbed feeding, and irritability. As the meningitis worsens, hyperthermia, respiratory distress or apnea, and seizures are present in about half of newborns, but bulging of the fontanelle occurs in only a quarter, and nuchal rigidity is unusual. Shock is the usual cause of death.

DIAGNOSIS. The diagnosis of septicemia and meningitis in the newborn is often difficult to establish on the basis of symptoms. Lumbar puncture must be prompted by the first suspicion of septicemia. Even in the absence of infection the cerebrospinal fluid of febrile newborns contains an average of 11 leukocytes/mm^3, with a range of 0 to 20. Less than 6% are polymorphonuclear leukocytes. The protein concentration has a mean value of 84 mg/dl (0.84 g/L), with a range from 40 to 130 mg/dl (0.4 to 1.3 g/L), and the glucose concentration has a mean value of 46 mg/dl (0.46 g/L), with a range from 36 to 56 mg/dl (0.36 to 0.56 g/L) (Bonadio et al, 1992).

In newborns with meningitis the leukocyte count is usually in the thousands and protein concentration may vary from less than 30 mg/dl (0.3 g/L) to more than 1,000 mg/dl (10 g/L). A Gram-stained smear of cerebrospinal fluid permits identification of an organism in less than half of cases (Hristeva et al 1993). Even when the smear is positive, identification may be inaccurate.

TREATMENT. Treatment is initiated with the first suspicion of sepsis. Laboratory confirmation is not required. The choice of initial antibiotic coverage varies, but usually includes ampicillin and either gentamicin or cefotaxime (Feigin et al, 1992). All antibiotics are administered intravenously in divided doses (Table 4–8). If an organism is grown on culture, specific therapy is initiated.

E. coli is best treated with ampicillin and cefotaxime, group B *Streptococcus* with penicillin or ampicillin, and *Klebsiella pneumoniae* with cefotaxime and an aminoglycoside. *Pseudomonas* is difficult to eradicate, and combined intravenous and intrathecal therapy

may be required. Carbenicillin and gentamicin are preferred for intravenous use.

Neonatal meningitis is treated for at least 2 weeks beyond the time the cerebrospinal fluid becomes sterile. Two days after antibiotic therapy is discontinued, the cerebrospinal fluid should be cultured again. If the culture is positive for bacteria, a second course of therapy is indicated.

Citrobacter diversus infections often cause a hemorrhagic necrosis of the brain with liquefaction of the cerebral white matter and abscess formation. These abscesses are readily identified on CT. Surgical drainage is seldom indicated and could cause further damage to the overlying preserved cortex.

Although the overall mortality rate for neonatal bacterial meningitis is less than 50%, significant neurologic sequelae are immediately evident in 50% of survivors. The more common sequelae include mental and motor disabilities, hydrocephalus, convulsive disorders, deafness, and vision loss. Even when the head circumference is normal, follow-up CT is often needed to exclude completely underlying hydrocephalus.

Meningitis in Infants and Young Children

For children 6 weeks to 3 months of age, group B *Streptococcus* remains a leading cause of meningitis and *E. coli* becomes less common. The other important organism is *Neisseria meningitidis* (Riordan et al, 1995). *Haemophilus influenzae*, which had been an important pathogen after 3 months of age, has almost disappeared because of routine immunization. The predominant organisms from 3 months to 5 years are now *S. pneumoniae* and *Neisseria meningitidis*.

CLINICAL FEATURES. The onset of meningitis may be insidious or fulminating. The typical clinical findings include fever, irritability, and neck stiffness. A bulging fontanelle is noted in young infants. Headache, vomiting, and lethargy are the initial features after the fontanelle has closed. Seizures occur in about a third of children with meningitis. They usually occur during the first 24 hours of illness and may be the initial feature that brings the child to medical attention. Once seizures have occurred, the state of consciousness declines. Seizures can be focal or generalized and may be difficult to control.

Examination reveals a sick and irritable child who resists being touched or moved. Ophthal-

■ TABLE 4-8
Intravenous Antibiotic Dosages for Newborns

DRUG	0-7 DAYS	8-28 DAYS
Ampicillin	100-150 mg/kg/day (q12h)	150-200 mg/kg/day (q8h)
Cefotaxime	100 mg/kg/day (q8h)	150-200 mg/kg/day (q8h)
Ceftaxidime	60 mg/kg/day (q12h)	90 mg/kg/day (q8h)
Gentamicin	5 mg/kg/day (q12h)	7.5 mg/kg/day (q8h)
Methacillin	100-150 mg/kg/day (q8h)	15-200 mg/kg/day (q6h)
Penicillin G	100,000-150,000 U/kg (q12h)	150,000-400,000 U/kg/day (q8h)
Vancomycin	20 mg/kg/day (q12h)	40-60 mg/kg/day (q6h)

moscopic findings are usually normal or show only minimal papilledema. Focal neurologic signs are unusual except in tuberculous meningitis or in cases when abscess formation has occurred.

The rapidity with which neurologic function declines depends on the severity of cerebral edema and cerebral vasculitis. Death may ensue from brainstem compression caused by transtentorial herniation. Peripheral vascular collapse can result from brainstem herniation, endotoxic shock, or adrenal failure. Sixty percent of children with meningococcemia have a characteristic petechial or hemorrhagic rash. The rash, although generalized, is most prominent below the waist.

Neck stiffness, characterized by limited mobility and pain on attempted flexion of the head, is caused by meningeal irritation. Other signs of meningeal irritation are those of Kernig and Brudzinski. Both are tested with the patient supine. The *Kernig sign* is marked by pain and resistance to extending the knee with the leg flexed at the hip; the *Brudzinski sign* is spontaneous flexion at the hips when the neck is passively flexed. These signs of meningeal irritation can be noted in subarachnoid hemorrhage as well as in infectious meningitis.

DIAGNOSIS. Lumbar puncture and examination of the cerebrospinal fluid are essential for the diagnosis of bacterial meningitis. However, because bacterial meningitis is often associated with septicemia, cultures of the blood, urine, and nasopharynx are indicated as well. The peripheral white blood cell count, especially immature granulocytes, is usually increased. Peripheral leukocytosis is much more common in bacterial than in viral infections but does not rule out viral meningitis. The platelet count is important because some infections are associated with thrombocytopenia. Blood glucose concentration must be measured concurrently for proper evaluation of the cerebrospinal fluid

concentration of glucose. Serum electrolytes, especially sodium, should be measured as well. Inappropriate antidiuretic hormone secretion is present in the majority of patients with acute bacterial meningitis. A tuberculin skin test should be administered to every child at risk for tuberculous meningitis.

Lumbar puncture must be performed as quickly as possible when bacterial meningitis is suspected. It has become routine to perform a cranial CT before doing a lumbar puncture, a routine that is of questionable value medically and adds considerably to the cost of care. Generalized increased intracranial pressure is always part of acute bacterial meningitis and is not a contraindication to lumbar puncture.

Information to be derived from the procedure includes opening and closing pressures, appearance, white blood cell count with differential count, red blood cell count, concentrations of glucose and protein, and identification of microorganisms as shown by Gram stain and culture. The characteristic findings are increased pressure, a cloudy appearance, a cellular response of several thousand polymorphonuclear leukocytes, a reduction in the concentration of glucose to less than half of that in the plasma, and an elevated protein concentration. However, the expected findings of bacterial meningitis may vary with the organism, the timing of the lumbar puncture, the prior use of antibiotics, and the immunocompetence of the host.

TREATMENT. Antimicrobials and dexamethasone should be administered immediately. Treatment should not be delayed until after lumbar puncture results are obtained, especially when lumbar puncture is preceded by CT. Dexamethasone is administered as 0.15 mg/kg every 6 hours for 4 days. Children treated with dexamethasone become afebrile more quickly and have an improved neurologic outcome and a lower incidence of postmeningitic deafness (Odio et al, 1991).

Ampicillin and chloramphenicol had been the standard initial therapy for infants and children younger than 5 years of age in whom bacterial meningitis was suspected before identification of the offending organism. However, newer cephalosporins (cefotaxime, ceftriaxone, and cefuroxime) are now considered the therapy of choice in the initial treatment of meningitis (Feigin et al, 1992). Gram-stain identification is useful, but can be misleading, and the final choice of antibiotic therapy should await the results of culture and antibiotic sensitivity.

Several special cases exist in the choice of initial antimicrobials to treat bacterial meningitis. Meningitis in children with a ventricular shunt in place is usually caused by a staphylococcal species and nafcillin may be added to the preceding choices or given alone if gram-positive cocci are present on smear. Meningitis secondary to chronic sinusitis or dental infection is frequently caused by anaerobic and aerobic organisms. Penicillin G and chloramphenicol are therefore reasonable choices for initial therapy, although cefotaxime may be needed for some gram-negative organisms not covered by chloramphenicol. Meningitis following trauma is usually caused by *S. pneumoniae,* whereas meningitis following neurosurgical procedures may be due to either streptococcal or staphylococcal organisms. Gram-negative organisms may be responsible as well, and a combination of penicillin G and cefotaxime is recommended.

Once a specific organism is identified, an appropriate antibiotic or combination of antibiotics is then chosen (Table 4–9).

The outcome for infants and children with bacterial meningitis depends on the infecting organism and the speed with which appropriate antibiotic therapy is initiated. Ten percent of children have persistent bilateral or unilateral hearing loss following bacterial meningitis, and 4% have neurologic deficits. The incidence of hearing loss is 31% following infection with *S. pneumoniae* and 6% with *H. influenzae.* Hearing loss occurs early and is probably not related to the choice of antibiotic. Children with neurologic deficits are at risk for epilepsy (Pomeroy et al, 1990).

Meningitis in School-Age Children

S. pneumoniae, and *N. meningitidis,* and *H. influenzae* account for most cases of bacterial meningitis in previously healthy school-age children in the United States, whereas *Mycobacterium tuberculosis* is a leading cause of menin-

■ TABLE 4–9
Intravenous Antibiotic Dosages for Children

DRUG	DOSAGE
Amikacin	20-30 mg/kg/day (q8h)
Ampicillin	200-300 mg/kg/day (q6h)
Cefotaxime	200 mg/kg/day (q6h)
Ceftriaxone	80-100 mg/kg/day (q12h)
Ceftrazidime	125-150 mg/kg/day (q8h)
Chloramphenicol	75-100 mg/kg/day (q6h)
Gentamicin	7.5 mg/kg/day (q8h)
Penicillin G	250,000 units/kg/day (q6h)
Tobramycin	6 mg/kg/day (q8h)
Vancomycin	40-60 mg/kg/day (q6h)

gitis in economically deprived populations. The symptoms of bacterial meningitis in school-age children do not differ substantially from those encountered in preschool children. The reader is referred to the previous section on clinical features and treatment.

Penicillin G is the treatment of choice for *S. pneumoniae* or *N. meningitidis.*

In one retrospective study of children who had been treated for bacterial meningitis in the 1980s, 8.5% had major neurologic deficits (mental retardation, seizures, hydrocephalus, cerebral palsy, blindness, or hearing loss) and 18.5% had learning disabilities (Grimwood et al, 1995).

Tuberculous Meningitis

Worldwide, tuberculosis remains a leading cause of morbidity and death in children. In the United States, it represents less than 5% of bacterial meningitis cases in children but occurs with higher frequency where sanitation is poor. Children are infected by inhalation of the organism from adults. Tuberculosis occurs first in the lungs and is then disseminated to other organs within 6 months.

CLINICAL FEATURES. The peak incidence of tuberculous meningitis is between 6 months and 2 years of age. First symptoms tend to be more insidious than with other bacterial meningitides, but they sometimes progress in a fulminating fashion. Tuberculous meningitis, unlike fungal meningitis, is not a cause of chronic meningitis. If not treated the child with tuberculous meningitis will die within 3 to 5 weeks.

Most often, fever develops first and the child becomes listless and irritable. Irritability may be caused in part by headache, which is a common feature. Vomiting and abdominal pain are sometimes associated. Headache and vomiting increase in frequency and severity and are accompanied by signs of meningismus during the second week after onset of fever. Cerebral infarction occurs in 30% to 40% of affected children. Seizures may occur early, but more often occur after meningismus is established. Consciousness declines progressively, and focal neurologic deficits are noted. Most common are cranial neuropathies and hemipareses. Papilledema occurs relatively early in the course.

DIAGNOSIS. Tuberculosis must be considered in any child with a household contact. General use of tuberculin skin testing in children is critical to early detection. In the early stages, children with tuberculous meningitis may have only fever. The peripheral white blood cell count is generally elevated to between 10,000 and 20,000 cells/mm^3. Hyponatremia and hypochloremia are frequently present because of inappropriate secretion of antidiuretic hormone. The cerebrospinal fluid is usually cloudy and increased in pressure. The leukocyte count in the cerebrospinal fluid may range from 10 to 250 cells/mm^3 and rarely exceeds 500. Lymphocytes predominate. The glucose concentration declines throughout the course of the illness and is generally less than 35 mg/dl (1.8 mmol/L). Conversely, the protein concentration increases steadily and is usually greater than 100 mg/dl (1 g/L).

Smears of cerebrospinal fluid stained by the acid-fast technique generally demonstrate the bacillus. Recovery of the organism from the cerebrospinal fluid is not always successful even when guinea pig inoculation is used.

Cranial CT is useful to show basilar enhancement, cerebral infarction, hydrocephalus, and tuberculoma (Curless and Mitchell, 1991).

TREATMENT. The prognosis for survival and for neurologic recovery is enhanced by early treatment. Once a child's skin test is positive for the organism, isoniazid therapy is initiated even if the child is asymptomatic. Complete neurologic recovery is unlikely once the child becomes comatose. Mortality rates of 20% are recorded even when treatment is initiated early.

The recommended initial drug regimen for treatment of tuberculous meningitis in the first 2 months is isoniazid, 20 mg/kg/day orally up to 500 mg/day; streptomycin, 20 mg/kg/day intramuscularly up to 1 g/day until drug susceptibility is known; rifampin, 15 mg/kg/day orally up to 600 mg/day, and pyrazinamide 30 mg/kg/day. Isoniazid and rifampin are continued for an additional 10 months (Committee on Infectious Disease, 1994a). The use of corticosteroids to reduce inflammation is an appropriate method to reduce inflammation and cerebral edema.

Communicating hydrocephalus is a common complication of tuberculous meningitis because of impaired reabsorption of cerebrospinal fluid. The size of the ventricles must be assessed by CT at periodic intervals and whenever unexplained deterioration of mental function occurs. Before the infection is brought under control, communicating hydrocephalus may be treated by repeated lumbar punctures and acetazolamide. In many cases obstructive hydrocephalus develops later; in those cases a surgical shunt is required.

Brain Abscess

The factors commonly predisposing to pyogenic brain abscess in children are meningitis, chronic otitis media, sinusitis, and congenital heart disease (Brook, 1992; Tekkok and Erbengi, 1992). Brain abscesses in the newborn are almost always the result of meningitis caused by *C. diversus* and other species of Enterobacteriaceae. Pyogenic abscesses in children younger than 5 months but beyond the neonatal period are uncommon and most often occur in children with hydrocephalus and shunt infection. The organisms most often responsible are species of *Staphylococcus.*

After 5 months of age the infecting organisms are diverse, and many abscesses contain a mixed flora. Coagulase-positive *S. aureus* and anaerobic *Streptococcus* are the organisms most frequently recovered, but no organism is recovered in up to 20% of cases.

CLINICAL FEATURES. The clinical features of brain abscess, like those of any other space-occupying lesion, depend on the age of the child and the location of the mass. Encapsulation of the abscess is preceded by a period of cerebritis characterized by fever, headache, and lethargy. Seizures may also occur but in the absence of seizures the initial symptoms may not be severe enough to arouse suspicion of cerebral infection. If the period of cerebritis is not recognized, the initial clinical manifestations are the same as with other mass lesions. Infants have abnormal head growth, a bulging fontanelle, failure to thrive, and sometimes seizures. Older children show signs of increased intracranial pressure and focal neurologic dysfunction. Fever is present in only 60% of cases, and meningeal irritation is relatively uncommon. Therefore, on the basis of clinical features alone, pyogenic brain abscess is difficult to separate from other mass lesions such as brain tumor. About 80% of abscesses are in the cerebral hemispheres. Hemiparesis, hemianopia, and seizures are the usual clinical features.

Cerebellar abscess most often results from chronic otitis and is manifest as nystagmus and ataxia.

DIAGNOSIS. The combination of headache and papilledema, with or without focal neurologic dysfunction, suggests the possibility of a mass lesion and calls for CT. Most abscesses appear as an area of decreased density surrounded by a rim of intense enhancement referred to as *a ring lesion.* This lesion, although characteristic, is not diagnostic. Malignant brain tumors may have a similar appearance. Ring enhancement occurs during the late stages of cerebritis, just before capsule formation. After the capsule forms, the diameter of the ring decreases and the center becomes more hypodense. Multiple abscesses may be present.

TREATMENT. The development of CT has altered the management of cerebral abscess. Previously, surgical drainage was initiated as soon as abscess formation was identified. Now even encapsulated abscesses are treated medically and the progress followed with serial scans.

The initial step in treatment is to reduce brain swelling by the use of corticosteroids. This is followed by an intravenous antibiotic regimen that generally includes a penicillinase-resistant penicillin such as methicillin, 300 mg/kg/day, and chloramphenicol, 100 mg/kg/day. This combination is selected for its effectiveness against *Staphylococcus* and mixed gram-negative organisms. If an organism can be identified by culture of spinal fluid or blood, more specific antibiotic therapy is selected. In general, penicillin G is preferable to ampicillin if penicillin-sensitive organisms are recovered.

If medical therapy does not resolve the abscess, surgical drainage is necessary. Even in such cases, prolonged medical therapy before surgery increases the success of total excision.

Subdural and Epidural Empyema

Meningitis in infants and sinusitis in older children are the most common factors causing infection in the subdural space. The subdural space is sterile in children with bacterial meningitis but can become contaminated by organisms if a subdural tap is performed before the subarachnoid space is sterilized with antibiotics or by secondary thrombophlebitis of perforating cerebral veins. In older children subdural and epidural abscesses are usually caused by penetrating head injuries or chronic mastoiditis.

Infections of the subdural space are difficult to contain and may extend over an entire hemisphere.

CLINICAL FEATURES. Subdural empyema produces increased intracranial pressure because of mass effect, cerebral edema, and vasculitis. Vasculitis leads to thrombosis of cortical veins, resulting in focal neurologic dysfunction as well as increased intracranial pressure. Children with subdural infections are very sick. They have headache, fever, vomiting, seizures, and states of decreasing consciousness. Unilateral and alternating hemipareses are common. Children who are comatose have papilledema.

DIAGNOSIS. Subdural empyema should be suspected in children with meningitis whose condition declines after an initial period of recovery or in children who continue to have increased intracranial pressure of uncertain cause. Examination of the cerebrospinal fluid may not be helpful; sometimes the fluid is normal. The usual abnormality is a mixed cellular response, generally less than 100 cells/mm^3, with a lymphocytic predominance. The glucose concentration is normal, and the protein concentration is only mildly elevated.

CT is particularly helpful in showing a subdural or epidural abscess. The infected collection appears as a lens-shaped mass of increased lucency just beneath the skull. A shift of midline structures is generally present.

In infants, subdural puncture can provide a specimen of the abscess for identification of the organism. Subdural puncture can also be used to drain much of the abscess.

TREATMENT. The child with subdural or epidural empyema must be treated with corticosteroids to decrease intracranial pressure, antibiotics to eradicate the organisms, and anticonvulsants for seizures. Surgical drainage of subdural empyema had been considered an absolute necessity; it now appears that some can be treated medically, using CT to monitor progress.

FUNGAL INFECTIONS

Fungi exist in two forms: molds and yeasts. Molds are filamentous and divided into segments by hyphae. Yeasts are unicellular organisms surrounded by a thick cell wall and sometimes a capsule. Several fungi exist as yeast in tissue but are filamentous when grown in culture. Such fungi are said to be dimorphic. The common fungal pathogens are listed in Table 4–10.

Fungal infections of the central nervous system may cause an acute, subacute, or chronic

■ TABLE 4-10
Common Fungal Pathogens

Yeast Forms
Cryptococcus neoformans
Candida
Dimorphic Forms
Histoplasma capsulatum
Blastomyces dermatitidis
Coccidioides immitis
Mold Forms
Aspergillus species

meningitis; solitary or multiple abscesses; and granulomas. Fungal infections of the nervous system are most common in children who are immunosuppressed, especially those with leukemia or acidosis. Fungal infections also occur in children who are immunocompetent. *Cryptococcus neoformans* and *Coccidioides immitis* are the leading causes of fungal meningitis in immunocompetent children.

Candidal Meningoencephalitis

Candida is a common inhabitant of the mouth, vagina, and intestinal tract. Ordinarily it causes no symptoms; however, it can multiply and become an important pathogen in children who are immunosuppressed, taking multiple antibiotics, suffering from debilitating diseases, and being treated with long-term vascular catheters. The most common sites of infection are the mouth (thrush), skin, and vagina. Candidal meningitis is almost unheard of in normal, non-hospitalized children.

CLINICAL FEATURES. *Candida* reaches the brain and other organs by vascular dissemination. The brain is less often involved than other organs, and the prominent features of candidal sepsis include fever, lethargy, and vomiting. Hepatosplenomegaly and arthritis may be present.

Cerebral involvement can be in the form of meningitis, abscess formation, or both. The clinical features of meningoencephalitis are fever, vomiting, meningismus, papilledema, and seizures leading to states of decreased consciousness. In some individuals a single large cerebral abscess forms that causes focal neurologic dysfunction and papilledema.

DIAGNOSIS. Cerebral candidiasis should be suspected when unexplained fever develops in children with risk factors for disseminated disease. The organism can be isolated from blood,

joint effusion fluid, or cerebrospinal fluid. When meningitis is present, a predominantly neutrophilic response is present in the cerebrospinal fluid associated with a protein concentration that is generally 100 mg/dl (1 g/L). The glucose concentration is only slightly reduced. Children who have a candidal abscess rather than meningitis are likely to have normal or near-normal cerebrospinal fluid. A mass lesion resembling a pyogenic abscess or tumor is seen on CT.

TREATMENT. When candidal infections develop in children because of indwelling vascular catheters, the catheter must be removed. Amphotericin B and flucytosine are used together and are thought to have a synergistic effect. Dosages are the same as for other fungal infections, and the drugs should be administered for 6 to 12 weeks, depending on the efficacy of therapy and presence of adverse reactions.

Coccidioidomycosis

C. immitis is endemic in the San Joaquin Valley of California and all southwestern states. Infection is by inhalation; almost 90% of individuals become infected within 10 years of moving into an endemic area. Only 40% of patients become symptomatic, the other 60% are identified only by positive skin test.

CLINICAL FEATURES. Malaise, fever, cough, myalgia, and chest pain follow respiratory infection.

The pulmonary infection is self-limited. The fungus is disseminated from the lung to other organs in only 1 person in 400. The dissemination rate is considerably higher in infants than in older children and adults.

Coccidioidal meningitis is almost always caused by hematogenous spread from lung to meninges but sometimes occurs by direct extension following infection of the skull. Symptoms of meningitis develop 2 to 4 weeks after respiratory symptoms begin. The main features are headache, apathy, and confusion. These symptoms may persist for weeks or months without concurrent seizures, meningismus, or focal neurologic disturbances. If the meningitis is allowed to become chronic, hydrocephalus eventually develops because the basilar meningitis prevents reabsorption of cerebrospinal fluid.

DIAGNOSIS. Coccidioidal meningitis should be suspected in patients living in endemic areas when headache develops following an acute respiratory infection. Skin hypersensitivity among individuals living in an endemic area is not helpful, because a large percentage of the population is exposed and has a skin test positive for the organism. The cerebrospinal fluid generally demonstrates increased pressure and a lymphocytic cellular response of 50 to 500 cells/mm^3. Eosinophils are frequently present as well. The protein concentration ranges from 100 to 500 mg/dl (1 to 5 g/L), and the glucose concentration is less than 35 mg/dl (1.8 mmol/L). The diagnosis is confirmed by isolation of the fungus, but this is often difficult to accomplish. Complement-fixing antibodies appear in the blood and in the cerebrospinal fluid. A positive serologic test in the cerebrospinal fluid is diagnostic, but false-negative results are possible.

TREATMENT. Amphotericin B is the drug of choice for coccidioidal meningitis. It must be administered both intravenously (Table 4–11) and intrathecally. The initial intrathecal dose is 0.1 mg for the first three injections and is then increased to 0.25 to 0.5 mg three or four times each week. Treatment must be prolonged, and some recommend that weekly intrathecal injections be continued indefinitely. Adverse reactions to intrathecal administration include aseptic meningitis and pain in the back and legs.

Miconazole may be administered intravenously and intrathecally to patients unable to tolerate high doses of amphotericin B. Ketoconazole, a synthetic antifungal agent, has excellent activity against *C. immitis* in culture, but penetrates the cerebrospinal fluid poorly. It is not recommended for systemic treatment of coccidioidal meningitis.

Cryptococcal Meningitis

C. neoformans is carried by birds, especially pigeons, and is widely disseminated in soil. Human infection is acquired by inhalation. The organism is disseminated in the blood but has a predilection for the central nervous system. It is an important cause of subacute and chronic meningoencephalitis.

CLINICAL FEATURES. Cryptococcal meningitis is uncommon before age 10 and perhaps only 10% of cases occur before age 20. Males are affected more often than females. Most children with cryptococcal meningitis are immunocompetent.

First symptoms are usually insidious; chronic headache is the major feature. The headache waxes and wanes, but eventually becomes continuous and associated with nausea, vomit-

■ T A B L E   4 – 11
Dosage Schedule for Amphotericin B

Amphotericin B is first administered intravenously in a single test dose of 0.1 mg/kg (not to exceed 1 mg) over at least 20 minutes to assess the child's temperature and blood pressure responses. If the response is acceptable, the first therapeutic dose of 0.25 mg/kg is administered over 2 hours the same day as the test dose. The dose is increased in daily increments of 0.1 to 0.25 mg/kg, depending on the severity of infection, until the daily maintenance dose of 1 mg/kg is achieved. In life-threatening situations, daily dosages of 1.25 to 1.5 mg/kg may be needed.

ing, and lethargy. Body temperature may remain normal, especially in older children and adults, but younger children often have low-grade fever. Personality and behavioral changes are relatively common. The child becomes moody, listless, and sometimes frankly psychotic. Increased intracranial pressure is characterized by blurred vision, diplopia, and papilledema. Seizures and focal neurologic dysfunction are not early features but are signs of vasculitis, hydrocephalus, and granuloma formation.

DIAGNOSIS. The diagnosis of cryptococcal meningitis is often missed even when suspected. The cerebrospinal fluid may be normal but more often shows an increased opening pressure and a lymphocytic leukocytosis that generally averages fewer than 100 cells/mm^3. The protein concentration is almost always elevated, generally greater than 100 mg/dl (1 g/L), and the glucose concentration is usually less than 40 mg/dl (2 mmol/L). Rapid diagnosis is possible by showing the fungus on cerebrospinal fluid sediment by the India ink technique. The cryptococcus is the only encapsulated fungus to invade the central nervous system and has a characteristic appearance on smear. However, the organism is not usually present in the lumbar subarachnoid space and must be obtained from cerebrospinal fluid at the base of the brain. This can be achieved either by removing large volumes of cerebrospinal fluid by lumbar puncture or by cisternal puncture.

Diagnosis has been made easier by the development of a latex agglutination test that reacts to the polysaccharide capsule of the organism. The test is reasonably accurate but may produce false-negative results, and serologic studies do not replace the actual demonstration of the organism. The latex agglutination technique can also be performed on the cerebrospinal fluid, and titers of 1:8 or greater are considered significant and support the diagnosis of cryptococcal meningitis.

TREATMENT. The treatment of choice is intravenous amphotericin B combined with oral flucytosine (Committee on Infectious Disease, 1994b). Amphotericin B is given intravenously diluted with 5% dextrose and water in a drug concentration no greater than 1 mg/10 ml of fluid. Nephrotoxicity is the limiting factor in achieving desirable blood levels. The intravenous regimen is generally the same for all fungal infections of the nervous system and is summarized in Table 4-11. The total dose varies with the response and the side effects, but is usually in the range of 1500 to 2000 mg/1.7 m^2 of body surface.

The toxic effects include chills, fever, nausea, and vomiting. Anemia and nephrotoxicity must be monitored with frequent blood counts and urinalyses. Renal impairment is manifested by the appearance of cells or casts in the urine, elevated blood urea nitrogen concentration, and decreased creatinine clearance. When renal impairment occurs, the drug must be discontinued and restarted at a lower dose.

Flucytosine is given orally at a dosage of 50 to 150 mg/kg/day in four divided doses at 6-hour intervals. Cytopenia limits its use. Seriously ill patients, treated late in the course of the disease, should also be given intrathecally administered amphotericin B and miconazole.

The efficacy of therapy can be followed by showing a decline of the agglutination titer in the cerebrospinal fluid. Periodic CT is necessary to monitor the development of hydrocephalus.

Other Fungal Infections

Histoplasmosis is endemic in the central United States and causes pulmonary infection. Miliary spread is unusual. Neurologic histoplasmosis may take the form of leptomeningitis, focal abscess, or multiple granulomas. Blastomycosis is primarily a disease of North America. It reaches the brain by hematogenous spread from the lungs and produces multiple abscesses that give the appearance of metastatic disease on CT. Cellular response in the cerebrospinal fluid is markedly increased when fungi produce meningitis and may be normal or only mildly increased when abscess formation occurs. Amphotericin B is the mainstay of therapy for fungal infections; miconazole is used in combination with amphotericin B against *Histoplasma capsulatum*.

■ TABLE 4-12
Causes of Pseudotumor Cerebri

Drugs
Corticosteroid withdrawal
Nalidixic acid
Oral contraceptives
Tetracycline
Thyroid replacement
Vitamin A

Systemic Disorders
Guillain-Barré syndrome
Iron deficiency anemia
Leukemia
Polycythemia vera
Protein malnutrition
Systemic lupus erythematosus
Vitamin A deficiency
Vitamin D deficiency

Head Trauma

Infections
Otitis media
Sinusitis

Metabolic Disorders
Adrenal insufficiency
Diabetic ketoacidosis (treatment)
Galactosemia
Hyperadrenalism
Hyperthyroidism
Hypoparathyroidism
Pregnancy

 ## Idiopathic Intracranial Hypertension (Pseudotumor Cerebri)

The term *pseudotumor cerebri* is used to characterize a syndrome of increased intracranial pressure, normal cerebrospinal fluid content, and a normal brain with normal or small ventricles on brain imaging studies. The syndrome may have an identifiable underlying cause or may be idiopathic. A specific cause can usually be found in children younger than 6 years of age, while most idiopathic cases occur after age 11. Some causes of pseudotumor are listed in Table 4-12. A cause-and-effect relationship has not been established in all of these conditions. The most frequent causes are otitis media, head trauma, the use of certain drugs and vitamins, and feeding following malnutrition.

CLINICAL FEATURES. Both sexes are affected equally and many affected children are overweight (Babikian et al, 1994). The initial features are headache (63%), vomiting (43%), and diplopia (36%). Young children may have only irritability, somnolence, or apathy. Less common symptoms are transient visual obscurations, neck stiffness, tinnitus, paresthesias, and ataxia. Most children are not acutely ill, and mentation is normal.

Neurologic examination is unremarkable except for papilledema and abducens nerve palsy. No signs of focal neurologic dysfunction are observed. The major concern is for vision. If the syndrome is left untreated, some children have progressive papilledema and optic atrophy. Loss of vision may be rapid and severe. Early diagnosis and treatment are therefore essential to preserve vision.

DIAGNOSIS. Pseudotumor cerebri is a diagnosis of exclusion. If a child has headache and papilledema, a brain imaging study is needed to exclude a mass lesion or hydrocephalus. Results of imaging studies are usually normal in children with pseudotumor cerebri. In some the ventricles are small and the normal sulcal markings may be obliterated by the increased cerebral volume.

Underlying causes of pseudotumor cerebri must be excluded by careful history and physical examination. Ordinarily these are easily identified.

TREATMENT. The goals of therapy are to relieve headache and preserve vision. A single lumbar puncture, with the closing pressure reduced to half of the opening pressure, is sufficient to reverse the process in many cases. The mechanism by which this is effective is unknown, but a transitory change in cerebrospinal fluid dynamics seem to sufficient to readjust the pressure.

Children with pseudotumor cerebri are commonly treated with acetazolamide, 10 mg/kg/day, following the initial lumbar puncture. Whether this is an important addition to lumbar puncture is not clear. If symptoms return, lumbar puncture should be repeated on subsequent days. Serial lumbar punctures are rarely needed.

Occasionally children continue to have increased intracranial pressure and evidence of progressive optic neuropathy despite the use of lumbar puncture and acetazolamide. In such patients studies should be repeated to look for a cause other than idiopathic pseudotumor cerebri. If none is found, a 2-week course of dexamethasone is appropriate. If this fails to relieve symptoms, optic nerve fenestration or lumboperitoneal shunt may be needed.

REFERENCES

Babikian P, Corbett J, Bell W. Idiopathic intracranial hypertension in children: The Iowa experience. J Child Neurol 1994;9:144-149.

Bonadio WA, Stanco L, Bruce R, et al. Reference values of normal cerebrospinal fluid composition in infants ages 0 to 8 weeks. Pediatr Infect Dis J 1992;11:589-591.

Brook I. Aerobic and anaerobic bacteriology of intracranial abscesses. Pediatr Neurol 1992;8:210-214.

Committee on Infectious Disease. Tuberculosis. The Redbook. 23rd edition. American Academy of Pediatrics, Elk Grove Village, IL, 1994a;480-500.

Committee on Infectious Disease. Ampoteracin B. The Redbook. 23rd edition. American Academy of Pediatrics, Elk Grove Village, IL, 1994b;562-564.

Curless RG, Mitchell CD. Central nervous system tuberculosis in children. Pediatr Neurol 1991;7:270-274.

De Volder AG, Michel CH, Thauvoy C, et al. Brain glucose utilisation in acquired childhood aphasia associated with a sylvan arachnoid cyst: Recovery after shunting as demonstrated by PET. J Neurol Neurosurg Psychiatry 1994;57:296-300.

Dykes FD, Dunbar B, Lazarra A, et al. Posthemorrhagic hydrocephalus in high-risk premature infants: Natural history, management and long-term outcome. J Pediatr 1989;114:611-618.

Ellenbogen RG, Winston KR, Kupsky WJ. Tumors of the choroid plexus in children. Neurosurgery 1989;25:327-335.

Feigin RD, McCracken GH Jr, Klein JO. Diagnosis and management of meningitis. Pediatr Infect Dis 1992;11:785-814.

Germano IM, Edwards MSB, Davis RL, et al. Intracranial meningiomas of the first two decades of life. J Neurosurg 1994;80:447-453.

Grimwood K, Anderson VA, Bond L, et al. Adverse outcome of bacterial meningitis in school-age survivors. Pediatrics 1995;95:646-656.

Hristeva L, Bowler I, Booy R, et al. Value of cerebrospinal fluid examination in the diagnosis of meningitis in the newborn. Arch Dis Child 1993;69:514-517.

Hudgins RJ, Boydston WR, Hudgins PA, et al. Treatment of intraventricular hemorrhage in the premature infant with urokinase. A preliminary report. Pediatr Neurosurg 1994;20:190-197.

Ito M, Yoshihara M, Ishii M, et al. Cerebral aneurysms in children. Brain Dev 1992;14:263-268.

Lasjaunias P, Hui F, Zerah M, et al. Cerebral arteriovenous malformations in children. Management of 179 consecutive cases and review of literature. Child Nerv Syst 1995;11:66-79.

Le Roux PD, Jardine DS, Loeser JD. Pediatric intracranial pressure monitoring in hypoxic and nonhypoxic brain injury. Child Nerv Syst 1991;7:34-39.

Mangiardi JR, Daras M, Geller ME, et al. Cocaine-related intracranial hemorrhage. Report of nine cases and review. Acta Neurol Scand 1988;77:177-180.

Marro PJ, Dransfield DA, Mott SM, et al. Posthemorrhagic hydrocephalus. Use of an intravenous-type catheter for cerebrospinal fluid drainage. Am J Dis Child 1991;145:1141-1146.

Oberbauer RW, Haase J, Pucher R. Arachnoid cysts in children: A European co-operative study. Child Nerv Syst 1992;8:281-286.

Odio CM, Faingezicht I, Paris M, et al. The beneficial effects of early dexamethasone administration in infants and children with bacterial meningitis. N Engl J Med 1991;324:1525-1531.

Philip AG, Allen WC, Tito AM, et al. Intraventricular hemorrhage in premature infants: Declining incidence in the 1980s. Pediatrics 1989;84:797-801.

Pollack IF. Brain tumors in children. N Engl J Med 1994;331:1500-1507.

Pollack IF, Claassen D, al-Shboul Q, et al. Low-grade gliomas of the cerebral hemispheres in children: An analysis of 71 cases. J Neurosurg 1995;82:536-547.

Pomeroy SL, Holmes SJ, Dodge PR, et al. Seizures and other neurologic sequelae of bacterial meningitis in children. N Engl J Med 1990;323:1651-1657.

Raps EC, Rogers JD, Galetta SL, et al. The clinical spectrum of unruptured intracranial aneurysms. Arch Neurol 1993; 50:265-268.

Riordan FAI, Thomson APJ, Sills Ja, et al. Bacterial meningitis in the first three months of life. Postgrad Med J 1995;71: 36-38.

Sposto R, Ertel IJ, Jenkins RDT, et al. The effectiveness of chemotherapy for treatment of high grade astrocytomas in children: Results of a randomized trial. A report of the Children's Cancer Study Group. J Neurooncol 1989;7: 433-440.

Tekkok IH, Erbengi A. Management of brain abscess in children: Review of 130 cases over a period of 21 years. Child Nerv Syst 1992;8:411-416.

Tomita T, McLone DG, Yasue M. Cerebral primitive neuroectodermal tumors in childhood. Neurooncol 1988;6: 233-243.

Vannucci RC: Current and potentially new management strategies for perinatal hypoxicischemic encephalopathy. Pediatrics 1990;85:961-968.

Vanuytsel IJ, Bessell EM, Ashley SE, et al. Intracranial ependymoma: Long-term results of a policy of surgery and radiotherapy. Int J Radiat Oncol Biol Phys 1992;23:313-319.

Volpe JJ. Intraventricular hemorrhage in the premature infant: Current concepts. Part II. Ann Neurol 1989;25:3, 109-116.

5

Psychomotor Retardation and Regression

The diagnosis of psychomotor retardation differential (developmental delay) is quite different from that of psychomotor regression. Slow progress in the attainment of developmental milestones may be caused by either a static (Table 5-1) or a progressive (Table 5-2) encephalopathy. In contrast, the loss of developmental milestones previously attained usually indicates a progressive disease of the nervous system but may also be caused by a parental misperception of attained milestones or the development of new clinical features from an established static disorder as the brain matures (Table 5-3).

 Developmental Delay

Delayed achievement of developmental milestones is one of the more common problems evaluated by child neurologists. Two important questions must be asked: (1) Is delay restricted to specific areas of development or is it global? (2) Is there only developmental delay, or is there also developmental regression?

The second question is often difficult to answer in regard to infants. Even in static encephalopathies, new symptoms such as involuntary movements and seizures may occur as the child gets older, and delayed acquisition of milestones without other neurologic deficits is

sometimes the initial feature of progressive disorders. However, once it is clear that milestones previously achieved have been lost or that focal neurologic deficits are evolving, a progressive disease of the nervous system must be considered.

The Denver Developmental Screening Test (DDST) is an efficient and reliable method for assessing development in the physician's office. It rapidly assesses four different components of development: personal-social, fine motor adaptive, language, and gross motor. The results can be amplified by several psychometric tests, but the DDST in combination with neurologic assessment provides sufficient information to initiate further diagnostic studies.

LANGUAGE DELAY

Normal infants and children have a remarkable facility for acquiring language. Infants and young children who are concurrently exposed to two languages usually learn both. Vocalization of vowels occurs in the first month, and laughing and squealing are well established by 5 months. At 6 months infants begin articulating consonants, usually M, D, and B. Parents translate these to mean "mama," "dada," and bottle or baby, although this is certainly not the infant's intention. These first attempts at vowels and conso-

■ T A B L E 5 – 1

Diagnosis of Developmental Delay: No Regression

Predominant Speech Delay
1. Hearing loss
2. Infantile autism
3. Pseudobulbar palsy (see Chapter 17)

Predominant Motor Delay
1. Ataxia (see Chapter 10)
2. Hemiplegia (see Chapter 11)
3. Hypotonia (see Chapter 6)
4. Paraplegia (see Chapter 12)

Global Delay
1. Cerebral malformations
2. Chromosomal disturbances
3. Intrauterine infection
4. Perinatal disorders
5. Progressive encephalopathies (see Table 5–2)

■ T A B L E 5 – 2

Progressive Encephalopathy: Onset Before Age 2

Acquired Immune Deficiency Disease Encephalopathy

Disorders of Amino Acid Metabolism
Homocystinuria
Maple syrup urine disease
  Intermediate form
  Thiamine-responsive form
Phenylketonuria

Disorders of Enzymes
Ganglioside storage disorders
  GM_1 gangliosidosis (types I and II)
  GM_2 gangliosidosis (Tay-Sachs disease, Sandhoff disease)
Gaucher disease type II (glucosylceramide lipidosis)
Globoid cell leukodystrophy (Krabbe disease)
Glycoprotein degradation disorders
  Mannosidosis type I
  Fucosidoses types I and II
  Sialidosis type II (infantile form)
I-cell disease
Mucopolysaccharidoses
  Type I (Hurler syndrome)
  Type II (Sanfilippo disease)
Niemann-Pick disease type A
Sulfatase-deficiency disorders
  Metachromatic leukodystrophy (sulfatide lipidoses)
  Multiple sulfatase deficiency

Hypothyroidism

Mitochondrial Disorders
Mitochondrial myopathy, encephalopathy, lactic acidosis, and stroke (see Chapter 11)
Progressive infantile poliodystrophy (Alpers disease)
Subacute necrotizing encephalomyelopathy (Leigh disease)
Trichopoliodystrophy (Menkes disease)

Neurocutaneous Syndromes
Chediak-Higashi syndrome
Neurofibromatosis
Tuberous sclerosis

Other Disorders of Gray Matter
Infantile ceroid lipofuscinosis (Santavuori disease)
Infantile neuroaxonal dystrophy
Lesch-Nyhan disease
Progressive neuronal degeneration with liver disease
Rett syndrome

Other Disorders of White Matter
Alexander disease
Aspartoacylase deficiency (Canavan disease)
Galactosemia: transferase deficiency
Neonatal adrenoleukodystrophy (see Chapter 6)
Pelizaeus-Merzbacher disease

Progressive Hydrocephalus

nants are automatic and sometimes occur even in deaf children. In the months that follow, the infant imitates many speech sounds, babbles and coos, and finally learns the specific use of "mama" and "dada" by 1 year of age. Receptive skills are always more highly developed than expressive skills, because it is necessary to decode language before it can be encoded. By 2 years of age children have learned to combine at least two words, understand more than 250 words, and follow many simple verbal directions.

Hearing Impairment

The major cause of isolated delay in speech development is a hearing impairment (see Chapter 17). Hearing loss may occur concomitantly with global developmental retardation, as in rubella embryopathy, cytomegalic inclusion disease, neonatal meningitis, kernicterus, and several genetic disorders. Hearing loss need not be profound; it can be insidious, yet delay speech development. The loss of high-frequency tones inherent in telephone conversation prevents the clear distinction of many consonants that we learn to fill in through experience; infants do not have experience in supplying missing sounds.

The hearing of any infant with isolated delay in speech development should be tested by audiometry. Crude testing in the office by slamming objects and ringing bells is inadequate. Hearing loss should be suspected in children with global retardation caused by disorders ordinarily associated with hearing loss or in retarded children who fail to imitate sounds. Other clues to hearing loss in children are excessive gesturing and staring at the lips of people who are talking.

Infantile Autism

Infantile autism is now conceptualized as a behavioral disorder caused by abnormal brain development from many different causes. Migrational defects are sometimes identified by

■ T A B L E 5 – 3
Causes of Apparent Regression in Static Encephalopathy

Parental misperception of attained milestones
New-onset seizures
Increasing spasticity (usually during the first year)
New-onset movement disorders (usually during the
 second year)
Progressive hydrocephalus

positron emission tomography in children with typical autism (Schifter et al, 1994), and some children with tuberous sclerosis and with the fragile X syndrome display autistic behavior (Tuchman 1991).

CLINICAL FEATURES. The major diagnostic criteria are failure of language development, severe impairment of interpersonal relationships, a restricted repertoire of activities, and onset before 3 years of age. Failure of language development is the feature most likely to bring autistic infants to medical attention and correlates best with outcome; children who fail to develop language before age 5 have the worst outcome. The IQ is less than 70 in most children with autism. Autistic children show no affection to their parents or other care providers but treat people as if they were inanimate objects. Some children show a morbid preoccupation with spinning objects, stereotyped behavior such as rocking and spinning, and relative insensitivity to pain.

DIAGNOSIS. Infantile autism is a clinical diagnosis and cannot be confirmed by laboratory tests. Infants with profound hearing impairment may display autistic behavior, and hearing must always be tested.

TREATMENT. Naltrexone improved behavior in one small study of autistic children (Kolmen et al, 1995), and trials of several other psychoactive drugs are in progress. These are more likely to act by relieving symptoms than by altering underlying mechanisms of disease.

Some aspects of the severely aberrant behavior can be improved by behavior modification techniques. However, despite the best program of treatment, these children function in a moderately to severely retarded range, even though some individuals have islands of normal ability (idiot savant).

DELAYED MOTOR DEVELOPMENT

Infants with delayed gross motor development but normal language and social skills are often

hypotonic and may have a neuromuscular disease (see Chapter 6). Isolated delay in motor function is also caused by ataxia (see Chapter 10), mild hemiplegia (see Chapter 11), and mild paraplegia (see Chapter 12). Many such children have a mild form of cerebral palsy, sufficient to delay the achievement of motor milestones but not severe enough to cause a recognizable disturbance of cognitive function during infancy. Mild disturbances in cognitive function are more often detected when the child enters school.

GLOBAL DEVELOPMENTAL DELAY

Most infants with global developmental delay have a static encephalopathy caused by an antenatal or perinatal disturbance. However, a small percentage of infants with developmental delay and no evidence of regression have an underlying genetic disease. An exhaustive search to find an underlying cause in every infant whose development is slow but not regressing is not cost effective. Factors that increase the likelihood of finding a progressive disease are an affected family member, parental consanguinity, organomegaly, and absent tendon reflexes. Unenhanced cranial magnetic resonance imaging (MRI) is a reasonable screening test in all infants with global developmental delay. It often detects a malformation or other evidence of prenatal disease and provides a diagnosis that ends uncertainty.

Chromosomal Disturbances

Abnormalities in chromosome structure or number are the single most common cause of severe mental retardation but still comprise only one third of the total. Abnormalities of autosomal chromosomes are always associated with infantile hypotonia (see Chapter 6). In addition, multiple minor face and limb abnormalities are usually associated that in themselves are not unusual but assume diagnostic significance in combination. Clinical features that suggest chromosomal aberrations are summarized in Table 5-4, and some of the more common chromosome syndromes in Table 5-5.

Fragile X Syndrome

The fragile X syndrome is the most common chromosomal cause of mental retardation. The name derives from a fragile site (constriction)

■ T A B L E   5 – 4
Clinical Indications for Chromosome Analysis

Genitourinary
Ambiguous genitalia
Polycystic kidney

Head and Neck
High nasal bridge
Hypertelorism or hypotelorism
Microphthalmia
Mongoloid slant (in non-Asians)
Occipital scalp defect
Small mandible
Small or fish mouth (hard to open)
Small or low-set ears
Upward slant of eyes
Webbed neck

Limbs
Abnormal dermatoglyphics
Low-set thumb
Overlapping fingers
Polydactyly
Radial hypoplasia
Rocker-bottom feet

■ T A B L E   5 – 5
Selected Autosomal Syndromes*,†

Defect	Features
5p monosomy	Characteristic "cri du chat" cry
	Moonlike face
	Hypertelorism
	Microcephaly
10p trisomy	Dolichocephaly
	"Turtle's beak"
	Osteoarticular anomalies
Partial 12p monosomy	Microcephaly
	Narrow forehead
	Pointed nose
	Micrognathia
18 trisomy	Pointed ears
	Micrognathia
	Occipital protuberance
	Narrow pelvis
	Rocker-bottom feet
21 trisomy	Hypotonia
	Round flat (mongoloid) facies
	Brushfield spots
	Flat nape of neck

*Modified from de Grouchy J, Turleau J. Autosomal disorders. In Emery AEH, Rimoin DL (eds): Principles and Practice of Medical Genetics, 2nd edition, Churchill Livingstone, New York, 1990, p. 247.
†Growth retardation and mental retardation are features of all autosomal chromosome disorders.

☐ F I G U R E   5 – 1   Fragile X chromosome.

CLINICAL FEATURES. Approximately 20% of males with a fragile X chromosome are normal, while 30% of carrier females are mildly affected. An asymptomatic male can pass the abnormal chromosome to his daughter, who is usually asymptomatic as well. The daughter's children, both male and female, may be symptomatic.

The typical syndrome in males is moderate retardation (IQ 40 to 55), behavioral problems that may resemble autism or attention deficit disorder, and somatic abnormalities (long face, enlarged ears, and macro-orchidism). While autistic behavior is common in children with the fragile X syndrome, the clinical features of the syndrome do not usually meet the diagnostic criteria of infantile autism.

DIAGNOSIS. Chromosome analysis shows the characteristic abnormality of the X chromosome.

TREATMENT. High-dose folic acid has been used to treat children with the fragile X syndrome because folic acid antagonists must be

detectable in folate-free culture medium at the Xq 27.3 site called FAX A (Figure 5–1) (Laxova, 1994). The unstable fragment contains a trinucleotide repeat that becomes larger in successive generations *(DNA amplification),* causing more severe phenotypic expression.

added to the culture medium in order to demonstrate the fragile X site. Controlled studies have not confirmed an improvement of IQ, but do suggest a behavioral improvement.

Cerebral Malformations

Approximately 3% of all children have at least one major malformation but the responsible etiologic factors can be identified in only 20% of cases. Many intrauterine diseases cause destructive changes that cause malformation in the developing brain. The exposure of an embryo to infectious or toxic agents during the first weeks after conception can disorganize the delicate sequencing of neural development at a time when the brain is incapable of generating a cellular response. Alcohol, lead, prescription drugs, and substances of abuse have all been implicated in the production of cerebral malformations. Although a cause-and-effect relationship is difficult to establish in an individual case, maternal cocaine use is probably responsible for vascular insufficiency and infarction of many organs, including the brain (Dominguez et al, 1991).

Cerebral malformations should be suspected in any retarded child who is dysmorphic, has malformations of other organs, or has an abnormality of head size and shape (see Chapter 18). Noncontrast-enhanced computed tomography (CT) is satisfactory to show major malformations, but MRI is the better method to show migrational defects and is more cost effective for diagnosis of malformations.

Intrauterine Infections

The most common intrauterine infections are human immunodeficiency virus (HIV) and cytomegalovirus (Griffith and Booss, 1994). The acquired immune deficiency syndrome (AIDS) epidemic in adults is responsible for the re-emergence of congenital syphilis, but has not been associated with a concomitant increase in the incidence of intrauterine toxoplasmosis. Rubella embryopathy had almost disappeared because of mass immunization but is re-emerging as immunization rates decline.

Congenital Syphilis

Reported cases of congenital syphilis have increased since 1988, partly because of an actual increase in case number but also because the case definition has broadened. All stillbirths and live births born to a woman with a history of untreated or inadequately treated syphilis are considered to have congenital syphilis (Ikeda and Jenson, 1990).

CLINICAL FEATURES. Two thirds of infected newborns are asymptomatic and only identified on screening tests. The more common features in symptomatic newborns and infants are condylomata lata, periostitis or osteochondritis, persistent rhinorrhea, and maculopapular rash. The onset of neurologic disturbances is usually after age 2 and includes nerve deafness, and mental retardation. The combination of nerve deafness, interstitial keratitis, and peg-shaped upper incisors is the *Hutchinson triad.*

DIAGNOSIS. Nontreponemal antibody tests (Venereal Disease Research Laboratory and rapid plasma reagin card tests) are used for screening, and the fluorescent treponemal antibody test absorbed with nonpallidum treponemas (FTA-ABS) for confirmation. AIDS should be suspected in every child with congenital syphilis.

TREATMENT. Newborns and infants with confirmed or presumptive congenital infection should be treated intravenously with crystalline penicillin G, 100,000 to 150,000 units/kg/day in six divided doses every 8 to 12 hours for 10 to 14 days; or intramuscularly with procaine penicillin G, 50,000 units/kg once daily for 10 to 14 days.

Cytomegalic Inclusion Disease

The cytomegalovirus (CMV) is a member of the herpesvirus group and produces chronic infection characterized by long periods of latency punctuated by intervals of reactivation. Cytomegalic inclusion disease is sexually transmitted in adults and causes an inapparent cervical infection. Pregnancy may cause reactivation of maternal infection, and CMV can be cultured from the urine in 1% to 2% of live-born infants in the United States. Fortunately, less than 0.05% of newborns with viruria have symptoms of cytomegalic inclusion disease.

CLINICAL FEATURES. Cytomegalic inclusion disease of the newborn is difficult to differentiate from other intrauterine infections on the basis of clinical examination alone. The typical clinical features are skin rash, hepatosplenomegaly, jaundice, chorioretinitis, and microcephaly with cerebral calcification. Migrational defects (lissencephaly, polymicrogyria, and cerebellar agenesis) are the main consequence of fetal infection during the first trimester (Barkovich and Linden,

1994). Some infants have microcephaly secondary to intrauterine infection without evidence of systemic infection at birth.

DIAGNOSIS. Isolation of CMV from the urine or cerebrospinal fluid indicates active infection in the newborn. In infants with developmental delay and microcephaly, the diagnosis of cytomegalic inclusion disease is made by serologic demonstration of prior infection and a consistent pattern of intracranial calcification.

TREATMENT. Ganciclovir is the standard treatment for CMV infections in adults and is used in congenitally infected newborns. No treatment given postnatally can reverse the malformations caused by intrauterine infection.

Rubella Embryopathy

CLINICAL FEATURES. Rubella embryopathy is a multisystem disease characterized by intrauterine growth retardation, cataracts, chorioretinitis, congenital heart disease, sensorineural deafness, hepatosplenomegaly, jaundice, anemia, thrombocytopenia, and rash. The neurologic features are lethargy, hypotonia, and seizures. Seizures may be delayed until 3 months of age.

DIAGNOSIS. Rubella embryopathy should not be considered a cause of psychomotor retardation unless the newborn has other symptoms of rubella infection.

TREATMENT. No treatment is available for active infection.

Toxoplasmosis

Toxoplasma gondii is a protozoan that is estimated to infect 1 per 1,000 live births in the United States each year. The symptoms of toxoplasmosis infection in the mother usually go unnoticed. Transplacental transmission of toxoplasmosis is possible only if primary maternal infection occurs during pregnancy. The rate of placental transmission is highest during the last trimester, but fetuses infected at that time are least likely to have later symptoms. The transmission rate is lowest during the first trimester, but fetuses who are infected at that time have the most serious sequelae.

CLINICAL FEATURES. About 25% of infected newborns have multisystem involvement (fever, rash, hepatosplenomegaly, jaundice, and thrombocytopenia) at birth. Neurologic dysfunction is manifested as seizures, altered states of consciousness, and increased intracranial pressure. The triad of hydrocephalus, chorioretinitis, and intracranial calcification is the hallmark of con-

genital toxoplasmosis in older children. About 8% of infected newborns, asymptomatic at birth, later show neurologic sequelae, especially psychomotor retardation.

DIAGNOSIS. The Sabin-Feldman dye test had been the standard for diagnosis, but another useful serologic test for the diagnosis of congenital toxoplasmosis in the newborn is an enzyme-linked immunosorbent assay (ELISA) that shows IgM-specific antibody to *Toxoplasma* in umbilical cord blood. The demonstration of IgM-specific antibody is essential to prove active infection in the newborn. IgM-specific antibody appears in the newborn's serum by passive transfer from the mother and does not indicate active infection. Persistence of IgG-specific antibody correlates with active infection.

In older children the diagnosis requires not only serologic evidence of prior infection but also compatible clinical features.

TREATMENT. A combined prenatal and postnatal treatment program for congenital toxoplasmosis can reduce the neurologic morbidity (Roizen et al, 1995). When maternal acute infection is recognized by seroconversion, fetal blood and amniotic fluid are cultured and fetal blood is tested for *Toxoplasma*-specific IgM. The mother is then treated with spiramycin; if fetal infection is documented, pyrimethamine and either sulfadoxine or sulfadiazine are added to the regimen. In newborns with clinical evidence of toxoplasmosis, pyrimethamine (Daraprim), 0.5 mg/kg, and sulfadiazine, 25 mg/kg, are administered orally every 12 hours for 1 year. Because pyrimethamine is a folic acid antagonist, folic acid, 0.1 mg/kg/day, is also given. The peripheral platelet count must be monitored regularly. Prednisone, 1 to 2 mg/kg/day, should be added to the therapy in newborns with a high protein concentration in the cerebrospinal fluid or chorioretinitis.

Perinatal Disorders

Perinatal infection, asphyxia, maternal drug use, and trauma are the main perinatal events that cause psychomotor retardation (see Chapter 1). The important infectious diseases are bacterial meningitis (see Chapter 4) and herpes encephalitis (see Chapter 1). Although the overall mortality rate for bacterial meningitis is now less than 50%, significant neurologic sequelae are noted almost immediately in 50% of survivors. The most common sequelae are mental and motor disabilities, hydrocephalus, epilepsy, deafness, and visual loss. Psychomotor retardation may be the only or the most prominent sequela. Progressive mental deterioration can occur if meningitis causes a secondary hydrocephalus.

TELLING PARENTS BAD NEWS

It is not possible to make bad news sound good, or even half bad. The goal of telling parents that their child will be mentally retarded or otherwise neurologically impaired is that they hear and understand what you are saying. The mind must be prepared to hear bad news. It is a mistake to tell people more than they are ready to accept. Too often, parents bring their child for a second or third opinion because previous doctors "didn't tell us anything." In fact, they said too much too fast and were tuned out.

My goal for the first visit is to establish that the child's development is not normal (not a normal variation), that something is wrong with the brain, and that I share their concern. Unfortunately, mothers often come alone for this critical visit and must later restate your comments to doubting fathers and grandparents. Most parents cannot handle more information than "the child is not normal" at the first consultation and further discussion is saved for a later visit. However, probing questions should always be answered fully. Parents must never lose confidence in your willingness to be forthright. The timing of the next visit depends on the age of the child and the severity of the retardation. The more the child falls behind in reaching developmental milestones, the more ready parents will be to accept the diagnosis of mental retardation.

When the time comes that you tell a mother that her child is retarded, she will cry. If she does not cry, she has not heard what you were saying or understood its implications and you have failed to communicate effectively. It is not helpful to describe mental retardation as mild, moderate, or severe. Parents want to know what the child will do: will he walk? Need special schools? Live alone? The next question is "What can I do to help my child?" Parents must do something, and should be directed to programs that provide developmental specialists and other parents who can help them learn how to live with a chronic handicapping disorder and to gain access to community resources.

Progressive Encephalopathies with Onset Before Age 2

The differential diagnosis of progressive diseases of the nervous system that start before age 2 years is somewhat different from those that begin during childhood (Table 5-6; also see Table 5-2). Three questions must be answered in the history and physical examination before laboratory diagnosis is initiated:

1. Are the clinical features referable only to the central nervous system or are other organs involved (Figure 5-2)?

2. Are the clinical features referable only to the central nervous system or is the peripheral nervous system (nerves or muscles) involved (see Chapters 6, 7, and 9)?

3. Does the disease affect primarily the gray matter or the white matter?

Early features of gray matter disease are personality change, seizures, and dementia. White matter disease is characterized by focal

■ TABLE 5-6
Progressive Encephalopathy: Onset After Age 2

Disorders of Lysosomal Enzymes
GM₂ gangliosidosis (juvenile Tay-Sachs disease)
Gaucher disease type III (glucosylceramide lipisosis)
Globoid cell leukodystrophy (late-onset Krabbe disease)
Glycoprotein degradation disorders
    Aspartylglycosaminuria
    Mannosidosis type II
Metachromatic leukodystrophy (late-onset sulfatide lipidoses)
Mucopolysaccharidoses types II and VII
Niemann-Pick type C (sphingomyelin lipidosis)

Infectious Disease
Acquired immune deficiency syndrome encephalopathy
Congenital syphilis
Subacute sclerosing panencephalitis

Other Disorders of Gray Matter
Ceroid lipofuscinosis
    Late infantile (Bielschowsky-Jansky disease)
    Juvenile
Heller syndrome
Huntington disease
Mitochondrial disorders
    Late-onset poliodystrophy
    Myoclonic epilepsy and ragged-red fibers (MERRF)
Progressive neuronal degeneration with liver disease
Xeroderma pigmentosum

Other Disorders of White Matter
Adrenoleukodystrophy
Alexander disease
Cerebrotendinous xanthomatosis

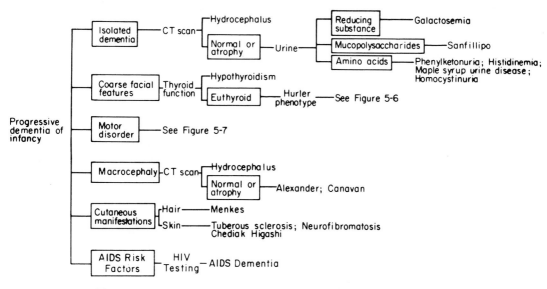

☐ F I G U R E 5 – 2 Evaluation of infants with progressive dementia.

neurologic deficits, spasticity, and blindness. Whether the process begins in the gray matter or the white matter, eventually clinical features of dysfunction develop in both. The electroencephalogram (EEG) is usually abnormal early in the course of gray matter disease and late in the course of white matter disease. MRI shows cortical atrophy in gray matter disease and cerebral demyelination in white matter disease (Figure 5-3). Visual evoked responses and motor conduction velocities are useful in documenting demyelination, even subclinical, in the optic and peripheral nerves, respectively.

ACQUIRED IMMUNE DEFICIENCY SYNDROME ENCEPHALOPATHY

Acquired immune deficiency syndrome (AIDS) is a human retroviral disease caused by the lentivirus subfamily now designated as human immunodeficiency virus (HIV). HIV is spread in adults by sexual contact, intravenous drug abuse, and blood transfusion. Most pediatric AIDS cases result from transplacental or perinatal transmission of HIV from mothers who are intravenous drug users and prostitutes. The mother may be asymptomatic when the infection is noted in the child. A smaller number of cases involve children receiving blood products, such as premature newborns and hemophiliacs. Approximately 30% of children born to AIDS-infected mothers show evidence of infection during the first year.

☐ F I G U R E 5 – 3 Krabbe disease. MRI demonstrates extensive demyelination of cerebral hemispheres.

CLINICAL FEATURES. As a rule, outcome is worse when the onset of symptoms is early, and the rate of progression in the child relates directly with the severity of disease in the mother (Blanche et al, 1994).

Children with AIDS fail to thrive and have

an increased incidence of bacterial infections, but only 10% acquire opportunistic infections. The most common opportunistic infections are *Pneumocystis carinii* pneumonia, disseminated candidiasis, and disseminated *Mycobacterium avium intracellulare*. Toxoplasmosis, a common complication in adults with AIDS, is uncommon in pediatric AIDS. An immunocompromised state should be suspected in every child with an opportunistic infection.

The possible spectrum of neurologic outcome in children infected with HIV includes a static encephalopathy resulting from other prenatal and perinatal risk factors associated with drug abuse in the mother; opportunistic infection of the nervous system; HIV infection of the brain, causing a subacute encephalopathy; and HIV infection of the spinal cord, causing a transverse myelitis (see Chapter 12) (Butler et al, 1991). AIDS experts now believe that the disease will develop in all children with HIV infection.

AIDS encephalopathy may be subacute or indolent and is not necessarily associated with failure to thrive or opportunistic infections. The onset of encephalopathy may occur from 2 months to 5 years after exposure to the virus. Ninety percent of affected infants show symptoms by 18 months of age. The encephalopathy is characterized by progressive loss of developmental milestones, microcephaly, dementia, and spasticity. Other features in less than 50% of children are ataxia, pseudobulbar palsy, involuntary movement disorders, myoclonus, and seizures. Death usually occurs a few months after the onset of AIDS encephalopathy.

DIAGNOSIS. The diagnosis of AIDS in infants born to infected mothers is complicated because all such newborns are HIV-antibody positive from passive transfer, but only 15% to 30% are HIV infected. The diagnosis of AIDS in a child less than 18 months of age who is HIV seropositive or born to an HIV-infected mother is established by a positive result on two separate determinations from one or more of the following tests: HIV culture, HIV polymerase chain reaction, or HIV antigen (Centers for Disease Control and Prevention, 1994). Children 18 months of age or older are diagnosed as HIV infected when the HIV-antibody tests are positive by reactive enzyme immunoassay and confirmed by Western blot or immunofluorescence assay.

Treatable infections (cryptococcal meningitis, *Candida* meningitis) must be excluded before HIV encephalitis is diagnosed. The cerebrospinal fluid abnormalities are minimal and vary from patient to patient. Protein concentration is 50 to 100 mg/dl (0.5 to 1 g/L), glucose concentration is normal or slightly decreased, but monocytic pleocytosis is uncommon. In some children progressive calcification of the basal ganglia is seen on CT.

The mortality rate in symptomatic children is 100%.

TREATMENT. Oral zidovudine (azidothymidine, AZT), 180 mg/m^2 every 6 hours, improves neurologic development in children with HIV infection. Continuous intravenous infusion of AZT may actually improve cognition (DeCarli et al, 1991). Bone marrow suppression is the only important evidence of toxicity.

In symptomatic children an intravenous infusion of immune globulin, 400 mg/kg/28 days, decreases the frequency of bacterial infections (Mofenson and Moye, 1993).

DISORDERS OF AMINO ACID METABOLISM

Disorders of amino acid metabolism impair neuronal function by the excessive production of toxic intermediary metabolites and the reduced production of neurotransmitters. The clinical syndromes are either an acute neonatal encephalopathy with seizures and cerebral edema (see Chapter 1) or mental retardation and dementia. Some disorders of amino acid metabolism cause cerebral malformations, such as agenesis of the corpus callosum. Although the main clinical features of aminoaciduria are referable to gray matter dysfunction (mental retardation, seizures), myelination is often profoundly delayed or defective.

Homocystinuria

The main defect responsible for mental retardation is almost complete deficiency of the enzyme cystathionine beta-synthase (Mudd et al, 1995). Transmission is by autosomal recessive inheritance. Heterozygotes have partial deficiencies. Cystathionine beta-synthase catalyzes the condensation of serine and homocysteine to form cystathionine (Figure 5–4). When the enzyme is deficient, the blood and urine concentrations of homocysteine, homocystine, and methionine are increased. It is hypermethioninemia that is detected in newborn screening programs.

CLINICAL FEATURES. Affected individuals appear normal at birth. Global developmental

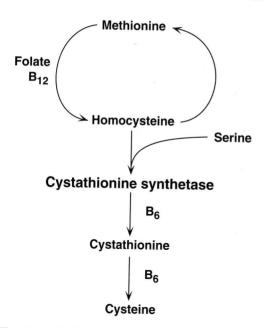

☐ F I G U R E 5 – 4 Metabolic disturbance in homocystinuria. Absence of cystathionine beta-synthase (cystathionine synthetase) blocks the metabolism of homocysteine, causing the accumulation of homocystine and methionine.

delay is usually the first clinical feature, and intelligence declines progressively with age in untreated children. Most eventually function in the mildly retarded range, but at least 20% have normal intelligence. Thromboembolism affecting large arteries, small arteries, and veins is a life-threatening complication of homocystinuria caused by hyperhomocyteinemia (Clarke et al, 1991). Emboli may occur in infancy or be delayed until adult life. Occlusion of the coronary or carotid arteries can lead to sudden death or severe neurologic handicap. Thromboembolism is the first clue to diagnosis in 15% of cases. Dislocation of the lens, an almost constant feature of homocystinuria, typically occurs between 2 and 10 years of age but may be delayed until adult life. Ninety-seven percent of patients have lens dislocation by age 40. Older children have osteoporosis. The spine is affected first and most severely, resulting in scoliosis and sometimes vertebral collapse. Many children are tall and thin and have a Marfan syndrome habitus. This habitus does not develop until middle or late childhood and serves as a clue to diagnosis in less than 40% of cases.

The diagnosis should be suspected in any infant with isolated and unexplained developmental delay, because disease-specific features may not appear until later childhood. The presence of either thromboembolism or lens dislocation strongly suggests homocystinuria.

DIAGNOSIS. The concentrations of homocystine and methionine are increased in the blood and urine. Definitive diagnosis is established by showing a deficiency of cystathionine beta-synthase either in the liver or in cultured fibroblasts.

TREATMENT. The administration of pyridoxine, 500 to 1000 mg/day, reduces or eliminates the biochemical abnormalities in one third of patients. An equal number are not pyridoxine responsive, and the remainder have an intermediate response. Folate must be given concomitantly. Most patients who respond to pyridoxine probably have a low-level or mutant form of cystathionine beta-synthase activity that is enhanced by the addition of cofactor.

The most widely used dietary treatment for homocystinuria is methionine restriction and cystine supplementation. Unfortunately, cystine is not palatable and long-term use is difficult to achieve even though it prevents mental retardation when started shortly after birth. Betaine, a methyl donor that recycles homocysteine to methionine, is recommended at a dose of 6 to 9 g/day for children who neither respond to pyridoxine or tolerate a methionine-restricted diet.

Maple Syrup Urine Disease (Intermediate)

The three major branched-chain amino acids are leucine, isoleucine, and valine. In the course of their metabolism, they are first transaminated to alpha-ketoacids and then further catabolized by oxidative decarboxylation (see Figure 1–4). Branched-chain ketoacid dehydrogenase is the enzyme responsible for oxidative decarboxylation. Its deficiency is associated with at least three different phenotypes: classic, intermittent, and intermediate maple syrup urine disease (Chuang and Shih, 1995). The classic and intermittent forms are characterized by acute encephalopathies with ketoacidosis (see Chapters 1 and 10). The main feature of the intermediate form is progressive mental retardation without ketoacidosis. The levels of dehydrogenase enzyme activity in the intermediate and intermittent forms are approximately the same (5% to 40%), whereas activity in the classic form is zero to 2% of normal. Phenotypic differences between the intermediate and intermittent

□ FIGURE 5–5 Phenylalanine metabolism. *1*, Phenylalanine hydroxylase. *2*, Dihydropteridine reductase. *3*, Tetrahydrobiopterin. *4*, Phenylalanine transaminase. *5*, Tyrosine transaminase.

forms may be related to protein intake. Some infants with the intermediate form are thiamine responsive. The enzyme defect in these cases may be unique.

CLINICAL FEATURES. Infants with intermediate maple syrup urine disease are normal at birth, slow in achieving milestones, and hyperactive. As children, they generally function in the moderately retarded range of intelligence. Physical development is normal except for coarse, brittle hair. The urine may have the odor of maple syrup. Acute mental changes, seizures, and focal neurologic deficits do not occur.

DIAGNOSIS. The diagnosis is established either by showing an increased blood and urine concentration of branched-chain ketoacids or by quantitation of enzyme activity in leukocytes or cultured fibroblasts.

TREATMENT. All infants with intermediate maple syrup urine disease should be put on a protein-restricted diet. In addition, a trial of thiamine, 100 mg/day, is given to determine whether the biochemical error is thiamine responsive. If 100 mg is not effective, daily dosages up to 1 g of thiamine should be tried before the condition is designated as thiamine-refractory.

Phenylketonuria

Phenylketonuria is a disorder of phenylalanine metabolism caused by partial or total deficiency of the hepatic enzyme phenylalanine hydroxylase. The deficiency is transmitted by autosomal recessive inheritance and occurs in approximately 1 per 16,000 live births. Because phenylalanine cannot be adequately hydroxylated to tyrosine, phenylalanine accumulates and is transaminated to phenylpyruvic acid (Figure

5-5). Phenylpyruvic acid is oxidized to phenylacetic acid, which is excreted in the urine and causes a musty odor.

CLINICAL FEATURES. Affected children are normal at birth and would not be detected in the absence of compulsory mass screening. The screening test detects hyperphenylalaninemia, which is not synonymous with phenylketonuria (Table 5-7). Blood phenylalanine and tyrosine concentrations must be precisely determined in every newborn whose abnormality is detected by the screening test in order to differentiate classic phenylketonuria from other conditions. In newborns with classic phenylketonuria, hyperphenylalaninemia develops 48 to 72 hours after initiation of milk feeding. Blood phenylalanine concentrations are 20 mg/dl (1,200 μmol/L) or greater and serum tyrosine levels are less than 5 mg/dl (275 μmol/L). When blood phenylalanine concentrations reach 15 mg/dl (900 μmol/L), phenylalanine spills over into the urine and the addition of ferric chloride solution (5 to 10 drops of FeCl to 1 ml of urine) produces a green color.

Untreated infants appear normal during the first months, but the skin may have a musty odor because of phenylacetic acid in the sweat. Developmental delay is sometimes obvious by the third month and always before the end of the first year. By the beginning of the second year, developmental regression is evident. Behavioral disturbances characterized by hyperactivity and aggressiveness are common; focal neurologic deficits are unusual. Approximately 25% of affected infants have seizures. Some have infantile spasms and hypsarrhythmia; others have tonic-clonic seizures. Infants with phenylketonuria frequently have blond hair, pale skin, and blue eyes owing to diminished pigment production.

■ TABLE 5-7
■ TABLE 5-7
Differential Diagnosis of
Hyperphenylalaninemia

Classic Phenylketonuria
Complete hydroxylase deficiency (zero to 6%)
Benign Variants
Partial hydroxylase deficiency (6% to 30%)
Transitory hydroxylase deficiency
Phenylalanine transaminase deficiency
Other
Malignant Variants
Dihydropteridine reductase deficiency
Tetrahydrobiopterin synthesis deficiency
Tyrosinemia
Transitory tyrosinemia
Tyrosinosis
Liver Disease
Galactose-1-phosphate uridylyl transferase deficiency

Eczema is common. These skin changes are the only non-neurologic features of phenylketonuria.

DIAGNOSIS. The existence of several mutant alleles for the phenylalanine hydroxylase enzyme probably account for the clinical heterogeneity of classic phenylketonuria (Svensson et al, 1993). Benign variants of phenylketonuria are generally characterized by blood phenylalanine levels less than 25 mg/dl (1,500 μmol/L), and frequently less than 15 mg/dl (900 μmol/L) and a normal concentration of tyrosine. The malignant forms of phenylketonuria are caused by disturbances in tetrahydrobiopterin. Seizures are the initial symptom and are followed by mental retardation and motor deficits. Progressive calcification of the basal ganglia occurs in untreated children.

Transitory tyrosinemia is estimated to occur in 2% of full-term newborns and in 25% of premature newborns. It is caused by a transitory deficiency of the enzyme p-hydroxyphenylpyruvic acid. It is a benign condition and can be distinguished from phenylketonuria because the blood concentrations of both tyrosine and phenylalanine are elevated.

TREATMENT. Experts agree that a phenylalanine-restricted diet should be started immediately in newborns with a blood phenylalanine concentration of 30 mg/dl (1,800 μmol/L) or greater; some would recommend diet therapy at a concentration of 20 mg/dl (1,200 μmol/L). After 3 months of therapy a 3-day challenge of phenylalanine, 180 mg/kg/day, is indicated to distinguish mild variants from classic phenylke-

tonuria. Children with phenylketonuria have a blood phenylalanine concentration of 20 mg/dl (1,200 μmol/L) or greater and need to continue restricted diets. Those with a blood concentration lower than 20 mg/dl (1,200 μmol/L) probably have a benign variant and do not require further dietary restriction of phenylalanine. The goal of therapy is to maintain blood phenylalanine concentrations between 5 and 10 mg/dl (300 and 600 μmol/L). Diet therapy is probably needed throughout life to prevent intellectual deterioration (Thompson et al, 1993).

Tetrahydrobiopterin is a cofactor for the enzymes phenylalanine hydroxylase, tyrosine hydroxylase, and tryptophan hydroxylase. Deficiency of tetrahydrobiopterin can be caused by defective recycling or defective synthesis. In infants with cofactor deficiency, a phenylalanine-restricted diet reduces the blood phenylalanine concentration but does not prevent neurologic deterioration. For these children, tetrahydrobiopterin administration is the therapy of choice.

DISORDERS OF LYSOSOMAL ENZYMES

Lysosomes are cytoplasmic vesicles containing hydrolytic enzymes that degrade the products of cellular catabolism. Lysosomal enzyme disorders are caused by impaired enzyme synthesis, abnormal enzyme targeting, or a defective accessory factor needed for enzymatic processing. When lysosomal enzymes are impaired, abnormal storage of materials occurs that causes cell injury and death. One or several organs may be affected and the clinical features depends on the organ(s) involved. Mental retardation and regression are features of many lysosomal enzyme storage diseases. In some, such as acid lipase deficiency (Wolman disease) and ceramide deficiency (Farber lipogranulomatosis), mental retardation occurs, but it is neither a prominent nor an initial feature. Such disorders are omitted from this discussion.

GM₁ Ganglioside Storage Disorders

Deficiency of the lysosomal enzyme beta-galactosidase causes GM₁ gangliosidosis and Morquio B disease (Suzuki et al, 1995b). The beta-galactosidase gene is on chromosome 3 and the deficiency state is transmitted by autosomal recessive inheritance. In GM₁ gangliosidosis, gangliosides are stored in the brain and viscera.

■ TABLE 5-8
The Hurler Phenotype

Abdominal hernia
Coarse facial features
Corneal opacity
Deafness
Dysostosis multiplex
Mental retardation
Stiff joints
Visceromegaly

■ TABLE 5-9
Lysosomal Enzyme Disorders with a Cherry-Red Spot

Cherry-red spot myoclonus (see Chapter 1)
Farber lipogranulomatosis
GM$_1$ gangliosidosis
GM$_2$ gangliosidosis
Metachromatic leukodystrophy
Niemann-Pick disease
Sialidosis type III

Morquio B disease is mainly a disorder of bone and is not discussed here.

GM$_1$ Gangliosidosis Type I

CLINICAL FEATURES. Difficulty in feeding and failure to thrive are noted shortly after birth. Edema of the limbs may be present as well. Psychomotor development is first slow and then regresses. Affected newborns are poorly responsive, hypotonic, and hypoactive. The Hurler phenotype is present (Table 5-8), except that the cornea is clear and a cherry-red spot of the macula is present in 50% of patients (Table 5-9). Symptoms are rapidly progressive, and many infants die within 1 year. Those who survive the first year are in a vegetative state.

DIAGNOSIS. Infantile GM$_1$ gangliosidosis can be distinguished from Hurler syndrome by the absence of mucopolysacchariduria and the presence of a cherry-red spot. The diagnosis is established by showing enzyme deficiency in leukocytes, cultured fibroblasts, or serum.

TREATMENT. No treatment is available.

GM$_1$ Gangliosidosis Type II

CLINICAL FEATURES. Children with GM$_1$ gangliosidosis type II are normal during infancy, but then develop ataxia, dysarthria, and strabismus. These motor disturbances are followed by men-

tal regression, lethargy, spasticity, and seizures. The Hurler phenotype is not present: corneal clouding and hepatosplenomegaly do not occur, and skeletal radiographs show only mild beaking of vertebral bodies and metacarpal bones.

DIAGNOSIS. The diagnosis is established by showing deficient enzyme in leukocytes, cultured fibroblasts, or serum.

TREATMENT. No treatment is available.

GM$_2$ Ganglioside Storage Disorders

These are a group of related disorders in which GM$_2$ gangliosides are stored because of deficiency of hexosaminidase A, hexosaminidase B, or the GM$_2$ activator of hexosaminidase A or B (Gravel et al, 1995). The gene for hexosaminidase A maps to chromosome 15 and hexosaminidase B and the GM$_2$ activator to chromosome 5.

Tay-Sachs Disease

Tay-Sachs disease is transmitted by autosomal recessive inheritance and is caused by deficiency of the enzyme hexosaminidase A or the GM$_2$ activator of hexosaminidase A. Gene frequency is 1:30 in Ashkenazi Jews and 1:300 in gentiles. The central nervous system is the only affected organ.

CLINICAL FEATURES. The typical initial symptom, between 3 and 6 months of age, is an abnormal startle reaction (Moro reflex) to noise or light. Motor regression begins between 4 and 6 months of age. The infant may be brought for medical attention because of either delayed achievement of motor milestones or loss of milestones previously attained. A cherry-red spot of the macula is present in almost every patient but is not specific for Tay-Sachs disease, because it can be seen in several storage diseases and in central retinal artery occlusion (Table 5-9). The cherry-red spot develops as retinal ganglion cells in the parafoveal region accumulate stored material, swell, and burst. The red color of the normal fundus can then be seen. Optic atrophy and blindness follow.

By 1 year of age, the infant is severely retarded, unresponsive, and spastic. During the second year the head enlarges and seizures develop. Most children die by 5 years of age.

DIAGNOSIS. The diagnosis should be strongly suspected in any Jewish child with psychomotor retardation and a cherry-red spot of the macula. The diagnosis is established by showing deficient activity of hexosaminidase A in white blood cells or serum. Heterozygotes can be detected by the same assay. Prenatal diagnosis is possible by amniocentesis.

TREATMENT. No treatment is available.

Sandhoff Disease

Sandhoff disease is a rare disorder of neurovisceral storage that occurs in non-Jewish children. It is transmitted by autosomal recessive inheritance and is caused by deficiency of both hexosaminidase A and B or their activators.

CLINICAL FEATURES. The clinical features and course of Sandhoff disease are identical to those of Tay-Sachs disease. The only difference is that organs other than the central nervous system are sometimes involved. Moderate hepatosplenomegaly may be present, and occasionally patients have bony deformities similar to those of infantile GM_1 gangliosidosis.

DIAGNOSIS. The disease should be suspected in every non-Jewish infant with a Tay-Sachs phenotype. Peripheral lymphocytes are not vacuolated, but foamy histocytes may be present in the bone marrow. The diagnosis is established in patients and carriers by showing hexosaminidase deficiency in leukocytes, cultured fibroblasts, or serum. Prenatal diagnosis can be made by the detection of *N*-acetylglucosaminyl-oligosaccharides in amniotic fluid.

TREATMENT. No treatment is available.

Gaucher Disease Type II (Glucosylceramine Lipidosis)

Gaucher disease type II, caused by a deficiency of the enzyme glucocerebrosidase, is transmitted by autosomal recessive inheritance (Beutler and Gelbart, 1994). Type I, the most common form of Gaucher disease, does not affect the nervous system. Type II is an acute and devastating infantile disorder affecting the brain and viscera. Type III, like type II, is characterized by neurovisceral storage, but the onset is in childhood and the course is slow.

CLINICAL FEATURES. Infants with Gaucher disease type II usually have symptoms of neurovisceral dysfunction before 6 months of age, and frequently before 3 months of age. The initial symptoms are motor regression and cranial nerve dysfunction. Children are first hypotonic and then spastic. Head retraction is an early and characteristic sign that probably is due to meningeal irritation. Difficulties in sucking and swallowing, trismus, and oculomotor palsies are typical. Mental deterioration is rapid, but seizures are uncommon. Splenomegaly is more prominent than hepatomegaly, and jaundice is unexpected. Hypersplenism results in anemia, thrombocytopenia, and leukopenia. Death usually occurs during the first year and always by the second.

DIAGNOSIS. The presence of Gaucher cells in the reticuloendothelial system establishes the diagnosis. These cells are altered macrophages measuring 20 to 100 μm. The cytoplasm has the appearance of wrinkled tissue paper, and the nucleus is eccentric. The cells are best identified from bone marrow aspirate stained by periodic acid-Schiff (PAS) reaction. Heterozygotes can be identified by a partial decrease in enzyme activity in leukocytes. No reliable method for prenatal diagnosis has been established.

TREATMENT. Enzyme replacement therapy is available by the intravenous administration of macrophage-targeted human placental glucocerebrosidase, but its use is limited by its high cost. Splenectomy may improve the hematologic abnormalities but does not provide long-term relief of symptoms. The role of bone marrow transplantation is not established (Beutler and Grabowski, 1995).

Globoid Cell Leukodystrophy (Krabbe Disease)

Krabbe disease is a rapidly progressive demyelinating disorder of infants caused by deficient activity of the enzyme galactosylceramidase (galactosylceramide beta-galactosidase). A juvenile and an adult form of the disease also occur. The defect is transmitted by autosomal recessive inheritance (Suzuki et al, 1995a).

CLINICAL FEATURES. The median age of onset is 4 months, with a range of 1 to 7 months. Initial symptoms are irritability and hyperreactivity to stimuli. These are followed by progressive hypertonicity in the skeletal muscles. Unexplained low-grade fever is common. Psychomotor development arrests and then regresses. Within 2 to 4 months, the infant is in a permanent position of opisthotonos and has lost all previously achieved milestones. Tendon reflexes become hypoactive and disappear. Startle myoclonus and seizures develop. The infant becomes blind, and before 1 year 90% are either dead or in a chronic vegetative state.

Several variant forms of globoid leukodystrophy with different clinical features are described: infantile spasm syndrome (see Chapter 1), focal neurologic deficits (see Chapters 10 and 11), and polyneuropathy (see Chapter 7). The juvenile form is discussed later in this chapter.

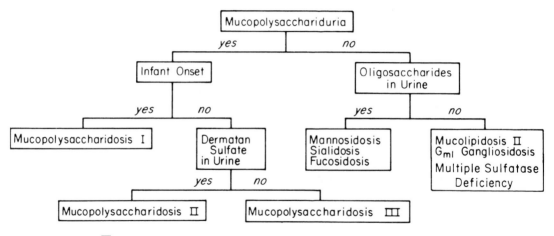

☐ FIGURE 5-6 Evaluation of infants with a Hurler phenotype.

DIAGNOSIS. MRI shows diffuse demyelination of the cerebral hemispheres (Figure 5-3). Motor nerve conduction velocity of peripheral nerves is usually prolonged, and the protein content of cerebrospinal fluid is elevated. The diagnosis is established by showing deficient activity of galactosylceramide beta-galactosidase in leukocytes or cultured fibroblasts.

TREATMENT. No treatment is available.

Glycoprotein Degradation Disorders

Glycoproteins are complex molecules composed of oligosaccharides attached to protein. Disorders of glycoprotein degradation are uncommon and resemble mild forms of mucopolysaccharidoses (Thomas and Beaudet, 1995). All are transmitted as autosomal recessive traits.

Mannosidosis Type I

The more common form of mannosidosis is caused by deficiency of the enzyme alpha-mannosidase coded on chromosome 19p. Type I has an infantile onset, and type II a juvenile onset. A less common form of mannosidosis is caused by deficiency of beta-mannosidase. It causes status epilepticus, quadriplegia, and death by 15 months of age.

CLINICAL FEATURES. All patients have mental retardation, dysostosis multiplex, hepatosplenomegaly, and coarse facial features. Deafness, corneal opacities, and recurrent bacterial infection are not constant features. Progression is rapid, and death occurs between 3 and 10 years of age.

DIAGNOSIS. The diagnosis is suspected in infants with a Hurler phenotype but without mucopolysacchariduria (Figure 5-6). Vacuolated lymphocytes are present in the peripheral blood. Demonstration of mannosidase deficiency in leukocytes or fibroblasts provides definitive diagnosis.

TREATMENT. Treatment is not available.

Fucosidosis Types I and II

Fucosidosis is caused by deficiency of the lysosomal enzyme alpha-fucosidase coded on chromosome 1p. Two clinical types are recognized; both have their onset during infancy. Type II progresses more slowly and allows longer survival.

CLINICAL FEATURES. The onset of psychomotor retardation and regression occurs between 3 and 18 months in type I and between 1 and 2 years in type II. In both types a Hurler phenotype (Table 5-8) develops, except that corneal opacities are not present and skeletal abnormalities are restricted to the spine. Infants with fucosidosis type II survive to early adult life. A distinctive feature is that patients with type I experience increased sweating while those with type II have anhidrosis and angiokeratoma.

DIAGNOSIS. The diagnosis is suspected in infants with a Hurler phenotype but without mucopolysacchariduria (Figure 5-6). Vacuolated lymphocytes are present in the peripheral blood. Demonstration of fucosidase deficiency in leukocytes or fibroblasts provides definitive diagnosis.

TREATMENT. No treatment is available.

Sialidosis Type II

Type II sialidosis is a rare disorder caused by a deficiency of the glycoprotein-specific alphaneuraminidase (sialidase). Three different clinical syndromes are associated with sialidosis: a congenital form (type I) with hydrops fetalis, an infantile form (type II) with Hurler phenotype, and a juvenile form (type III) characterized only by myoclonus and a cherry-red spot of the macula (Table 5-9).

CLINICAL FEATURES. Infants with sialidosis type II look like they have a mucopolysaccharidosis. Toward the end of the first decade, ataxia, myoclonus, and seizures develop, sometimes associated with a cherry-red spot of the macula. Mental retardation is present, but progressive dementia is not a feature.

DIAGNOSIS. Vacuolated lymphocytes are present in the peripheral blood, and the urine contains oligosaccharides. Definitive diagnosis requires demonstration of the enzyme deficiency in cultured fibroblasts.

TREATMENT. No treatment is available.

Carbohydrate-Deficient Glycoprotein Syndromes

Three metabolic disorders affecting the carbohydrate moiety of glycoproteins (carbohydrate-deficient glycoprotein [CDG] syndrome types I, II, and III), are described mainly in northern Europeans (Hagberg et al, 1993; Jaeken et al, 1994). All are multisystem diseases transmitted by autosomal recessive inheritance. The affected organelles are not lysosomes but may be the Golgi apparatus or the endoplasmic reticulum.

CLINICAL FEATURES. Affected newborns with CDG syndrome type I seem normal except for the appearance of dysmaturity. Early infancy is characterized by failure to thrive, developmental delay, hypotonia, and multisystem failure. Neurologic deterioration follows in later infancy. The main features are mental deficiency, ataxia, retinitis pigmentosa, hypotonia, and weakness. Childhood and adolescence are characterized by short stature, failure of sexual maturation, skeletal abnormalities, liver dysfunction, and polyneuropathy.

Children with CDG syndrome type II have a more profound mental retardation but no cerebellar ataxia or peripheral neuropathy, and those with type III have severe neurologic impairment and seizures from birth.

DIAGNOSIS. Several serum glycoproteins are deficient in their carbohydrate moiety. Abnormal serum transferrin isoform patterns are the most constant abnormality in CDG syndrome type I and serves as the basis for diagnosis. The abnormal serum transferrin patterns in types II and III are different from those found in type I.

TREATMENT. No treatment is available.

I-Cell Disease

I-cell disease (mucolipidosis II) is caused by the abnormal transport of lysosomal enzymes in cells of mesenchymal origin. Newly synthesized lysosomal enzymes are secreted into the extracellular medium instead of into lysosymes (Kornfeld and Sly, 1995). The lysosomal enzyme N-acetylglucosamine-1-phosphotransferase is defective. The trait is transmitted by autosomal recessive inheritance.

CLINICAL FEATURES. I-cell disease resembles Hurler syndrome except that symptoms appear earlier, the neurologic deterioration is more rapid, and mucopolysacchariduria is not present. Affected newborns are small for gestational age and may have hyperplastic gums. Coarsening of facial features and limitation of joint movements occur within the first months. The complete Hurler phenotype is present within the first year, except that corneal opacification is not seen in all cases. Death from congestive heart failure usually occurs before age 5.

DIAGNOSIS. I-cell disease should be considered in infants with Hurler phenotype and a screening test negative for mucopolysacchariduria (Figure 5-6). The diagnosis is established by showing a specific pattern of lysosomal enzyme deficiency in fibroblasts. Phosphotransferase activity can also be measured.

TREATMENT. No treatment is available.

Mucopolysaccharidoses

The mucopolysaccharidoses (MPS) are caused by a deficiency of those lysosomal enzymes responsible for catalyzing the degradation of glycosaminoglycans (mucopolysaccharides) (Neufeld and Muenzer, 1995). Mucopolysaccharides are a normal component of cornea, cartilage, bone, connective tissue, and the reticuloendothelial system, and all may be affected by excessive storage. All mucopolysaccharidoses are transmitted by autosomal recessive inheritance except type II, which is X linked.

Type I MPS (Hurler Syndrome)

The Hurler syndrome is caused by absence of the lysosomal hydrolase alpha-L-iduronidase.

The defective gene is located on chromosome 4. Dermatan sulfate and heparan sulfate cannot be fully degraded and appear in the urine. Mucopolysaccharides are stored in the cornea, collagen, and leptomeninges, and gangliosides are stored in cortical neurons.

CLINICAL FEATURES. Affected children are normal during the first year. In the second year, development is arrested and slow regression occurs. Motor dysfunction affects the corticospinal tracts and peripheral nerves. A distinctive Hurler phenotype evolves that is common to many lysosomal enzyme disorders (Table 5-8). Clouding of the cornea is present in all cases, sometimes causing complete blindness. Facial features become coarse. The child has progressive hepatosplenomegaly, umbilical hernia, and skeletal deformities that produce dwarfism, kyphoscoliosis, and limited movement of the joints. The skeletal deformities, termed *dysostosis multiplex,* produce characteristic radiographic features: hypoplasia of the lateral clavicle, rounding and sometimes hypoplasia of the thoracolumbar vertebral bodies, flaring of the pelvis with hypoplasia of the acetabula, broadening of the ribs, and widening of the diaphyses of long bones. The skull loses its convolutional markings, the sella turcica is enlarged, and the orbits are shallow. Communicating hydrocephalus may result from thickening of the leptomeninges. Death usually occurs by age 10.

DIAGNOSIS. The diagnosis is suggested by the physical and radiographic appearance, the presence of vacuolated lymphocytes, and mucopolysacchariduria. A simple screening test is the appearance of a metachromatic spot when a drop of urine is placed on paper impregnated with toluidine blue. The diagnosis is only established by showing the enzyme deficiency in leukocytes or cultured fibroblasts.

TREATMENT. Bone marrow transplantation is being tried, with variable success, in all MPS types.

Type III MPS (Sanfilippo Disease)

Type III MPS is distinct from other mucopolysaccharidoses because only heparan sulfate is stored in viscera and appears in the urine. Gangliosides are stored in neurons. Four different, but related, enzyme deficiencies have been implicated. All are transmitted by autosomal recessive inheritance.

CLINICAL FEATURES. The Hurler phenotype is not prominent, but hepatomegaly is present in two thirds of cases. Dwarfism does not occur. The major feature is neurologic deterioration characterized by delayed motor development beginning toward the end of the second year, followed by an interval of arrested mental development and progressive dementia. Hyperactivity and sleep disorders are relatively common between the ages of 2 and 4. Most affected children are severely retarded by age 11 and dead before age 20. However, considerable variability exists, and type III MPS should be considered even when the onset of mental regression occurs after age 5.

DIAGNOSIS. The diagnosis should be suspected in infants and children with progressive psychomotor regression and a screening test positive for mucopolysacchariduria. The presence of heparan sulfate, but not dermatan sulfate, in the urine is presumptive evidence of the disease. Definitive diagnosis requires the demonstration of enzyme deficiency in cultured fibroblasts.

TREATMENT. Bone marrow transplantation is being tried, with variable success, in all MPS types.

Niemann-Pick Disease Type A (Sphingomyelin Lipidosis)

Niemann-Pick disease type A is caused by a deficiency of the enzyme sphingomyelinase. The trait is transmitted by autosomal recessive inheritance. Type A is the acute infantile form of Niemann-Pick disease.

CLINICAL FEATURES. The onset of the acute infantile form occurs in the first months of life. The features are feeding difficulty, failure to thrive, and hepatomegaly. Splenomegaly occurs later and is not prominent. A cherry-red spot is present in 50% of cases (Table 5-9). Psychomotor regression, characterized by postural hypotonia and loss of reactivity to the environment, occurs during the first year but may be overlooked because of the child's failure to thrive. With time, emaciation, a tendency for opisthotonos, exaggerated tendon reflexes, and blindness develop. Seizures are uncommon.

DIAGNOSIS. The diagnosis is suggested by the clinical course (Figure 5-7). Vacuolated histiocytes are present in the bone marrow and vacuolated lymphocytes in the peripheral blood. The diagnosis is established by showing a deficiency of sphingomyelinase in leukocytes or cultured fibroblasts.

TREATMENT. No treatment is available.

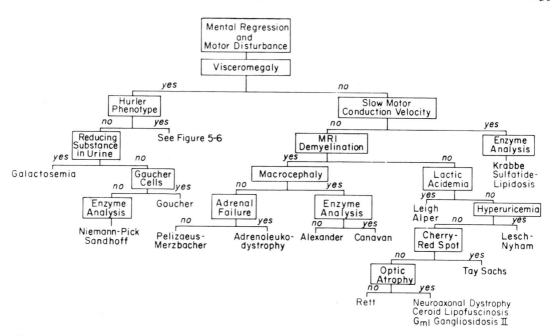

☐ FIGURE 5–7 Evaluation of infants with progressive mental regression and motor disturbances.

Sulfatase-Deficiency Disorders

Metachromatic Leukodystrophy (Sulfatide Lipidoses)

Metachromatic leukodystrophy is a disorder of central and peripheral myelin metabolism caused by deficient activity of the enzyme arylsulfatase A. The disease is transmitted by autosomal recessive inheritance. An infantile, juvenile, and adult form are recognized Two groups of mutations in the gene encoding arylsulfatase A are identified as I and A. The I group generates no active enzyme and the A group generates small amounts. The late-infantile form is associated with an I-I genotype, and the later onset forms with I-A or A-A genotypes (Kolodny and Fluharty, 1995).

Because peripheral neuropathy is a prominent feature of the late-infantile form of metachromatic leukodystrophy, the condition is discussed in Chapter 7. The juvenile form affects primarily the brain and is discussed later in this chapter.

Multiple Sulfatase Deficiency

Multiple sulfatase deficiency is a rare disorder characterized by deficiency of several sulfatases (arylsulfatase A, arylsulfatase B, iduronate sulfatase, N-acetylgalactosamine-6-sulfate sulfatase, and heparan-N-sulfatase) and the accumula-

tion of sulfatides, glycosaminoglycans, sphingolipids, and steroid sulfates in tissue and body fluids.

CLINICAL FEATURES. Development during the first year is normal, but in the second year developmental arrest and regression occur. Ataxia and speech disturbances are also noted during the second year. Neurologic deterioration is progressive. The appearance suggests a mucopolysaccharidosis: short stature, microcephaly, and facial dysmorphism. Retinal degeneration can occur as well and suggests a neuronal ceroid lipofuscinosis (Harbord et al, 1991).

DIAGNOSIS. Sulfatase activity is deficient, but not absent, in cultured skin fibroblasts and leukocytes. If only arylsulfatase A is measured, an improper diagnosis of juvenile sulfatide lipidosis may be considered because peripheral neuropathy is not present. However, the facial dysmorphism is not consistent with either the infantile or the juvenile form of sulfatide lipidosis.

TREATMENT. No treatment is available.

HYPOTHYROIDISM

Congenital hypothyroidism resulting from thyroid dysgenesis occurs in 1 per 4,000 live births. The cause is unknown, but the occasional familial occurrence in siblings has suggested either a genetic basis or an underlying maternal factor. Early diagnosis and treatment are imperative to ensure a favorable outcome. Fortunately, newborn screening is universal in the United States and detects virtually all cases.

CLINICAL FEATURES. Affected infants are usually asymptomatic at birth. Clinical features evolve insidiously during the first weeks postpartum, and their significance is not always appreciated. Frequently the gestation lasts for more than 42 weeks and birth weight is greater than 4 kg. Early clinical features include a wide-open posterior fontanelle, constipation, jaundice, poor temperature control, and umbilical hernia. The tongue is sometimes large, which makes feeding difficult. Edema of the eyes, hands, and feet may be present at birth but is often unrecognized in early infancy.

DIAGNOSIS. Radiographs of the long bones show delayed maturation, and radiographs of the skull show excessive numbers of wormian bones. The diagnosis is established by showing low serum concentrations of thyroxine (T_4) and high serum concentrations of thyroid stimulating hormone (TSH).

TREATMENT. Once the diagnosis of congenital hypothyroidism is confirmed, treatment is initiated with sodium-1-thyroxine, 24 to 50 μg/day. Most, if not all, of the sequelae of congenital hypothyroidism can be prevented by early treatment (Fisher and Foley, 1989). The ultimate intelligence of the hypothyroid infant declines with each month of delay.

MITOCHONDRIAL DISORDERS

Mitochondrial disorders involve pyruvate metabolism, the Krebs cycle, and respiratory complexes (DiMauro and Moraes, 1993). Figure 8–5 depicts the five respiratory complexes, and Table 8–7 lists the disorders assigned to abnormalities in each of these complexes.

Subacute Necrotizing Encephalomyelopathy (Leigh Disease)

Leigh isease is a syndrome of progressive poliodystrophy primarily affecting neurons of the brainstem, thalamus, basal ganglia, and cerebellum. These pathologic features can be caused by more than one enzyme deficiency in pyruvate metabolism or by abnormalities in respiratory chain complexes I and IV. Usually the disease is transmitted by autosomal recessive inheritance, but X-linked inheritance occurs as well (Matthews et al, 1993).

CLINICAL FEATURES. Onset occurs during the first year in 60%, during the second year in 20%, and after infancy in 20%. Children who have symptoms in early infancy have a steadily progressive course with severe disability and death. The initial symptoms are some combination of developmental delay, failure to thrive because of poor feeding or vomiting, hypotonia, and seizures. Symptoms are made worse by intercurrent infection or ingestion of a heavy-carbohydrate meal. Three typical, but not constant, features during infancy are respiratory disturbances, abnormal ocular motility, and hypotonia. Respiratory disturbances are at first episodic and can be characterized by Cheyne-Stokes breathing, ataxic breathing, or central hyperventilation. Respiratory distress is the usual cause of death. Ocular motility dysfunction varies from nystagmus to ophthalmoplegia. Hypotonia results from a combination of peripheral neuropathy and disturbed cerebellar function.

Children with Leigh disease caused by cytochrome *c* oxidase deficiency are normal during the first 8 to 12 months and then develop diarrhea, vomiting, and failure to thrive. Symptoms of neurologic deterioration, similar to those described above, occur in late infancy or early childhood. The course is less rapidly progressive and symptoms are more intermittent, with exacerbations at time of infection (Van Coster et al, 1991).

DIAGNOSIS. Blood concentrations of lactate and pyruvate are usually elevated and rise even higher at the time of clinical exacerbation. An oral glucose load causes blood lactate concentrations to double after 60 minutes (Chi et al, 1992).

Lesions in the brainstem and around the third ventricle may be visualized on CT and MRI and the interpeak latency of waves V to III is prolonged on brainstem auditory evoked response. Motor nerve conduction velocities are usually slowed. When peripheral neuropathy is present, the protein content of the cerebrospinal fluid is elevated. Studies should search for cytochrome-oxidase deficiency and for disturbances in pyruvate utilization caused by deficiencies in pyruvate decarboxylase, multiple carboxylases, or pyruvate dehydrogenase. Muscle biopsy specimens have been useful for enzyme analysis in several patients.

TREATMENT. Patients with disorders of pyruvate utilization are less likely to have acute exacerbations of illness on a carbohydrate-restricted diet. Calories should be provided primarily as lipid. Large doses of thiamine are helpful in some patients.

Oral acetazolamide is useful in the treatment of cases transmitted by X-linked recessive inheritance. The mechanism of action is unknown. Whether acetazolamide is also effective in cases transmitted by autosomal recessive inheritance is not established.

Progressive Infantile Poliodystrophy (Alpers Disease)

Alpers disease was described originally as a progressive degeneration of cerebral gray matter and probably encompassed several disease processes. Deficiencies in pyruvate carboxylase activity and respiratory chain complexes I and IV have been identified in familial cases of progressive infantile poliodystrophy associated with mitochondrial myopathy (DiMauro and Moraes, 1993). A transmissible agent may be responsible for some sporadic cases; a poliodystrophy has been serially transmitted to hamsters with brain tissue from an affected child (Manuelidis and Rorke, 1989).

CLINICAL FEATURES. The onset of symptoms is either during infancy or childhood. The disorder with infantile onset tends to be sporadic and is characterized first by delay in the achievement of developmental milestones and then by either myoclonic or tonic-clonic seizures. Status epilepticus can be the first seizure. Prolonged seizures are sometimes followed by transitory hemiplegia. Psychomotor regression becomes evident, and blindness may occur.

DIAGNOSIS. Definitive diagnosis can be established only by postmortem examination. However, an elevated blood lactate concentration should suggest disturbed pyruvate utilization and prompt investigation of mitochondrial enzymes in liver and skeletal muscle. A carbohydrate load in the form of an oral glucose tolerance test may raise the blood lactate concentration to two or three times normal and worsen symptoms.

TREATMENT. A low-carbohydrate diet is recommended for children with disorders of pyruvate utilization. However, no specific treatment has proved effective in Alpers disease.

Trichopoliodystrophy (Menkes Syndrome)

Menkes syndrome is believed to be a primary defect in the intestinal transport of copper. The symptoms are attributed to a secondary defi-

ciency of copper-dependent enzymes, especially cytochrome c oxidase. Some patients show enzyme deficiency in muscle, brain, and liver mitochondria; others show decreased copper concentration only in the brain.

CLINICAL FEATURES. The initial symptoms usually develop in the first 3 months. Development is first arrested and then regresses. The infant becomes lethargic and less reactive. Myoclonic seizures, provoked by stimulation, are an early and almost constant feature. By the end of the first year the infant is in a chronic vegetative state, and most die before 18 months.

The appearance of the scalp hair and eyebrows is almost pathognomonic. The hair is sparse, poorly pigmented, and wiry. The shafts break easily forming short stubble (kinky hair). Radiographs of the long bones suggest osteogenesis imperfecta. Other facial abnormalities include abnormal fullness of the cheeks, a high-arched palate, and micrognathia.

DIAGNOSIS. A carbohydrate load in the form of an oral glucose tolerance test may raise the blood lactate concentration to two or three times normal (Chi et al, 1992). In infants with clinical features of Menkes disease the diagnosis can be established by the microscopic appearance of the hair shaft and by showing a decreased plasma concentrations of copper.

TREATMENT. One patient, treated from an early age with intramuscular copper histidine and oral D-penicillamine, developed much less severe neurologic dysfunction than did his maternal uncle (Nadal and Baerlocher, 1988).

NEUROCUTANEOUS SYNDROMES

Chédiak-Higashi Syndrome

Chédiak-Higashi syndrome is a rare disorder transmitted by autosomal recessive inheritance. The postulated mechanism is lack of regulation of fusion of primary lymphocytes.

CLINICAL FEATURES. Affected children are born with deficient pigment of the skin and hair. Areas of skin depigmentation form bizarre patterns that resemble giant fingerprints. Recurrent infections are prominent during infancy.

Developmental retardation, seizures, and severe peripheral neuropathy develop during the first 2 years. Symptoms of autonomic dysfunction, increased perspiration and failure to produce overflow tears, are common and may suggest dysautonomia.

DIAGNOSIS. The diagnosis is primarily based on the typical neurologic features and pigmentary changes. Examination of the peripheral blood smear is confirmatory. The nuclei of polymorphonuclear leukocytes are pyknotic and their cytoplasm contains large oval and fusiform granules that stain for myeloperoxidase.

TREATMENT. No treatment is available.

Neurofibromatosis Type 1

The neurofibromatoses are divided into a peripheral type (type 1) and a central type (type 2) (NIH Conference, 1990). Both are transmitted by autosomal dominant inheritance and show considerable variation in expression. The abnormal gene for neurofibromatosis type 1 is located on chromosome 17q (Gutmann and Collins, 1993). Almost 50% of patients with neurofibromatosis type 1 are new mutations. New mutations are associated with increased paternal age.

Neurofibromatosis type 2 is characterized by bilateral acoustic neuromas as well as other intracranial and intraspinal tumors (see Chapter 17).

CLINICAL FEATURES. Type 1 disease is believed to be the most common single-gene disorder of the nervous system, affecting 1 in 4,000 individuals. Mild cases are characterized by café au lait spots and subcutaneous neurofibromas. Axillary freckles are common.

Severely affected individuals have developmental and neoplastic disorders of the nervous system. The main central nervous system tumors are optic pathway glioma, hamartoma, plexiform neurofibroma, intraspinal neurofibromas, and megalencephaly. Acoustic neuromas are not part of neurofibromatosis type 1. The usual cognitive defect is a learning disability (Hofman et al, 1994). No more than 10% of patients with type 1 disease are retarded. Those who are retarded are more likely to have seizures than developmental delay as their initial manifestation. Nevertheless, neurofibromatosis should be suspected in any infant with psychomotor retardation and café au lait spots.

DIAGNOSIS. Two or more of the following features are considered diagnostic: (1) six café au lait spots greater than 5 mm in diameter in prepubertal individuals, or greater than 15 mm in postpubertal individuals, (2) two or more neurofibromas or one plexiform neurofibroma, (3) freckling in the axillary or inguinal region, (4) optic glioma, (5) two or more iris hamartomas (Lisch nodules), (6) a distinctive osseous lesion such as sphenoid dysplasia or thinning of long bones, and (7) a first-degree relative with neurofibromatosis type 1.

MRI may provide additional diagnostic information. Areas of increased T_2 signal intensity are often present in the basal ganglia, cerebellum, brainstem, and subcortical white matter. The histology of these areas is not established but the total burden of such areas correlates with intellectual impairment (North et al, 1994).

TREATMENT. Management is primarily symptomatic: anticonvulsant drugs for seizures, surgery for accessible tumors, and orthopedic procedures for bony deformities. Routine MRI studies to screen for optic gliomas in nonsymptomatic children is not recommended.

Tuberous Sclerosis

Tuberous sclerosis is transmitted by autosomal dominant inheritance and has variable phenotypic expression (Aicardi, 1993). Genetic linkage to chromosome 9 has been established in some families, and to chromosome 16 in others (Kandt, 1993). Two different genetic disorders are therefore encompassed by the term *tuberous sclerosis*.

CLINICAL FEATURES. The most common initial symptom of neurologic dysfunction during infancy is seizures, especially infantile spasms (see Chapter 1). Some infants have evidence of developmental delay before the onset of seizures. The delay is often insufficient to prompt medical consultation. Most children with tuberous sclerosis who are mentally retarded eventually have seizures, and all children who have intractable seizures during the first year will be mentally retarded.

Life expectancy is shortened by the disease. The causes of death during childhood are renal disease, cardiovascular disorders, brain tumors, and status epilepticus.

DIAGNOSIS. Tuberous sclerosis should be suspected in infants with developmental delay when hypopigmented areas are present in the skin. These hypochromic nevi are usually lance shaped or oval, and are scattered on the trunk and limbs. Only 18% of patients have "characteristic" leaf-shaped hypochromic nevi. Depigmented areas are readily delineated by illumination with a Wood light.

In late infancy and early childhood, café au lait spots develop and an isolated raised plaque in the skin over the lower back or buttocks (Shagreen patch) is present by 15 years in 50% of affected children. During childhood, adenomata sebaceum (actually angiokeratomas) appear on the face, usually in a butterfly distribution. Other organ involvement includes retinal tumors, rhabdomyoma of the heart, renal tumors, and cysts of the kidney, bone, and lung. Seizures and mental retardation are due to disturbed histogenesis of the brain. Neurons are decreased in number, and astrocytes are large and bizarrely shaped. Glial tumors are common in the subependymal region and may cause obstructive hydrocephalus.

TREATMENT. Anticonvulsants are helpful in reducing seizure frequency but rarely provide complete control. Mental retardation is not reversible. Genetic counseling is an important aspect of patient management. Although the disease is transmitted by autosomal dominant inheritance, gene expression is so variable that neither parent may appear affected. Sporadic cases were thought to be common. However, 25% of parents without personal or family history of tuberous sclerosis are shown to be affected by careful history and physical examination, including Wood light examination of the skin, funduscopic examination, renal ultrasound, and cranial CT.

OTHER DISORDERS OF GRAY MATTER

Infantile Neuronal Ceroid Lipofuscinosis (Santavuori Disease)

In this group of genetic disorders, lipopigment is deposited in neurons and some visceral tissues. These disorders are usually classified by age at onset and rapidity of progression. The more common types occur after age 2 (see "Progressive Encephalopathies of Childhood" later in this chapter). The early infantile type (Santavuori disease) occurs primarily in Finnish people and is transmitted by autosomal recessive inheritance.

CLINICAL FEATURES. Onset is usually in the second year, but may be in the first. Visual impairment and myoclonus are initial features. Rapid deterioration follows and is characterized by psychomotor regression, hypotonia, ataxia, and hyperkinesia. Seizures are not prominent.

Total blindness develops between the ages of 2 and 3 years. The macula has degenerated and has a brownish color, the optic disk is atrophic, and the peripheral retina is hypopigmented.

DIAGNOSIS. Antemortem diagnosis can be established by ultrastructural studies of leukocytes, skin, or conjunctiva. Between 15% and 21% of lymphocytes or monocytes contain granular, osmiophilic membrane-bound cytoplasmic inclusions. Skin and conjunctival biopsies reveal similar granular inclusions in endothelial and neuronal cells.

TREATMENT. Seizures and myoclonus should be treated with a combination of valproate, clonazepam, and phenobarbital (see Chapter 1). No treatment for the underlying metabolic error is available.

Infantile Neuroaxonal Dystrophy

Infantile neuroaxonal dystrophy (Seitelberger disease) is a disorder of axon terminals transmitted by autosomal recessive inheritance. It shares many pathologic features with Hallervorden-Spatz disease (see Chapter 14) and may be an infantile form.

CLINICAL FEATURES. Affected children usually develop normally during the first year, but most do not walk independently. Toward the end of the first year, motor regression is evidenced by clumsiness and frequent falling. The infant is first hypotonic and hyporeflexic. Muscle atrophy may be present as well. At this stage a peripheral neuropathy is suspected, but motor nerve conduction velocity and the protein content of the cerebrospinal fluid are normal.

After the initial phase of hypotonia, symptoms of cerebral degeneration become prominent. Increasing spastic quadriparesis, optic atrophy, involuntary movements, and mental regression are evident. By 2 years of age, most children are severely handicapped. They deteriorate to a vegetative state, and death usually occurs by age 10 years.

DIAGNOSIS. The cerebrospinal fluid is usually normal. Electromyography shows a denervation pattern consistent with anterior horn cell disease. Motor nerve conduction velocities are normal. T_2-weighted MRI shows marked cerebellar atrophy with diffuse hyperintensity of the cerebellar cortex (Tanabe et al, 1993). The hyperintensity is probably due to extensive gliosis.

A definitive diagnosis requires showing neuroaxonal spheroids in peripheral nerve endings, conjunctiva, or brain. Neuroaxonal spheroids are large eosinophilic spheroids, caused by axonal swelling, throughout the gray matter. They are not unique to neuroaxonal dystrophy and are also seen in Hallervorden-Spatz disease, infantile GM_2 gangliosidosis, Niemann-Pick disease type C, and several other neurodegenerative conditions.

TREATMENT. No treatment is available.

Lesch-Nyhan Disease

Lesch-Nyhan disease is caused by a deficiency of the enzyme hypoxanthine guanine phosphoribosyltransferase. The trait is transmitted by X-linked inheritance.

CLINICAL FEATURES. Affected newborns appear normal at birth, except for mild hypotonia. Delayed motor development and poor head control are present during the first 3 months. These are followed by progressive limb rigidity and torticollis or retrocollis. The progression of neurologic disturbance is insidious, and many affected patients are thought to have cerebral palsy. During the second year, facial grimacing, corticospinal tract dysfunction, and involuntary movements (usually chorea but sometimes athetosis) develop.

It is not until after age 2, and sometimes considerably later, that affected children begin biting their fingers, lips, and cheeks. Compulsive self-mutilation is characteristic, but not invariable, and causes severe disfigurement. Often wrapping the hands or removing teeth is necessary to prevent further harm. In addition to self-directed aggressive behavior, aggressive behavior toward caretakers may be present. Mental retardation is constant but of variable severity. Intelligence is difficult to evaluate because of behavioral and motor disturbances.

DIAGNOSIS. Uric acid concentrations are increased in the blood and urine. Indeed, some parents note a reddish discoloration of diapers caused by uric acid. The diagnosis is established by showing that hypoxanthine guanine phosphoribosyltransferase activity is absent in erythrocytes or cultured fibroblasts.

TREATMENT. Allopurinol decreases the urinary concentration of uric acid and prevents the development of nephropathy. Self-mutilatory behavior may be abated by the use of levodopa or tetrabenazine (Jankovic et al, 1988). However, no treatment is available to prevent progressive degeneration of the nervous system.

Progressive Neuronal Degeneration with Liver Disease

This syndrome probably encompasses several different conditions and is sometimes referred to as *Alpers disease* or *Alpers-Huttenlocher disease* (Harding et al, 1995). It is not the same disorder as progressive infantile poliodystrophy (Alpers) listed in this chapter as a mitochondrial disorder.

CLINICAL FEATURES. Hypotonia, failure to thrive, and developmental delay during infancy are followed by intractable seizures and liver failure. Status epilepticus is common. Death from liver failure usually occurs by age 3.

In addition to the infantile form, a similar syndrome has been described in children and adolescents. Among older children, visual hallucinations may be in initial features. Status epilepticus and liver failure are common. Death is invariable.

DIAGNOSIS. MRI shows lesions in the deep gray matter as well as the cortex. The occipital lobes are selectively involved. The diagnosis is suspected by the combination of encephalopathy and liver failure. The encephalopathy is not caused by the liver failure, and the liver disease is not caused by drugs used to treat seizures. The definitive diagnosis requires postmortem examination to show a patchy destruction of the cerebral cortex with predominant involvement in the occipital lobes.

TREATMENT. Anticonvulsant drugs are used to treat seizures, but no treatment is available for the underlying disease.

Rett Syndrome

Rett syndrome occurs only in girls and the prevalence is estimated to be 1:10,000. Most cases are sporadic, but a few families with more than one affected sibling have been reported, suggesting a genetic mode of transmission. X-linked dominant inheritance with lethality in male fetuses is suspected.

CLINICAL FEATURES. Affected girls are normal during the first year. Developmental arrest usually begins at 12 months, but may appear as early as 5 months or as late as 18 months. Within a few months rapid developmental regression occurs and is characterized by loss of language skills, decreased use of the hands, gait ataxia, and autistic behavior. Head growth is arrested, with eventual microcephaly. Dementia is usually severe. Although affected girls are unable to sustain interest in the environment, stimulation produces an exaggerated, stereotyped reaction consisting of jerking movements of the trunk and limbs with episodes of disorganized breathing and apnea, followed by hyperpnea. During these episodes circumoral cyanosis and diffuse perspiration may occur. Similar episodes may also occur without stimulation but not during sleep. Such episodes are frequently interpreted as seizures, although it is not clear that they are epileptic in nature. Typical tonic-clonic seizures, partial complex seizures, or myoclonic seizures occur in most children between the ages of 2 and 4 years.

■ TABLE 5–10
Diagnostic Criteria for Rett Syndrome

Necessary Criteria
Apparently normal prenatal and perinatal period and development in first 6 months
Normal head circumference at birth and deceleration of head growth between 5 months and 4 years
Loss of acquired purposeful hand movements between 6 and 30 months
Development of stereotyped hand movements
Severe progressive dementia
Appearance of gait apraxia and truncal apraxia and ataxia between 1 and 4 years of age

Supportive Criteria
Breathing dysfunction
Electroencephalographic abnormalities and seizures
Growth retardation and hypotrophic small feet
Spasticity and dystonia
Peripheral vasomotor disturbances
Scoliosis

Exclusion Criteria
Intrauterine growth retardation or microcephaly at birth
Organomegaly or signs of storage disease
Retinopathy or optic atrophy
Evidence of an identifiable, acquired neurologic disease

A characteristic feature of the syndrome is loss of purposeful hand movements before the age of 3. They are replaced by stereotyped activity that looks like hand wringing or washing. Repetitive blows to the face are another form of stereotyped hand movement.

The initial rapid progression is followed by a continued slower progression of neurologic deterioration. Spastic paraparesis and quadriparesis are frequent endpoints.

DIAGNOSIS. Diagnosis is based entirely on the clinical features. Laboratory tests are not helpful. The Rett Syndrome Diagnostic Criteria Work Group (1988) established the diagnostic criteria that are summarized in Table 5–10.

TREATMENT. Seizures often respond to standard anticonvulsant drugs. Naltrexone, 1 to 2 mg/kg/day, has been tried to treat the underlying disease, but its value is not established.

OTHER DISORDERS OF WHITE MATTER

Alexander Disease

Alexander disease is a rare disorder believed to be caused by astrocytic dysfunction (Pridmore et al, 1993). All cases are sporadic, and a genetic basis is only suspected. Rosenthal fibers, the pathologic hallmark of disease, are rod-shaped or round bodies that stain red with hematoxylin and eosin and black with myelin stains. They appear as small granules within the cytoplasm of astrocytes. Rosenthal fibers are scattered diffusely in the cerebral cortex and the white matter, but have a predilection for the subpial, subependymal, and perivascular regions.

CLINICAL FEATURES. Rosenthal fibers are pathologic features of three clinical syndromes. First and most common is the *infantile form,* which affects primarily males. The onset may be anytime from birth to early childhood. These infants show arrest and regression of psychomotor development, enlargement of the head owing to megalencephaly, spasticity, and seizures. Megalencephaly may be the initial feature. Optic atrophy does not occur. Death by the second or third year is the rule.

The *juvenile form* is characterized by bulbar symptoms, and the *adult form* has a course that suggests multiple sclerosis.

DIAGNOSIS. The cerebrospinal fluid is normal. The disease should be suspected in infants with macrocephaly and MRI evidence of progressive leukodystrophy affecting the deep white matter and sparing the periventricular region. Definitive diagnosis relies entirely on the postmortem demonstration of Rosenthal fibers.

TREATMENT. No treatment is available.

Aspartoacylase Deficiency (Canavan Disease)

Canavan disease (also spongy degeneration of infancy) is transmitted by autosomal recessive inheritance. It is caused by deficiency of aspartoacylase. Different mutations account for Jewish and non-Jewish cases (Kaul et al, 1994).

CLINICAL FEATURES. Psychomotor arrest and regression occur during the first 6 months postpartum. Clinical features include decreased awareness of the environment, difficulty in feeding, irritability, and hypotonia. The initial flaccidity is eventually replaced by spasticity. A characteristic posture, with leg extension, arm flexion, and head retraction, is assumed, especially when the child is stimulated. Macrocephaly is noted by 6 months of age. The head continues to enlarge throughout infancy and reaches a plateau by the third year. Optic atrophy leading to blindness is noted between 6 and 10 months.

DIAGNOSIS. Abnormal excretion of N-acetylaspartic acid can be detected in the urine, and aspartoacylase activity in cultured fibroblasts is less than 40% of normal. MRI shows diffuse symmetric leukoencephalopathy even before neurologic symptoms are evident. Demyelination of peripheral nerves does not occur, and the cerebrospinal fluid is normal.

TREATMENT. No treatment is available.

Galactosemia: Transferase Deficiency

Three separate inborn errors of galactose metabolism are known to produce galactosemia in the newborn, but only galactose-1-phosphate uridyltransferase deficiency produces mental retardation. The defect is transmitted by autosomal recessive inheritance.

CLINICAL FEATURES. Affected newborns appear normal, but cataracts are already developing. The initial symptoms are provoked by the first milk feeding and include failure to thrive, vomiting, diarrhea, jaundice, and hepatomegaly. During this time some newborns have clinical features of increased intracranial pressure, probably resulting from cerebral edema. The combination of a tense fontanelle and vomiting suggests a primary intracranial disturbance and can delay the diagnosis and treatment of the metabolic error.

DIAGNOSIS. Galactosemia should be considered in any newborn with vomiting and hepatomegaly, especially when cataracts are present. The best time to test the urine for reducing substances (by use of Clinitest tablets) is after feeding. Specific tests for glucose (Testape, Clinistix) show no abnormality. Most cases of galactosemia in newborns are now detected by routine screening tests.

TREATMENT. Symptoms are usually reversed by providing a galactose-free diet. The diet must be started early to optimize intellectual outcome, and even then some children have mental retardation. In children who do not respond fully to diet, the achievement of developmental milestones is delayed during the first year and intellectual function is moderately retarded by age 5. After age 5, truncal ataxia develops and progresses in severity. Associated with ataxia is a coarse resting tremor of the limbs. Because of the restricted diet, cataracts and hepatomegaly are not present. The enzyme deficiency in children who deteriorate neurologically does not appear different from the deficiency in those who respond favorably to diet therapy.

Pelizaeus-Merzbacher Disease

Pelizaeus-Merzbacher disease is a rare demyelinating disorder transmitted by X-linked recessive inheritance. It is caused by defective bio-synthesis of a proteolipid protein that comprises half of the myelin sheath protein (Pratt et al, 1995). An infantile, a neonatal, and a transitional phenotype are differentiated.

CLINICAL FEATURES. The first symptoms of the neonatal form suggest spasmus nutans (see Chapter 15). The neonate has an intermittent nodding movement of the head and pendular nystagmus. Chorea or athetosis develops, psychomotor development is arrested by the third month, and regression follows. Limb movements become ataxic and tone becomes spastic, first in the legs and then in the arms. Optic atrophy and seizures are a late occurrence. Death occurs by 5 to 7 years of age.

When the onset of disease is at the end of the first month or later, the symptoms are the same as in the neonatal form but the course is more prolonged and survival to adult life is relatively common.

DIAGNOSIS. MRI shows diffuse demyelination of the hemispheres with sparing of scattered small areas. Diagnosis is established by showing a deletion of the exon coding the proteolipid protein on the X chromosome. Postmortem examination shows diffuse demyelination of the cerebral and cerebellar hemispheres with patches of normal myelin remaining. Nerve cells and axons appear normal. When survival is prolonged, myelin is completely absent in the cerebral hemispheres.

TREATMENT. No treatment is available.

PROGRESSIVE HYDROCEPHALUS

CLINICAL FEATURES. Progressive dilatation of the ventricular system may be a consequence of congenital malformations, infectious diseases, intracranial hemorrhage, or connatal tumors. Whatever the cause, the clinical features of increasing intracranial pressure are much the same. Head circumference enlarges, the anterior fontanelle feels full, and the child becomes lethargic, has difficulty feeding, and vomits. Ataxia and a spastic gait are common.

DIAGNOSIS. Progressive hydrocephalus is often insidious in premature newborns with intraventricular hemorrhage, especially when delayed progression follows initial arrest. Hydrocephalus should always be suspected in newborns and infants with excessive head growth; the diagnosis is readily confirmed by CT.

TREATMENT. Ventriculoperitoneal shunt is the usual procedure to relieve hydrocephalus in newborns and small infants with primary dilatation of the lateral ventricles (see Chapter 18).

⮕ Progressive Encephalopathies with Onset After Age 2

DISORDERS OF LYSOSOMAL ENZYMES

GM$_2$ Gangliosidosis (Juvenile Tay-Sachs Disease)

The juvenile form of Tay-Sachs disease, like the infantile form, is caused by deficiency of N-acetyl-beta-hexosaminidase. The enzymatic basis of the phenotypic variability is incompletely understood (Specola et al, 1990).

CLINICAL FEATURES. There is no ethnic predilection. Affected children appear normal until age 3 years but then dysarthria, language retardation, and gait disturbances develop. The gait is first ataxic and then spastic. Progressive dementia follows, and death usually occurs within the first decade. Seizures and involuntary movements may occur in some patients.

DIAGNOSIS. Enzyme deficiency is demonstrated in leukocytes and fibroblasts.

TREATMENT. No treatment is available.

Gaucher Disease Type III (Glucosylceramide Lipidosis)

The late-onset type of Gaucher disease, like other types, is caused by deficiency of the enzyme glucocerebrosidase and transmitted by autosomal recessive inheritance.

CLINICAL FEATURES. Age at onset ranges from early childhood to adult life. Hepatosplenomegaly usually precedes neurologic deterioration. The most common neurologic manifestations are seizures and mental regression. Mental regression varies from mild memory loss to severe dementia. Myoclonus and myoclonic seizures develop in many patients. Some combination of spasticity, ataxia, and cranial nerve dysfunction may be present as well. Vertical oculomotor apraxia, as described in Niemann-Pick disease, may occur in late-onset Gaucher disease as well.

DIAGNOSIS. Gaucher cells are present in the bone marrow and are virtually diagnostic. Confirmation requires the demonstration of deficient glucocerebrosidase activity in hepatocytes or leukocytes.

TREATMENT. Repeated infusions of modified acid beta-glucosidase reverses the clinical fea-

tures, but its use is limited by its expense. Bone marrow transplantation may prevent progression of neurologic disease but its long-term usefulness is not established (Beutler and Grabowski, 1995).

Globoid Cell Leukodystrophy (Late-Onset Krabbe Disease)

Globoid cell leukodystrophy is caused by deficiency of the enzyme galactosylceramide beta-galactosidase. The defect is transmitted by autosomal recessive inheritance. The onset of symptoms in late infancy and in adolescence can occur in the same family (Verdru et al, 1991). The severity of enzyme deficiency is similar in all phenotypes from early infancy to adolescence.

CLINICAL FEATURES. Neurologic deterioration usually begins between the ages of 2 and 6, but may start as early as the second year or as late as adolescence. The major features are mental regression, cortical blindness, and generalized or unilateral spasticity. The initial feature may be progressive spasticity rather than dementia. Unlike the infantile form, peripheral neuropathy is not a feature of the juvenile form, and the protein content of the cerebrospinal fluid is normal. Progressive neurologic deterioration results in a vegetative state.

DIAGNOSIS. MRI shows diffuse demyelination of the cerebral hemispheres. The diagnosis is established by showing enzyme deficiency in leukocytes or cultured fibroblasts.

TREATMENT. No treatment is available.

Glycoprotein Degradation Disorders

Aspartylglycosaminuria

Aspartylglycosaminuria is a very rare condition that occurs primarily in Finnish individuals. The defect, a deficiency of the enzyme N-aspartyl-beta-glucosaminidase, is transmitted by autosomal recessive inheritance.

CLINICAL FEATURES. Affected individuals are healthy in early infancy but later have recurrent infection, diarrhea, and inguinal hernia (Thomas and Beaudet, 1995). During early childhood, the facial features become coarse and hepatomegaly occasionally develops. Lens opacities occur after age 10. Speech may be delayed, but mental development is otherwise normal until age 5. Afterward, a slowly progressive regression of mental and motor skills results in severe retardation and generalized weakness.

DIAGNOSIS. Vacuolated lymphocytes are present in the peripheral blood of most patients, and a mild form of dysostosis multiplex is demonstrated radiographically. The urine does not contain mucopolysaccharides but does contain oligosaccharides. The diagnosis is established by showing enzyme deficiency in leukocytes or cultured fibroblasts.

TREATMENT. No treatment is available.

Mannosidosis Type II

CLINICAL FEATURES. The late-onset, juvenile and adult form of mannosidosis is characterized by normal early development followed by mental regression during childhood or adolescence. Dysostosis multiplex is not a prominent feature, but deafness occurs in all cases.

DIAGNOSIS. Vacuolated lymphocytes are present in peripheral blood. The urine contains oligosaccharides, but not mucopolysaccharides. The diagnosis is established by showing deficient activity of beta-mannosidase in cultured fibroblasts.

TREATMENT. No treatment is available.

Metachromatic Leukodystrophy (Late-Onset Lipidosis)

The juvenile form of sulfatide lipidosis, like the infantile form, is caused by a deficiency of the enzyme arylsulfatase A and is transmitted by autosomal recessive inheritance. Two groups of mutations in the gene encoding arylsulfatase A are identified as I and A. The I group generates no active enzyme and the A group generates small amounts. Late-onset disease is associated with an I-A genotype, and the adult form with an A-A genotype (Kolodny and Fluharty, 1995), correlate with the clinical phenotype.

CLINICAL FEATURES. The onset of symptoms is generally between 5 and 10 years, but may be delayed until adolescence or occur as early as late infancy. The early-onset juvenile form is clinically different from the infantile form despite the age overlap. No clinical symptoms of peripheral neuropathy occur, progression is slow, and the protein content of the cerebrospinal fluid is normal.

Mental regression, speech disturbances, and clumsiness of gait are the prominent initial features. The dementia usually progresses slowly over a period 3 to 5 years, but sometimes progresses rapidly to a vegetative state. A delay of several years may separate the onset of dementia from the appearance of other neurologic disturbances. Ataxia may be an early and prominent manifestation. A spastic quadriplegia

eventually develops in all affected children, and most have seizures. Death usually occurs during the second decade.

DIAGNOSIS. The juvenile form can overlap in age with a late-onset form that usually is manifest as psychosis or dementia. MRI demonstrates demyelination in the cerebral hemispheres. Motor nerve conduction velocities may be normal early in the course. The diagnosis is established by showing arylsulfatase A deficiency in leukocytes or cultured fibroblasts.

TREATMENT. No treatment is available.

Mucopolysaccharidoses

The mucopolysaccharidoses (MPS) result from deficiencies of enzymes involved in the catabolism of dermatan sulfate, heparan sulfate, or keratin sulfate. There are at least seven major types of mucopolysaccharidoses. Four of these, types I, II, III, and VII, affect the nervous system and cause mental retardation. Types I and III have their onset in infancy and are discussed in the prior section. Types II and VII ordinarily have their onset in childhood following 2 or more years of normal development (Figure 5–8).

Type II MPS (Hunter Syndrome)

This is the only MPS transmitted by X-linked inheritance.

CLINICAL FEATURES. Patients with the Hunter syndrome have a Hurler phenotype (Table 5–8), but lack corneal clouding (Neufeld and Muenzer, 1995). Iduronate sulfatase is the deficient enzyme; dermatan sulfate and heparan sulfate are stored in the viscera and appear in the urine.

The Hurler phenotype may develop rapidly or evolve slowly during childhood and may not be recognized until the second decade or later. A prominent feature is the appearance of a nodular, ivory-colored lesion on the back, usually around the shoulders and upper arms. Mental regression caused by neuronal storage of gangliosides is slowly progressive, but many patients come to medical attention because of chronic hydrocephalus. Affected children survive into adult life. The accumulation of storage materials in collagen causes the entrapment of peripheral nerves, especially the median and ulnar.

DIAGNOSIS. Diagnosis is suggested by the presence of mucopolysacchariduria with equal excretion of dermatan sulfate and heparan sulfate. The diagnosis is established by showing

☐ FIGURE 5 – 8 Evaluation of children with progressive dementia.

enzyme deficiency in cultured fibroblasts or serum. Prenatal diagnosis is accomplished by detecting iduronate sulfatase activity in amniotic fluid.

TREATMENT. Nerve entrapment and hydrocephalus can be relieved by appropriate surgical procedures. No treatment is available for the underlying storage disease.

Type VII MPS (Sly Disease)

Sly disease is a rare disorder caused by deficiency of the enzyme beta-glucuronidase. It is transmitted by autosomal recessive inheritance.

CLINICAL FEATURES. The patient has an incomplete Hurler phenotype, with hepatosplenomegaly, inguinal hernias, and dysostosis multiplex as the major features. Corneal clouding does not occur, and the face, although unusual, is not typical of the Hurler phenotype. Psychomotor retardation develops after age 2, but not in all cases.

DIAGNOSIS. Both dermatan sulfate and heparan sulfate are present in the urine, causing a screening test to be positive for mucopolysacchariduria. Specific diagnosis requires the demonstration of beta-glucuronidase deficiency in leukocytes or cultured fibroblasts.

TREATMENT. No treatment is available.

Niemann-Pick Disease Type C (Sphingomyelin Lipidosis)

The chronic neuronopathic form of Niemann-Pick disease is similar to the acute infantile form except that onset is usually after age 2, progression is slower, and there is no specific racial predilection. Sphingomyelinase is the deficient enzyme in all forms of Niemann-Pick disease. The defect is transmitted by autosomal recessive inheritance.

CLINICAL FEATURES. Three phenotypes are distinguished by age of onset and predominant symptoms (Fink et al, 1989):

1. The early-onset form is characterized by organomegaly and rapidly progressive hepatic dysfunction during the first year, often in the first 6 months. Developmental delay is noted during the first year, and neurologic deterioration (ataxia, vertical gaze apraxia, dementia) occurs between 1 and 3 years of age.

2. The delayed-onset form is more common than the other two and has the most stereotyped clinical features. Early development is normal. Cerebellar ataxia or dystonia are the initial features, mean age 3 years, and apraxia of vertical gaze and cognitive difficulties follow, mean age 6 years (Higgins et al, 1992). Oculomotor

apraxia, in which the eyes move reflexively but not voluntarily, is unusual in children (see Chapter 15). Vertical gaze apraxia is particularly uncommon and always suggests Niemann-Pick disease type C. Progressive neurologic degeneration is relentless. Dementia, seizures, spasticity, dysphasia, and dystonia develop after age 6 and cause severe disability during the second decade. Organomegaly is seldom prominent early in the course.

3.   The late-onset form begins in adolescence or adult life and is similar to the delayed-onset form except that the progression is considerably slower.

DIAGNOSIS. Examination of bone marrow reveals two unusual storage cells. One is large and vacuolated, the other is smaller. Both contain dark, granular material. Definitive diagnosis requires demonstration of sphingomyelinase deficiency in leukocytes or cultured fibroblasts. Heterozygote detection and prenatal diagnosis are possible.

TREATMENT. A regimen of lovastatin, cholestyramine, and niacin lower plasma and hepatic lipid concentrations, but its effect on neurologic progression is not established (Patterson et al, 1993).

INFECTIOUS DISEASES

Infectious diseases are an uncommon cause of progressive dementia in childhood. Several fungal species may produce a chronic meningitis characterized by personality change and some decline in higher intellectual function. *Cryptococcus* infection is especially notorious for its long indolent course. However, the major features of these infections are fever and headache. Chronic meningitis is not a serious consideration in the differential diagnosis of isolated psychomotor regression.

In contrast, chronic viral infections, especially HIV (see previous discussion of AIDS encephalopathy), may produce a clinical picture similar to many genetic disorders in which dementia is a prominent feature.

Subacute Sclerosing Panencephalitis

Subacute sclerosing panencephalitis (SSPE) is a form of chronic measles encephalitis that was once endemic in several parts of the world but has almost disappeared in countries that require routine measles immunization. In a nonimmunized population the average age at onset is 8 years. As a rule, children with SSPE have experienced natural infection with the rubeola virus at an early age, half before age 2. A concomitant infection with a second virus at the time of initial exposure to measles and immunosuppression are additional risk factors for SSPE. In the United States incidence rates were highest in rural areas, especially in the southeastern states and the Ohio River valley.

CLINICAL FEATURES. The first symptoms of disease are personality change and declining school performance. Personality change may be aggressive behavior or withdrawal, and psychological rather than medical services may be sought. However, retinal examination during this early stage already shows pigmentary changes in the macula. Generalized seizures, usually myoclonic, develop next. An EEG at this time shows the characteristic pattern of periodic bursts of spike-wave complexes (approximately every 5 to 7 seconds) occurring synchronously with the myoclonic jerk. After the onset of seizures, the child shows a rapid neurologic deterioration characterized by spasticity, dementia, and involuntary movements. Within 1 to 6 years from the onset of symptoms, the child is in a chronic vegetative state.

DIAGNOSIS. The diagnosis can be suspected from the clinical course and characteristic EEG. Confirmation requires demonstration of an elevated antibody titer against rubeola, usually associated with elevated gamma globulin concentrations, in the cerebrospinal fluid. The cerebrospinal fluid is otherwise normal. Plasma rubeola antibody titers are also markedly elevated.

A similar progressive disorder of the nervous system may occur in children who were born with rubella embryopathy (chronic rubella panencephalitis).

TREATMENT. No drug is effective in treating the disease, but it can be prevented by measles immunization.

OTHER DISORDERS OF GRAY MATTER

Ceroid Lipofuscinosis

Several disorders characterized by dementia and blindness are now considered to be forms of ceroid lipofuscinosis (Boustany and Kolodny, 1989). When these disorders were first described, different eponymic designations were used depending on age at onset. The common pathologic feature is the accumulation of autofluorescent lipopigments, ceroid and lipofuscin, within the brain, retina, and some visceral tissues. Juvenile-onset disease is thought to be transmitted by autosomal recessive inheritance localized to chromosome 16 (Yan et al, 1993), but some adult-onset disorders are transmitted as an autosomal dominant trait.

An early-infantile form was described in the previous section. In addition, there are an infantile or childhood form (*Bielschowsky-Jansky disease*), a juvenile form (*Spielmeyer-Vogt-Sjögren disease*), and several adult forms.

Late Infantile Type (Bielschowsky-Jansky Disease)

CLINICAL FEATURES. Age at onset is 2 to 4 years. Seizures rather than blindness are the initial feature. The seizures are myoclonic, akinetic, and tonic-clonic and are usually refractory to anticonvulsant drugs. Severe ataxia develops, owing in part to seizures and in part to motor system deterioration. This is followed by myoclonus, involuntary movements, and dementia. Dementia sometimes precedes the first seizure.

Ophthalmoscopic findings are abnormal before visual symptoms occur. They include attenuation of vessels, early optic atrophy, and pigmentary degeneration of the macula. The loss of motor, mental, and visual function is relentlessly progressive, and within months the child is in a chronic vegetative state. Death is usually in the first decade.

DIAGNOSIS. Antemortem diagnosis is accomplished by skin and conjunctival biopsy (Santavuori et al, 1991). Curvilinear inclusions are observed by electron microscopy within the cytoplasm of endothelial and neuronal cells. In addition, azurophilic granules are present in neutrophilic leukocytes stained by the Giemsa method.

TREATMENT. Seizures are difficult to control, but may respond in part to a combination of valproate, clonazepam, and phenobarbital (see Chapter 1). No treatment is available for the underlying metabolic error.

Juvenile Type (Spielmeyer-Vogt-Sjögren Disease)

CLINICAL FEATURES. The mean age at onset of the juvenile type is 6 years, with a range from 4 to 9 years. Unlike patients with the late-infantile type, these children frequently have decreasing visual acuity. Ophthalmoscopic examination shows attenuation of retinal vessels, a patchy retinal atrophy that resembles retinitis pigmentosa, mild optic atrophy, and a granular discoloration of the macula that may have a bull's-eye appearance with a dull red spot in the center.

The dementia is characterized by declining school performance and behavioral disturbances. Delusions and hallucinations are common. Blindness and dementia are the only symptoms for many years. Late in the course, speech becomes slurred and Parkinson-like rigidity develops. Myoclonic jerks and tonic-clonic seizures begin some years after onset but are not usually severe. Death usually occurs within 15 years of onset.

DIAGNOSIS. Antemortem diagnosis is reasonably certain because of the characteristic retinal changes and confirmed by skin and conjunctival biopsy. Fingerprint bodies are present in the cytoplasm of several cell types. The electroretinogram shows depression or absence of retinal potentials early in the course. Leukocytes in the peripheral blood are frequently abnormal. Translucent vacuoles are present in lymphocytes, and azurophilic granules occur in neutrophils.

TREATMENT. No treatment is available for the underlying metabolic defect. Seizures usually respond to standard anticonvulsant drugs.

Heller Syndrome

Heller syndrome was originally described as a progressive dementia of childhood affecting males and females between the ages of 1 and 4 years. The early-onset female cases are now believed to be Rett syndrome.

CLINICAL FEATURES. Heller syndrome probably has a male predominance of cases. Affected children develop normally to at least 30 months of age. Dementia progresses for 1 to 3 years and results in profound mental retardation with marked autistic features but no affect on motor skills (Burd et al, 1989).

DIAGNOSIS. The diagnosis is based on clinical symptoms. The syndrome is differentiated from Rett syndrome by the age at onset, male predominance, and lack of motor disturbances; and from infantile autism by the age at onset. All other causes of progressive dementia of childhood must be excluded (Table 5-4).

TREATMENT. No treatment is available.

Huntington Disease

Huntington disease is a chronic degenerative disease of the nervous system transmitted by autosomal dominant inheritance. It is associated with an expanded trinucleotide repeat on chromosome 4 (Kremer et al, 1994). The prevalence is 5 to 10:100,000.

CLINICAL FEATURES. The age of onset is usually between 35 and 55, but may be as early as 2 years. Approximately 10% of affected children show symptoms before 20 years of age, and 5% before 14 years. When Huntington disease begins in childhood, the father is the affected parent in 83% of cases and may be asymptomatic when the child is born. Extrachromosomal organelles, such as mitochondria, are inherited exclusively from the mother and may delay the expression of the gene when the mother is the affected individual.

The initial features are usually progressive dementia and behavioral disturbances. Declining school performance often brings the child to medical attention. Rigidity, with loss of facial expression and associative movements, is more common than choreoathetosis and hyperkinesis in early-onset cases. Cerebellar dysfunction occurs in approximately 20% of cases and can be a major cause of disability. Ocular motor apraxia may also be present (see Chapter 15). Seizures, which are rare in adult-onset cases, are present in 50% of affected children. The course in childhood is relentlessly progressive, and the average duration from onset to death is 8 years.

DIAGNOSIS. Diagnosis depends upon disease in one parent. Striatal hyperintensity on T_2-weighted MRI is characteristic of the akinetic-rigid form of Huntington disease (Oliva et al, 1993).

TREATMENT. Rigidity may be temporarily relieved with levodopa, bromocriptine, and amantadine. Neuroleptics are useful for behavioral control, but no treatment is available for the dementia.

Mitochondrial Encephalomyopathies

The mitochondrial encephalomyopathies are a diverse group of disorders with defects in oxidative metabolism. Three such disorders are described in the section on progressive encephalopathies of infancy. Later-onset mitochondrial disorders are characterized by progressive external ophthalmoplegia or myopathy. However, a late-onset form of poliodystrophy and a syndrome of myoclonic epilepsy associated with ragged-red fibers in skeletal muscle cause childhood dementia as the initial feature. Genetic transmission is by maternal inheritance.

Late-Onset Poliodystrophy

CLINICAL FEATURES. The clinical features are similar to those of progressive infantile poliodystrophy except that the onset of dementia is delayed until 6 years of age or later. The dementia may be preceded by years of intermittent vomiting, lethargy, and headaches. Generalized tonic-clonic seizures can precede the onset of dementia or at least bring the child, who is already demonstrating poor school performance, to medical attention. The subsequent course is variable and probably depends on the underlying defect in mitochondrial metabolism. In many children a myopathy develops; others have spasticity and blindness.

DIAGNOSIS. Many children with mitochondrial enzyme defects have an increased blood concentration of lactate. However, the blood lactate concentration may vary with diet and a glucose-lactate tolerance test is useful to screening test for disturbances in mitochondrial function. An ordinary glucose tolerance test is administered except that both blood lactate and glucose concentrations are measured concurrently. Lactate levels do not rise significantly in normal children but may reach two or three times the upper limit of normal in children with defective mitochondrial metabolism. The elevated glucose concentration is slow in returning to normal. When myopathy is present in addition to dementia, muscle biopsy usually demonstrates ragged red fibers (see Figure 8–6).

TREATMENT. Children with defects in mitochondrial enzymes may benefit from a low-carbohydrate, high-fat diet to prevent lactic acidosis. Several vitamins that serve as cofactors for mitochondrial metabolism have been tried without proven benefit.

Myoclonic Epilepsy and Ragged-Red Fibers

Myoclonic epilepsy and ragged-red fibers (MERRF) is caused by a point mutation in mitochondrial DNA (mtDNA). The severity of the clinical phenotype is proportional to the amount of mutant mtDNA (Graf et al, 1993).

CLINICAL FEATURES. Clinical heterogeneity is common even among members of the same family. Onset may be anytime during childhood or up until the fourth decade. An insidious decline in school performance is often the initial feature, but generalized tonic-clonic seizures or myoclonus may be the symptoms that first prompt medical consultation. The seizures may be induced by flickering light or watching television. Brief myoclonic twitching develops, often induced by action (action myoclonus), that may interfere with hand movement and posture. Ataxia is a constant feature as the disease progresses, and this may be due to action myoclonus rather than cerebellar dysfunction. Some patients have hearing loss, short stature, and endocrine dysfunction.

Neurologic deterioration is progressive and may include spasticity, sensory loss, and central hypoventilation. Clinical evidence of myopathy is not always present.

DIAGNOSIS. Blood concentrations of pyruvate and lactate may be elevated. EEG shows slowing of the background rhythms and a photoconvulsive response. Ragged-red fibers are seen on muscle biopsy (see Figure 8-4).

TREATMENT. Anticonvulsant therapy may provide seizure control early in the course but often fails as the disease progresses. Glucose loads should be avoided. No treatment is available for the underlying defect.

Xeroderma Pigmentosum

Xeroderma pigmentosa is a genetic disorder characterized by defective deoxyribonucleic acid (DNA) repair. Ten genetic subtypes have been defined. Group A is the most common form and is associated with neurologic deterioration (Robbins et al, 1991).

CLINICAL FEATURES. A photosensitive dermatitis develops during the first year, and skin cancer may develop as well. Progressive psychomotor retardation and poor head growth leading to microcephaly are noted after age 3. Sensorineural hearing loss and spinocerebellar degeneration may develop after age 7. Approximately one third of patients are short in stature and some have a phenotype suggesting Cockayne syndrome, which is a separate genetic error (see Chapter 7), but also involves defective DNA repair (Broughton et al, 1995).

DIAGNOSIS. The diagnosis is suggested by the typical skin rash and neurologic deterioration in both the central and peripheral nervous systems, and is confirmed by showing abnormal DNA repair in cultured fibroblasts.

TREATMENT. No treatment is available. Radiation must be avoided.

OTHER DISEASES OF WHITE MATTER
Adrenoleukodystrophy

Adrenoleukodystrophy is a progressive demyelination of the central nervous system associated with adrenal cortical failure. It is transmitted by X-linked inheritance. Affected children have an impaired ability to oxidize very-long-chain fatty acids, especially hexacosanoic acid, because of deficiency of a peroxisomal acyl coenzyme A (CoA) synthetase. Very-long-chain fatty acids accumulate in tissues and plasma. Many cases previously designated as Schilder disease were probably the juvenile form of adrenoleukodystrophy.

Four phenotypes may coexist in the same family. The cerebral form accounts for approximately 56% of cases and is discussed in this section, a slowly progressive adrenomyeloneuropathy accounts for 25% of cases (see Chapter 12), and the remainder have only Addison disease or are asymptomatic (Moser et al, 1992).

CLINICAL FEATURES. The onset of the cerebral form is usually between 5 and 10 years of age, but can be delayed until adolescence or adult life. The first symptoms are usually an alteration in behavior ranging from a withdrawn state to aggressive outbursts. Poor school performance follows invariably and may lead parents to seek psychological services. Neurologic deterioration is then relentlessly progressive and includes disturbances of gait and coordination, loss of vision and hearing, and ultimate deterioration to a vegetative state. Seizures are a late manifestation. The average interval from onset to a vegetative state or death is 3 years.

DIAGNOSIS. The protein concentration of cerebrospinal fluid is generally increased. T_2-weighted MRI shows high signal intensity in the periventricular white matter even in asymptomatic individuals (Aubourg et al, 1989). Adrenal insufficiency may be shown in asymptomatic children by a subnormal response to the stimulation by adrenocorticotropic hormone (ACTH). However, up to 15% have a normal response, and definitive diagnosis requires a plasma assay of very-long-chain fatty acids. The assay also permits identification of carrier females and the prenatal diagnosis of affected fetuses by measuring long-chain fatty acid concentrations in amniocytes.

TREATMENT. Corticosteroids reverse clinical symptoms of adrenal insufficiency, and a diet restricted in very-long-chain fatty acids and enriched with monounsaturated fatty acids

(Lorenzo's oil) normalizes the level of very-long-chain fatty acids in 4 weeks. Lorenzo's oil does not alter the rate of progression of disease in childhood with the cerebral form; its utility in preventing neurologic deterioration in presymptomatic cases is being tested (Moser, 1993).

Cerebrotendinous Xanthomatosis

Cerebrotendinous xanthomatosis is a rare disorder transmitted as an autosomal recessive trait. Deficiency of a liver mitochondrial enzyme blocks the oxidation of cholesterol to bile acids, causing the accumulation of cholestanol and bile alcohols in serum and the storage of sterols in all tissues, but especially the central nervous system (Meiner et al, 1994).

CLINICAL FEATURES. Dementia begins in early childhood but is insidious in its progression so that affected children seem mildly retarded rather than actively deteriorating. By age 15, cataracts are present and tendinous xanthomas begin to form. They are small at first and may go unnoticed until adult life. Progressive spasticity and ataxia develop during adolescence, and the patient becomes incapacitated in early adult life. A demyelinating neuropathy may be present as well. Speech and swallowing are impaired, and death occurs from brainstem dysfunction or myocardial infarction.

DIAGNOSIS. The triad of cataracts, tendon xanthomas, and progressive neurologic deterioration establishes the diagnosis, but all three features are not expressed completely until late in the course. Biochemical screening should be carried out in every child with cataracts or Achilles tendon xanthoma (Wevers et al, 1992). The diagnosis is established by showing increased concentrations of cholestanol in plasma or xanthomas.

TREATMENT. Oral chenodeoxycholic acid, lovastatin, and simvastin decrease cholestanol plasma and tissue concentrations by expanding the deficient bile pool. However, the biochemical improvement does not have a clinical benefit.

REFERENCES

Aicardi J. Tuberous sclerosis. Int Pediatr 1993;8:171-175.
Aubourg P, Sellier N, Chaussain JL, et al. MRI detects cerebral involvement in neurologically asymptomatic patients with adrenoleukodystrophy. Neurology 1989;39:1619-1621.
Barkovich AJ, Linden CE. Congenital cytomegalovirus infections of the brain: Imaging analysis and embryologic considerations. Am J Neuroradiol 1994;15:703-715.
Beutler E, Gelbart T. Two new Gaucher disease mutations. Hum Genet 1994;93:209-210.
Beutler E, Grabowski GA. Gaucher disease. In Scriver CR, Beaudet AL, Sly WS, et al (eds): The Metabolic and Molecular Basis of Inherited Disorders, 7th edition. New York, McGraw-Hill, 1995;2641-2670.
Blanche S, Mayaux M-J, Rouzioux C, et al. Relation of the course of HIV infection in children to the severity of the disease in their mother at delivery. N Engl J Med 1994;330:308-312.
Boustany RM, Kolodny EH. The neuronal ceroid lipofuscinosis: A review. Rev Neurol 1989;145:105-110.
Broughton BC, Thompson AF, Harcourt SA, et al. Molecular and cellular analysis of the DNA repair defect in a patient in xeroderma pigmentosum complementation group D who has the clinical features of xeroderma pigmentosum and Cockayne syndrome. Am J Hum Genet 1995;56:167-174.
Burd L, Fisher W, Kerbeshian J. Pervasive disintegrative disorder: Are Rett syndrome and Heller dementia infantilis subtypes? Dev Med Child Neurol 1989;31:609-616.
Butler C, Hittelman J, Hauger SB. Approach to neurodevelopmental and neurologic complications in pediatric HIV infection. J Pediatr 1991;119 (suppl):S41-S46.
Centers for Disease Control and Prevention. 1994 Revised classification system for human immunodeficiency virus infection in children less than 13 years of age. MMWR 1994;43:1-12.
Chi, C-S, Mak S-C, Shian W-J, et al. Oral glucose lactate stimulation test in mitochondrial diseases. Pediatr Neurol 1992;8:445-449.
Chuang DT, Shih VE. Disorders of branched chain amino acid and keto acid metabolism. In Scriver CR, Beaudet AL, Sly WS, et al (eds): The Metabolic and Molecular Basis of Inherited Disorders, 7th edition. New York, McGraw-Hill, 1995;1239-1278.
Clarke R, Daly L, Robinson K, et al. Hyperhomocysteinemia: An independent risk factor for vascular disease. N Engl J Med 1991;324:1149-1155.
DeCarli C, Fugate L, Falloon J, et al. Brain growth and cognitive improvement in children with human immunodeficiency virus-induced encephalopathy after six months of continuous infusion zidovudine therapy. J Acquir Immune Defic Syndr 1991;4:585-592.
de Grouchy J, Turleau J. Autosomal disorders. In Emery AEH, Rimoin DL (eds): Principles and Practice of Medical Genetics, 2nd edition. Churchill Livingstone, New York, 1990;247.
DiMauro S, Moraes CT. Mitochondrial encephalomyopathies. Arch Neurol 1993;50:1197-1208.
Dominguez R, Vila-Coro AA, Slopis JM, et al. Brain and ocular abnormalities in infants with in utero exposure to cocaine and other street drugs. Am J Dis Child 1991;145:688-695.
Fink JK, Filling-Katz MR, Sokol J, et al. Clinical spectrum of Niemann-Pick disease type C. Neurology 1989;39:1040-1049.
Fisher DA, Foley BL. Early treatment of congenital hypothyroidism. Pediatrics 1989;83:785-789.
Graf WD, Sumi SM, Copass MK, et al. Phenotypic heterogeneity in families with the myoclonic epilepsy and ragged-red fiber disease point mutation in mitochondrial DNA. Ann Neurol 1993;33:640-645.
Gravel RA, Clarke JTR, Kaback MM, et al. The G$_{M2}$ gangliosidoses. In Scriver CR, Beaudet AL, Sly WS, et al (eds): The Metabolic and Molecular Basis of Inherited Disorders, 7th edition. New York, McGraw-Hill, 1995;2839-2879.
Griffith BP, Booss J. Neurologic infections of the fetus and newborn. Neurol Clin 1994;12:541-564.

Gutmann DH, Collins FS: Neurofibromatosis type 1: Beyond positional cloning. Arch Neurol 1993;50:1185-1193.

Hagberg BA, Blennow G, Kristiansson B, et al. Carbohydrate-deficient glycoprotein syndromes: Peculiar group of new disorders. Pediatr Neurol 1993;9:255-262.

Harbord M, Buncic JR, Chuang SA, et al. Multiple sulfatase deficiency with early severe retinal degeneration. J Child Neurol 1991;6:229-235.

Harding BN, Alsanjari N, Smith SJM, et al. Progressive neuronal degeneration of childhood with liver disease (Alpers' disease) presenting in young adults. J Neurol Neurosurg Psychiatry 1995;58:320-325.

Higgins JJ, Patterson MC, Dambrosia JM, et al. A clinical staging classification for type C Niemann-Pick disease. Neurology 1992;42:2286-2290.

Hofman KJ, Harris EL, Bryan N, et al. Neurofibromatosis type 1: The cognitive phenotype. J Pediatr 1994;124:S1-S8.

Ikeda MK, Jensen HB. Evaluation and treatment of congenital syphillis. J Pediatr 1990;117:843.

Jaeken J, Schachter H, Carchon H, et al. Carbohydrate deficient glycoprotein syndrome type II: A deficiency in Golgi localized n-acetyl-glucosaminyltransferase II. Arch Dis Child 1994;71:123-127.

Jankovic J, Caskey TC, Stout JT, et al. Lesch-Nyhan syndrome: A study of motor behavior and cerebrospinal fluid transmitters. Ann Neurol 1988;23:466-469.

Kandt RS. Tuberous sclerosis: The next step. J Child Neurol 1993;8:107-110.

Kaul R, Gao GP, Aloya M, et al. Canavan disease: Mutations among Jewish and non-Jewish patients. Am J Hum Genet 1994;55:34-41.

Kolmen BK, Feldman HM, Handen BL, et al. Naltrexone in young autistic children: A double-blind, placebo-controlled crossover study. J Am Acad Child Adolesc Psychiatry 1995;34:223-231.

Kolodny EH, Fluharty AL. Metachromatic leukodystrophy and multiple sulfatase deficiency: Sulfatide lipidosis. In Scriver CR, Beaudet AL, Sly WS, et al (eds): The Metabolic and Molecular Basis of Inherited Disorders, 7th edition. New York, McGraw-Hill, 1995;2693-2739.

Kornfeld S, Sly WS. I-cell disease and pseudohurler polydystrophy: Disorders of lysosomal enzyme phosphorylation and localization. In Scriver CR, Beaudet AL, Sly WS, et al (eds): The Metabolic and Molecular Basis of Inherited Disorders, 7th edition. New York, McGraw-Hill, 1995; 2495-2508.

Kremer B, Goldberg P, Andrew SE, et al. A worldwide study of the Huntington disease mutation: The sensitivity and specificity of measuring CAG repeats. N Eng J Med 1994;330:1401-1406.

Laxova R. Fragile X syndrome. Adv Pediatr 1994;41:305-342.

Manuelidis EE, Rorke LB. Transmission of Alpers' disease (chronic progressive encephalopathy) produces experimental Creutzfeldt-Jacob disease in hamsters. Neurology 1989;39:615-621.

Matthews PM, Marchington DR, Squier M, et al. Molecular genetic characterization of an X-linked form of Leigh's syndrome. Ann Neurol 1993;33:652-655.

Meiner V, Meiner Z, Reshef A, et al. Cerebrotendinous xanthomatosis: Molecular diagnosis enables presymptomatic detection of a treatable disease. Neurology 1994;44: 288-290.

Mofenson LM, Moye J Jr. Intravenous immune globulin for the prevention of infections in children with symptomatic human immunodeficiency virus infection. Pediatr Res 1993;33:S87-S90.

Moser HW. Lorenzo oil therapy for adrenoleukodystrophy: A prematurely amplified hope. Ann Neurol 1993;34:121-122.

Moser HW, Moser AB, Smith KD, et al. Adrenoleukodystrophy: Phenotypic variability and implications for therapy. J Inherited Metab Dis 1992;15:645-654.

Mudd SH, Levy HL, Skovby F. Disorders of transsulfuration. In Scriver CR, Beaudet AL, Sly WS, et al (eds): The Metabolic and Molecular Basis of Inherited Disorders, 7th Edition, New York, McGraw-Hill, 1995;1279-1327.

Nadal D, Baerlocher K. Menkes' disease. Long-term treatment with copper and D-penicillamine. Eur J Pediatr 1988;147:621.

National Institutes of Health Conference: Neurofibromatosis 1 (Recklinghausen Disease) and neurofibromatosis 2 (bilateral acoustic neurofibromatosis): An update. Ann Intern Med 1990;113:39-52.

Neufeld EF, Muenzer J. The mucopolysaccharidoses. In Scriver CR, Beaudet AL, Sly WS, et al (eds): The Metabolic and Molecular Basis of Inherited Disorders, 7th edition. New York, McGraw-Hill, 1995;2465-2494.

North K, Joy P, Yuille D, et al. Specific learning disability in children with neurofibromatosis type 1: Significance of MRI abnormalities. Neurology 1994;44:878-883.

Oliva D, Carella F, Savoiardo M, et al. Clinical and magnetic resonance features of the classic and akinetic-rigid variants of Huntington's disease. Arch Neurol 1993;50:17-19.

Patterson MC, Di Bisceglie AM, Higgins JJ, et al. The effect of cholesterol-lowering agents on hepatic and plasma cholesterol in Niemann-Pick disease type C. Neurology 1993;43:61-64.

Pratt VM, Naidu S, Dlouhy SR, et al. A novel mutation in exon 3 of the proteolipid protein gene in Pelizaeus-Merzbacher disease. Neurology 1995;45:394-395.

Pridmore CL, Baraitser M, Harding B, et al. Alexander's disease: Clues to diagnosis. J Child Neurol 1993;8:134-144.

Rett Syndrome Diagnostic Criteria Work Group. Diagnostic criteria for Rett syndrome. Ann Neurol 1988;23:425-428.

Robbins JH, Brumback RA, Mendiones M, et al. Neurological disease in xeroderma pigmentosum. Documentation of a late onset type of the juvenile onset form. Brain 1991;114: 1335-1361.

Roizen N, Swisher CN, Stein MA, et al. Neurologic and developmental outcome in treated congenital toxoplasmosis. Pediatrics 1995;95:11-20.

Santavuori P, Rapola J, Nuutila A, et al. The spectrum of Jansky-Bielschowsky disease. Neuropediatrics 1991;22: 92-96.

Schifter T, Hoffman JM, Hatten Jr P, et al. Neuroimaging in infantile autism. J Child Neurol 1994;9:155-161.

Specola N, Vanier MT, Goutiéres F, et al. The juvenile and chronic forms of G_{M2} gangliosidosis: Clinical and genetic heterogeneity. Neurology 1990;40:145-150.

Suzuki K, Suzuki Y, Suzuki K. Galactosylceramide lipidosis: Globoid cell leukodystrophy (Krabbe disease). In Scriver CR, Beaudet AL, Sly WS, et al (eds): The Metabolic and Molecular Basis of Inherited Disorders, 7th edition. New York, McGraw-Hill, 1995a;2671-2692.

Suzuki Y, Sakaraba H, Oshima A. β-galactosidase deficiency (β-galactosidosis): G_{M1} gangliosidosis and Morquio B disease. In Scriver CR, Beaudet AL, Sly WS, et al (eds): The Metabolic and Molecular Basis of Inherited Disorders, 7th edition. New York, McGraw-Hill, 1995b;2785-2823.

Svensson E, von Dobeln U, Eisensmith RC, et al. Relation between genotype and phenotype in Swedish phenylketonuria and hyperphenylalaninemia patients. Eur J Pediatr 1993;152:132-139.

Tanabe Y, Iai M, Ishii M, et al. The use of magnetic resonance imaging in diagnosing infantile neuroaxonal dystrophy. Neurology 1993;43:110-113.

Thomas GH, Beaudet AL. Disorders of glycoprotein degradation and structure: α mannosidosis, β mannosidosis, fucosidoses, sialidosis, aspartylglycosaminuria, and carbohydrate deficient glycoprotein syndrome. In Scriver CR, Beaudet AL, Sly WS, et al (eds): The Metabolic and Molecular Basis of Inherited Disorders, 7th edition. New York, McGraw-Hill, 1995;2529-2562.

Thompson AJ, Tillotson S, Smith I, et al. Brain MRI changes in phenylketonuria: Associations with dietary status. Brain 1993;116:811-821.

Tuchman RE. Autism: Delineating the spectrum. Int Pediatr 1991;6:161-169.

Van Coster R, Lombes A, De Vivo D, et al. Cytochrome c oxidase-associated Leigh syndrome: Phenotypic features

and pathogenetic speculations. J Neurol Sci 1991;104: 97-111.

Verdru P, Lammens M, Dom R, et al. Globoid cell leukodystrophy: A family with both late-infantile and adult type. Neurology 1991;41:1382-1384.

Wevers RA, Cruysberg JRM, Heijst AFV, et al. Paediatric cerebrotendinous xanthomatosis. J Inherited Metab Dis 1992;15:374-376.

Yan W, Boustany R-M N, Konradi C, et al. Localization of juvenile, but not late-infantile, neuronal ceroid lipofuscinosis on chromosome 16. Am J Hum Genet 1993;52:89-95.

6

The Hypotonic Infant

Definitions

Tone is the resistance of muscle to stretch. Two kinds of tone are measured clinically: phasic and postural. *Phasic tone* is a rapid contraction in response to a high-intensity stretch. It is examined by testing the tendon reflexes. When a hammer strikes the patellar tendon, the quadriceps muscle is stretched and the spindle apparatus, sensing the stretch, sends an impulse through the sensory nerve to the spinal cord. This information is transmitted to the alpha motor neuron and the quadriceps muscle contracts (the monosynaptic reflex). *Postural tone* is the prolonged contraction of antigravity muscles in response to the low-intensity stretch of gravity. When postural tone is depressed, the trunk and limbs cannot be maintained against gravity and the infant is hypotonic.

The maintenance of normal tone requires an intact central and peripheral nervous system. Not surprisingly, hypotonia is a common symptom of neurologic dysfunction and is encountered in diseases of the brain, spinal cord, nerves, and muscles (Table 6-1). One anterior horn cell and all the muscle fibers that it innervates make up a *motor unit.* A primary disorder of the anterior horn cell body is a *neuronopathy,* a primary disorder of the axon or its myelin covering is a *neuropathy,* and a primary disorder of the muscle fiber is a *myopathy.* In infancy and childhood, diseases of the brain are far more common than diseases of the motor unit. The term *cerebral hypotonia* is used to encompass all causes of postural hypotonia caused by a cerebral disease or defect.

The Appearance of Hypotonia

When lying supine, all hypotonic infants look much the same regardless of the underlying cause or the location of abnormality within the nervous system. Spontaneous movement is lacking, the legs are fully abducted with the lateral surface of the thighs against the examining table, and the arms lie either extended at the sides of the body or flexed at the elbow with the hands beside the head. Pectus excavatum is present when the infant has long-standing weakness in the muscles of the chest wall. Infants who lie motionless eventually develop flattening of the occiput and loss of hair on the portion of the scalp that is in constant contact with the crib sheet. When the infant is placed in a sitting posture, the head falls forward, the shoulders droop, and the limbs hang limply.

Newborns who are hypotonic in utero may be born with dislocation of the hips, arthrogryposis, or both. Hip dislocation is a common feature of intrauterine hypotonia because the formation of a normal hip joint requires the forceful contraction of muscles to pull the head of the femur into the acetabulum. Arthrogryposis varies in severity from clubfoot, the most common manifestation, to symmetric flexion deformities of all limb joints. Joint contractures are believed to be a nonspecific consequence of intrauterine immobilization. However, among the several disorders that equally decrease fetal movement, some commonly produce arthrogryposis and others never do. The differential diagnosis of arthrogryposis is summarized in Table 6-2. As a rule, newborns with arthrogryposis who require

■ T A B L E   6 – 1
Differential Diagnosis of Infantile Hypotonia [Gene Location]

Cerebral Hypotonia

"Benign" congenital hypotonia
Chromosome disorders
   Prader-Willi syndrome [15q11-13]
   Trisomy
Chronic nonprogressive encephalopathy
   Cerebral malformation
   Perinatal distress
   Postnatal disorders
Peroxisomal disorders
   Cerebrohepatorenal syndrome (Zellweger syndrome)
   Neonatal adrenoleukodystrophy
Other genetic defects
   Familial dysautonomia
   Oculocerebrorenal syndrome (Lowe syndrome)
Other metabolic defects
   Acid maltase deficiency (see "Metabolic Myopathies")
   Infantile GM_1 gangliosidosis (see Chapter 5)

Spinal Cord Disorders

Hypoxic-ischemia myelopathy
Injuries

Spinal Muscular Atrophies

Acute infantile
   Autosomal recessive [5q11-13]
   Autosomal dominant
   X-linked
Chronic infantile
   Autosomal recessive [5q11-13]
   Autosomal dominant
Congenital cervical spinal muscular atrophy
Infantile neuronal degeneration
Neurogenic arthrogryposis
Pelizaeus-Merzbacher disease (connatal form)

Polyneuropathies

Congential hypomyelinating neuropathy
Giant axonal neuropathy (see Chapter 7)
Hereditary motor-sensory neuropathies (see Chapter 7)

Disorders of Neuromuscular Transmission

Infantile botulism
Familial infantile myasthenia
Transitory myasthenia gravis

Fiber-Type Disproportion Myopathies

Central core disease [19q13]
Congenital fiber-type disproportion myopathy
[translocation 10p11:17q25]
Myotubular (centronuclear) myopathy
   Acute [Xq28]
   Chronic
Nemaline (rod) myopathy [1q21-23]

Infantile Myositis

Metabolic Myopathies

Acid maltase deficiency [17q23]
Cytochrome c oxidase deficiency
Phosphofructokinase deficiency [1cenq32]
Phosphorylase deficiency [11q13]

Muscular Dystrophies

Congenital muscular dystrophy
   Cerebro-ocular dystrophy
   Fukuyama type [9q31-33]
   Leukodystrophy [9q31-33]
Merosin deficiency [6q2]
Congenital myotonic dystrophy [19q13]

---

respiratory assistance do not survive extubation unless the underlying disorder is myasthenia (Bianchi and Van Marter, 1994).

The tone of infants who appear hypotonic at rest can be further evaluated by the traction response, by vertical suspension, and by horizontal suspension.

THE TRACTION RESPONSE

The traction response is the most sensitive measure of postural tone and can be tested in premature newborns within an isolette. The response is initiated by grasping the hands and pulling the infant to a sitting position. In a normal infant the head lifts from the surface immediately with the body. When the sitting position is attained, the head is held erect in the midline. During traction the examiner should feel the infant pulling back against traction and observe flexion at the elbow, knee, and ankle.

The traction response cannot be elicited in premature newborns less than 33 weeks' gestation. After 33 weeks, the neck flexors show increasing success in lifting the head. At term only minimal head lag is present; when the sitting posture is attained, the head may continue to lag or may become erect momentarily and then fall forward.

The presence of more than minimal head lag and of failure to counter traction by flexion of the limbs in the term newborn is abnormal and indicates hypotonia.

VERTICAL SUSPENSION

To perform vertical suspension, the examiner places both hands in the infant's axillae and, without grasping the thorax, lifts straight up. The muscles of the shoulders should be strong enough to press down against the examiner's hands and allow the infant to suspend vertically

■ T A B L E   6 – 2
Differential Diagnosis of Arthrogryposis

Cerebrohepatorenal syndrome
Cerebral malformations
Chromosomal disorders
Fetal, non-nervous system causes
Motor unit disorders
   Congenital benign spinal muscular atrophy
   Congenital cervical spinal muscular atrophy
   Congenital fiber-type disproportion myopathy
   Congenital hypomyelinating neuropathy
   Congenital muscular dystrophy
   Genetic myasthenic syndromes
   Infantile neuronal degeneration
   Myotonic dystrophy
   Neurogenic arthrogryposis
   Phosphofructokinase deficiency
   Transitory neonatal myasthenia
Nonfetal causes

■ T A B L E   6 – 3
Combined Cerebral and Motor Unit Hypotonia

Acid maltase deficiency
Familial dysautonomia
Giant axonal neuropathy
Hypoxic-ischemic encephalomyopathy
Infantile neuronal degeneration
Lipid storage diseases
Mitochondrial (respiratory chain) disorders
Neonatal myotonic dystrophy
Perinatal asphyxia secondary to motor unit disease

■ T A B L E   6 – 4
Motor Unit Disorders with Perinatal Respiratory Distress

Acute infantile spinal muscular atrophy
Congenital hypomyelinating neuropathy
Congenital myotonic dystrophy
Familial infantile myasthenia
Neurogenic arthrogryposis
X-linked myotubular myopathy

without falling through. While the infant is in vertical suspension, the head is held erect in the midline and the legs are kept flexed at the knee, hip, and ankle. When a hypotonic infant is suspended vertically, the head falls forward, the legs dangle, and the infant may slip through the examiner's hands because of weakness in the shoulder muscles.

HORIZONTAL SUSPENSION

When suspended horizontally, a normal infant keeps the head erect, maintains the back straight, and flexes the elbow, hip, knee, and ankle joints. A healthy full-term newborn makes intermittent efforts to maintain the head erect, the back straight, and the limbs flexed against gravity. Hypotonic newborns and infants drape over the examiner's hands with the head and legs hanging limply.

 Approach to Diagnosis

The first step in diagnosis is to determine whether the disease is sited in the cerebrum, spine, or motor unit. More than one site may be involved (Table 6-3). The brain and the peripheral nerves are concomitantly involved in some lysosomal and mitochondrial disorders. Both brain and skeletal muscles are abnormal in acid maltase deficiency and neonatal myotonic dystrophy. Newborns with severe hypoxic-ischemic encephalopathy may have hypoxic injury to the spinal cord as well. Several motor unit disorders produce sufficient hypotonia at birth to impair

respiration and cause perinatal asphyxia (Table 6-4). Such infants may then have cerebral hypotonia as well. Newborns with spinal cord injuries are frequently the product of long, difficult deliveries in which brachial plexus injuries and hypoxic-ischemic encephalopathy are concomitant problems.

CLUES TO THE DIAGNOSIS OF CEREBRAL HYPOTONIA

Cerebral hypotonia in newborns usually does not pose diagnostic difficulty and can be identified by history and physical examination. Many clues to the diagnosis of cerebral hypotonia exist (Table 6-5), but most important is the presence of other abnormal brain functions: decreased consciousness and seizures. Cerebral malformation is the likely explanation for hypotonia in an infant with dysmorphic features or with malformations in other organs.

A tightly fisted hand in which the thumb is constantly enclosed by the other fingers and does not open spontaneously *(fisting)*, and adduction of the thigh so that the legs are crossed when the infant is suspended vertically *(scissoring)* are considered precursors of spasticity and indicate cerebral dysfunction. Postural reflexes may be elicited in newborns and infants with cerebral hypotonia even when spontaneous movement is lacking. In some acute en-

■ TABLE 6-5
Clues to Cerebral Hypotonia

Abnormalities of other brain function
Dysmorphic features
Fisting of the hands
Malformations of other organs
Movement through postural reflexes
Normal or brisk tendon reflexes
Scissoring on vertical suspension

■ TABLE 6-6
Clues to Motor Unit Disorders

Absent or depressed tendon reflexes
Failure of movement on postural reflexes
Fasciculations
Muscle atrophy
No abnormalities of other organs

cephalopathies, and especially in metabolic disorders, the Moro reflex may be exaggerated. The tonic neck reflex is an important indicator of cerebral abnormality if the responses are excessive and obligatory and persist beyond 6 months of age. When hemispheric damage is severe but the brainstem is intact, turning the head produces full extension of both ipsilateral limbs and tight flexion on the contralateral side. An obligatory reflex is one in which these postures are maintained for as long as the head is kept rotated. Tendon reflexes are generally normal or brisk, and clonus may be present.

CLUES TO MOTOR UNIT DISORDERS

Disorders of the motor unit are not associated with malformations of other organs except for joint deformities and the maldevelopment of bony structures. The face sometimes looks dysmorphic when facial muscles are weak or when the jaw is underdeveloped.

Tendon reflexes are absent or depressed. Total loss of reflexes in muscles with residual movement is more likely caused by neuropathy than myopathy, whereas diminished reflexes consistent with the degree of weakness are more often caused by myopathy than neuropathy (Table 6-6). Muscle atrophy suggests motor unit disease but does not exclude the possibility of cerebral hypotonia. Failure of growth and even atrophy can be considerable in brain-damaged infants. The combination of atrophy and fasciculations is strong evidence for denervation. However, the observation of fasciculations in newborns and infants is often restricted to the tongue, and distinguishing fasciculations from normal random movements of the tongue is difficult unless atrophy is present.

Postural reflexes, such as the tonic-neck and positive supporting reaction, cannot be superimposed on weak muscles. The motor unit is the final common pathway of tone; limbs that will not move voluntarily cannot be moved reflexively.

 Cerebral Hypotonia

Hypotonia is a feature of almost every cerebral disorder in newborns and infants. This section does not deal with conditions in which the major symptoms are states of decreased consciousness, seizures, and progressive psychomotor retardation. Rather, the discussion is limited to conditions in which hypotonia is so prominent a feature that the examining physician may consider the possibility of motor unit disease.

BENIGN CONGENITAL HYPOTONIA

The term *benign congenital hypotonia* is retrospective and refers to infants who are hypotonic at birth or shortly thereafter and later have normal tone. It encompasses many different pathologic processes affecting either the brain, the motor unit, or both. The majority of affected children have cerebral hypotonia. An increased incidence of mental retardation, learning disabilities, and other sequelae of cerebral abnormality is evident later in life, despite the recovery of normal muscle tone.

CHROMOSOME DISORDERS

Despite considerable syndrome diversity, common characteristics of autosomal chromosome aberrations in the newborn are dysmorphic features of the hands and face and profound hypotonia (see Table 5-4). For this reason chromosome studies are indicated for any hypotonic newborn with dysmorphic features of the hands and face, with or without other organ malformation (Table 6-7).

Prader-Willi Syndrome

The Prader-Willi syndrome is characterized by hypotonia, hypogonadism, mental retardation, short stature, and obesity (Holm et al, 1993). Approximately 70% of children with this syn-

■ TABLE 6–7
Hypotonia and Dysmorphic Features

Cerebral dysgenesis
Cerebrohepatorenal syndrome
Congenital myotonic dystrophy
Chromosomal aberrations
Fiber-type disproportion myopathies
Neonatal adrenoleukodystrophy
Prader-Willi syndrome

■ TABLE 6–8
Difficulty of Feeding in the Alert Newborn

Congenital myotonic dystrophy
Familial dysautonomia
Genetic myasthenic syndromes
Hypoplasia of bulbar motor nuclei (see Chapter 17)
Infantile neuronal degeneration
Myophosphorylase deficiency
Neurogenic arthrogryposis
Prader-Willi syndrome
Transitory neonatal myasthenia

drome have an interstitial deletion of the proximal long arm of chromosome 15 (q11-13). A majority of nondeletion patients have the syndrome on the basis of maternal disomy (both chromosomes 15 are from the mother). Paternal disomy of chromosome 15 causes Angelman syndrome.

CLINICAL FEATURES. Decreased fetal activity is reported in 75% of pregnancies and is associated with a 10% incidence of congenital hip dislocation and a 6% incidence of clubfoot. At birth the hypotonia is profound and tendon reflexes are absent or greatly depressed. Feeding problems are invariable, and prolonged nasogastric tube feeding is common (Table 6–8). Cryptorchidism is present in 84% and hypogenitalism in 100%.

Both hypotonia and feeding difficulty persist until 8 to 11 months of age and are later replaced by relatively normal muscle tone and insatiable hunger. Developmental milestones are delayed, and mental retardation is a constant feature. Minor abnormalities that become more obvious during infancy include a narrow bifrontal diameter of the skull, strabismus, almond-shaped eyes, enamel hypoplasia, and small hands and feet. Obesity is the rule during childhood. The combination of obesity and minor abnormalities of the face and limbs produces a "resemblance" among children with this syndrome.

DIAGNOSIS. The combination of hypotonia, difficulty feeding, and cryptorchidism in the newborn warrants chromosome analysis with special reference to chromosome 15. Other studies are not helpful and without chromosome analysis the diagnosis is delayed until obesity develops.

TREATMENT. Dietary supervision is needed to control obesity. No specific treatment is available.

CHRONIC NONPROGRESSIVE ENCEPHALOPATHY

Cerebral dysgenesis may be due to known or unknown noxious environmental agents, chromosomal disorders, or genetic defects. In the absence of an acute encephalopathy, hypotonia may be the only symptom at birth or during early infancy. Hypotonia is usually worse at birth and gets better with time. Cerebral dysgenesis should be suspected when hypotonia is coupled with malformations in other organs or abnormalities in head size and shape. Magnetic resonance imaging (MRI) of the head is advisable when cerebral malformation is suspected. The identification of a cerebral malformation provides useful information not only for prognosis but also on the feasibility of aggressive therapy to correct malformations in other organs.

Brain injuries occur in the perinatal period and less commonly throughout infancy as a result of anoxia, hemorrhage, infection, and trauma. The sudden onset of hypotonia in a previously well newborn or infant, with or without signs of encephalopathy, should always suggest a cerebral cause. The premature newborn who shows a decline in spontaneous movement and tone may have an intraventricular hemorrhage. Hypotonia is an early feature of meningitis in full-term and premature newborns. Tendon reflexes may be diminished or absent during the acute phase.

PEROXISOMAL DISORDERS

Peroxisomes are subcellular organelles that participate in the biosynthesis of ether phospholipids and bile acids; the oxidation of very-long-chain fatty acids, prostaglandins, and unsaturated long-chain fatty acids; and the catabolism of phytanate, pipecolate, and glycolate. Peroxide is generated in the course of several oxidation reactions and catabolized by the enzyme catalase. The chemical abnormalities usually associated with peroxisomal defects include elevated concentrations of very-long-chain fatty acids in

■ TABLE 6-9
Phenotype Features of Peroxisomal Disorders*

Aberrant bone calcification
Adrenal insufficiency (rare)
Dysmorphic features
Hepatomegaly with impaired function
Hypotonia
Impaired hearing
Psychmotor retardation
Renal cysts
Retinal pigmentary degeneration
Seizures

*Modified from Naidu et al. Phenotypic and genotypic variability of generalized peroxisomal disorders. Pediatr Neurol 4:5, 1988.

tissue and plasma, secretion of abnormal bile acid precursors, hyperpipecolic acidemia and aciduria, and decreased concentrations of tissue plasmalogens. Table 6-9 lists the clinical features that suggest peroxisomal disorders; only mental retardation is an obligatory criterion (Naidu et al, 1988).

The three infantile syndromes of peroxisomal dysfunction are cerebrohepatorenal (Zellweger) syndrome, neonatal adrenoleukodystrophy, and infantile Refsum disease. Infantile hypotonia is a prominent feature of the first two disorders whereas infantile Refsum disease is characterized mainly by impaired vision and hearing (see Chapter 16).

Cerebrohepatorenal Syndrome (Zellweger Syndrome)

Cerebrohepatorenal syndrome is a defect in peroxisomal biogenesis; the intrinsic protein membrane can be identified, but all matrix enzymes are missing (Santos et al, 1988). The defect is probably transmitted by autosomal recessive inheritance. Biochemical disturbances include nonspecific aminoaciduria, increased serum levels of iron and copper, alterations in bile acid synthesis, pipecolic acidemia, and the accumulation of very-long-chain fatty acids in ocular tissue.

CLINICAL FEATURES. Affected newborns are poorly responsive and have severe hypotonia, arthrogryposis, and dysmorphic features. The arthrogryposis is characterized by limited extension of the fingers (*camptodactyly*) and flexion deformities of the knee and ankle. Suck and cry are weak, and tendon reflexes are diminished or absent. Characteristic craniofacial abnormalities include a pear-shaped head owing to a high forehead and an unusual fullness of the cheeks, widened sutures, micrognathia, a high-arched

palate, flattening of the bridge of the nose, and hypertelorism. Abnormalities of other organs include biliary cirrhosis, polycystic kidneys, retinal degeneration, and cerebral malformation.

Seizures usually begin shortly after birth but may begin anytime during infancy. They are difficult to control. Death from aspiration, gastrointestinal bleeding, or liver failure usually occurs within 6 months and almost always within 1 year.

DIAGNOSIS. Clinical diagnosis can be made on the basis of specific organ involvement. Muscle biopsy reveals large aggregates of mitochondria and increased lipid in subsarcolemmal intermyofibrillary spaces. Liver biopsy specimens show biliary dysgenesis and iron storage.

TREATMENT. Experimental diet therapy has had limited success and is being refined and tested.

Neonatal Adrenoleukodystrophy

The neonatal form of adrenoleukodystrophy is transmitted by autosomal recessive inheritance. The childhood form, discussed in Chapter 5, is transmitted by X-linked inheritance.

CLINICAL FEATURES. In some newborns with adrenoleukodystrophy, the disease shows phenotypic resemblance to the cerebrohepatorenal syndrome. The initial clinical features are hypotonia and failure to thrive. Tendon reflexes are present and often brisk. Abnormal facial features, hepatomegaly, and retinitis pigmentosa are constant features. Progressive neurologic deterioration is characterized by seizures, blindness, psychomotor retardation, and spasticity. The adrenal glands are hypoplastic, but no symptoms of adrenal failure are present. Death usually occurs during early childhood.

DIAGNOSIS. The diagnosis is established by demonstrating poor adrenal function and increased concentrations of very-long-chain fatty acids in the plasma. Increased concentrations of phytanic acid and trihydroxycoprostanic acid may be present as well.

TREATMENT. Dietary treatment has been attempted in the X-linked childhood form (see Chapter 5) but has not been reported in the neonatal form.

OTHER GENETIC DEFECTS
Familial Dysautonomia

Familial dysautonomia, the *Riley-Day syndrome,* was originally described as a genetic disorder transmitted by autosomal recessive inheritance in Ashkenazi Jews. Similar clinical syndromes also occur in non-Jewish infants; these are often sporadic and the mode of inheritance is not clear.

CLINICAL FEATURES. In the newborn the important clinical features are meconium aspiration, poor or no suck reflex, and hypotonia. Hypotonia is caused by disturbances in the brain, the dorsal root ganglia, and the peripheral nerves. Tendon reflexes are hypoactive or absent. The feeding difficulty is unusual and provides a clue to diagnosis. Sucking and swallowing are normal separately but cannot be coordinated for effective feeding. Other clinical features that may be noted either in the newborn or later in infancy are pallor, temperature instability, absence of fungiform papillae of the tongue, diarrhea, abdominal distention, poor weight gain, lethargy, episodes of irritability, absence of corneal reflexes, a labile blood pressure, and failure to produce overflow tears.

DIAGNOSIS. Diagnosis should be suspected from the constellation of clinical symptoms and can be confirmed by the pilocarpine or histamine test. The instillation of 1 drop of 0.0625% pilocarpine solution into the conjunctival sac has no effect on a normal pupil but causes immediate pupillary constriction in infants with dysautonomia. This reaction is an example of denervation hypersensitivity. An intradermal injection of 0.1 ml of histamine sulfate (1:10,000) produces an erythematous wheal followed by a painful flare that extends more than 5 cm and lasts for more than an hour in normal children. In infants with dysautonomia the same injection produces a wheal 2 to 3 cm in diameter with a sharp red border, but the axon flare, an axon reflex, is lacking.

TREATMENT. Treatment is directed at symptoms. Bethanechol (Urecholine), 1 to 2 mg/kg/day orally, is thought to be helpful. Its use is based on the observation that injections of acetylcholine produce a transient relief of some symptoms. Longevity has increased because of improved treatment of symptoms.

Oculocerebrorenal Syndrome (Lowe Syndrome)

Oculocerebrorenal syndrome is transmitted by X-linked recessive inheritance. Partial expression in the form of minor lenticular opacities is seen in female carriers. The primary abnormality of this disease has not been established, but a mitochondrial disorder causing multiple organ dysfunction is likely.

CLINICAL FEATURES. The important features at birth are hypotonia and hyporeflexia, sometimes associated with congenital cataracts and glaucoma. The differential diagnosis of cataracts in newborns and young infants is listed in Table 16–3. Features that appear later in infancy are mental retardation and a progressive disorder of the renal tubules resulting in metabolic acidosis, proteinuria, aminoaciduria, and defective acidification of the urine. Many infants die after failing to thrive. Others have mild symptoms, including growth retardation, borderline intellectual function, mild renal disturbances, and late-onset cataract formation. Life expectancy is normal in the milder cases.

DIAGNOSIS. Diagnosis depends on recognition of the clinical constellation. MRI shows diffuse and irregular foci of increased signal consistent with demyelination.

TREATMENT. Most patients require alkinization therapy, and many benefit from supplements of potassium, phosphate, calcium, and carnitine (Charnas et al, 1991).

OTHER METABOLIC DEFECTS

Inborn errors of metabolism, other than peroxisomal disorders, are rarely manifested by hypotonia alone. However, two disorders with onset in newborns or infants are sometimes exceptions to the rule: acid maltase deficiency and generalized GM$_1$ gangliosidosis. Acid maltase deficiency, the more common of the two, causes a severe myopathy and is discussed with other metabolic myopathies. Generalized GM$_1$ gangliosidosis is discussed in Chapter 5.

 Spinal Cord Disorders

HYPOXIC-ISCHEMIC MYELOPATHY

Hypoxic-ischemic encephalopathy is an expected outcome in severe perinatal asphyxia (see Chapter 1). Affected newborns are hypotonic and areflexic. These features have been attributed exclusively to the cerebral injury but also may be caused by spinal cord dysfunction. Concurrent ischemic necrosis of gray matter occurs in the spinal cord as well as in the brain (Clancy et al, 1989). The spinal cord component is often found on postmortem examination but may also be shown in nonfatal cases by electromyography (EMG).

SPINAL CORD INJURY

Only in the newborn does spinal cord injury enter the differential diagnosis of hypotonia. Injuries to the cervical spinal cord occur almost exclusively during vaginal delivery; approximately 75% are associated with breech presentation, and 25% with cephalic presentation. Because the injuries are always associated with a difficult and prolonged delivery, decreased consciousness is common and hypotonia may be falsely attributed to asphyxia or cerebral trauma. However, the presence of impaired sphincter function and loss of sensation below the mid-chest should suggest myelopathy.

Injuries in Breech Presentation

Traction injuries to the lower cervical and upper thoracic regions of the cord occur almost exclusively when the angle of extension of the fetal head exceeds 90%. Indeed, the risk of spinal cord injury to a fetus in breech position whose head is hyperextended is greater than 70%. In such cases delivery should always be by cesarean section. The tractional forces applied to the extended head are sufficient not only to stretch the cord but also to herniate the brainstem through the foramen magnum. In addition, the hyperextended position compromises the vertebral arteries as they enter the skull.

The spectrum of pathologic findings varies from edema of the cord without loss of anatomic continuity to massive hemorrhage (epidural, subdural, and intramedullary), which is most pronounced in the lower cervical and upper thoracic segments but may extend the entire length of the cord. Concurrent hemorrhage in the posterior fossa and laceration of the cerebellum may be present as well.

CLINICAL FEATURES. Mild tractional injuries, in which there is edema of the cord but not intraparenchymal hemorrhage or loss of anatomic continuity, produce few or no clinical features. The main feature is hypotonia, which may be falsely attributed to asphyxia.

Severe tractional injuries are accompanied by hemorrhage into the posterior fossa. Affected newborns are unconscious and atonic at birth. They have flaccid quadriplegia with diaphragmatic breathing. Most do not survive the neonatal period. Injuries restricted to the low cervical and high thoracic segments produce near-normal strength in the biceps muscles and weakness of the triceps muscles. The result is flexion of the arms at the elbows and flaccid paraplegia. Spontaneous movement and tendon reflexes in the legs are absent, but foot withdrawal from pinprick may occur as a spinal reflex. The infant has a distended bladder and dribbling of urine. Sensory levels are difficult to measure but may be deduced by the absence of sweating below the injury.

DIAGNOSIS. Radiographs of the vertebrae show no abnormalities because bony displacement does not occur. MRI of the spine shows intraspinal edema and hemorrhage (Adams et al, 1988).

Unconscious newborns are generally thought to have intracerebral hemorrhage or asphyxia (see Chapter 2), and the diagnosis of spinal cord injury may not be considered until consciousness is regained and the typical motor deficits observed. Even then, a neuromuscular disorder may be suspected. The disturbance in bladder function and the development of progressive spastic paraplegia should alert the physician to the correct diagnosis.

TREATMENT. The treatment of spinal cord traction injuries of the newborn is similar to the management of cord injuries in older children (see Chapter 12).

Injuries in Cephalic Presentation

Injuries in cephalic presentation are high cervical cord injuries caused by twisting of the neck during midforceps rotation when the trunk fails to rotate with the head. The risk is greatest when amniotic fluid is absent because of delay from time of membrane rupture to application of forceps. The spectrum of injury varies from intraparenchymal hemorrhage to complete transection. Transection usually occurs at the level of a fractured odontoid process with atlantoaxial dislocation.

CLINICAL FEATURES. Newborns are flaccid and fail to breathe spontaneously. Those with milder injuries may have shallow, labored respirations, but all require assisted ventilation at birth. Most are unconscious at birth owing to edema in the brainstem. When consciousness is regained, eye movements, sucking, and the withdrawal reflex are the only movements observed. Tendon reflexes are at first absent but later become exaggerated if the child survives. The bladder becomes distended, and overflow incontinence occurs. Priapism may be present.

Sensation is difficult to assess because the withdrawal reflex is present.

Death from sepsis or respiratory complications generally occurs in the first week. Occasional children have survived for several years.

DIAGNOSIS. Most children with high cervical cord injuries are thought to have neuromuscular disorders, especially infantile spinal muscular atrophy, because the limbs are flaccid but the eye movements are normal. EMG of the limbs should exclude that possibility. Radiographs of the cervical vertebrae usually do not show abnormalities, but MRI shows marked thinning or disruption of the cord at the site of injury (Lanska et al, 1990).

TREATMENT. Newborns with high cervical cord injuries are intubated and provided with respiratory assistance before the diagnosis is established. Further management of spinal cord transection is discussed in Chapter 12.

 Motor Unit Disorders

EVALUATION OF MOTOR UNIT DISORDERS

In the diagnosis of cerebral hypotonia in infants, the choice of laboratory tests varies considerably depending on the disease entity. This is not the case with motor unit hypotonia. A battery of tests is available that readily define the anatomy and cause of pathologic processes affecting the motor unit (Table 6-10). The sequence in which the tests are done is important.

Serum Creatine Kinase

Increased serum concentrations of creatine kinase reflect skeletal or cardiac muscle necrosis. Blood should be drawn for creatine kinase determination before the performance of EMG or muscle biopsy because either procedure transiently elevates the serum concentration of creatine kinase. Laboratory reference values for the normal serum concentration are usually based on nonambulatory patients. Normal values tend to be higher in an ambulatory population, especially after exercise. The total concentration of creatine kinase and its isoenzymes increases significantly with acidosis. Levels as high as 1,000 IU/L may be recorded in severely asphyxiated newborns, but even normal newborns have a higher than normal concentration during the first 24 hours postpartum. A normal creatine kinase level in a hypotonic infant is strong evidence against a rapidly progressive myopathy, but it does not exclude fiber-type disproportion myopathies and some metabolic myopathies from the diagnosis. Conversely, a mild elevation in the creatine kinase concentration is sometimes encountered in rapidly progressive spinal muscular atrophies.

Electrodiagnosis

EMG is extremely useful in the diagnosis of infantile hypotonia when the study is performed by an experienced physician. It enables the prediction of the final diagnosis in most infants younger than 3 months of age with hypotonia of motor unit origin. Hypotonic infants with normal EMG findings rarely show abnormalities on muscle biopsy. The needle portion of the study helps to distinguish myopathic from neuropathic processes. Myopathies are generally characterized by the appearance of brief, small-amplitude, polyphasic potentials. Neuropathies are characterized by the presence of denervation potentials at rest (fibrillations, fasciculations, sharp waves) and motor unit potentials that are large, prolonged, and polyphasic. Studies of nerve conduction velocity are useful in distinguishing axonal from demyelinating neuropathies; demyelinating neuropathies cause greater slowing of conduction velocity. Repetitive nerve stimulation studies demonstrate disturbances in neuromuscular transmission.

Muscle Biopsy

Muscle biopsy should not be undertaken unless the tissue can be processed by histochemical techniques. The muscle selected for biopsy should be weak but still able to contract. When weakness is symmetric, the muscles of one limb should be studied by EMG and the muscles of the other limb reserved for biopsy. Histochemical analysis is essential for the complete evaluation of muscle histology because special techniques are needed to demonstrate fiber types and storage materials. Human skeletal muscle can be arbitrarily divided into two fiber types on the basis of the intensity of reaction to myosin adenosine triphosphatase (ATPase) at pH 9.4. Type I fibers react weakly to ATPase, are characterized by oxidative metabolism, and serve a tonic function. Type II fibers react intensely to ATPase, utilize glycolytic metabolism, and serve a phasic function. Type I and II fibers are generally equal in number and randomly distributed in each fascicle. Disorders may be characterized by abnormalities in fiber type number, fiber type size, or both.

The important storage materials identified in skeletal muscle are glycogen and lipid. In most storage disorders vacuoles are present in the fibers that contain the abnormal material. The vacuoles are seen with light microscopy, and the specific material is identified by its histochemical reaction.

Nerve Biopsy

Sural nerve biopsy is rarely needed in the diagnosis of infantile hypotonia and should only be done if sural neuropathy has been shown by electrodiagnosis. Its main use is in the diagnosis of hypomyelinating neuropathies.

The Tensilon Test

Edrophonium chloride (Tensilon) is a rapidly acting anticholinesterase that temporarily reverses weakness in patients with myasthenia. Ptosis and oculomotor paresis are the only functions that are reliably tested. Rare patients are supersensitive to edrophonium chloride and may stop breathing because of depolarization of endplates or an abnormal vagal response. Equipment for mechanical ventilation should always be available when the test is performed. In newborns, a subcutaneous injection of 0.15 mg/kg produces a response within 10 minutes. In infants, the drug is given intravenously at a dose of 0.2 mg/kg and reverses weakness within 1 minute.

SPINAL MUSCULAR ATROPHIES

Spinal muscular atrophies (SMA) are usually genetic disorders in which anterior horn cells in the spinal cord and motor nuclei of the brainstem are progressively lost. The mechanism is probably a defect in programmed cell death,

wherein the deletion of cells, a normal process during gestation, continues after birth. At some point, the process usually ends and weakness becomes static (Iannaccone et al, 1993). The onset of weakness may be any age from birth to adult life. Some spinal muscular atrophies are marked by a generalized distribution of weakness, and others affect specific muscle groups. Those with onset in infancy usually cause generalized weakness and hypotonia. Infantile spinal muscular atrophy is one of the more common motor unit disorders causing infantile hypotonia.

Two clinical syndromes of infantile spinal muscular atrophy, both transmitted by autosomal inheritance, can be distinguished. One is an acute fulminating form that begins at birth or within the first 6 months (type I), and the other is a more chronic form that usually begins after 3 to 6 months of age (type II). Both types, as well as a juvenile type (III), described in Chapter 7, are caused by a genetic defect on chromosome 5q. The overlap in clinical features between the three types is considerable, and even adult onset cases may occur in families where other members are affected in childhood (Shaw et al, 1992).

An X-linked form also exists with clinical features that are indistinguishable from the more prevalent autosomal recessive type I. Arthrogryposis is often present. Some with this syndrome may have the connatal form of Pelizaeus-Merzbacher disease, discussed later in this section.

Two dominantly inherited types of spinal muscular atrophy occur in newborns. One is an acute fulminating disorder that may be part of the phenotypic variability of the juvenile distal form described in Chapter 7, and the other is a benign disorder characterized by arthrogryposis and nonprogressive weakness (Frijns et al, 1994).

Acute Infantile Spinal Muscular Atrophy (SMA Type I)

CLINICAL FEATURES. Age at onset is birth to 6 months. Reduced fetal movement may be reported when neuronal degeneration begins in utero. Affected newborns have generalized weakness involving proximal more than distal muscles, hypotonia, and areflexia. Newborns who are hypotonic in utero and weak at birth may have difficulty adapting to extrauterine life and experience postnatal asphyxia and encephalopathy. The majority breathe adequately at first and appear alert despite the generalized weakness because facial expression is relatively well preserved and extraocular movement is normal. Some newborns have paradoxic respiration because intercostal paralysis and thoracic collapse occur before diaphragmatic movement is impaired while others have diaphragmatic paralysis as an initial feature. Despite intrauterine hypotonia, arthrogryposis is not present. Neurogenic arthrogryposis is probably a distinct entity and is described separately in this chapter.

When weakness begins in infancy, the decline in strength can be sudden or decremental. At times, the child seems to improve because of normal cerebral development, but the progression of weakness is relentless. Atrophy and fasciculations may be observed in the tongue. After the gag reflex is lost, feeding becomes difficult and death results from aspiration and pneumonia. When weakness is present at birth, death usually occurs by 6 months of age, but the course is variable when symptoms develop after 3 months of age. Some infants will attain sitting balance but will not walk. Survival should not be predicted.

DIAGNOSIS. The diagnosis is readily established by laboratory investigation. Serum concentration of creatine kinase is usually normal but may be mildly elevated in infants with rapidly progressive weakness. EMG studies show fibrillations and fasciculations at rest and an increased mean amplitude of motor unit potentials. Motor nerve conduction velocities may be slowed but are usually normal.

The histopathologic findings in muscle establish the diagnosis. Routine histologic stains demonstrate groups of small fibers adjacent to groups of normal-sized or hypertrophied fibers. The diagnostic features of acute infantile spinal muscular atrophy are revealed by the myosin ATPase reaction. All hypertrophied fibers are type I, whereas fibers of medium and small size are a mixture of types I and II (Figure 6-1). The normal random arrangement of fiber types is replaced by type grouping, a sign of reinnervation in which large numbers of fibers of the same type are contiguous. Some biopsy specimens show uniform small fibers of both fiber types.

TREATMENT. No treatment is available for this disorder. However, prenatal diagnosis can be accomplished by DNA analysis of chorion villus biopsies (Cobben et al, 1993).

Chronic Infantile Spinal Muscular Atrophy (SMA Type II)

CLINICAL FEATURES. The onset of weakness is usually between 6 and 24 months but can be

□ FIGURE 6 – 1 Infantile spinal muscular atrophy (ATPase reaction). The normal checkerboard pattern is lost. Groups of large type I fibers *(light shade)* are adjacent to groups of small type II fibers *(dark shade).*

as early as 3 months. Therefore, when weakness begins between 3 and 6 months, the course of illness is even more unpredictable. Initial weakness is usually symmetric and affects the proximal muscles of the legs, the arms, or all limbs. Initial hip weakness is the most common pattern. Distal muscles are affected little or not at all during early infancy. Tendon reflexes of weak muscles are depressed or unobtainable. Almost all attain sitting balance, most will stand alone, and some will walk. Facial muscles are not affected early in the course, and extraocular muscles are spared.

The weakness is slowly progressive during infancy but eventually ceases and may remain stable for many years; eventually slow progression of weakness resumes. Survival to adult life is expected. Improvement never occurs, and even during periods of stabilization the EMG continues to show fibrillations and fasciculations.

Contractures commonly develop during childhood. Pseudohypertrophy of the calves and gluteal muscles is common and may suggest Duchenne muscular dystrophy. As the plantar flexor muscles become weaker, the foot everts into an equinovarus posture. Some children have hand tremors.

An unusual form of SMA type II is one that begins with neck weakness (Goutiéres et al, 1991). The initial feature is head droop and generalized weakness with respiratory insufficiency. Children with this variant die by 3 years of age.

DIAGNOSIS. The serum concentration of creatine kinase is normal. EMG findings are identical to those described for the acute infantile form. Muscle biopsy shows groups of small fibers adjacent to fibers of normal size. Type grouping is usually present, but type I fiber hypertrophy is not seen.

TREATMENT. Although curative treatment is not available, physical therapy and other rehabilitative measures may prevent contractures and maintain function.

Congenital Cervical Spinal Muscular Atrophy

This is a rare sporadic disorder characterized by severe weakness and wasting confined to the arms (Hageman et al, 1993). Contractures of the shoulder, elbow, and wrist joints are present at birth. The legs are normal. Postnatal progression of weakness does not occur. Central nervous system function is normal.

Infantile Neuronal Degeneration

CLINICAL FEATURES. Infantile neuronal degeneration is a rare disorder in which the typical features of infantile spinal muscular atrophy are combined with degenerative changes in the cerebellum, thalamus, and peripheral sensory nerves. The defect is thought to be transmitted as an autosomal recessive trait because of three families with two or more affected siblings. All had hypotonia and areflexia, and one had arthrogryposis as well. The hypotonia is primarily caused by denervation but probably has a cerebral component. Half of children have symptoms at birth, and the remainder during infancy. Dyspnea, weak cry, and difficulty in feeding are prominent features in the newborns, all of whom die within 5 months. The symptoms are the same when the onset is delayed until early infancy, but survival beyond 2 years of age is recorded.

DIAGNOSIS. Infantile neuronal degeneration can be differentiated from infantile spinal muscular atrophy by electrophysiologic studies. Motor nerve conduction velocities are slow, and sensory nerve responses are absent or reduced.

TREATMENT. No treatment is available.

Neurogenic Arthrogryposis

The term *neurogenic arthrogryposis* was originally used to denote the association of arthrogryposis with infantile spinal muscular atrophy. Most cases are sporadic. Transmission occurs by autosomal recessive inheritance in some families and by X-linked inheritance in others. I am aware of two sets of identical twins in which one twin was born with neurogenic arthrogryposis and the other remained normal. This suggests that some sporadic cases may have nongenetic causes.

Families in whom neurogenic arthrogryposis is transmitted as an autosomal dominant trait tend to have clinical or pathologic features that distinguish them from the sporadic cases and those transmitted as an autosomal recessive trait. Arthrogryposis may not occur in every affected family member, weakness or joint deformity may be limited to the legs or arms, and progression is minimal.

CLINICAL FEATURES. In neurogenic arthrogryposis the most active phase of disease occurs in utero. Severely affected newborns have respiratory and feeding difficulties, and some die of aspiration. The less severely affected survive and have little or no progression of their weakness. Indeed, the respiratory and feeding difficulties lessen with time. Contractures are present in both proximal and distal joints. Micrognathia and a high-arched palate may be associated features, and a pattern of facial anomalies suggesting trisomy 18 is present in some newborns.

Newborns with respiratory distress at birth may not have a fatal course. Limb weakness may be minimal and long intervals of stability occur. Some children with neurogenic arthrogryposis have malformations of the prosencephalon (Fedrizzi et al, 1993). Microcephaly and mental retardation are associated.

DIAGNOSIS. The diagnosis is suspected in newborns with arthrogryposis who have a normal serum concentration of creatine kinase and EMG findings compatible with a neuropathic process. Muscle histologic examination reveals the typical pattern of denervation and reinnervation. However, the histology may also have myopathic features: increased collagen and adipose tissue, structural derangements in medium-sized fibers, and fibrosis of the muscle spindle capsule.

MRI of the head to look for cerebral malformations should be done in children with microcephaly.

TREATMENT. The joint deformities respond to physical therapy, and an intensive program of rehabilitation should be initiated as soon after birth as possible.

Pelizaeus-Merzbacher Disease (Connatal)

Pelizaeus-Merzbacher disease is a disorder of proteolipid protein expression that is usually expressed as progressive dementia and choreoathetosis during childhood (see Chapter 5). It also has a connatal form with hypotonia as the main feature (Kaye et al, 1994).

CLINICAL FEATURES. Affected newborns are hypotonic and may require respiratory assistance. Tendon reflexes are absent, fasciculations are seen in the tongue, and sensation is normal. Abnormal eye movements develop shortly after birth; spasticity and movement disorders follow during the first year. The subsequent course is characterized by progressive features of cerebral and motor neuron dysfunction and early death.

DIAGNOSIS. MRI shows diffuse cerebral demyelination and EMG is consistent with motor neuron disease. Nerve conduction velocity does not slow until later in childhood.

POLYNEUROPATHIES

Polyneuropathies are uncommon in childhood and even more uncommon during infancy. Table 6–11 lists the polyneuropathies that begin during infancy. They are divided into those that affect primarily the myelin (demyelinating) and those that affect primarily the axon (axonal). In newborns and infants, the term *demyelinating* also refers to disorders in which myelin has failed to form (hypomyelinating neuropathy). Only with congenital hypomyelinating neuropathy is infantile hypotonia the initial feature. The others are more likely to start as progressive gait disturbance or psychomotor retardation. A complete discussion of the clinical approach to neuropathy is given in Chapter 7.

Congenital Hypomyelinating Neuropathy

The term *congenital hypomyelinating neuropathy* encompasses several disorders with similar clinical and pathologic features. Sporadic occurrence is the rule, but autosomal recessive inheritance is suggested by reports of disease in cousins and in siblings of both sexes. Some cases, especially those with a family history of the disease, may represent an infantile form of hereditary motor and sensory neuropathy type III (Balestrini et al, 1991) (see Chapter 7).

CLINICAL FEATURES. The clinical features are indistinguishable from those of acute infantile

■ TABLE 6–11
Polyneuropathies with Possible Onset in Infancy

Axonal
Familial dysautonomia
Hereditary motor-sensory neuropathy type II (see Chapter 7)
Idiopathic with encephalopathy (see Chapter 7)
Infantile neuronal degeneration
Subacute necrotizing encephalopathy (see Chapters 5 and 10)

Demyelinating
Acute inflammatory demyelinating polyneuropathy (Guillain-Barré syndrome) (see Chapter 7)
Chronic inflammatory demyelinating polyneuropathy (see Chapter 7)
Congenital hypomyelinating neuropathy
Globoid cell leukodystrophy (see Chapter 5)
Hereditary motor-sensory neuropathy type I (see Chapter 7)
Hereditary motor-sensory neuropathy type II (see Chapter 7)
Metachromatic leukodystrophy (see Chapter 5)

spinal muscular atrophy. Arthrogryposis may be present. Newborns have progressive flaccid weakness and atrophy of the skeletal muscles, a bulbar palsy that spares extraocular motility, and areflexia. Respiratory insufficiency causes death during infancy.

Some children are not identified as abnormal until they fail to meet motor milestones. Examination shows diffuse weakness, distal atrophy, and areflexia. Weakness progresses slowly and is not life threatening during childhood. Sensation remains intact. These late-onset cases may represent demyelinating-remyelinating neuropathies, with subsequent enlargement of the peripheral nerves.

DIAGNOSIS. The serum concentration of creatine kinase is normal, EMG findings are consistent with denervation, and motor nerve conduction velocities are usually less than 10 m/sec. The protein concentration of the cerebrospinal fluid is markedly elevated in almost every case. Muscle biopsy reveals groups of atrophic fibers adjacent to groups of normal fibers, without fiber hypertrophy.

Definitive antemortem diagnosis is established by sural nerve biopsy, which shows naked axons without evidence of myelin formation (Vital et al, 1989). No evidence of inflammation or lipid storage is seen. However, the possibility of a prednisone-responsive hypomyelinating neuropathy cannot be eliminated by laboratory investigation.

TREATMENT. Some infants with hypomyelinating neuropathies respond to treatment with oral prednisone. I have treated one newborn who became normal, both clinically and electrophysiologically, by 1 year of age, but relapsed several times later in childhood and then responded to prednisone and to intravenous immunoglobulin. Such children may have a connatal form of chronic inflammatory demyelinating neuropathy (see Chapter 7). Whatever the mechanism, every affected child should be given a course of oral prednisone, 2 mg/kg/day. Those who respond become stronger within 4 weeks of starting therapy. Following the initial response the children should be maintained on alternate-day therapy, 0.5 mg/kg, for at least one year.

DISORDERS OF NEUROMUSCULAR TRANSMISSION

Infantile Botulism

Human botulism ordinarily results from eating food contaminated by preformed exotoxin of the organism *Clostridium botulinum*. The exotoxin prevents the release of acetylcholine, causing a cholinergic blockade of skeletal muscle and end organs innervated by autonomic nerves. Infantile botulism is an age-limited disorder in which *C. botulinum* is ingested, colonizes the intestinal tract, and produces toxin in situ. Dietary contamination with honey or corn syrup accounts for almost 20% of cases, but in most the source is not defined (Spika et al, 1989).

CLINICAL FEATURES. The clinical spectrum of infantile botulism includes asymptomatic carriers of organisms, mild hypotonia and failure to thrive, severe, progressive, life-threatening paralysis, and sudden infant death. Infected infants are between 2 and 26 weeks of age and usually live in a dusty environment adjacent to construction or agricultural soil disruption. The incidence is mainly between March and October. Most infants experience a prodromal syndrome of constipation and poor feeding. Progressive bulbar and skeletal muscle weakness and loss of tendon reflexes develop 4 to 5 days later. Typical features on examination include diffuse hypotonia, ptosis, dysphagia, weak cry, and dilated pupils that react sluggishly to light.

Infantile botulism is a self-limited disease generally lasting 2 to 6 weeks. Recovery is complete, but relapse occurs in as many as 5% of babies (Glauser et al, 1990).

DIAGNOSIS. The syndrome suggests postinfectious polyradiculoneuropathy (Guillain-Barré syndrome), infantile spinal muscular atrophy, or generalized myasthenia gravis. Clinical differentiation of infantile botulism from Guillain-Barré syndrome is difficult, and some reported cases of Guillain-Barré syndrome during infancy may actually have been infantile botulism. Infantile botulism differs from infantile spinal muscular atrophy by the early appearance of facial and pharyngeal weakness, the presence of ptosis and dilated pupils, and the occurrence of severe constipation. Infants with generalized myasthenia do not have dilated pupils, absent reflexes, or severe constipation.

Electrophysiologic studies provide the first clue to diagnosis. Repetitive stimulation between 20 and 50 Hz reverses the presynaptic block and produces an incremental increase in the size of the motor unit potentials in 90% of cases. The EMG shows short-duration, low-amplitude motor unit potentials. The diagnosis is confirmed by the isolation of organisms from the stool.

TREATMENT. The use of antitoxin and antibiotics does not influence the course of the disease. Indeed, gentamicin, an agent that produces presynaptic neuromuscular blockade, may worsen the condition. Intensive care is necessary throughout the period of profound hypotonia, and many infants require ventilator support. Sudden apnea and death are a constant danger.

Familial Infantile Myasthenia

Several genetic defects causing myasthenic syndromes have been identified (Table 6–12) (Engel, 1993). All are known or presumed to be transmitted by autosomal recessive transmission except for the slow channel syndrome, which is transmitted as an autosomal dominant trait (see Chapter 7). All genetic myasthenic syndromes are seronegative for antibodies that bind the acetylcholine receptor (AChR).

Despite considerable phenotypic diversity, two clinical syndromes are recognized in the newborn: familial infantile myasthenia with prominent respiratory and feeding difficulty at birth, and congenital myasthenia with predominantly ocular findings (see Chapter 15). Familial infantile myasthenia can be caused by a presynaptic defect in acetylcholine resynthesis and packaging or by several postsynaptic defects involving the kinetics of the AChR or

■ T A B L E 6 – 1 2
Genetic Myasthenic Syndromes

Presynaptic Defects
Defect in acetylcholine resynthesis or mobilization
Paucity of synaptic vesicles and reduced quantal release
Postsynaptic Defects
Endplate acetylcholinesterase deficiency
Primary acetylcholine receptor (AChR) deficiency
  Congenital paucity of secondary synaptic clefts
  Deficiency and short-open time of the acetylcholine receptor
Kinetic abnormalities of the receptor without primary AChRP deficiency
  Abnormal interaction of acetylcholine and receptor
  High conductance and fast closure of the acetylcholine receptor channel
  Slow-channel syndrome

congenital endplate acetylcholinesterase deficiency.

CLINICAL FEATURES. Respiratory insufficiency and feeding difficulty may be present at birth. Many affected newborns require mechanical ventilation. Ptosis and generalized weakness either are present at birth or develop during infancy. Arthrogryposis may also be present (Vajsar et al, 1995). Although facial and skeletal muscles are weak, extraocular motility is usually normal. Within weeks the infants become stronger and no longer need mechanical ventilation. However, episodes of weakness and life-threatening apnea occur repeatedly throughout infancy and childhood, sometimes even into adult life.

DIAGNOSIS. The diagnosis is established by the intravenous or subcutaneous injection of edrophonium chloride, 0.15 mg/kg. The weakness and the respiratory distress are reversed almost immediately after intravenous injection and within 10 minutes of subcutaneous injection. Further confirmation can be accomplished by showing a decrement in the amplitude of successive motor unit potentials with repetitive nerve stimulation at low frequency. Identification of the precise defect requires special laboratory techniques (Engel, 1993).

TREATMENT. Long-term treatment with neostigmine or pyridostigmine is needed to prevent sudden episodes of apnea at the time of intercurrent illness. Treatment should be continued throughout childhood. Thymectomy and immunosuppressive therapy are not beneficial.

Transitory Neonatal Myasthenia

A transitory myasthenic syndrome is observed in 10% to 15% of offspring of myasthenic mothers. The syndrome is believed to be due to the passive transfer of antibody directed against AChRP from the myasthenic mother to her normal fetus. Passive transfer of antibody from mother to fetus clearly occurs, but this does not fully explain why only a small percentage of newborns are affected or why symptoms are delayed. The severity of symptoms in the newborn correlates with the newborn's antibody concentration but not with the severity or duration of weakness in the mother (Morel et al, 1988).

CLINICAL FEATURES. Difficulty feeding and generalized hypotonia are the major clinical features. Affected children are eager to feed, but the ability to suck fatigues quickly and nutrition is inadequate. Symptoms usually arise within hours of birth but can be delayed until the third day. Some newborns have had intrauterine hypotonia and are born with arthrogryposis. Weakness of cry and facial expression is present in 50%, but only 15% have limitation of extraocular movement and ptosis. Respiratory insufficiency is uncommon. Weakness becomes progressively worse in the first few days and then improves. The mean duration of symptoms is 18 days, with a range of 5 days to 2 months. Recovery is complete, and transitory neonatal myasthenia does not develop into myasthenia gravis later in life.

DIAGNOSIS. The diagnosis of transitory neonatal myasthenia is accomplished by showing high serum concentrations of AChR binding antibody in the newborn and temporary reversal of weakness by the subcutaneous or intravenous injection of edrophonium chloride, 0.15 mg/kg.

TREATMENT. Newborns with severe generalized weakness and respiratory distress should be treated with exchange transfusion. For those who are less impaired, an intramuscular injection of 0.1% neostigmine methylsulfate before feeding sufficiently improves sucking and swallowing to allow adequate nutrition. The dose is progressively reduced as symptoms remit. Neostigmine may also be administered through a nasogastric tube at a dose 10 times the parenteral level.

CONGENITAL MYOPATHIES

Congenital myopathies are developmental disorders of skeletal muscle (Sarnat, 1994). The

☐ F I G U R E 6 – 2 Fiber-type disproportion myopathy (ATPase reaction). Type I fibers (*light shade*) are more numerous than type II fibers (*dark shade*). Type II fibers are generally larger in diameter than type I fibers.

main clinical feature is infantile hypotonia. Diagnosis is only established by muscle biopsy. The common histologic feature is that type I fibers are greater in number, but smaller in size, than type II fibers (Figure 6-2). Many infants with hypotonia and type I fiber predominance are later shown to have a cerebral abnormality; cerebellar aplasia is particularly common (Kyriakides et al, 1993).

The term *congenital fiber-type disproportion myopathy* is used to describe newborns with hypotonia, and sometimes arthrogryposis, whose muscle biopsy specimens show type I predominance as the only histologic abnormality. The biopsy specimens in some infants have not only a type I fiber predominance but also a unique histologic feature for which their condition is named: central core disease, myotubular myopathy, and nemaline myopathy. Several other congenital myopathies, reported in one child or one family, are not discussed. These include *multicore/minicore disease, trilaminar myopathy, lysis of myofibrils in type I fibers, "cap" disease, spheroid body myopathy, fingerprint body myopathy, reducing body myopathy,* and *tubular aggregate myopathy* (Bodensteiner, 1994).

Central Core Disease

Central core disease is a rare but distinct genetic entity transmitted by autosomal dominant inheritance. The gene locus is on chromosome 19q13 and may be allelic with the gene for malignant hyperthermia.

CLINICAL FEATURES. Mild hypotonia is noted immediately after birth or during infancy. Congenital dislocation of the hips is relatively common. Weakness is greater in proximal than in distal limb muscles, and greater in the arms than in the legs. Tendon reflexes of weak muscles are depressed or absent. Extraocular motility, facial expression, and swallowing are normal. Some children become progressively weaker, have motor impairment, and develop kyphoscoliosis. In others, weakness remains mild and never causes disability.

All children with central core disease are at risk for malignant hyperthermia and should not be administered anesthetics without appropriate caution (see Chapter 8).

DIAGNOSIS. The serum concentration of creatine kinase is normal, and the EMG findings may be normal as well. More frequently the EMG suggests a myopathic process. Diagnosis depends on muscle biopsy. Sharply demarcated cores of closely packed myofibrils undergoing varying degrees of degeneration are present in the center of all type I fibers (Figure 6-3). Because of the tight packing of myofibrils, the cores are deficient in sarcoplasmic reticulum, glycogen, and mitochondria.

TREATMENT. No treatment is available, nor is there a method for prenatal diagnosis.

Congenital Fiber-Type Disproportion Myopathy

The congenital fiber-type disproportion myopathies are a heterogeneous group of diseases that have a similar pattern of muscle histology. The initial feature of all these diseases is infantile hypotonia. Both sexes are involved equally. Most cases are sporadic, some are clearly transmitted by autosomal dominant inheritance, and others are familial but without a definite pattern of genetic transmission. A balanced chromosomal translocation of loci on chromosomes 10 and 17 (p11.2:q25) transmitted by the asymptomatic mother was identified in one affected infant (Gerdes et al, 1995). The affected breakpoints are therefore candidate regions for some congenital myopathies. Despite the label "congenital," an identical pattern of fiber-type disproportion may be present in patients who are asymptomatic at birth and first have weakness during childhood.

CLINICAL FEATURES. The severity of weakness in the newborn varies from mild hypotonia to respiratory insufficiency. Many had intrauter-

☐ F I G U R E 6 – 3 Central core disease (DPNH reaction). The center of every fiber has a central core that appears clear when oxidative enzyme reactions are applied.

ine hypotonia and show congenital hip dislocation, dysmorphic features, and joint contractures. Proximal muscles are weaker than distal
muscles. Facial weakness, high arched palate,
ptosis, and disturbances of ocular motility may
be present. When axial weakness is present in
infancy, kyphoscoliosis often develops during
childhood. Tendon reflexes are depressed or
absent. Intellectual function is normal.

Weakness is most severe during the first 2
years and then becomes relatively stable or
progresses slowly.

DIAGNOSIS. The essential feature seen in
muscle specimens is type I fiber predominance
and hypotrophy. Type I fibers are 15% smaller
than type II fibers. Other laboratory studies are
not helpful. The serum concentration of creatine kinase may be slightly elevated or normal,
and the EMG may be consistent with a neuropathic process, a myopathic process, or both.
Nerve conduction velocities are normal.

TREATMENT. Physical therapy should be initiated immediately, not only to relieve existing
contractures but also to prevent new contractures from developing.

Myotubular (Centronuclear) Myopathy

Several clinical syndromes are included in the
category of myotubular (centronuclear) myopathy. Some are clearly transmitted by X-linked inheritance, others by autosomal dominant inheritance, and still others are sporadic and possibly
transmitted by autosomal recessive inheritance.
The common histologic feature on muscle biopsy is an arrest in the morphogenesis of the
muscle fiber at the myotube stage (Sarnat, 1994).

Acute Myotubular Myopathy

CLINICAL FEATURES. The abnormal gene that
causes acute myotubular myopathy has been
mapped to the long arm of the X chromosome
(Xq28) (Thomas et al, 1990). The clinical features in the newborn are generalized hypotonia
and respiratory distress. Decreased fetal movement during pregnancy, polyhydramnios, and
fetal cardiac arrhythmias are common (Tyson et
al, 1992). Sucking, swallowing, and tendon reflexes are depressed or absent. Ptosis, and sometimes complete ophthalmoplegia, may be present. Repeated episodes of apnea, asphyxia, and
pneumonia usually cause death during early
infancy.

DIAGNOSIS. The serum concentration of creatine kinase is normal. The EMG may suggest a
neuropathic process, a myopathic process, or
both. Muscle biopsy shows type I fiber predominance and hypotrophy, the presence of many
internal nuclei, and a central area of increased
oxidative enzyme and decreased myosin ATPase
activity.

TREATMENT. No treatment is available for
this disorder, nor is there a method for prenatal
diagnosis.

Chronic Myotubular Myopathy

CLINICAL FEATURES. Chronic myotubular myopathy is usually transmitted by autosomal
dominant inheritance. Sporadic cases may represent families in which the phenotype is not
fully expressed in other generations. Some
children with the disease have hypotonia at
birth; others come to attention because of
delayed motor development. Limb weakness

may be predominantly proximal or distal. The axial and neck flexor muscles are weak as well. Ptosis, but not ophthalmoplegia, is sometimes present at birth. Infants have a slowly progressive ophthalmoplegia, loss of facial expression, continuing weakness of limb muscles, and loss of tendon reflexes. Many patients have seizures and mental deficiency.

DIAGNOSIS. The serum concentration of creatine kinase is normal, and EMG findings are abnormal but do not establish the diagnosis. Muscle biopsy is essential for diagnosis, and the histologic features are identical to those of the acute form.

TREATMENT. No treatment is available, nor is there a method for prenatal diagnosis.

Nemaline (Rod) Myopathy

Nemaline myopathy is probably transmitted by autosomal dominant inheritance. Penetrance is variable, and affected parents may be asymptomatic.

CLINICAL FEATURES. Hypotonia is usually mild but can be so severe as to cause immediate respiratory insufficiency and neonatal death. Affected newborns often appear normal, and attention is not sought until infancy, when achievement of motor milestones is delayed. The infant is hypotonic with greater weakness in proximal than distal muscles. Weakness of facial muscles causes a dysmorphic appearance in which the face appears long and narrow and the palate is high and arched. Axial weakness leads to scoliosis. Weakness is not progressive and tends to stabilize, but some residual handicap remains.

DIAGNOSIS. The serum concentration of creatine kinase is either normal or only mildly elevated. EMG findings may be normal, and when abnormal they are not the basis for diagnosis. Muscle biopsy is essential for diagnosis. Multiple small rodlike particles, thought to be structural protein, are present within most, if not all, muscle fibers (Figure 6-4). Similar rodlike structures are a nonspecific histologic feature in some inflammatory myopathies, but only in nemaline myopathy is type I fiber predominance an associated feature.

TREATMENT. No treatment is available, nor is there a method for prenatal diagnosis. Parents who have the abnormal gene but are not weak may have rod bodies and fiber-type predominance in their muscle.

□ F I G U R E 6 – 4 Nemaline (rod) myopathy (trichrome). A spectrum of fiber sizes is present. The small fibers are all type I and contain rodlike bodies in a subsarcolemmal position.

MUSCULAR DYSTROPHIES

Congenital Muscular Dystrophy

The term *congenital muscular dystrophy* (CMD) is often used generically for any muscular disorder present at birth or shortly thereafter. These are probably all genetic disorders, but the abnormal gene sites and the abnormal gene products are just beginning to be recognized. Merosin deficiency has been shown in some forms of CMD with brain malformations (Sunada et al, 1995). The abnormal gene site for merosin deficient CMD is 6q2 and transmission is by autosomal recesive inheritance. Merosin is an important linking protein for the dystrophin-glycoprotein complex in skeletal muscle and is also expressed in the nervous system where it has biologic activity on neurite outgrowth. Therefore, its absence could cause brain malformations. Some cases of CMD are merosin positive and others are merosin negative.

Until further abnormal gene locations and gene products are determined, the classification of CMD relies mainly on clinical features (Table 6-1). A satisfying definition and classification of CMD are not possible at present, but for purposes of this discussion CMD may be defined by the following criteria (Fenichel, 1988).

1. Hypotonia, weakness, or arthrogryposis is present at birth.

2. The muscle biopsy is consistent with myopathy (i.e., spectrum of fiber sizes, degeneration of medium-sized muscle fibers, fat and collagen replacement of muscle

fibers) and specifically excludes denervation.

3. Other myopathies of the newborn with recognizable clinical or pathologic features are excluded.

In most cases the defect appears to be transmitted by autosomal recessive inheritance; siblings are frequently affected and many instances of parental consanguinity have been reported. Autosomal dominant transmission has been identified in two families.

Several phenotypes are considered variants of CMD, depending on the involvement of other organs, especially the brain and eye.

CLINICAL FEATURES. Hypotonia and arthrogryposis are present at birth. The infant has generalized limb weakness; proximal muscles are affected earlier and more severely than distal muscles. Facial and neck weakness is common, but extraocular motility is normal. Tendon reflexes may be present or absent and are often difficult to test because of joint contractures. Contractures at birth may involve any joint, but torticollis and clubfoot are particularly common and congenital dislocation of the hips is often an associated feature.

Weakness progresses little or remains stable, but new joint contractures may continue to form at the ankles, hips, knees, and elbows. Muscles are not hypertrophied. Motor development is delayed because of weakness and contractures, but intelligence is normal. Because approximately 15% of children with CMD die, a more severe form of the disease than described in the preceding section must be recognized. The neck muscles are especially weak and head control is impaired. Contractures are often absent at birth but may develop during infancy. Intercostal and diaphragmatic muscle weakness may be present at birth or develop during infancy. Chronic hypoventilation leading to respiratory failure is the usual cause of death.

DIAGNOSIS. The serum concentration of creatine kinase may be normal or elevated in the newborn and tends to decline with age; however, it does not correlate with the severity of weakness. Asymptomatic siblings and parents may have elevated serum concentrations of creatine kinase. EMG findings are consistent with a myopathic process.

Muscle histologic appearance is characteristic. Features include a variation in fiber size with occasional central nucleation, extensive fibrosis and proliferation of adipose tissue, fibers undergoing regeneration and degeneration, and thickening of the muscle spindle capsule. MRI is mandatory to look for demyelination or cerebral malformation.

TREATMENT. Physical therapy is important to prevent further contractures. Antenatal diagnosis is not available.

Fukuyama Type CMD

A clinical syndrome of congenital muscular dystrophy associated with cerebral dysplasia is the second most prevalent form of muscular dystrophy in Japan. The abnormal gene site is 9q31-33, and transmission is by autosomal recessive inheritance. The high prevalence of the disease in Japan, but not among ethnic Japanese living outside Japan, suggests that an environmental factor acting on a genetically predisposed population may be important.

The major feature is a disturbance of cellular migration to the cortex between the fourth and fifth gestational months, resulting in polymicrogyria, lissencephaly, and heterotopia. Other abnormalities may include fusion of the frontal lobes, hydrocephalus, periventricular cysts, optic nerve atrophy, hypoplasia of the pyramidal tracts, reduction in the number of anterior horn cells, and inflammation of the leptomeninges.

Myelination may be delayed. MRI shows hypomyelination of the centrum semiovale in 50% of children with Fukuyama-type CMD. This probably represents delayed myelination rather than demyelination because it becomes less prominent as the child gets older.

CLINICAL FEATURES. A history of spontaneous abortion is recorded for 25% of mothers who have affected children. Affected newborns are often normal at birth but soon develop hypotonia, an expressionless face, a weak cry, and an ineffective suck. Weakness affects the proximal more than distal limb muscles. Mild contractures of the elbow and knee joints may be present at birth or develop later. Tendon reflexes are usually absent. Pseudohypertrophy of the calves develops in half of cases.

Symptoms of cerebral involvement are present early in infancy. Febrile or nonfebrile generalized seizures are usually the first manifestation. Development is always globally delayed, and microcephaly is the rule. Weakness and atrophy are progressive and result in severe disability, cachexia, and death before 10 years of age.

DIAGNOSIS. The serum concentration of creatine kinase is generally elevated, and the EMG indicates a myopathy. Muscle biopsy specimens show excessive proliferation of adipose tissue and collagen out of proportion to the degree of fiber degeneration. Typical MRI abnormalities are dilatation of the cerebral ventricles and subarachnoid space and lucency of cortical white matter.

TREATMENT. No treatment is available for this disorder, nor is there a method for prenatal diagnosis.

Leukodystrophy

Demyelination of the cerebral hemispheres is often associated with CMD in European children (Trevisan et al, 1991). However, the combination of leukodystrophy and migrational malformations as seen in Fukuyama-type CMD is unusual. Several affected sibling pairs have been reported, suggesting autosomal recessive inheritance.

CLINICAL FEATURES. Affected newborns are hypotonic, and some have arthrogryposis as well. Feeding disturbances and apnea may be associated symptoms. Tendon reflexes are diminished or absent. Intelligence is normal at first, and some children never show clinical evidence of cerebral abnormality. Others have progressive dementia and epilepsy during childhood.

DIAGNOSIS. The serum concentration of creatine kinase is elevated, and the EMG is consistent with a myopathic process. Nerve conduction velocity is normal. The electroencephalogram may show epileptiform activity. Antemortem diagnosis is established by MRI evidence of cerebral demyelination.

TREATMENT. No treatment is available for this disorder, nor is there a method for prenatal diagnosis.

Cerebro-ocular Muscular Dystrophy

Cerebro-ocular dysplasia is characterized by the combination of CMD, cerebral malformations, and ocular anomalies. The cerebral and the muscle abnormalities are the same as in Fukuyama-type CMD. The major differences from Fukuyama-type CMD are the presence of ocular abnormalities and the occurrence of this syndrome in non-Japanese children (Leyton et al, 1993).

CLINICAL FEATURES. Hypotonia and generalized weakness are present at birth. Severe mental retardation is evident in the first year, and most children die during infancy or early childhood. Several different cerebral and cerebellar malformations may be present: abnormal gyral patterns, heterotopias, hypomyelination, and agenesis of tracts. Hydrocephalus occurs in most cases (see discussion of Warburg syndrome in Chapter 18). Ocular abnormalities include corneal clouding, cataracts, retinal dysplasia or detachment, and optic nerve hypoplasia.

DIAGNOSIS. All newborns with muscular dystrophy and eye-brain abnormalities, no matter how mild any one element may be, should be considered to have cerebro-ocular dysplasia.

TREATMENT. No treatment is available, nor is there a method for prenatal diagnosis

Congenital Myotonic Dystrophy

Myotonic dystrophy is a multisystem disorder transmitted by autosomal dominant inheritance. Symptoms usually begin in young adult life (see Chapter 7). The disease is caused by an unstable DNA triplet on chromosome 19 that repeats 50 to several thousand times in successive generations; the number of repeats correlates with severity of disease (Pizzuti et al, 1993). Repeat size changes from mother to child are greater than from father to child, and for this reason the mother is always the affected parent when a child has congenital myotonic dystrophy. A mother with repeats of 100 units has a 90% chance that her child will have repeats of 400 units or greater.

The main features during pregnancy are reduced fetal movement and polyhydramnios (Hageman et al, 1993). Fifty percent of babies are born prematurely. Labor may be prolonged because of inadequate uterine contraction, and forceps assistance is frequently needed. Severely affected newborns have inadequate diaphragmatic and intercostal muscle function and are incapable of spontaneous respiration. In the absence of prompt intubation and mechanical ventilation, many will die immediately after birth.

Prominent clinical features in the newborn include facial diplegia, in which the mouth is oddly shaped so that the upper lip forms an inverted V; generalized muscular hypotonia; joint deformities ranging from bilateral clubfoot to generalized arthrogryposis; and gastrointestinal dysfunction, including choking, regurgitation, aspiration, swallowing difficulties, and gastroparesis. Limb weakness in the newborn is more often proximal than distal. Tendon reflexes are usually absent in weak muscles. Myotonia, an abnormality in muscle relaxation after contraction, is not elicited by percussion and may not be demonstrable on EMG.

Neonatal mortality is 16%, a frequent cause of death being cardiomyopathy. Survivors usually gain strength and become able to feed and breathe normally within the first month. The long-term prognosis is poor; all are mentally retarded and have features of severe myotonic dystrophy (Roig et al, 1994).

DIAGNOSIS. The diagnosis of congenital myotonic dystrophy in the newborn requires the diagnosis of myotonic dystrophy in the mother. She is likely to have many clinical features of the disease and myotonia on EMG. The diagnosis can be confirmed by showing DNA amplification on chromosome 19 in both mother and child. Nonsymptomatic family members at risk should be tested for the carrier state.

TREATMENT. The immediate treatment is intubation and mechanical ventilation. Fixed joints respond to physical therapy and casting. Gastroparesis may be alleviated by metoclopramide therapy.

METABOLIC MYOPATHIES

Acid Maltase Deficiency (Pompe Disease)

Acid maltase is a lysosomal enzyme, present in all tissues, that hydrolyzes maltose and other branches of glycogen to yield glucose. It has no function in maintaining blood glucose concentrations. Three distinct clinical forms of deficiency are recognized: infantile, childhood (see Chapter 7), and adult. All are transmitted by autosomal recessive inheritance. The defective gene is located on chromosome 17q.

CLINICAL FEATURES. The infantile form may begin immediately after birth but usually appears during the second month. Profound generalized hypotonia without atrophy and congestive heart failure are the initial symptoms. Hypotonia is the result of glycogen storage in the brain, spinal cord, and skeletal muscles, causing mixed signs of cerebral and motor unit dysfunction: decreased awareness and depressed tendon reflexes. The mixed signs may be confusing, but the presence of cardiomegaly is almost diagnostic. The electrocardiogram shows abnormalities, including short P-R intervals and high QRS complexes on all leads. Most patients die of cardiac failure by 1 year of age.

DIAGNOSIS. Diagnosis is established by muscle biopsy. Large vacuoles containing glycogen are observed in muscle fibers. The diagnosis is established by showing deficient acid maltase activity in fibroblasts or other tissues.

TREATMENT. A high-protein diet has been found helpful in childhood form of the disease but has not yet proved useful in the infantile form.

Cytochrome c Oxidase Deficiency

The electron transfer chain and oxidative phosphorylation are the principal sources of adenosine triphosphate (ATP) synthesis (see Chapter 8). Deficiencies of mitochondrial enzymes that comprise the electron transfer chain in skeletal muscle may cause hypotonia in newborns or infants and exercise intolerance in older children. Deficiency of complex IV (cytochrome c oxidase) is often associated with infantile hypotonia (Oldfors et al, 1989). Most cases are sporadic. Both a fatal and a benign form of infantile cytochrome c oxidase deficiency are recognized. Early in their course these forms are indistinguishable, but in the benign form a spontaneous increase in cytochrome c oxidase activity associated with increased strength occurs during infancy. Different abnormalities in subunits of cytochrome c oxidase account for the phenotypic difference (Tritschler et al, 1991).

CLINICAL FEATURES. Clinical features vary with the number of enzyme deficiencies, the percentage reduction in enzyme activity, and the presence of mitochondrial enzyme deficiencies in organs other than muscle. The typical syndrome is characterized by profound generalized weakness, causing difficulty in feeding, early respiratory failure, and death; severe lactic acidosis; and the *De Toni-Fanconi-Debré syndrome* (glycosuria, proteinuria, phosphaturia, and generalized aminoaciduria). Onset is anytime within the first 6 months. Ptosis, ophthalmoplegia, and macroglossia may be present. Newborns with multiple enzyme deficiencies in multiple organs die within 6 months.

DIAGNOSIS. A deficiency in respiratory chain enzymes should be suspected in any hypotonic infant with lactic acidosis. The serum concentration of creatine kinase is elevated, but EMG findings may be normal. Muscle biopsy reveals vacuoles, mainly in type I fibers, with abnormal glycogen and lipid accumulations. Mitochondria are large, increased in number, and abnormal in structure (ragged-red fibers).

TREATMENT. No effective treatment is available for infants with overwhelming disease caused by multiorgan enzyme deficiency. Coenzyme Q therapy may be tried, although the evidence supporting efficacy is not compelling (Nishikawa et al, 1989). The fatal and the benign form of the deficiency should be distinguished by immunohistochemical findings and supportive care should be provided for newborns with the transitory form.

Phosphofructokinase Deficiency

The usual manifestations of muscle phosphofructokinase deficiency are cramps on exercise and myoglobinuria (see Chapter 8). Symptoms usually begin in childhood, and patients are otherwise asymptomatic. A rare neonatal form of phosphofructokinase deficiency exists and is transmitted by autosomal recessive inheritance.

CLINICAL FEATURES. The neonatal form is characterized by hypotonia, weakness, respiratory deficiency, and joint deformities. The tendon reflexes are diminished or absent. Cerebral and corneal abnormalities may be present. Death occurs during infancy or early childhood.

DIAGNOSIS. The serum concentration of creatine kinase is normal. The EMG, at least late in the disease, is consistent with a myopathic process. Muscle biopsy is critical for diagnosis. Light microscopy shows only nonspecific myopathy, but electron microscopy shows an abnormal accumulation of subsarcolemmal and intramyofibrillary glycogen. Large cytoplasmic vacuoles, as in acid maltase deficiency, are not present. Phosphofructokinase activity is absent in skeletal muscle but present in red blood cells and fibroblasts.

TREATMENT. No treatment is available for this disorder.

Phosphorylase Deficiency

Myophosphorylase deficiency (McArdle disease) is characterized by exercise intolerance in young adults and progressive myopathy in middle life (see Chapter 8). A rare neonatal form of variable severity has been recognized. It is reported in siblings and is probably transmitted, like the older onset forms, by autosomal recessive inheritance. Indeed, the enzyme deficiency appears identical at all ages, and the reason for clinical heterogeneity is not understood.

CLINICAL FEATURES. Newborns with myophosphorylase deficiency have difficulty with sucking and swallowing immediately postpartum or in the early neonatal period. In some, weakness is so profound that it produces imme-diate respiratory insufficiency. In others, weakness is progressive over several months or years. The child appears alert and has normal cranial nerve function. The tongue and heart are not affected. Tendon reflexes are depressed or absent.

DIAGNOSIS. The serum concentration of creatine kinase is elevated, and the EMG findings are abnormal, with features of both neuropathy and myopathy. Muscle biopsy is diagnostic. Fibers vary in size from atrophic to normal and contain peripheral vacuoles that react intensely for glycogen. The glycogen concentration of muscle is greatly elevated, and phosphorylase activity cannot be detected.

TREATMENT. A high-protein diet is useful in older patients with phosphorylase deficiency, but has not yet been tried in newborns.

REFERENCES

Adams C, Babyn PS, Logan WJ. Spinal cord birth injury: Value of computed tomographic myelography. Pediatr Neurol 1988;4:105-109.

Balestrini MR, Cavaletti G, D'Angelo A, et al. Infantile hereditary neuropathy with hypomyelination: Report of two siblings with different expressivity. Neuropediatrics 1991;22:65-70.

Bianchi DW, Van Marter LJ. An approach to ventilator-dependent neonates with arthrogryposis. Pediatrics 1994; 94:682-686.

Bodensteiner JB. Congenital myopathies. Muscle Nerve 1994;17:131-144.

Charnas LR, Bernardini I, Rader D, et al. Clinical and laboratory findings in the oculocerebrorenal syndrome of Lowe, with special reference to growth and renal function. N Engl J Med 1991;324:1318-1325.

Clancy RR, Sladky JT, Rorke LB. Hypoxic-ischemic spinal cord injury following perinatal asphyxia. Ann Neurol 1989;25:185-189.

Cobben JM, de Visser, M, Scheffer H, et al. Confirmation of clinical diagnosis in requests for prenatal prediction of SMA type I. J Neurol Neurosurg Psychiatry 1993;56:319-321.

Engel AG. The investigation of congenital myasthenic syndromes. Ann NY Acad Sci 1993;681:425-434.

Fedrizzi E, Botteon G, Inverno M, et al. Neurogenic arthrogryposis multiplex congenita: Clinical and MRI findings. Pediatr Neurol 1993;9:343-348.

Fenichel GM. Congenital muscular dystrophies. Neurol Clin 1988;6:519-528.

Frijns CJM, Deutekom JV, Frants RR, et al. Dominant congenital benign spinal muscular atrophy. Muscle Nerve 1994;17:192-197.

Gerdes AM, Petersen MB, Schroder HD, et al. Congenital myopathy with fiber type disproportion: A family with a chromosomal translocation t(10;17) may indicate candidate gene regions. Clin Genet 1994;45:11-16.

Glauser TA, Maguire HC, Sladky JT. Relapse of infant botulism. Ann Neurol 1989;28:187-189.

Goutiéres F, Bogicevic D, Aicardi J. A predominantly cervical form of spinal muscular atrophy. J Neurol Neurosurg Psychiatry 1991;54:223-225.

Hageman ATM, Gabreels FJM, Liem KD, et al. Congenital

myotonic dystrophy; a report on thirteen cases and a review of the literature. J Neurol Sci 1993;115:95-101.

Holm VA, Cassidy SB, Butler MG, et al. Prader-Willi syndrome: Consensus diagnostic criteria. Pediatrics 1993;91: 398-402.

Iannaccone ST, Browne RH, Samaha FJ, et al. Prospective study of spinal muscular atrophy before age 6 years. Pediatr Neurol 1993;9:187-193.

Kaye EM, Doll RF, Natowicz MR, et al. Pelizaeus-Merzbacher disease presenting as spinal muscular atrophy: Clinical and molecular studies. Ann Neurol 1994;36:916-919.

Kyriakides T, Silberstein JM, Jongpiputvanich S, et al. The clinical significance of type 1 fiber predominance. Muscle Nerve 1993;16:418-423.

Lanska MJ, Roessmann U, Wiznitzer M. Magnetic resonance imaging in cervical cord birth injury. Pediatrics 1990;85: 760-764.

Leyton QH, Gabreëls FJM, Renier WO, et al. Congenital muscular dystrophy with eye and brain malformations in six Dutch patients. Neuropediatrics 1993;23:316-320.

Morel E, Eymard B, Garabedian BV, et al. Neonatal myasthenia gravis: A new clinical and immunologic appraisal on 30 cases. Neurology 1988;38:138-142.

Naidu S, Moser AE, Moser HW. Phenotypic and genotypic variability of generalized peroxisomal disorders. Pediatr Neurol 1988;4:5-12.

Nishikawa Y, Takahashi M, Nakamura Y, et al. Long-term coenzyme Q10 therapy for a mitochondrial encephalomyopathy with cytochrome c oxidase deficiency: A31P NMR study. Neurology 1989;39:399-403.

Oldfors A, Sommerland H, Holme E, et al. Cytochrome c oxidase deficiency in infancy. Acta Neuropathol 1989;77: 267-275.

Pizzuti A, Friedman DL, Caskey T. The myotonic dystrophy gene. Arch Neurol 1993;50:1173-1179.

Roig M, Balliu P-R, Navarro C, et al. Presentation, clinical course, and outcome of the congential form of myotonic dystrophy. Pediatr Neurol 1994;11:208-213.

Santos MJ, Imanaka T, Shio H, et al. Peroxisomal membrane ghosts in Zellweger syndrome-aberrant organelle assembly. Science 1988;239:1536-1538.

Sarnat HB. New insights into the pathogenesis of congenital myopathies. J Child Neurol 1994;9:193-201.

Shaw PJ, Ince PG, Goodship J, et al. Adult-onset motor neuron disease and infantile Werdnig-Hoffmann disease (spinal muscular atrophy type 1) in the same family. Neurology 1992;42:1477-1480.

Spika JC, Shaffer N, Hargrett-Bean N. Risk factors for infant botulism in the United States. Am J Dis Child 1989;143: 828-832.

Sunada Y, Edgar TS, Lotz BP, et al. Merosin-negative congenital muscular dystrophy associated with extensive brain abnormalities. Neurology 1995;45:2084-2089.

Thomas NS, Williams H, Cole G, et al. X-linked neonatal centronuclear/myotubular myopathy: Evidence for linkage to Xq28 DNA marker loci. J Med Genet 1990;27:284-287.

Trevisan CP, Carollo C, Angelini C, et al. Congenital muscular dystrophy: Brain alterations in an unselected series of Western patients. J Neurol Neurosurg Psychiatry 1991;54: 330-334.

Tritschler HJ, Bonilla E, Lombes A, et al. Differential diagnosis of fatal and benign cytochrome c oxidase deficient myopathies of infancy. An immunohistochemical approach. Neurology 1991;41:300-305.

Tyson RW, Ringel SP, Manchester DK, et al. X-linked myotubular myopathy: A case report of prenatal and perinatal aspects. Pediatr Pathol 1992;12:535-543.

Vajsar J, Sloane A, MacGregor DL, et al. Arthrogryposis multiplex congenita due to congenital myasthenic syndrome. Pediatr Neurol 1995;12:237-241.

Vital A, Vital C, Coquet M, et al. Congenital hypomyelination with axonopathy. Eur J Pediatr 1989;148:470-472.

7

Flaccid Limb Weakness in Childhood

Most children with acute or chronic flaccid limb weakness have a disorder of the motor unit. Flaccid leg weakness may be the initial feature of disturbances in the lumbosacral region, but other symptoms of spinal cord dysfunction are usually present. Table 12-1 should also be consulted when considering the differential diagnosis of flaccid leg weakness without arm impairment. Cerebral disorders may cause flaccid weakness, but dementia (see Chapter 5) or seizures (see Chapter 1) are usually concomitant features.

⇒ Clinical Features of Neuromuscular Disease

Weakness is decreased strength as measured by the force of a maximal contraction. Fatigue is inability to maintain a less than maximal contraction as measured by exercise tolerance. Weak muscles are always more easily fatigued than normal muscles, but fatigue may occur in the absence of weakness. Conditions in which strength is normal at rest but fatigue or cramps occur on exercise are discussed in Chapter 8.

THE INITIAL COMPLAINT

Limb weakness in children is almost always noted first in the legs and then in the arms (Table 7-1). This is because many neuromuscular disorders affect the legs before the arms and symptoms of mild leg weakness are more obvious than mild arm weakness, because walking is impaired. Delayed development of motor skills is often an initial complaint or a prominent feature in the history of children with neuromuscular disorders. Marginal motor delay in a child whose other developmental skills are normal is often overlooked as part of the spectrum of normal development. Older children with neuromuscular disorders are frequently referred for neurologic examination because they are unable to keep up with peers or because they tire easily.

An abnormal gait can be the initial symptom of either proximal or distal leg weakness. With proximal weakness, the pelvis is not stabilized and waddles from side to side as the child walks. Running is especially difficult and accentuates the hip waddle. Descending stairs is particularly difficult in children with quadriceps weakness; the knee must be kept locked and stiff. Difficulty with ascending stairs suggests hip extensor weakness. Rising from the floor or a deep chair is difficult and the hands are used to push off.

Stumbling is an early complaint when there is distal leg weakness, especially weakness of the evertors and dorsiflexors of the foot. Falling is first noted when the child is walking on uneven surfaces. The child is thought to be clumsy, but after a while parents realize that the child is "tripping on nothing at all." Repeated ankle

■ T A B L E 7 – 1
Symptoms of Neuromuscular Disease

Abnormal gait
  Steppage
  Toe-walking
  Waddle
Easy fatigability
Frequent falls
Slow motor development
Specific disability
  Arm elevation
  Climbing stairs
  Hand grip
  Rising from floor

☐ F I G U R E 7 – 1 Gower sign. The child rises from the floor by pushing off with the hands to overcome proximal pelvic weakness.

spraining occurs because of lateral instability. Children with footdrop tend to lift the knee high in the air so the foot will clear the ground. The weak foot then comes down with a slapping motion (steppage gait).

Toe-walking is commonly encountered in Duchenne muscular dystrophy because the pelvis is thrust forward to shift the center of gravity and the gastrocnemius muscle is replaced by collagen and fat. Toe-walking is seen also in upper motor neuron disorders that cause spasticity and in children who have tight heel cords but no identifiable neurologic disease. Muscular dystrophy is usually associated with hyporeflexia and spasticity with hyperreflexia. However, the ankle tendon reflex may be difficult to elicit when the tendon is tight for any reason.

Adolescents, but usually not children, with weakness complain of specific disabilities. A young woman with proximal weakness may have difficulty keeping her arms elevated to groom her hair or rotating the shoulder to get into and out of garments that have a zipper or hook in the back. Weakness in hand muscles is frequently spotted by teachers who become upset with the child's handwriting. Adolescents may notice difficulty in unscrewing jar tops or working with tools. Teachers report to parents when children are slower than classmates in climbing stairs, getting up from the floor, and skipping and jumping. Parents may report a specific complaint to the physician, but more often they say that the child's problem is an inability to keep up with peers.

A child whose limbs are weak also may have weakness in the muscles of the head and neck. Specific questions should be asked about double vision, drooping eyelids, difficulty chewing and swallowing, change of facial expression and strength (whistling, sucking, chewing, blowing), and the clarity and tone of speech.

Weakness of neck muscles is frequently noticed when the child is a passenger in a car that suddenly accelerates or decelerates. The neck muscles are unable to stabilize the head, which snaps backward or forward.

PHYSICAL FINDINGS

The examination begins by watching the child sit, stand, and walk. A normal child sitting cross-legged on the floor can rise to standing in a single movement without using the hands. This remarkable feat is lost sometime after age 10 in most children, and proximal leg strength can then be tested by rising from a low stool. The child with weak pelvic muscles uses the hands for assistance (Figure 7–1), and with progressive weakness, the hands are used to climb up the legs (Gower sign).

After observing normal gait, the child is asked to walk first on toes and then on heels (Table 7–2). Inability to walk on toes indicates gastrocnemius weakness and inability to walk on heels indicates weakness of the anterior compartment muscles.

Push-ups are a quick test of strength in almost all arm muscles. Most normal children can do at least one push-up. The child is then asked to touch the tip of the shoulder blade with the ipsilateral thumb, an impossible task when the rhomboids are weak.

■ T A B L E   7 – 2
Signs of Neuromuscular Disease

Observation
Atrophy and hypertrophy
Fasciculations
Functional ability
Palpation
Muscle texture
Tenderness
Examination
Joint contractures
Myotonia
Strength
Tendon reflexes

■ T A B L E   7 – 3
Progressive Proximal Weakness [Gene Location]

Spinal Cord Disorders (see Chapter 12)
Juvenile Spinal Muscular Atrophies
Autosomal recessive [5q11-13]
Autosomal dominant
GM$_2$ gangliosidosis (hexosaminidase A deficiency) [15q23-24]
Myasthenic Syndromes
Acquired limb-girdle myasthenia
Slow-channel syndrome
Myopathies
Muscular dystrophies
  Bethlem myopathy
  Duchenne/Becker dystrophy [Xp21.2]
  Facioscapulohumeral syndrome [4q35]
  Limb-girdle dystrophy [2, 5, 13, 15q, 17]
  Severe childhood autosomal recessive muscular dystrophy [13q12]
  X-linked vacuolated myopathy
Inflammatory myopathies
  Dermatomyositis
  Polymyositis
  Inclusion-body myositis
Metabolic myopathies
  Acid maltase deficiency [17q23]
  Carnitine deficiency
  Debrancher enzyme deficiency (see Chapter 8)
  Lipid storage myopathies
  Mitochondrial myopathies (see Chapter 8)
  Myophosphorylase deficiency (see Chapter 8)
Endocrine myopathies
  Adrenal cortex
  Parathyroid
  Thyroid

Finally, the face and eye movements are tested. The best test of facial strength is to blow out the cheeks and hold air against compression. Normally the lips are smooth. Wrinkling of the perioral tissues and failure to hold air indicate facial weakness. During this period of observation and again during muscle strength testing, the physician should look for atrophy or hypertrophy. Wasting of muscles in the shoulder is easily seen because bony prominences stand out even further. Wasting of hand muscles causes flattening of the thenar and hypothenar eminences. Wasting of the quadriceps muscles causes a tapering appearance to the thigh that is exaggerated when the patient is asked to tense the thigh by straightening the knee. Atrophy of the anterior tibial and peroneal muscles gives the anterior border of the tibia a sharp appearance, and atrophy of the gastrocnemius muscle diminishes the normal contour of the calf.

Individual muscles should be palpated for texture and tenderness when they are tested individually for strength. The texture of normal muscle is quite different from the flabby texture of denervated muscle and the rubbery consistency of dystrophic muscle infiltrated with collagen and fat. Tenderness generally suggests an inflammatory process.

Loss of tendon reflexes occurs early in denervation, especially when sensory nerves are involved, but tends to parallel the degree of weakness in myopathy. Tendon reflexes are usually normal even during times of weakness in patients with myasthenia gravis and may be normal between episodes of recurrent weakness in metabolic myopathies.

Myotonia, a disturbance in muscle relaxation following contraction, is described in the section on myotonic dystrophy.

 Progressive Proximal Weakness

Progressive proximal weakness in childhood is most often due to myopathy, usually a muscular dystrophy (Table 7–3). Juvenile spinal muscular atrophy is the only chronic denervating disease in which weakness is more proximal than distal. It is readily distinguished from myopathic disorders by electromyography (EMG) and muscle biopsy. Limb-girdle myasthenia is rare but is an important consideration because specific treatment is available (Table 7–4).

SPINAL MUSCULAR ATROPHIES

The juvenile form of spinal muscular atrophy was initially thought to be genetically distinct from infantile spinal muscular atrophy (see Chapter 6). However, despite considerable phenotypic heterogeneity, most cases of infantile and juvenile spinal muscular atrophy are caused

■ TABLE 7-4
Distinguishing Features in Proximal Weakness

	NEURONOPATHY	MYOPATHY	MYASTHENIA
Tendon reflexes	Absent	Depressed or absent	Normal
Electromyography	Fasciculations; denervation potentials; high-amplitude, polyphasic motor units	Brief, small-amplitude, polyphasic motor units	Normal
Nerve conduction studies	Normal or mildly slow	Normal	Abnormal repetitive stimulation
Creatine kinase concentration	Normal or mildly elevated	Elevated	Normal
Muscle biopsy	Group atrophy; group typing	Fiber necrosis, fatty replacement; excessive collagen	Normal

by defects on chromosome 5 (Gilliam et al, 1990; Munsat et al, 1990). The only genetic distinction possible at this time is between an autosomal recessive and an autosomal dominant form of juvenile spinal muscular atrophy.

The prevalence of juvenile spinal muscular atrophy is estimated at 1.2 per 100,000 general population (Emery, 1991) but is higher in some inbred populations. Almost all cases are the autosomal recessive type.

Autosomal Recessive Type

Fetal movements are normal and the child is normal at birth. Three subtypes of spinal muscular atrophy (SMA) are distinguished by age at onset. The severe type (SMA I) begins before 6 months of age and is described in Chapter 6. A mild type (SMA III) begins after 18 months and an intermediate type (SMA II) begins between 7 and 18 months. The age at onset does not consistently predict the degree of eventual disability, and outcome should not be predicted at the time of initial diagnosis.

CLINICAL FEATURES. The initial feature of SMA II is delayed motor development, and affected children do not usually stand alone. The initial feature of SMA III is gait instability caused by proximal weakness. Calf hypertrophy may occur and suggests the erroneous diagnosis of Duchenne muscular dystrophy. Disease progression is very slow, sometimes in a stepwise fashion, and often seems arrested. The progression of weakness may be either to the distal muscles of the legs or to the proximal muscles of the arms. The hands are affected last. Facial muscles may be weak, but extraocular motility is always spared. Cases with ophthalmoplegia are probably genetically distinct. Tendon reflexes of weak muscles are absent or greatly diminished.

An exaggerated physiologic tremor of the hands, of unknown cause, is sometimes associated. Some children have more profound weakness of the arms than the legs, and are likely to have facial weakness as well. Within a family, some children may have predominant leg weakness, whereas their siblings have predominant arm weakness. The pattern of progression in other family members is a clue to prognosis but cannot predict the future with assurance in a specific patient.

DIAGNOSIS. The serum concentration of creatine kinase may be 2 to 4 times the upper limit of normal and the increase in concentration correlates directly with the duration of illness. Needle EMG is the most useful investigation. Spontaneous discharges (fasciculations, fibrillations, and positive sharp waves) are seen in half of patients. With exertion, motor unit potentials are consistently of large amplitude and often polyphasic, prolonged in duration, and reduced in number. Sensory nerve conduction is always normal, but motor nerve conduction velocity is occasionally prolonged late in the course.

Muscle biopsy reveals a pattern of denervation similar to that observed in the infantile form (SMA type I) described in Chapter 6. Groups of atrophic fibers are adjacent to groups of fibers that are normal in size or hypertrophied. Hypertrophied fibers are always type I. Myopathic changes may be seen in children with chronic denervation. Because of sampling error, occasional biopsy specimens show only myopathic features. Therefore, confirmation by muscle biopsy is not essential if the EMG results are clearly consistent with spinal muscular atrophy.

TREATMENT. Proper management of spinal muscular atrophy in children increases longevity and decreases disability. The goals are to maintain function and prevent contractures. Children who quickly take to a wheelchair develop disuse atrophy. Dietary counseling is usually needed to prevent obesity, which only increases the strain on weak muscles. The prevention of contractures usually requires range of motion exercise and the early use of splints, especially at night.

Families need genetic counseling. Antenatal diagnosis and tests to detect the carrier state are not yet available.

Autosomal Dominant Type

The gene for the autosomal dominant type does not link to chromosome 5. A juvenile-onset type and an adult-onset type were thought to be genetically distinct but are probably not; variability in age of onset from childhood to adult life occurs within families. The onset of weakness is before age 10 years in most children, but some have mild joint contractures at birth (Frijns et al, 1994). A new dominant mutation would be difficult to distinguish from the autosomal recessive form.

CLINICAL FEATURES. The pattern of weakness in the autosomal dominant type is somewhat more generalized than in the autosomal recessive type, but proximal muscles are still affected more severely than distal muscles. Symptoms progress slowly, and some patients report no worsening of weakness after adolescence. Most patients walk and function well into middle and late adult life. Bulbar weakness is unusual and is mild when present. Extraocular muscles are not affected. Tendon reflexes are depressed or absent in weak muscles. Joint contractures are uncommon.

DIAGNOSIS. The serum concentration of creatine kinase is normal or only mildly elevated. The EMG is the basis for diagnosis, as in the autosomal recessive type. Muscle biopsy provides further confirmation of diagnosis.

TREATMENT. Treatment for the dominant type is the same as for the recessive type. Genetic counseling should stress the complete penetrance of the phenotype. Antenatal diagnosis is not available. When the family has no history of spinal muscular atrophy, genetic counseling is difficult, but autosomal dominant inheritance should be considered if the onset is after 3 years of age.

GM$_2$ Gangliosidosis

The typical clinical expression of *hexosaminidase A deficiency* is Tay-Sachs disease (see Chapter 5). Several phenotypic variants of the enzyme deficiency with onset throughout childhood and adult life are described. All are transmitted by autosomal recessive inheritance. Most patients are of Ashkenazi Jewish origin. The initial features of the juvenile-onset type mimic juvenile spinal muscular atrophy.

CLINICAL FEATURES. Weakness, wasting, and cramps of the proximal leg muscles begin after infancy and frequently not until adolescence. These are followed by distal leg weakness, proximal and distal arm weakness, and tremor. Symptoms of cerebral degeneration (personality change, intermittent psychosis, dementia) become evident after motor neuron dysfunction is established.

Examination shows a mixture of upper and lower motor neuron signs. The macula is usually normal and the cranial nerves are intact, with the exception of atrophy and fasciculations in the tongue. Fasciculations also may be present in the limbs. Tendon reflexes are absent or exaggerated, depending on the relative severity of upper and lower motor neuron dysfunction. Plantar responses are sometimes extensor and sometimes flexor. Tremor, but not dysmetria, is present in the outstretched arms, and sensation is intact.

Some children never develop cerebral symptoms and only have motor neuron disease; some adults have only dementia and psychosis. The course is variable and compatible with prolonged survival.

DIAGNOSIS. The serum concentration of creatine kinase is normal or only mildly elevated. Motor and sensory nerve conduction velocities are normal, but needle EMG shows neuropathic motor units. The diagnosis is established by showing a severe deficiency or absence of hexosaminidase A activity in leukocytes or cultured fibroblasts.

TREATMENT. No treatment is available. Heterozygote detection is possible because enzyme activity is partially deficient. Prenatal diagnosis is available.

MYASTHENIC SYNDROMES

Proximal weakness and sometimes wasting may occur in acquired immune-mediated myasthenia and in a genetic myasthenic syndrome.

Limb-Girdle Myasthenia

Immune-mediated myasthenia gravis that begins as progressive proximal weakness of the limbs and spares ocular motility is called *limb-girdle myasthenia* (Oh and Kuruoglu, 1992).

CLINICAL FEATURES. Onset is after 10 years of age, and girls are more often affected than boys. Weakness does not fluctuate with exercise. Muscles of facial expression may be affected, but other bulbar function is spared. Tendon reflexes are usually present but may be hypoactive. The clinical features suggest limb-girdle dystrophy or polymyositis.

DIAGNOSIS. Limb-girdle myasthenia should be suspected in every child with proximal weakness and preserved tendon reflexes. Repetitive nerve stimulation shows a decremental response and the serum concentration of antibodies that bind the acetylcholine receptor is increased.

Families with limb-girdle myasthenia affecting two or more siblings have been reported in the past but none in recent years. Some of these families may have had the slow-channel syndrome or another genetic myasthenia.

TREATMENT. The treatment is the same as for other forms of antibody-positive myasthenia (see Chapter 15).

Slow-Channel Syndrome

The slow-channel syndrome is an inherited disorder of the ion channel of the skeletal muscle acetylcholine receptor (Gomez and Gammack, 1995). It is transmitted by autosomal dominant inheritance. Some individuals have EMG evidence of disease without clinical symptoms.

CLINICAL FEATURES. No symptoms are present at birth. Onset is usually during infancy but can be delayed until adult life. Weakness of the cervical and scapular muscles is often the initial feature. Other common features are exercise intolerance, ophthalmoparesis, and muscle atrophy. Ptosis, bulbar dysfunction, and leg weakness are unusual. The syndrome progresses slowly, and many patients do not come to medical attention until after the first decade.

DIAGNOSIS. Weakness does not respond either to injection or to oral administration of anticholinesterase medication. Two patients were hypersensitive to edrophonium (Tensilon) and responded with muscarinic side effects. Repetitive nerve stimulation at 3 stimuli per second causes an abnormal decremental response and single-nerve stimulation causes a repetitive muscle potential. Muscle biopsy shows type I fiber predominance. Group atrophy, tubular aggregates, and an abnormal endplate configuration are present in some specimens.

TREATMENT. No treatment is available.

MUSCULAR DYSTROPHIES

The dystrophies are a group of genetic myopathies that are usually caused by defects in structural proteins. Enzyme deficiencies, such as acid maltase deficiency, are not classified as dystrophies. The abnormal gene product is known for Duchenne and Becker muscular dystrophies and severe childhood autosomal recessive muscular dystrophy, but not for facioscapulohumeral dystrophy, myotonic dystrophy, or most forms of limb-girdle dystrophy.

Bethlem Myopathy

Bethlem myopathy is a benign muscular dystrophy transmitted by autosomal dominant inheritance (Merlini et al, 1994).

CLINICAL FEATURES. The onset of pelvic weakness is in infancy or early childhood but is often so mild that families are unaware of abnormality. The weakness progresses slowly and usually does not produce disability or shorten life span. Flexion contractures form early in the elbows, ankles, and interphalangeal joints of the last four fingers, but spare the spine. Shortening of the Achilles tendon causes toe-walking. Tendon reflexes are normal or depressed. Cardiomyopathy does not occur.

DIAGNOSIS. The serum concentration of creatine kinase is normal or slightly elevated, EMG is usually myopathic, and muscle biopsy shows a nonspecific myopathy.

TREATMENT. Physical therapy for contractures is the only treatment available.

Duchenne and Becker Muscular Dystrophies

Duchenne and Becker muscular dystrophies are variable phenotypic expressions of a gene defect at the Xp21 site. Several different phenotypes are associated with abnormalities at the Xp21 site (Table 7-5). The abnormal gene product in both Duchenne and Becker muscular dystrophies is a reduced muscle content of the structural protein *dystrophin.* In Duchenne muscular dystrophy, the dystrophin content is less than 3% of normal, whereas in Becker muscular dystrophy, the dystrophin content is 3% to 20% of normal (Hoffman and Wang, 1993). Duchenne dystrophy has a worldwide distribution, with a mean incidence of 1 per 3,500 male births

■ TABLE 7-5
Phenotypes Associated with the Xp21 Gene Site

Becker muscular dystrophy
Duchenne muscular dystrophy
Familial X-linked myalgia and cramps (see Chapter 8)
McLeod syndrome (elevated serum creatine kinase
  concentration, acanthocytosis, and absence of Kell
  antigen)
Quadriceps myopathy

(Emery, 1991). The phenotypic difference between the two dystrophies is that the Becker form has a later age of onset (after age 5), unassisted ambulation after age 15, and survival into adult life. The mildest form is *quadriceps myopathy,* characterized by slowly progressive weakness of the quadriceps muscle, calf enlargement, and an elevated serum concentrations of creatine kinase (Sunohara et al, 1990).

CLINICAL FEATURES. The initial feature in most boys with Duchenne muscular dystrophy is a gait disturbance; onset is always before age 5 and is often before age 3. Toe-walking and frequent falling are typical complaints. A history of delayed achievement of motor milestones is often recalled in retrospect. Early symptoms are insidious and likely to be dismissed by both parents and physicians. Children may not be brought to medical attention until proximal weakness is sufficiently severe to cause difficulty in rising from the floor and an obvious waddling gait. At this stage, mild proximal weakness is present in the pelvic muscles and the Gower sign (Figure 7-1) is present. The calf muscles are large and feel rubbery (Figure 7-2). The ankle tendon is shortened, and the heels do not quite touch the floor. Tendon reflexes may still be present at the ankle and knee, but are difficult to obtain.

The decline in motor strength is linear throughout childhood. Motor function usually appears static between the ages of 3 and 6 years because of cerebral maturation. Most maintain their ability to walk and climb stairs until 8 years of age. Between ages 3 and 8 the child shows progressive contracture of the ankle tendon and the iliotibial band, increased lordosis, a more pronounced waddling gait, and increased toe-walking. Gait is more precarious, and the child falls more often. Tendon reflexes at the knees and ankles are lost, and proximal weakness develops in the arms.

Considerable variability of expression occurs even within the Duchenne phenotype (Brooke

□ FIGURE 7-2 Enlarged calf muscles in Duchenne muscular dystrophy. Enlarged calves may be seen in other neuromuscular disorders.

et al, 1989). On average, functional ability declines rapidly after 8 years of age because of increasing muscle weakness and contractures. By 9 years of age, some children require a wheelchair, but most can remain ambulatory until age 12 and may continue to stand in braces until age 16.

Scoliosis occurs in some boys and is not caused by early use of a wheelchair. Deterioration of vital capacity to less than 20% of normal leads to symptoms of nocturnal hypoventilation. The child awakens frequently and is afraid of sleep.

The immediate cause of death is not always clear, but respiratory insufficiency is a contributing factor in almost every case. Arrhythmia caused by cardiomyopathy can be documented in some boys. In others with chronic hypoxia, intercurrent infection or aspiration causes respiratory arrest.

DIAGNOSIS. Before 5 years of age the serum concentration of creatine kinase is 10 times the upper limit of normal. The concentration then declines with age at an approximate rate of 20% per year.

Mutation analysis using restriction fragment length polymorphism linkage studies is the standard for diagnosis, carrier detection, and fetal diagnosis. Intragenic deletions can be identified in 60% of affected boys, and duplications in another 6%. Dystrophin analysis is useful to distinguish Duchenne from Becker dystrophy.

TREATMENT. Although Duchenne muscular dystrophy is not curable, it is treatable. Prednisone, 0.75 mg/kg/day, increases strength and function (Fenichel et al, 1991). Treatment goals are to maintain function, prevent contractures, and provide psychological support not only for the child but also for the family. Every effort should be made to keep children standing and walking as long as possible. This is best accomplished by passive stretching exercises to prevent contractures, use of a lightweight plastic ankle-foot orthosis to maintain the foot in a neutral position during sleep, and the use of long-leg braces when walking becomes precarious. Scoliosis can not be prevented or reversed by external appliances; only surgery is effective to straighten the spine.

Facioscapulohumeral Syndrome

Progressive facioscapulohumeral (FSH) weakness was originally considered a muscular dystrophy. Later, similar patterns of weakness were described in spinal muscular atrophy and polymyositis. It is now recognized that patients with genetic FSH weakness may have histologic evidence of myopathy, neuropathy, and inflammation. Therefore, the term *facioscapulohumeral syndrome* is used to designate this entity that, although predominantly a dystrophy, has elements of denervation.

The gene responsible for FSH syndrome has been localized to chromosome 4q35 (Lee et al, 1995). The genetic abnormality has complete penetrance but variable expression.

CLINICAL FEATURES. Weakness usually begins in the second decade. Initial involvement is often in the shoulder girdle with subsequent spread to the face, but the reverse also occurs. The progression of weakness is insidious and diagnosis is often delayed. Family history of the syndrome may not be elicited because affected family members are unaware they have a problem. Patients eventually notice a change in facial expression. Late in the course, speech becomes indistinct and leg muscles are sometimes involved. Anterior tibial weakness is most prominent, but proximal weakness may occur as well. In patients with only minimal facial weakness,

the combination of proximal weakness in the arms and distal weakness in the legs may suggest a scapuloperoneal syndrome. FSH syndrome and scapuloperoneal syndrome are probably allelic disorders at the same gene locus (Jardine et al, 1994).

The course of FSH syndrome is variable. Many patients do not become disabled, and their life expectancy is normal. Others are confined to a wheelchair in adult life. In the infantile form, progression is always rapid and disability is always severe (see Chapter 17).

Retinal vascular abnormalities can be shown by angiography in the majority of people with FSH syndrome and should be considered part of the phenotype (Padberg et al, 1995). The most severe manifestations are retinal telangiectasia, exudation, and detachment *(Coates disease).* Hearing loss and mental retardation may also be present.

DIAGNOSIS. The serum concentration of creatine kinase can be normal or increased to 5 times normal. The EMG may show denervation potentials, myopathic motor units, or both. Histologic changes are minimal in many limb muscles; the supraspinatus muscle yields the highest abnormal return. Occasional fibers are noted undergoing degeneration, small angulated denervated fibers may be seen, and inflammatory cells may be present.

TREATMENT. No treatment for the weakness is available. The retina should be carefully examined for Coates disease. Retinal telangiectasia can be treated by coagulation to prevent blindness.

Limb-Girdle Dystrophy

The term *limb-girdle dystrophy* is used to describe proximal muscle weakness beginning in the second or third decade and progressing slowly to severe disability after 20 years. Both sexes are affected, and although the disease occurs sporadically, autosomal recessive inheritance is the rule. Limb-girdle muscular dystrophy is not a single entity, and at least six different genetic defects have been identified. A deficiency of *adhalin,* a component of the dystrophin-glycoprotein complex, is now established as one cause of autosomal recessive limb-girdle muscular dystrophy (Ljunggren et al, 1995).

CLINICAL FEATURES. Patients with slowly progressive symmetric proximal weakness, with or without facial involvement, and diminished or absent tendon reflexes should be considered to have limb-girdle dystrophy if other specific entities can be excluded. Either the pelvic or the shoulder girdle muscles can be affected first.

DIAGNOSIS. The most common problem in differential diagnosis is distinguishing limb-girdle dystrophy from Becker muscular dystrophy, and, indeed, many males in whom a limb-girdle dystrophy is diagnosed prove to have Becker muscular dystrophy when dystrophin is measured. The distinction between these dystrophies is important for accurate genetic counseling. In addition to Duchenne and Becker muscular dystrophies, conditions to be considered in the differential diagnosis include juvenile spinal muscular atrophy, glycogen storage myopathies, endocrine myopathies, polymyositis, and inclusion-body myositis.

The serum concentration of creatine kinase is elevated, but not to the extent seen in early Duchenne muscular dystrophy. The EMG findings are consistent with a myopathy. Muscle histologic findings vary with the stage of disease. The earliest changes are variation in fiber size and increase in internal nuclei. Later, fiber splitting and an uneven distribution of mitochondria produce a moth-eaten appearance when histochemical reagents for oxidative enzymes are applied. Both fiber types are affected equally (Figure 7-3).

TREATMENT. The treatment goals in limb-girdle muscular dystrophy are the same as those for Duchenne muscular dystrophy. The only difference is that contractures are not as serious a problem.

Severe Childhood Autosomal Recessive Muscular Dystrophy

Severe childhood autosomal recessive muscular dystrophy (SCARMD) is caused by deficiency of the 50-kd dystrophin associated glycoprotein (50DAG). This is one of the five glycoproteins attaching dystrophin to the sarcolemmal membrane (Matsumura and Campbell, 1994). The responsible gene is on chromosome 13q.

CLINICAL FEATURES. Both sexes are affected equally. The severity of disease is intermediate between Duchenne and Becker dystrophies. Proximal leg weakness begins between 5 and 10 years of age and calf hypertrophy is common. Some children are wheelchair confined by age 10. Death often results from cardiomyopathy.

DIAGNOSIS. SCARMD should be suspected in all girls with a Duchenne phenotype and in boys who appear to have Duchenne dystrophy but show normal dystrophin content in muscle.

□ F I G U R E   7 – 3 Moth-eaten appearance in limb-girdle dystrophy (DPNH reaction). The usual lace-like appearance of the mitochondria is replaced by mitochondrial clumping.

Serum creatine kinase concentration is 10 times the upper limit of normal.

TREATMENT. Management is the same as for Duchenne muscular dystrophy.

X-Linked Vacuolated Myopathy

This is a genetic disorder with an immune-mediated attack on the muscle fiber surface.

CLINICAL FEATURES. A slowly proximal leg weakness begins during childhood but does not become clinically apparent until adolescence. Disability does not occur until middle adult life. Tendon reflexes are depressed or absent.

DIAGNOSIS. The serum concentration of creatine kinase is normal. EMG findings are consistent with myopathy. Muscle biopsy findings show an increased variation in fiber size and increased interstitial connective tissue. Up to 50% of the fibers contain vacuoles that sometimes show intense reactivity for acid phosphatase. All fibers show sarcolemmal immunolabeling with anti-major histocompatibility complex I, suggesting that the membrane attack complex is part of the pathogenesis of muscle degeneration.

TREATMENT. No treatment is available and none is needed during childhood.

INFLAMMATORY MYOPATHIES

The inflammatory myopathies are a heterogeneous group of disorders whose causes are infectious or immune mediated, or both. A progressive proximal myopathy occurs in adults, but not in children, with acquired immune deficiency syndrome (AIDS). However, the concentration of serum creatine kinase is elevated in children with AIDS treated with zidovudine (Walter et al, 1991). Acute infectious myositis is described in the section on acute generalized weakness. The conditions discussed in this section are considered idiopathic.

Dermatomyositis

Dermatomyositis is a systemic angiopathy in which vascular occlusion and infarction account for all pathologic changes observed in muscle, connective tissue, skin, gastrointestinal tract, and small nerves. More than 30% of adults with dermatomyositis have an underlying malignancy, but cancer is not a factor before the age of 16 (Sigurgeirsson et al, 1992). The childhood form of dermatomyositis is a relatively homogeneous disease.

CLINICAL FEATURES. Peak incidence is generally between the ages of 5 and 10 years, but an onset as early as 4 months has been reported. The initial features may be insidious or fulminating. An insidious onset is characterized by fever, fatigue, and anorexia in the absence of rash or weakness. These symptoms may persist for weeks or months and suggest an underlying infection. Dermatitis precedes myositis in most children. The characteristic rash is marked by an erythematous discoloration and edema of the upper eyelids that spread to involve the entire periorbital and malar regions. Erythema and edema of the extensor surfaces overlying the joints of the knuckles, elbows, and knees develop later. With time the skin appears atrophic and scaly.

The myopathy is characterized by proximal weakness, stiffness, and pain. Weakness becomes generalized and flexion contractures develop rapidly and cause joint deformities. Ten-

□ F I G U R E 7 – 4 Perifascicular atrophy in childhood dermatomyositis (trichrome stain). The muscle fibers at the edge of each fascicle are atrophied.

don reflexes become increasingly difficult to obtain and finally disappear.

Calcinosis of subcutaneous tissue, especially under discolored areas of skin, occurs in 60% of children. When severe, it produces an armor-like appearance, termed *calcinosis universalis,* on radiographs. In some children stiffness is the main initial feature and skin and muscle symptoms are only minor.

In the past, gastrointestinal tract infarction was a leading cause of death. The mortality rate has fallen to less than 5% with modern treatment.

DIAGNOSIS. The combination of fever, rash, myalgia, and weakness is compelling evidence for the diagnosis of dermatomyositis. The serum concentration of creatine kinase is usually elevated early in the course. During the time of active myositis, the resting EMG shows increased insertional activity, fibrillations, and positive sharp waves; muscle contraction produces brief, small-amplitude polyphasic potentials. The diagnostic feature on muscle biopsy is perifascicular atrophy (Figure 7-4). Capillary necrosis usually starts at the periphery of the muscle fascicle and causes ischemia in the adjacent muscle fibers. The most profound atrophy occurs in fascicular borders that face large connective tissue septa. Type I and type II fibers are affected equally.

TREATMENT. The inflammatory process is thought to be active for approximately 2 years. Corticosteroids may suppress the inflammatory response and provide symptomatic relief but do not cure the underlying disease. The best results are obtained when corticosteroids are started early in high doses and are maintained for long periods of time.

Prednisone is initiated in a dosage of 2 mg/kg/day, not to exceed 100 mg/day. The response follows a predictable pattern. Temperature returns to normal within 48 hours. Serum concentrations of creatine kinase returns to normal by the second week, and muscle strength increases simultaneously. When these occur, prednisone should be given on alternate days in the same dosage to reduce the frequency and severity of corticosteroid-induced side effects. Alternate-day and every-day therapy are equally effective if the doses are large and the treatment is maintained. As muscle strength increases, the original dosage of alternate-day prednisone is tapered by 10% per month for 5 months. Further reductions are then at a rate of 5% per month. For most children the alternate-day maintenance dosage needed for normal muscle strength and normal serum concentrations of creatine kinase is 25% of the starting dosage. The response of the skin rash to prednisone is variable: in some children the rash heals completely, but most will have some permanent scarring from the disease.

Although most children show a dramatic improvement and seem normal in 3 months, prednisone must be continued for a full 2 years. If treatment is discontinued prematurely, relapse is invariable. Calcinosis and contractures are more likely to develop in children treated intermittently. Corticosteroids also are useful in the treatment of calcinosis universalis. In addition to prednisone, a well-structured program of physical therapy is needed to prevent contractures.

Eighty percent of children with dermatomyositis have a favorable outcome if high-dose prednisone is started within 4 months of the onset of symptoms. Children who do not respond immediately to high-dose prednisone should be started on oral methotrexate, 10 to 20 mg/m^2, given twice weekly. Regular monitoring of liver function and white blood cell count is required.

Plasmapheresis or courses of intravenous immunoglobulin may be used in children whose condition is refractory to corticosteroids or to reduce dosage when adverse side effects limit therapy. (Sansome and Dubowitz, 1995).

Once the disease becomes inactive, reactivation is unlikely. However, late progression or recurrence may occur and should be treated with an additional 1-year course of corticosteroids.

Polymyositis

Polymyositis without evidence of other target organ involvement is uncommon before puberty. Children with systemic lupus erythematosus may have myalgia and arthralgia as early symptoms, but generally do not have muscle weakness at onset. Skin, joint, and systemic manifestations are usually well established before the onset of myopathy. Polymyositis in children is similar to the disorder in adult life except that malignancy is not usually a causative factor (Sherry et al, 1993).

CLINICAL FEATURES. Polymyositis begins as a symmetric proximal weakness that develops insidiously and progresses to moderate handicap within weeks to months. The patient may have prolonged periods of stability or even remission that suggest the diagnosis of limb-girdle muscular dystrophy because of the slow progress. Tendon reflexes are present early in the course and become hypoactive as muscle bulk is lost. Cardiorespiratory complications are less common in childhood than in adult polymyositis.

DIAGNOSIS. The serum concentration of creatine kinase is not invariably elevated, but EMG almost always shows abnormalities that typically show both myopathic and neuropathic features. Muscle biopsy may show several different patterns of abnormality, and perivascular inflammation may not be present. Instead, features of myopathy, denervation, or both may be observed.

TREATMENT. The same treatment schedule suggested for childhood dermatomyositis should be used for children with polymyositis. Unfortunately, the response to corticosteroids is far less predictable in polymyositis than in dermatomyositis. Children who do not respond to corticosteroids should be treated with methotrexate. Plasmapheresis and intravenous immunoglobulins are reasonable alternatives when other remedies fail.

Inclusion Body Myositis

Inclusion body myositis is an insidiously progressive myopathy with characteristic clinical and histologic features. The onset ordinarily occurs after 50 years of age, but childhood onset is recognized as well (Riggs et al, 1989). Mitochondrial DNA deletions have been identified in three adult cases and may be involved in the pathogenesis of the disorder (Oldfors et al, 1993).

CLINICAL FEATURES. Males are affected more often than females. Painless weakness occurs first in the proximal muscles of the pelvis. The progression of weakness is slow. The biceps and triceps muscles are affected next, but the interval between leg and arm weakness may be as long as 10 years. Facial weakness may occur. Dysphagia, fatigue, myalgia, and paresthesias may occur later in the course. Tendon reflexes are either reduced or absent.

DIAGNOSIS. The serum concentration of creatine kinase is normal or only mildly elevated. EMG shows abnormal spontaneous electrical activity: increased insertion activity and fibrillations. Short-duration motor units and polyphasic potentials are the rule, but long-duration motor units are also observed. Motor and sensory conduction velocities are normal unless a concomitant neuropathy is present.

Light microscopy characteristically shows muscle fibers with single or multiple vacuoles rimmed with basophilic material, predominantly endomysial mononuclear inflammatory cells in necrotic or non-necrotic fibers, and atrophic fibers. Electron microscopy demonstrates filamentous inclusions, usually adjacent to vacuoles.

THERAPY. The weakness seldom responds to corticosteroid or immunosuppressive therapy. Progressive debilitation results in death from cardiac or respiratory failure.

METABOLIC MYOPATHIES

Acid Maltase Deficiency

The initial features of acid maltase deficiency may occur in infancy, childhood, or adult life. The enzyme defect appears to be the same regardless of the age of onset, and different ages of onset may occur within the same family. Why the age at onset varies so widely is unknown. The abnormal gene is on chromosome 17 and is transmitted by autosomal recessive inheritance.

CLINICAL FEATURES. Infants with acid maltase deficiency have glycogen storage in both skeletal and cardiac muscle. Death occurs from cardiac failure during infancy (see Chapter 6).

In the childhood form, only skeletal muscle is involved and the main clinical feature is slowly progressive proximal limb weakness. Tendon reflexes are hypoactive or unobtainable. Some children have mild hypertrophy of the calves simulating Duchenne muscular dystrophy. The weakness progresses steadily leading to disability and respiratory insufficiency by 20 years of age. The later the onset of symptoms, the longer and more benign the course.

DIAGNOSIS. The diagnosis of acid maltase deficiency is established by showing glycogen storage in muscle fibers and the absence of acid maltase in muscle or fibroblasts.

TREATMENT. No treatment is available.

Other Carbohydrate Myopathies

Slowly progressive proximal weakness is sometimes the initial features of McArdle disease and debrancher enzyme deficiency. Both disorders must at least be considered in the differential diagnosis. The initial symptoms of these disorders is usually exercise intolerance, and for this reason they are discussed in Chapter 8.

Muscle Carnitine Deficiency

Carnitine is an essential cofactor in the transfer of long-chain fatty acids across the inner mitochondrial membrane and modulates the ratio of acyl to acylcoenzyme A (Breningstall, 1990). Its deficiency causes a failure in the production of energy for metabolism and the storage of triglycerides. It occurs (1) in newborns receiving total parenteral alimentation, (2) in several systemic disorders (see Table 2-6), (3) as the result of several genetic disorders of organic acid metabolism, (4) in children treated with valproate, (5) and as a primary genetic defect that causes deficiency of the cellular carnitine transporter (DeVivo and Tein, 1990).

The primary genetic defect is transmitted by autosomal recessive inheritance. The clinical features may be restricted to skeletal muscle or may include systemic symptoms resembling Reye syndrome (see Chapter 2).

CLINICAL FEATURES. The main clinical feature of muscle carnitine deficiency is the childhood onset of progressive proximal weakness, affecting the legs before and more severely than the arms. Occasional patients have recurrent attacks of myoglobinuria and cardiomyopathy. The cardiomyopathy is usually asymptomatic but is recognized on electrocardiography (ECG) and echocardiography.

DIAGNOSIS. The serum concentration of creatine kinase is elevated. EMG findings may suggest a neuropathic process early in the course and later indicate a myopathy. Muscle biopsy specimens show a vacuolar myopathy with lipid storage mainly in type I fibers and a reduced carnitine content.

TREATMENT. Dietary therapy with L-carnitine is effective and safe. Diarrhea is the major side effect. The usual dosage is 100 mg/kg/day in three or four divided doses.

Other Lipid Myopathies

Children with progressive proximal weakness associated with lipid storage in muscle and a normal carnitine content usually have a disturbance of mitochondrial fatty acid oxidation. These disorders are genetically heterogeneous and difficult to distinguish from other mitochondrial myopathies.

CLINICAL FEATURES. Progressive proximal weakness begins anytime from early childhood to adolescence. The legs are affected first and then the arms. Exercise intolerance is noted, and in some cases the ingestion of fatty foods leads to nausea and vomiting. The pattern and progression of weakness may simulate Duchenne muscular dystrophy even to the presence of calf hypertrophy. Limb weakness is steadily progressive, and cardiomyopathy may develop.

DIAGNOSIS. The serum concentration of creatine kinase is markedly elevated. EMG findings are abnormal and consistent with a myopathic process. Muscle biopsy is critical to diagnosis. Type I muscle fibers contain fatty droplets. Carnitine and carnitine palmitoyl transferase levels are normal.

TREATMENT. Patients with fat intolerance may show improvement on a diet free of long-chain fatty acids.

ENDOCRINE MYOPATHIES

Progressive proximal limb weakness may occur in children with hyperthyroidism, hypothyroidism, hyperparathyroidism, hypoparathyroidism, hyperadrenalism, and hypoadrenalism.

CLINICAL FEATURES. Systemic features of endocrine disease usually predate the onset of weakness. However, weakness may be the initial feature in primary or secondary hypoparathyroidism and in thyroid disorders. Weakness is much more prominent in the legs than the arms. Tendon reflexes, even in weak muscles, are normal or diminished but generally are not absent.

DIAGNOSIS. The serum concentration of creatine kinase is typically normal. EMG is not useful for diagnosis; it may show normal results, myopathy, or neuropathy. Many endocrinopathies produce both neuropathy and myopathy. In Cushing disease and in hyperparathyroidism, muscle histologic studies show type II fiber atrophy. Other endocrinopathies show nonspecific myopathic changes that vary with the severity of disease.

TREATMENT. In all endocrine myopathies, weakness is reversed by treating the underlying endocrinopathy.

Progressive Distal Weakness

Progressive distal weakness in childhood is most often due to neuropathy (Table 7-6). Among the slowly progressive neuropathies of childhood, hereditary disorders are far more common than acquired disorders. The only common acquired neuropathy is acute inflammatory demyelinating polyradiculoneuropathy (Guillain-Barré syndrome), in which weakness evolves rapidly.

DIAGNOSIS IN NEUROPATHY

The typical initial features of neuropathy in children is progressive symmetric distal weakness affecting the legs and then the arms. When sensation is disturbed, dysesthesias consisting of tingling, "pins and needles," or burning sensations of the feet are felt. Dysesthesias usually occur in acquired neuropathies but not in hereditary neuropathies. The weakness and sensory loss move from distal to proximal in a glove-and-stocking distribution. Tendon reflexes are lost early in the course of disease, especially when sensory fibers are affected.

An important first step in diagnosis is to determine the primary site of the disorder: cell body (anterior horn cell), nerve axon, or myelin. This is accomplished by electrodiagnosis (Table 7-7). In primary disorders of the cell body

■ T A B L E   7 – 6
Progressive Distal Weakness [Gene Location]

Spinal Cord Disorders (see Chapter 12)
Motor Neuron Diseases
Juvenile amyotrophic lateral sclerosis
Spinal muscular atrophies
  Autosomal recessive forms
  Autosomal dominant forms
  Nonfamilial Asian (see Chapter 13)
Neuropathies
Hereditary motor sensory neuropathies
  Charcot-Marie-Tooth syndrome type 1 [17p; 1q; X]
  Charcot-Marie-Tooth syndrome type 2 [1p]
  Déjérine-Sottas disease [17p11]
  Refsum disease
Other genetic neuropathies
  Familial amyloid neuropathy (see Chapter 9)
  Giant axonal neuropathy
  Pyruvate dehydrogenase deficiency (see Chapter 10)
  Sulfatide lipidoses: metachromatic leukodystrophy
  Other leukodystrophies
Neuropathies with systemic diseases
  Drug-induced
  Systemic vasculitis
  Toxins
  Uremia
Idiopathic neuropathy
  Chronic axonal neuropathy
  Chronic demyelinating neuropathy
Myopathies
Autosomal dominant infantile myopathy
Autosomal dominant childhood myopathy [17p11]
Autosomal recessive distal (Miyoshi) myopathy
  [2p12-14]
Myotonic dystrophy [19q13]
Scapulo (Humeral) Peroneal Syndrome
Emery-Dreifuss syndrome [Xq28]
Scapulohumeral syndrome with dementia
Scapuloperoneal neuronopathy

(neuronopathy) fibrillations and fasciculations are seen in resting muscle. With voluntary contraction the number of motor unit potentials is reduced but the amplitude is normal or increased because of collateral reinnervation. Motor conduction nerve velocity is normal or only slightly diminished, and the amplitude of sensory action potentials is normal. In axonopathies the EMG shows fibrillations at rest and a reduced number of motor unit potentials that are normal or increased in amplitude. High-amplitude potentials may be polyphasic. Motor nerve conduction velocity is normal or mildly reduced, and the amplitude of sensory action potentials may also be reduced. Demyelinating neuropathies are characterized by marked slowing of motor conduction velocity and reduced amplitude of sensory evoked potentials. EMG findings may be normal early in the course.

JUVENILE AMYOTROPHIC LATERAL SCLEROSIS

This term *juvenile amyotrophic lateral sclerosis* describes a group of rare hereditary diseases characterized by some combination of upper and lower motor neuron dysfunction (Hamida et al, 1990). Genetic transmission may be by autosomal recessive or dominant inheritance. Onset usually occurs in the second decade, and progression is slow. The clinical features are some combination of spastic paraplegia and wasting of the hands or peroneal atrophy. Bulbar and pseudobulbar palsy may also be present. Clinical overlap exists between these conditions, the hereditary spinal muscular atrophies, and familial spastic paraplegia (see Chapter 12). Many of the hereditary motor neuron diseases may prove to have a similar genetic defect or abnormal gene product.

SPINAL MUSCULAR ATROPHY

The distal form of spinal muscular atrophy is genetically heterogeneous. Sometimes the disease is segmental (*juvenile progressive segmental spinal muscular atrophy*) and affects only the hands or only the feet. The trait may be transmitted by autosomal dominant or recessive inheritance. The dominant form is not linked to the spinal muscular atrophy locus on chromosome 5q11. Severe and mild forms exist for each type of inheritance.

CLINICAL FEATURES. These disorders usually begin with weakness and wasting in the anterior compartment of the legs associated with pes cavus deformities of the feet. Tendon reflexes may be preserved. The clinical picture can be indistinguishable from hereditary motor sensory neuropathy type I except that sensation is normal. In one family with dominantly inherited disease, the weakness began in the plantar flexors so that the first symptom was inability to stand on the toes (Boylan et al, 1995).

In the severe autosomal recessive form, weakness progresses to involve the proximal muscles of the legs and sometimes the hands. Weakness in the arms varies among families but shows concordance within an individual family. However, one family, in which transmission was by autosomal dominant inheritance, included a

■ TABLE 7–7
Electrodiagnosis in Neuropathy

	NEURONOPATHY	AXONAL	DEMYELINATING
Fasciculations	+++	+++	+
Denervation potentials	+++	+++	+
Reduced number of motor units	+++	+++	0
High-amplitude potentials	+++	+++	0
Slow motor velocity	0	+	+++
Reduced sensory potentials	0	+	+++

0, absent; +, rare; +++, common.

female infant with an acute fulminating disease, whereas her father and uncles had late onset hand weakness (Boylan and Cornblath, 1992). Approximately 25% of patients have scoliosis. Calf atrophy or hypertrophy may be present, even among members of the same family (Groen et al, 1993).

Juvenile segmental spinal muscular atrophy is primarily a disorder of teenage males, probably transmitted by autosomal recessive inheritance (Liu and Specht, 1993; Tandan et al, 1990). Atrophy of the hands, often asymmetric, progresses for 2 to 4 years, and sometimes involves the forearms. Fasciculations and cramps are common. The atrophy usually arrests but may progress to involve the legs and can be associated with hyperreflexia. Progressive atrophy with hyperreflexia in the legs suggests a link between juvenile segmental spinal muscular atrophy and familial amyotrophic lateral sclerosis.

DIAGNOSIS. Electrodiagnosis is critical to distinguish these disorders from peripheral neuropathies. Motor nerve conduction velocity is normal despite total denervation of the small muscles of the foot. Sensory evoked potentials are also normal. The serum concentration of creatine kinase is usually normal but may be mildly elevated. Muscle biopsy specimens show nonspecific changes of denervation, and the sural nerve is normal.

TREATMENT. No treatment is available, nor is there a method for antenatal diagnosis.

HEREDITARY MOTOR AND SENSORY NEUROPATHY

The term *hereditary motor and sensory neuropathy* (HMSN) encompasses several genetic neuropathies. The likelihood of identifying a genetic basis for an "idiopathic polyneuropathy" is increased when detailed family histories are taken and other family members are examined.

The *Charcot-Marie-Tooth* (CMT) phenotype, in which peroneal atrophy is the characteristic feature, is the prototype HMSN. It may be primarily a demyelinating (HMSN I or CMT1) or an axonal (HMSN II or CMT2) neuropathy (Chance and Pleasure, 1993). HMSN I and HMSN II are clinically distinguished by nerve conduction velocity studies. HMSN I is twice as common as HMSN II. As a group, the incidence of HMSN is estimated to be 10 per 100,000 population (Emery, 1991).

Hereditary Motor and Sensory Neuropathy Type I: Demyelinating Type

HMSN I is further divided into those cases with a DNA duplication on chromosome 17p (HMSN IA) and those in which the abnormal gene is mapped to chromosome 1q (HMSN IB). The 17p duplication accounts for more than 95% of cases and causes trisomic expression of the myelin protein, PMP-22 (Harding, 1995). Deletion in the 17p region with monosomic expression of PMP-22 causes hereditary polyneuropathy with liability to pressure palsies (see Chapter 13). Identical HMSN I syndromes are also transmitted by X-linked inheritance (HMSN IX) and on an unidentified autosome (HMSN IC).

CLINICAL FEATURES. The initial symptoms are either foot deformities or gait disturbances, beginning usually in the second decade or later but sometimes in early infancy (Feasby et al, 1992). Dysesthesias are never an early symptom, although some patients, because of foot deformity, may complain of pain from pressure by shoes. Pes cavus is typical, and hammer toes may be present. These deformities are caused by weakness of the intrinsic foot muscles and result in foreshortening of the foot and elevation of the arch. The initial gait disturbance is usually described as clumsiness, especially in running.

HMSN I is not usually a severe disorder in childhood. The main early features are pes cavus, weakness of the peroneal muscles, and diminished reactivity of the ankle tendon reflex. With time the anterior tibial, as well as the peroneal, muscles become weak, producing footdrop. The calf muscles become weak in some families, but calf hypertrophy may occur in some families with the 17p duplication (Uncini et al, 1994). Eventually, usually after 20 years of age, weakness spreads to the proximal muscles of the legs and the hands. Scoliosis is present in only a minority of patients. Cramps with exercise and fasciculations are present in weak muscles. Sensation is mildly impaired in the legs.

Peripheral nerves are enlarged in adults, but not in children. The enlargement is caused by repeated episodes of demyelination and remyelination.

DIAGNOSIS. Diagnosis relies on characteristic clinical findings and a family history of the disease. Motor nerve conduction velocities are less than 50% of normal in affected individuals. The cerebrospinal fluid protein content is usually normal in children, but may be elevated in adults. Muscle histologic appearance reveals nonspecific changes of denervation; myopathic changes may also be present in older individuals. "Onion bulb" formation is noted in peripheral nerves that have undergone repeated episodes of demyelination and remyelination but is not pathognomonic.

TREATMENT. No specific treatment is available, but proper foot care may minimize discomfort and maximize function. Shoes should be roomy and soft to prevent rubbing against bony prominences. Footwear that is molded to the shape of the foot is especially useful. When footdrop is present, a lightweight plastic ankle-foot orthosis that fits into the patient's own shoe not only lifts the foot but also prevents turning and injury of the ankle.

Hereditary Motor and Sensory Neuropathy Type II: Neuronal Type

HMSN II is transmitted by autosomal dominant inheritance and clinically resembles HMSN I, except that symptoms are considerably milder. Three forms are recognized: HMSN IIA, HMSN IIB, and HMSN IIC. Some families with HMSN II show linkage to markers on chromosome 1p, but none show linkage to the sites responsible for HMSN I (Othmane et al, 1993).

CLINICAL FEATURES. The peak age at onset of HMSN IIA and IIB is during the second decade.

Onset in early childhood may represent a genetically distinct form that is transmitted by autosomal recessive inheritance. Distal weakness begins in the legs and can be asymmetric. The hands are affected later. Tendon reflexes are generally absent at the ankle but may be preserved at the knee and elbow. Most children have mild distal sensory loss. In some children all modalities are affected; others experience loss of pain or vibration and position sense. Progression of symptoms is slow, and disability does not occur until middle adult life.

HMSN IIC is different from the other types because of prominent vocal cord and respiratory (intercostal and diaphragmatic) muscle paralysis (Dyck et al, 1994b). The onset is insidious and difficult to date precisely. The initial symptom may be hoarseness or frequent tripping, but neonatal respiratory disturbance also occurs. The course is one of progressive peroneal atrophy with minimal sensory deficit.

DIAGNOSIS. The cerebrospinal fluid protein content is normal as is the serum concentration of creatine kinase. Because the pathologic process is primarily axonal rather than demyelinating, motor nerve conduction velocities are either normal or only mildly slowed, 60% or more of normal. The EMG shows a denervation pattern in affected muscles.

TREATMENT. No specific treatment is available.

Hereditary Motor and Sensory Neuropathy Type III: Déjérine-Sottas Disease

HMSN III is a demyelinating and remyelinating neuropathy transmitted by autosomal recessive inheritance. Many cases are sporadic. Parenteral consanguinity is a factor in many families. The heterozygote parent is usually asymptomatic, but the same phenotype also occurs in children whose parents both have either HMSN I or HMSN II (Sghirlanzoni et al, 1992). Such cases suggest that HMSN III may be the homozygous expression of several different genetic neuropathies. Some infants with congenital hypomyelinating neuropathy (see Chapter 6) may actually have a severe form of the disease (Balestrini et al, 1991).

CLINICAL FEATURES. Slow motor development and hypotonia are common during the first year. Weakness begins distally in the limbs and progresses to involve the proximal muscles by the second decade. Distal sensory loss of all modalities is profound and sensory ataxia is always present. Tendon reflexes are absent. Peripheral nerves enlarge, and the great auricular, the median, and the ulnar nerves are often palpable.

Clubfoot and scoliosis are associated findings. Other features in some patients are miosis, sluggish pupillary responses to light, nystagmus, and choreiform movements of the fingers.

DIAGNOSIS. The cerebrospinal fluid protein content is generally elevated in proportion to the severity of weakness. Motor nerve conduction velocities are markedly prolonged, and sensory potentials are reduced in amplitude. Sural nerve biopsy shows massive interstitial hypertrophy and marked onion bulb formation.

TREATMENT. No treatment is available.

Hereditary Motor and Sensory Neuropathy Type IV: Refsum Disease

HMSN IV is an inborn error of phytanic acid metabolism reported mainly from Scandinavia, Great Britain, Germany, and France. Autosomal recessive transmission is suspected because of a high incidence of consanguinity in affected families and no evidence of disease in parents. In fibroblasts derived from homozygotes the rate of phytanic acid oxidation is 3% of that in control samples; in heterozygotes the rate is 50%.

CLINICAL FEATURES. The initial symptoms are insidious and difficult to date. Age at onset varies from the first to the third decades. The main features are retinitis pigmentosa, chronic or recurrent polyneuropathy, and cerebellar ataxia. Retinitis pigmentosa is a constant finding and is indispensable for diagnosis. Night blindness is often the first symptom. The neuropathy is hypertrophic, symmetric, and distal, affecting both motor and sensory fibers. Vibration and position sense are more diminished than are pain and temperature. Tendon reflexes become progressively hyporesponsive and are finally lost. The ataxia may be of cerebellar origin; nystagmus and intention tremor are sometimes present, but it could be caused by sensory neuropathy. Other symptoms include progressive loss of hearing, cataracts, cardiomyopathy, ichthyosis, and pes cavus.

The course is variable; there may be steady progression, long periods of stability, or remissions and exacerbations. Sudden death may occur from cardiac arrhythmia caused by cardiomyopathy.

DIAGNOSIS. The protein content of the cerebrospinal fluid is elevated to between 100 and 700 mg/dl (1 and 7 g/L). Motor and sensory nerve conduction velocities are markedly reduced. EMG results are consistent with denervation. Electroretinography shows a severe abnormality of the photoreceptors of the retina, involving both rods and cones. The diagnosis is established by showing reduced oxidation of phytanic acid in cultured fibroblasts. Antenatal diagnosis is accomplished by measuring phytanic acid oxidation in amniotic cells.

TREATMENT. Phytanic acid is not produced endogenously and must be derived completely from diet. Exacerbations of disease correlate well with blood levels of phytanic acid. Treatment is by a combination of diet and plasma exchange. This has proved successful in preventing progression of symptoms and in reversing symptoms already present.

OTHER GENETIC NEUROPATHIES

Giant Axonal Neuropathy

Giant axonal neuropathy is a rare disorder transmitted by autosomal recessive inheritance. It may be an inborn error of enzyme-linked sulfhydryl-containing enzymes. Both central and peripheral axons are affected.

CLINICAL FEATURES. Males and females are affected equally and 6 of 19 cases have been from consanguineous marriages (Donaghy et al, 1988). Affected children are pale and thin, and have curly scalp hair. Gait impairment usually begins by 3 years of age but can appear later. Symmetric distal atrophy of leg muscles is a constant early feature. Vibratory and proprioceptive sensations in the legs are profoundly impaired, and tendon reflexes are decreased or absent.

Central involvement may result in cerebellar dysfunction, dementia, optic atrophy, and cranial neuropathies.

DIAGNOSIS. Sural nerve biopsy shows enlarged axons filled with disrupted neurofilaments that are surrounded by a thin or fragmented myelin sheath. Large myelinated nerve fibers are mainly affected. Magnetic resonance imaging of the brain may show increased signal intensity of the white matter.

TREATMENT. No treatment is available.

Sulfatide Lipidosis: Metachromatic Leukodystrophy

Metachromatic leukodystrophy is an inherited disorder of myelin metabolism caused by deficient activity of the enzyme arylsulfatase A. The gene defect is transmitted by autosomal recessive inheritance. Three forms are recognized: late infantile, juvenile, and adult. The late infantile form is the most common. Juvenile- and adult-onset cases affect primarily the brain and are difficult to distinguish from each other (see Chapter 5). Metachromatic leukodystrophy is a disorder of central and peripheral myelin metabolism caused by deficient activity of the enzyme arylsulfatase A. The disease is transmitted by autosomal recessive inheritance. An infantile, juvenile, and adult form are recognized. Two groups of mutations in the gene encoding arylsulfatase A are identified as I and A. The I group generates no active enzyme and the A group generates small amounts. The late-infantile form is associated with an I-I genotype, and the later-onset forms with I-A or A-A genotypes (Kolodny and Fluharty, 1995). Heterozygosity and homozygosity of two alleles account for the different forms of the disease (Polten et al, 1991). Only the late infantile form is discussed in this section.

CLINICAL FEATURES. After a period of normal development, gait disturbances develop, usually by 2 years of age, but sometimes not until age 4. Initial examination shows distal weakness of the feet with loss of the ankle tendon reflex. Progressive weakness of all limbs results in generalized hypotonia and hyporeflexia. Cerebral demyelination follows causing dementia, spasticity, and blindness.

DIAGNOSIS. The protein content of the cerebrospinal fluid is elevated, and motor nerve conduction velocities are reduced at the time of initial leg weakness. The diagnosis is established by showing the absence of arylsulfatase A in white blood cells. Prenatal diagnosis is possible by analysis of arylsulfatase A in amniocytes.

TREATMENT. Bone marrow transplantation early in the course of disease may slow its progress (Krivit et al, 1990). No other treatment is available.

Other Leukodystrophies

Peripheral neuropathy occurs in *globoid cell leukodystrophy* (Krabbe disease), but it is not as prominent a feature as in metachromatic leukodystrophy. The usual initial features are psychomotor retardation and irritability rather than flaccid weakness (see Chapter 5). Tendon reflexes may be absent or hyperactive, and motor nerve conduction velocity is reduced in half of cases. Cerebrospinal fluid protein concentration is always elevated.

Cockayne syndrome is characterized by progeria, small stature, ataxia, retinitis pigmentosa, deafness, and mental retardation (see Chapter 16). A primary segmental demyelinating neuropathy is present in 10% to 20% of cases but is not an initial symptom. The main features are hyporeflexia and reduced motor nerve conduction velocity.

Other disorders of lipid metabolism in which demyelinating neuropathy is present, but not an important feature, include Niemann-Pick disease, Gaucher disease, and Farber disease.

NEUROPATHIES WITH SYSTEMIC DISEASE

Drug-Induced Neuropathy

Several drugs that are used widely in children, such as phenytoin, can cause neuropathy. Such neuropathies are usually subclinical, detected only by electrodiagnosis or because of loss of the ankle tendon reflex (Ouvrier et al, 1990a). Drugs that commonly produce clinical evidence of motor and sensory neuropathy are isoniazid, nitrofurantoin, vincristine, and zidovudine.

Isoniazid

CLINICAL FEATURES. The initial symptoms are numbness and paresthesias of the fingers and toes. If treatment is continued, superficial sensation is diminished in a glove-and-stocking pattern. Distal limb weakness follows and is associated with tenderness of the muscles and burning dysesthesias. The ankle tendon reflex is diminished or absent.

DIAGNOSIS. Isoniazid neuropathy should be suspected whenever a neuropathy develops in a child taking the drug.

TREATMENT. Isoniazid interferes with pyridoxine metabolism and produces neuropathy by causing a pyridoxine deficiency state. The administration of pyridoxine along with isoniazid prevents neuropathy without interfering with antituberculous activity. The longer that symptoms are allowed to progress, the longer the time until recovery. Although pyridoxine can prevent the development of neuropathy, it has little effect on the speed of recovery once neuropathy is established.

Nitrofurantoin

CLINICAL FEATURES. Nitrofurantoin neuropathy most often occurs in patients with impaired renal function. High blood concentrations of nitrofurantoin cause an axonal neuropathy. The initial features are usually paresthesias, followed within a few days or weeks by glove-and-stocking sensory loss and weakness of distal muscles. Pure motor neuropathy is occasionally present.

DIAGNOSIS. Nitrofurantoin neuropathy should be suspected in any child who has neuropathy and is taking the drug. It may be difficult to distinguish from uremic neuropathy.

TREATMENT. Recovery is usually complete when the drug is stopped. Occasional patients have developed complete paralysis and death despite discontinuation of nitrofurantoin.

Vincristine

CLINICAL FEATURES. Neuropathy is an expected complication of vincristine therapy. The ankle tendon reflex is lost first; later, other tendon reflexes become less reactive and may be lost. The first symptoms are paresthesias, often starting in the fingers rather than the feet, and then progressing to mild loss of superficial sensation, but not position sense. Weakness follows sensory loss and is evidenced by clumsiness in the hands and cramps in the feet. Distal muscles are affected more than proximal muscles and extensors more than flexors. Weakness may progress rapidly, with loss of ambulation in a few weeks. The initial weakness may be asymmetric and suggests mononeuropathy multiplex.

DIAGNOSIS. Electrodiagnostic features are consistent with axonal neuropathy; fibrillations and fasciculations are seen on the EMG, but motor nerve conduction velocity is normal.

TREATMENT. The neuropathy is dose related, and usually the patient recovers 1 to 3 months after the drug is discontinued.

Zidovudine

Postnatal infection of children with the human immunodeficiency virus (HIV) was caused by contamination of the blood supply before screening was implemented. Children with hemophilia were especially at risk. AIDS can cause neuropathy, as can its treatment with zidovudine.

Toxins

Several heavy metals, inorganic chemicals, and insecticides produce polyneuropathies in children (Ouvrier et al, 1990a). In adults, heavy metal poisoning is generally caused by industrial exposure, agricultural exposure, or attempted homicide. Small children who have a single accidental ingestion are more likely to have acute symptoms of systemic disease or central nervous system dysfunction than a slowly progressive neuropathy. Sometimes, progressive distal weakness is an early sign in older children addicted to sniffing glue or gasoline. Even in these cases symptoms of central nervous system dysfunction are usually present.

Uremia

Some degree of neuropathy occurs at one time or another in many children undergoing long-term periodic hemodialysis. Uremic neuropathy is more common in males than females, but the reason for the sex bias is unknown.

CLINICAL FEATURES. The earliest symptoms may be muscle cramps in the hands and feet, burning feet or restless legs, and loss of the ankle tendon reflex. After the initial sensory symptoms, the disorder progresses to a severe distal, symmetric, mixed motor, and sensory polyneuropathy affecting the legs more than the arms. The rate of progression is variable and may be fulminating or may evolve over several months.

A pure motor neuropathy develops in some children with uremia. Symptoms begin after hemodialysis is started. The rapid progression of distal weakness in all limbs does not respond to dialysis but may be reversed by renal transplantation.

DIAGNOSIS. Uremia causes an axonal neuropathy, but chronic renal failure causes segmental demyelination that is out of proportion to axonal changes (Ouvrier et al, 1990b). Therefore, motor nerve conduction velocity measurements are useful to monitor the severity of neuropathy. Slow conduction velocities are present even before clinical symptoms occur. Reduced creatine clearance correlates with slowing of the conduction velocity.

TREATMENT. Early neuropathy can be reversed by dialysis. Patients with severe neuropathy rarely recover fully despite adequate treatment.

Systemic Vasculitis and Vasculopathy

Polyneuropathy and mononeuropathy multiplex are relatively common neurologic complications of vasculitis in adults but not in children. Children with lupus erythematosus are generally sicker than adults, but peripheral neuropathy is neither an initial nor a prominent feature of their disease.

IDIOPATHIC NEUROPATHY

Chronic Axonal Neuropathy

CLINICAL FEATURES. Most axonal neuropathies are either hereditary or toxic. Glue sniffing is an example of a toxic cause. Some children have a progressive axonal neuropathy for which no cause can be determined. Progressive weakness of the feet, with or without sensory impairment, is often the initial feature. A hereditary basis can sometimes be established by electrodiagnostic studies in parents and siblings.

DIAGNOSIS. The EMG shows fibrillations and fasciculations, but motor nerve conduction velocity is normal or only mildly delayed. The protein content of the cerebrospinal fluid is normal.

TREATMENT. Children with idiopathic axonal neuropathies usually have a slowly progressive weakness that does not respond to corticosteroids. However, occasional patients do respond, and a 2-month trial of prednisone is indicated in patients with subacute progression of disease. These responsive cases may be variants of chronic inflammatory demyelinating neuropathy, in which both axonal involvement and demyelination are present.

Chronic Inflammatory Demyelinating Polyradiculoneuropathy

Acquired demyelinating neuropathies occur in both an acute and a chronic form. The acute form is called *Guillain-Barré syndrome* and is described in the section that follows (Table 7–8). The chronic form is called *chronic inflammatory demyelinating polyradiculoneuropathy* (CIDP). The acute and chronic forms may be difficult to distinguish from each other at the onset of symptoms but are identified by their subsequent course.

CIDP, like the Guillain-Barré syndrome, is generally believed to be immune mediated (van der Meché and van Doorn, 1995). However, although a clear relationship exists between the Guillain-Barré syndrome and a preceding infection, the provocative stimulus for CIDP is unknown.

CLINICAL FEATURES. CIDP affects adults more often than children, but a similar syndrome may be present even at birth (see Chapter 6).

■ T A B L E   7 – 8
Acute Generalized Weakness [Gene Location]

Infectious Disorders
Acute infectious myositis
Acute inflammatory polyradiculoneuropathy (Guillain-Barré syndrome)
Enterovirus infections
Metabolic Disorders
Acute intermittent porphyria (see Chapter 9)
Hereditary tyrosinemia (see Chapter 9)
Neuromuscular Blockade
Botulism
Corticosteroid-induced quadriplegia
Tick paralysis
Periodic Paralysis
Familial hyperkalemic [17q23-25]
Familial hypokalemic [1q31-32]
Familial normokalemic

The usual initial features are both weakness and paresthesias in the distal portions of the limbs; only rarely does motor involvement occur alone. Facial weakness occurs in only 13% of cases. Mandatory criteria for diagnosis are (1) progressive or relapsing motor and sensory dysfunction of more than one limb, of a peripheral nerve nature, developing over at least 2 months, and (2) areflexia or hyporeflexia, usually affecting all four limbs. The course is steadily progressive or stepwise in two thirds of cases, and is characterized by recurrent episodes of acute polyradiculoneuropathy with only partial or complete recovery between episodes in the remainder. Whichever the course of CIDP, progression occurs for at least 6 months and sometimes several years.

Children with CIDP may develop palpable nerves and pes cavus deformities that suggest a hereditary motor and sensory neuropathy (Baba et al, 1995).

DIAGNOSIS. Exclusionary criteria in establishing the diagnosis of CIDP are a family history of a similar disorder, a pure sensory neuropathy, other organ involvement, or an abnormal storage of material in nerves. The protein content of the cerebrospinal fluid is always greater than 0.45 g/L, and a small number of mononuclear cells may be present. Motor nerve conduction velocity is less than 70% of the lower limit of normal in at least two nerves. Sural nerve biopsy shows features of demyelination. Cellular infiltration of the nerve is uncommon and evidence of vasculitis excludes the diagnosis of CIDP.

Acquired demyelinating neuropathies in children can be differentiated from familial demyelinating neuropathies by electrodiagnosis. Acquired neuropathies show a multifocal disturbance of conduction velocity, whereas in hereditary disorders conduction is uniformly slowed throughout the length of the nerve.

TREATMENT. The ideal management of patients with CIDP is not established (Dyck et al, 1994a). The main choices are between a course of intravenous immune globulin (IVIG), chronic use of prednisone, or some combination of the two. I am now starting with IVIG, 1 g/kg/day on two successive days, because the results are more rapid than with prednisone. If relapse occurs after a beneficial response, I then repeat the course and follow it with prednisone, 0.5 mg/kg/qod, for 2 years.

The outcome is more favorable in children than in adults and full recovery is the rule, although some children have relapses in adult life.

MYOPATHIES

Hereditary Distal Myopathies

Three clinical forms of hereditary distal myopathy are described: two are transmitted by dominant inheritance and one by recessive inheritance. One of the dominant forms occurs in infancy and the other in childhood or later. The infantile dominant form may be a variant of Bethlem myopathy. The childhood dominant form shows linkage to chromosome 14 (Laing et al, 1995). The recessive form begins during adolescence or later and shows linkage to chromosome 2p12-14 (Bejaoui et al, 1995).

Autosomal Dominant Infantile-Onset Distal Myopathy

CLINICAL FEATURES. Hereditary distal myopathy with onset in infancy begins anytime during the first 2 years. The first signs are footdrop and weakness in the hand extensor muscles. Little or no progression occurs throughout the remainder of childhood. Some children have pseudohypertrophy of the calves, scoliosis, or pes cavus.

DIAGNOSIS. The creatine kinase concentration is usually normal, but EMG shows brief, small-amplitude polyphasic potentials, occasional fibrillations, and myotonia. Muscle biopsy specimens show fiber-type disproportion in which type I fibers are more numerous but smaller than type II fibers.

TREATMENT. No treatment is available.

Autosomal Dominant Childhood-Onset Distal Myopathy

This is the clinical phenotype that most resembles "Gower's distal myopathy" (Laing et al, 1995). The gene site is on chromosome 14.

CLINICAL FEATURES. Age at onset is after 4 years and may be delayed to the third decade. The initial weakness is in the toe and ankle extensors and the neck flexors. Weakness of the finger extensors develops years later, with relative sparing of the finger flexors and intrinsic hand muscles. Some proximal limb muscles are mildly affected late in life, but walking is usually preserved.

DIAGNOSIS. EMG findings are consistent with a myopathic process. Muscle biopsy specimens show variation in fiber size, nuclear clumps, moth-eaten type I fibers, and small angulated type II fibers. The serum concentration of creatine kinase is 1 to 3 times the upper limit of normal.

TREATMENT. No treatment is available.

Autosomal Recessive Distal (Miyoshi) Myopathy

The abnormal gene site is on chromosome 2p12-14 (Bejaoui et al, 1995).

CLINICAL FEATURES. Onset of weakness is between 15 and 25 years of age. Weakness and atrophy in the gastrocnemius muscle are the initial features, with relative sparing of the anterior compartment. The ankle jerk reflex is lost, but other tendon reflexes are normal. Slowly progressive weakness is the rule, with eventual involvement of the quadriceps muscle. However, ambulation is usually preserved.

DIAGNOSIS. The serum creatine kinase concentration is at least 10 times the upper limit of normal; this distinguishes Miyoshi myopathy from the other distal myopathies. EMG findings are consistent with a myopathy, and muscle biopsy shows a chronic active myopathy without vacuoles.

TREATMENT. Immunosuppressive therapy does not affect the course of disease.

Myotonic Dystrophy

Myotonic dystrophy is a multisystem disorder transmitted by autosomal dominant inheritance with variable penetrance. The disease is caused by an unstable DNA region on chromosome 19 that amplifies 50 to several thousand times (Pizzuti et al, 1993). Amplification increases in successive generations and correlates with more severe disease. A neonatal form, which occurs in children born to mothers with myotonic dystrophy, is described in Chapter 6.

CLINICAL FEATURES. The onset of symptoms is usually during adolescence or later. The major features are myotonia (a disturbance in muscle relaxation after contraction), weakness in the face and distal portion of the limbs, cataracts, frontal baldness, and multiple endocrinopathies. The pattern of muscle atrophy in the face is so stereotyped that all patients with the disease have a similar facies. The face is long and thin because of wasting of the temporal and masseter muscles, and the neck is thin because of atrophy of the sternocleidomastoid muscles. The eyelids and corners of the mouth droop, and the lower part of the face sags, producing the appearance of sadness.

Although medical treatment is rarely sought before adolescence, myotonia is usually present in childhood and can be detected by EMG, if not by clinical examination. Myotonia is demonstrated by percussion of muscle, usually the thenar eminence, which dimples and remains dimpled at the site of percussion. In addition, the thumb abducts and remains in that position for several seconds. The physician can also detect myotonia by shaking hands with the patient, who has difficulty in letting go and releases the grip in part by flexing the wrist to force the flexors of the fingers open.

Some patients have little or no evidence of muscle weakness, only cataracts, frontal baldness, or endocrine disturbances. However, when muscle weakness is present before age 20, it is likely to be relentlessly progressive, causing severe distal weakness in the hands and feet by adult life. Smooth and cardiac muscle involvement may be present and is characterized by disturbed gastrointestinal motility. Endocrine disturbances include testicular atrophy, infertility in women, hyperinsulinism, adrenal atrophy, and disturbances in growth hormone secretion.

DIAGNOSIS. The diagnosis of myotonic dystrophy is usually based on clinical features and family history. EMG studies show myotonia (the appearance of motor unit potentials that wax and wane in amplitude and frequency), myopathic potentials, and involvement of peripheral large-diameter motor and sensory fibers. Muscle biopsy is not needed to confirm the diagnosis. Studies to show the presence and number of trinucleotide repeats are now commercially available and can be used to detect asymptomatic individuals and for prenatal diagnosis.

TREATMENT. Myotonia frequently responds to drugs that stabilize membranes: quinidine, procainamide, phenytoin, and carbamazepine. However, it is weakness, for which no treatment is available, and not myotonia that disables the patient. Braces for footdrop are usually required as the disease progresses.

SCAPULO(HUMERAL)PERONEAL SYNDROMES

Progressive weakness and atrophy affecting the proximal muscles of the arms and the distal muscles of the legs may result from neuronopathy or myopathy. Many patients with dominantly inherited scapulo(humeral)peroneal syndromes have both muscle and nerve disease. Such patients probably have a variant phenotype of facioscapulohumeral syndrome.

Emery-Dreifuss Muscular Dystrophy

Emery-Dreifuss muscular dystrophy is transmitted by X-linked recessive inheritance.

CLINICAL FEATURES. The onset of symptoms is between 5 and 15 years of age. The earliest feature of disease is the development of contractures in the flexors of the elbows, the ankle tendon, and the extensors of the hand. This is followed by muscle weakness and wasting in the biceps and triceps muscles and then the deltoid and other shoulder muscles. The peroneal muscles are severely affected. Calf hypertrophy does not occur. The progression of symptoms is slow, and the condition usually stabilizes by 20 years of age. In some patients, however, weakness progresses into adult life and ambulation is lost. In all patients a cardiomyopathy leading to permanent atrial paralysis develops. Bradycardia and syncope may precede muscle weakness or be delayed until the third decade. The arrhythmia, if not treated by use of a permanent pacemaker, may cause stroke and death.

DIAGNOSIS. The EMG may show features of denervation and myopathy in the same patient or myopathy in one sibling and neuropathy in another. The most prominent feature on muscle biopsy is type I fiber atrophy. This histologic pattern is seen in many congenital myopathies in which it is uncertain whether the primary disease is in nerve or muscle (see Chapter 6). Molecular diagnosis has been accomplished but is not yet commercially available.

TREATMENT. No treatment is available for the muscle weakness and wasting, but cardiac arrhythmia should be treated early by implantation of a permanent pacemaker.

Scapulohumeral Syndrome with Dementia

Scapulohumeral syndrome with dementia is transmitted by X-linked inheritance and may be allelic with Emery-Dreifuss dystrophy.

CLINICAL FEATURES. Affected children appear normal until 5 years of age and then have mental deterioration, recognized first as a learning disability and then as mental retardation. Weakness and atrophy of the scapular or humeral muscles and peroneal muscles follow shortly thereafter. Contractures do not develop in affected muscles, and pseudohypertrophy is not present. Symptomatic cardiomyopathy occurs during adolescence and proves fatal.

DIAGNOSIS. Scapulohumeral syndrome with dementia is distinguished from Emery-Dreifuss dystrophy by the absence of contractures and the presence of mental deterioration. EMG shows a mixed myopathic-neuropathic pattern, and muscle biopsy reveals excessive internal nuclei and fiber splitting. The concentration of serum creatine kinase is elevated.

TREATMENT. No treatment is available for the underlying disease. Fatalities are only prevented by heart transplantation.

Scapuloperoneal Neuronopathy

A dominantly inherited neuronopathic scapuloperoneal syndrome with increasing severity in successive generations has been described in a French-Canadian family (DeLong and Siddique, 1992). This family validates the hypothesis that congenital absence of muscle and progressive spinal muscular atrophy are a continuum of disturbed programmed cell death. The anticipation in succeeding generations is best explained by DNA amplification.

CLINICAL FEATURES. Males are generally affected more severely than females. The phenotypic expression varies from congenital absence of muscle groups (congenital laryngeal abductor palsy, Möbius syndrome, clubfoot) to progressive neurogenic atrophy. Congenital absence of muscles may be noted at birth without progression of weakness, or scapuloperoneal weakness may develop during the first two decades. In later generations, weakness progresses to severe

disability that causes loss of ambulation, hand weakness, and laryngeal paralysis requiring tracheostomy by adolescence.

DIAGNOSIS. The concentration of serum creatine kinase is normal. EMG shows denervation potentials with normal conduction velocity, and muscle biopsy is consistent with chronic denervation atrophy.

TREATMENT. No treatment is available.

 ## Acute Generalized Weakness

The sudden onset or rapid evolution of generalized flaccid weakness, in the absence of symptoms of encephalopathy, is always due to disorders of the motor unit. Among the disorders listed in Table 7-8, acute inflammatory demyelinating polyradiculoneuropathy (Guillain-Barré syndrome) is by far the most common.

The combination of acute weakness and rhabdomyolysis, as evidenced by myoglobinuria, indicates that muscle is degenerating rapidly. This may occur in some disorders of carbohydrate metabolism (see Chapter 8), after intense and unusual exercise, in some cases of infectious and idiopathic polymyositis, and in intoxication with alcohol and cocaine (Roth et al, 1988). Death from renal failure is a possible outcome in patients with rhabdomyolysis.

INFECTIOUS DISEASE

Acute Infectious Myositis

Acute myositis in children most often follows influenza or other respiratory infections.

CLINICAL FEATURES. Ordinarily, prodromal respiratory symptoms persist for 1 to 7 days before the onset of severe symmetric muscle pain and weakness, which may cause severe disability within 24 hours. Proximal muscles are more severely affected than distal muscles, but generalized weakness may be present. The muscles are very tender to palpation. Tendon reflexes are present.

DIAGNOSIS. The serum concentration of creatine kinase is elevated, usually more than 10 times the upper limit of normal.

TREATMENT. Spontaneous resolution of the myositis occurs almost immediately. Bed rest is required for 2 to 7 days until pain subsides, after which the patient recovers completely.

Acute Inflammatory Demyelinating Polyradiculoneuropathy (Guillain-Barré Syndrome)

The Guillain-Barré syndrome is an acute, monophasic demyelinating neuropathy in which abnormal immune responses are directed against peripheral nerve (Hartung et al, 1995). More than half of patients describe an antecedent viral infection. Respiratory tract infections are most common, and the remainder are mainly gastrointestinal infections. Enteritis caused by specific strains of *Campylobacter jejuni* is the inciting disease in up to 18% of cases.

CLINICAL FEATURES. The natural history of the Guillain-Barré syndrome in children is substantially the same as in adults (Kleyweg et al, 1989). The clinical features are so stereotyped that the diagnosis is usually established without laboratory confirmation. This is especially important because the characteristic laboratory features of Guillain-Barré syndrome may not be present at the onset of clinical symptoms. The two essential features of Guillain-Barré syndrome are progressive motor weakness involving more than one limb and areflexia. Weakness is frequently preceded by insidious sensory symptoms that are usually ignored. These consist of fleeting dysesthesias and muscle tenderness in limbs that are soon to become paralytic. Weakness progresses rapidly, and approximately 50% of patients will reach a nadir by 2 weeks, 80% by 3 weeks, and the rest by 4 weeks. The weakness may be ascending or descending but is relatively symmetric qualitatively, if not quantitatively. Tendon reflexes are absent in all weak muscles and can be absent even before the muscle is weak. Bilateral facial weakness occurs in as many as half of cases. Autonomic dysfunction (arrhythmia, labile blood pressure, and gastrointestinal dysfunction) are commonly associated, and a syndrome of acute autonomic dysfunction without paralysis may be a variant of the Guillain-Barré syndrome (Zochodne, 1994).

Recovery of function usually begins 2 to 4 weeks after progression stops. In children recovery is almost always complete. The prognosis is best when recovery begins early. Respiratory paralysis occurs in 20% to 30% of children with the Guillain-Barré syndrome. If the patient's respiratory function can be supported during the critical time of profound paralysis, complete recovery can be expected.

DIAGNOSIS. The concentration of protein in the cerebrospinal fluid is elevated after the first week of symptoms. During the first week, the cerebrospinal fluid commonly contains 10 or fewer mononuclear leukocytes per cubic millimeter; however, these rapidly disappear and none are found in subsequent weeks. Electrophysiologic evidence of segmental demyelination is present in 50% of patients during the first 2 weeks of illness and in 85% during the third week (Albers and Kelly, 1989).

TREATMENT. Respiratory function must be carefully monitored in children with Guillain-Barré syndrome. If vital capacity falls rapidly to less than 50% of normal, an endotracheal tube should be inserted. Most children who require respiratory support need that support for several weeks, and many require tracheostomy. Adequate control of respiration should prevent death from the disorder. Corticosteroids are not helpful because, although they may produce some initial improvement, they tend to prolong the course.

Patients, too weak to walk without assistance, recover more quickly when five doses of intravenous immune globulin, 0.4 g/kg/day, are given within 2 weeks of the onset of symptoms (van der Meché and van Doorn, 1995).

Acute Motor Axonal Neuropathy

Annual epidemics of acute-onset flaccid paralysis have been recognized in China for at least 20 years. The syndrome is believed to be a postviral neuronopathy or motor axonal neuropathy. Similar cases of an acute "axonal" form of Guillain-Barré syndrome occur in the Western Hemisphere but not as epidemics (Reisin et al, 1993). Enteritis caused by specific strains of *C. jejuni* has been implicated in the pathogenesis of some cases (Yuki et al, 1992).

CLINICAL FEATURES. The clinical features are indistinguishable from the Guillain-Barré syndrome except that sensation is unaffected. Maximal weakness, symmetric quadriparesis and respiratory failure, usually occurs in 1 week. Tendon reflexes are absent early in the course, but parasthesias are rare. Distal atrophy occurs. Recovery is slow and the mean time to ambulation is 5 months.

DIAGNOSIS. The cerebrospinal fluid cell count is normal but the protein concentration is increased after 1 or 2 weeks. Electrophysiologic studies are consistent with an axonopathy rather than a demyelinating neuropathy and sensory nerve action potentials are normal.

TREATMENT. Respiratory support is often needed. Specific treatment is not available, but most children recover spontaneously.

Enterovirus Infections

Poliovirus, coxsackievirus, and the echovirus group are small RNA viruses that inhabit the intestinal tract of humans. They are neurotropic and produce paralytic disease by destroying the motor neurons of the brainstem and spinal cord. Of this group, poliovirus causes the most severe and devastating disease. Coxsackievirus and echoviruses are more likely to cause aseptic meningitis, although they can cause an acute paralytic syndrome similar to poliomyelitis.

CLINICAL FEATURES. Enterovirus infections occur in epidemics during the spring and summer. The most common syndrome associated with poliovirus infection is a brief illness characterized by fever, malaise, and gastrointestinal syndromes. Aseptic meningitis occurs in more severe cases. The extreme situation is paralytic poliomyelitis. It begins with fever, sore throat, and malaise lasting 1 to 2 days. After a brief period of apparent well-being, fever recurs in association with headache, vomiting, and signs of meningeal irritation. Pain in the limbs or over the spine is an antecedent symptom of limb paralysis. Flaccid muscle weakness develops rapidly thereafter. The pattern of muscle weakness varies, but it is generally asymmetric. One arm or leg is affected more than other limbs.

Bulbar polio may occur with or without spinal cord disease and is life threatening. Affected children have prolonged episodes of apnea and require respiratory assistance. Several motor cranial nerves may be involved as well, but the extraocular muscles are spared.

The introduction of inactivated poliomyelitis vaccine in 1954, followed by the use of attenuated live poliomyelitis vaccine in 1960, has abolished the disease in the Western Hemisphere. Nearly all recently reported cases are vaccine related. Paralytic poliomyelitis develops in approximately 1 healthy child in 1 million immunized with trivalent oral polio vaccine, almost always after the first immunization.

DIAGNOSIS. The diagnosis can be suspected from clinical findings and confirmed by isolation and viral typing from stool and nasopharyngeal specimens. The cerebrospinal fluid initially shows a polymorphonuclear reaction with the cell count ranging from 50 to 200/mm^3. After a week, lymphocytes predominate; after 2 to 3 weeks the total cell count decreases. The protein content is elevated early and remains elevated for several months.

TREATMENT. No treatment is available other than supportive care.

NEUROMUSCULAR BLOCKADE

A fulminating form of myasthenia gravis in which generalized weakness progresses to respiratory distress within 12 to 18 hours has been described in infants. Bulbar and limb paralysis are present. No recent reports have been published and earlier cases may have been infantile botulism (see Chapter 6).

Children treated for prolonged periods with neuromuscular blocking agents for assisted ventilation may remain in a flaccid state for days or weeks after the drug is discontinued (Benzing et al, 1990). This is especially true in newborns, who often receive several drugs that block the neuromuscular junction.

Botulism

Clostridium botulinum produces a toxin that interferes with the release of acetylcholine at the neuromuscular junction. An infantile form of botulism is described in Chapter 6, but most cases occur after infancy in people who eat food, usually preserved at home, contaminated with the organism.

CLINICAL FEATURES. The first symptoms are blurred vision, diplopia, dizziness, dysarthria, and dysphagia, which have their onset 12 to 36 hours after the ingestion of toxin. Some patients have only bulbar signs; in others, flaccid paralysis develops in all limbs. Patients with generalized weakness always have ophthalmoplegia, but the pupillary response is usually spared. Tendon reflexes may be present or absent.

DIAGNOSIS. Repetitive supermaximal nerve stimulation at a rate of 20 to 50 stimuli per second produces an incremental response characteristic of a presynaptic defect. The electrical abnormality evolves with time and may not be demonstrable in all limbs on any given day.

TREATMENT. Botulism can be fatal because of respiratory depression. Treatment relies primarily on supportive care, which is similar to the management of Guillain-Barré syndrome. Antitoxin does not influence the course of disease. Guanidine hydrochloride, a drug that enhances the release of acetylcholine from nerve terminals, may offer some benefit at an average dosage of 250 mg every 6 hours in adults. In both children and adults the dose should be titrated to the degree of weakness. Recovery is prolonged when paralysis has been severe, but all patients recover completely.

Corticosteroid-Induced Quadriplegia

The administration of high-dose intravenous corticosteroids, especially in combination with a neuromuscular blocking agent, causes acute generalized weakness (Hirano et al, 1992; Lacomis et al, 1993).

CLINICAL FEATURES. Most patients with this syndrome received corticosteroids to treat asthma. The onset of weakness is 4 to 14 days after treatment is started. The weakness is usually diffuse at onset but may be limited to proximal or distal muscles. Tendon reflexes are usually preserved. Complete recovery is the rule.

DIAGNOSIS. Serum creatine kinase concentration may be normal or elevated. EMG is normal or consistent with myopathy or neuropathy. Muscle biopsy usually shows a myopathic process.

TREATMENT. Respiratory assistance may be needed. Cessation of the offending drugs usually ends the disorder and allows the patient to recover spontaneously.

Tick Paralysis

The female of several species of North American ticks elaborates a salivary gland toxin that induces paralysis.

CLINICAL FEATURES. The clinical syndrome is similar to Guillain-Barré syndrome. A severe generalized flaccid weakness develops rapidly and is sometimes associated with bifacial palsy. Tendon reflexes are usually absent or greatly depressed. Dysesthesias may be present at the onset of weakness, but loss of sensation cannot be demonstrated on examination.

DIAGNOSIS. The cerebrospinal fluid protein concentration is normal. Electrophysiologic studies show slowing of conduction velocities. The possibility of tick paralysis should be considered during the spring and summer in any child who has Guillain-Barré syndrome and a normal protein content in the cerebrospinal fluid.

TREATMENT. Strength returns quickly once the tick is removed. However, the tick may be hard to find, because it is frequently hidden in body hair.

PERIODIC PARALYSES

The periodic paralyses are usually classified in relation to serum potassium: hyperkalemic, hypokalemic, or normokalemic. In addition, periodic paralysis may be primary (genetically transmitted) or secondary. Secondary hypokalemic periodic paralysis is caused by urinary or gastrointestinal loss of potassium. Urinary loss accompanies primary hyperaldosteronism, licorice intoxication, amphotericin B therapy, and several renal tubular defects. Gastrointestinal loss most often occurs with severe chronic diarrhea, prolonged gastrointestinal intubation and vomiting, and a draining gastrointestinal fistula. Either urinary or gastrointestinal loss, or both, may occur in children with anorexia nervosa who overuse diuretics or induce vomiting. Hypokalemic periodic paralysis is also seen with thyrotoxicoses, especially in Asians. Secondary hyperkalemic periodic paralysis is associated with renal or adrenal insufficiency.

Familial Hyperkalemic Periodic Paralysis

Familial hyperkalemic periodic paralysis is transmitted by autosomal dominant inheritance and occurs with equal frequency in both sexes. It is caused by a defect of the gene encoding the sodium channel on chromosome 17q23-25 (Hudson et al, 1995). Myotonia of the eyelids, face, and hands is sometimes an associated symptom, and such cases are referred to as *paramyotonia congenita* (de Silva et al, 1990).

CLINICAL FEATURES. The onset of weakness is in early childhood and sometimes in infancy. As in hypokalemic periodic paralysis, attacks may be provoked by rest shortly after exercise. However, only moderate exercise is required. Weakness begins with a sensation of heaviness in the back and leg muscles. Sometimes the patient can delay the paralysis by walking or moving about. In infants and small children, the attacks are characterized by an episode of floppiness in which the child lies around and can not move. In older children and adults, both mild and severe attacks may occur. Mild attacks last for less than an hour and do not produce complete paralysis. More than one mild attack may occur in a day. Severe attacks are similar to the complete flaccid paralysis seen in hypokalemic periodic paralysis and may last for several hours. Residual weakness may persist after several severe attacks.

DIAGNOSIS. Myotonia in patients with hyperkalemic periodic paralysis is mild and may only occur on exposure to cold. This can be shown by laying a towel soaked in ice water over the patient's eyes for a few minutes. After the towel is removed, the patient is asked to look upward briefly and then to look down quickly. When the eyelids are myotonic, the lids cannot come down quickly and a rim of sclera is exposed.

During attacks the serum concentration of potassium increases but may not increase sufficiently to be abnormal. When potassium concentrations are high, ECG changes are consistent with hyperkalemia. The oral administration of potassium chloride just after exercise in the fasting state provokes an attack. During the attack the muscles are electrically silent.

TREATMENT. Acute attacks seldom require treatment, because they are brief. Daily administration of acetazolamide may prevent recurrence of attacks. The mechanism by which acetazolamide is effective in preventing attacks of both hyperkalemic and hypokalemic periodic paralysis is unknown.

Familial Hypokalemic Periodic Paralysis

Familial hypokalemic periodic paralysis is transmitted by autosomal dominant inheritance with decreased penetrance in women. The abnormal gene maps to chromosome 1q31-32 (Fontaine et al, 1994).

CLINICAL FEATURES. The onset of symptoms occurs before 16 years of age in 60% of cases and by 20 years of age in the remainder. Attacks of paralysis are at first infrequent but then may occur several times a week. Factors that trigger an attack include rest after exercise (therefore many attacks occur early in the morning), a large meal with high carbohydrate content, emotional or physical stress, alcohol ingestion, and exposure to cold. Before and during the attack the patient may have excessive thirst and oliguria. The weakness begins with a sensation of aching in the proximal muscles. Sometimes only the proximal muscles are affected; at other times there is complete paralysis so that the patient cannot even raise the head. Facial muscles are rarely affected, and extraocular motility is always normal. Respiratory distress does not occur. When the weakness is most extreme, the muscles feel swollen and the tendon reflexes are absent. Most attacks last for 6 to 12 hours and some for the whole day. Strength recovers

rapidly, but after several attacks residual weakness may be present.

DIAGNOSIS. During the attack, serum potassium concentrations may fall to 1.5 mEq/L (1.5 mmol/L) and ECG changes occur, including: bradycardia, flattening of T waves, and prolongation of the P-R and Q-T intervals. The muscle is electrically silent and not excitable. Attacks can be provoked by the oral administration of glucose, 2 g/kg, with 10 to 20 units of crystalline insulin given subcutaneously. The serum potassium concentration falls, and an attack of paralysis is initiated within 2 to 3 hours.

TREATMENT. Acute attacks in patients with good renal function are treated by repeated oral doses of potassium. In adolescents 5 to 10 g is used. Smaller amounts should be considered for younger children. Daily use of acetazolamide is beneficial in many families to prevent attacks and lithium gluconate may be useful in refractory cases (Confavreux et al, 1991).

Familial Normokalemic Periodic Paralysis

Several families reported in the literature have an autosomal dominant inherited periodic paralysis in which no alteration in serum concentration of potassium can be detected. These may represent hyperkalemic periodic paralysis in which the flux of potassium into the serum was insufficient to be detected.

R E F E R E N C E S

Albers JW, Kelly JJ Jr. Acquired inflammatory demyelinating polyneuropathies: Clinical and electrodiagnostic features. Muscle Nerve 1989;12:435-451.

Baba M, Takeda H, Miura H, et al. "Pseudo" hypertrophic neuropathy of childhood. J Neurol Neurosurg Psychiatry 1995;58:236-237.

Balestrini MR, Cavaletti G, D'Angelo A, et al. Infantile hereditary neuropathy with hypomyelination: Report of two siblings with different expressivity. Neuropediatrics 1991;22:65-70.

Bejaoui K, Hirabayashi K, Hentati F, et al. Linkage of Miyoshi myopathy (distal autosomal recessive muscular dystrophy locus to chromosome 2p12-14. Neurology 1995;45:768-772.

Benzing G III, Iannaccone ST, Bove KE, et al. Prolonged myasthenic syndrome after one week of muscle relaxants. Pediatr Neurol 1990;6:190-196.

Boylan KB, Cornblath DR. Werdnig-Hoffmann disease and chronic distal spinal muscular atrophy with apparent autosomal dominant inheritance. Ann Neurol 1992;32:404-407.

Boylan KB, Cornblath DR, Glass JD, et al. Autosomal dominant distal spinal muscular atrophy in four generations. Neurology 1995;45:699-704.

Breningstall GN. Carnitine deficiency syndromes. Pediatr Neurol 1990;6:75-81.

Brooke MH, Fenichel GM, Griggs RC, et al. Duchenne muscular dystrophy: Patterns of clinical progression and effects of supportive therapy. Neurology 1989;39:475-481.

Chance PF, Pleasure D. Charcot-Marie-Tooth syndrome. Arch Neurol 1993;50:1180-1184.

Confavreux C, Garassus P, Vighetto A, et al. Familial hypokalemic periodic paralysis: Prevention of paralytic attacks with lithium gluconate. J Neurol Neurosurg Psychiatry 1991;54:87-88.

DeLong R, Siddique T. A large New England kindred with autosomal dominant neurogenic scapuloperoneal amyotrophy with unique features. Arch Neurol 1992;49:905-908.

de Silva SM, Kuncl RW, Griffin JW, et al. Paramyotonia congenita or hyperkalemic periodic paralysis? Clinical and electrophysiological features of each entity in one family. Muscle Nerve 1990;13:21,-26.

DeVivo DC, Tein I. Primary and secondary disorders of carnitine metabolism. Pediatrics 1990;5:134.

Donaghy M, Brett EM, Ormerod EC, et al. Giant axonal neuropathy: Observations on a further patient. J Neurol Neurosurg Psychiatry 1988;51:991-994.

Dyck PJ, Litchy WJ, Kratz KM, et al. A plasma exchange versus immune globulin infusion trial in chronic inflammatory demyelinating polyradiculoneuropathy. Ann Neurol 1994a;36:838-845.

Dyck PJ, Litchy WJ, Minnerath S, et al. Hereditary motor and sensory neuropathy with diaphragm and vocal cord paresis. Ann Neurol 1994b;35:608-615.

Emery AEH. Population frequencies of inherited neuromuscular diseases—a world survey. Neuromusc Dis 1991:1:19-29.

Feasby TE, Hahn AF, Bolton CF, et al. Detection of hereditary motor sensory neuropathy type I in childhood. J Neurol Neurosurg Psychiatry 1992;55:895-897.

Fenichel GM, Florence J, Pestronk A, et al. Long-term use of prednisone therapy in the treatment of Duchenne muscular dystrophy. Neurology 1991;41:1874-1877.

Fontaine B, Vale-Santos J, Jurkat-Rott K, et al. Mapping of the hypokalemic periodic paralysis (HypoPP) locus to chromosome 1q31-32 in three European families. Nature Genet 1994;6:267-272.

Frijns CJM, Van Deutekom J, Frants RR, et al. Dominant congenital benign spinal muscular atrophy. Muscle Nerve 1994;17:192-197.

Gilliam TC, Brzustowicz LM, Castilla LH, et al. Genetic homogeneity between acute (SMA I) and chronic (SMA II & III) forms of spinal muscular atrophy. Nature 1990;345:823-825.

Gomez CM, Gammack JT. A leucine-to-phenylalanine substitution in the acetylcholine receptor ion channel in a family with the slow-channel syndrome. Neurology 1995;45:982-985.

Groen RJM, Sie OG, van Weerden TW. Dominant inherited distal spinal muscular atrophy with atrophic and hypertrophic calves. J Neurol Sci 1993;114:81-84.

Hamida MB, Hentati F, Hamida CB. Hereditary motor system diseases (chronic juvenile amyotrophic lateral sclerosis): Conditions combining a bilateral pyramidal syndrome with limb and bulbar amyotrophy. Brain 1990;113:347-363.

Harding AE. From the syndrome of Charcot, Marie and Tooth to disorders of peripheral myelin proteins. Brain 1995;118:809-818.

Hartung H-P, Pollard JD, Harvey GK, et al. Immunopathogenesis and treatment of the Guillain-Barré syndrome—Part I. Muscle Nerve 1995;18:137-153.

Hirano M, Ott BR, Raps EC, et al. Acute quadriplegic myopathy: A complication of treatment with steroids, nondepolarizing blocking agents, or both. Neurology 1992;42:2082-2087.

Hoffman EP, Wang J. Duchenne-Becker muscular dystrophies and the nondystrophic myotonias: Paradigms for loss of function and change of function of gene products. Arch Neurol 1993;50:1227-1237.

Hudson AJ, Ebers GC, Bulman DE. The skeletal muscle sodium and chloride channel diseases. Brain 1995;118:547-563.

Jardine PE, Upadhyaya M, Maynard J, et al. A scapular onset muscular dystrophy without facial involvement: Possible allelism with facioscapulohumeral muscular dystrophy. Neuromusc Dis 1994;4:477-482.

Kleyweg RP, van der Meché FGA, Loonen MCB, et al. The natural history of the Guillain-Barré syndrome in 18 children and 50 adults. J Neurol Neurosurg Psychiatry 1989;52:853-856.

Kolodny EH, Fluharty AL. Metachromatic leukodystrophy and multiple sulfatase deficiency: Sulfatide lipidosis. In Scriver CR, Beaudet AL, Sly WS, et al (eds): The Metabolic and Molecular Basis of Inherited Disorders, 7th edition. New York, McGraw-Hill, 1995;2693-2739.

Krivit W, Shapiro E, Kennedy W, et al. Treatment of late infantile metachromatic leukodystrophy by bone marrow transplantation. N Engl J Med 1990;322:28-32.

Lacomis D, Smith TW, Chad DA. Acute myopathy and neuropathy in status asthmaticus: Case report and literature review. Muscle Nerve 1993;16:84-90.

Laing NG, Laing BA, Meredith C, et al. Autosomal dominant distal myopathy: Linkage to chromosome 14. Am J Hum Genet 1995;56:422-427.

Lee JH, Goto K, Matsuda C, et al. Characterization of a tandemly repeated 3.3-kb KpnI unit in the fascioscapulohumeral muscular dystrophy (FSHD) gene region on chromosome 4q35. Muscle Nerve 1995;Suppl 2:S6-S13.

Liu GT, Specht LA. Progressive juvenile segmental spinal muscular atrophy. Pediatr Neurol 1993;9:54-56.

Ljunggren A, Duggan D, McNally E, et al. Primary adhalin deficiency as a cause of muscular dystrophy in patients with normal dystrophin. Ann Neurol 1995;38:367-372.

Matsumura K, Campbell KP. Dystrophin-glycoprotein complex: Its role in the molecular pathogenesis of muscular dystrophies. Muscle Nerve 1994;17:2-15.

Merlini L, Morandi L, Granata C, et al. Bethlem myopathy. Early-onset benign autosomal dominant myopathy with contractures. Description of two new families. Neuromusc Dis 1994;4:503-511.

Munsat TL, Skerry L, Korf B, et al. Phenotypic heterogeneity of spinal muscular atrophy mapping to chromosome 5q11.2-13.3 (SMA 5q). Neurology 1990;40:1831-1836.

Oh SJ, Kuruoglu R. Chronic limb-girdle myasthenia gravis. Neurology 1992;42:1153-1156.

Oldfors A, Larsson N-G, Lindberg C, et al. Mitochondrial DNA deletions in inclusion body myositis. Brain 1993;116:325-336.

Othmane KB, Middleton LT, Loprest LJ, et al. Localization of a gene (CMT2A) for autosomal dominant Charcot-Marie-Tooth disease, type 2 to chromosome 1p and evidence of genetic heterogeneity. Genomics 1993;17:370-375.

Ouvrier R, McLeod JG, Pollard J. Toxic neuropathies. In Peripheral Neuropathy in Childhood. International Review of Child Neurology Series. Raven Press, New York, 1990a; 167.

Ouvrier R, McLeod JG, Pollard J. Neuropathies in systemic disease. In Peripheral Neuropathy in Childhood. International Review of Child Neurology Series. Raven Press, New York, 1990b; 181.

Padberg GW, Brouwer OF, de Keizer RJW, et al. On the significance of retinal vascular disease and hearing loss in facioscapulohumeral muscular dystrophy. Muscle Nerve 1995;Suppl 2:S73-S80.

Pizzuti A, Friedman DL, Caskey T. The myotonic dystrophy gene. Arch Neurol 1993;50:1173-1179.

Polten A, Fluharty AL, Fluharty CB, et al. Molecular basis of different forms of metachromatic leukodystrophy. N Engl J Med 1991;324:18-22.

Reisin RC, Cersosimo R, Alvarez MG, et al. Acute "axonal" Guillain-Barré syndrome in childhood. Muscle Nerve 1993; 16:1310-1316.

Riggs JE, Schochet SS, Gutman L, et al. Childhood onset inclusion body myositis mimicking limb-girdle muscular dystrophy. J Child Neurol 1989;4:283-285.

Roth D, Alarcon FJ, Fernandez JA, et al. Acute rhabdomyolysis associated with cocaine intoxication. N Engl J Med 1988;319:673-677.

Sansome A, Dubowitz V. Intravenous immunoglobulin in juvenile dermatomyositis—four year review of nine cases. Arch Dis Child 1995;72:25-28.

Sghirlanzoni A, Pareyson D, Balestrini MR, et al. HMSN III phenotype due to homozygous expression of a dominant HMSN II gene. Neurology 1992;42:2201-2204.

Sherry DD, Haas JE, Milstein JM. Childhood polymyositis as a paraneoplastic phenomenon. Pediatr Neurol 1993;9: 156-156.

Sigurgeirsson B, Lindelöf B, Edhag O, et al. Risk of cancer in patients with dermatomyositis or polymyositis. N Engl J Med 1992;326:363-367.

Sunohara N, Arahata K, Hoffman EP, et al. Quadriceps myopathy: forme fruste of Becker muscular dystrophy. Ann Neurol 1990;28:634-639.

Tandan R, Sharma KR, Bradley WG, et al. Chronic segmental spinal muscular atrophy of upper extremities in identical twins. Neurology 1990;40:236-239.

Uncini A, Di Muzio A, Chiavaroli F, et al. Hereditary motor and sensory neuropathy with calf hypertrophy is associated with 17p11.2 duplication. Ann Neurol 1994;35:552-558.

van der Meché FGA, van Doorn PA. Guillain-Barré syndrome and chronic demyelinating polyneuropathy: Immune mechanisms and update on current therapies. Ann Neurol 1995;37(S1):S14-S31.

Walter EB, Drucker RP, McKinney RE. Myopathy in human immunodeficiency virus-infected children receiving long-term zidovudine therapy. J Pediatr 1991;119:152-155.

Yuki N, Yoshino H, Sato S, et al. Severe acute axonal form of Guillain-Barré syndrome associated with IgG anti-GD_{1a} antibodies. Muscle Nerve 1992;15:899-903.

Zochodne DW. Autonomic involvement in Guillain-Barré syndrome: A review. Muscle Nerve 1994;17:1145-1155.

8

Cramps, Muscle Stiffness, and Exercise Intolerance

A cramp is an involuntary painful contraction of a muscle or part of a muscle. Cramps can occur in normal children during and after vigorous exercise and after excessive loss of fluid or electrolytes. Such cramps are characterized on electromyography (EMG) by the repetitive firing of normal motor unit potentials. Stretching the muscle relieves the cramp. Muscle that is partially denervated is particularly susceptible to cramping not only during exercise, but also during sleep. Night cramps may awaken patients with neuronopathies, neuropathies, or root compression. Cramps during exercise occur also in patients with several different disorders of muscle energy metabolism. These cramps differ from other cramps in that they are not detected by electrodiagnostic examination.

Muscle stiffness and spasms are sometimes called cramps by patients but are actually prolonged contractions of several muscles that are able to impose postures (Auger, 1994). Such contractions may or may not be painful. When painful, they lack the explosive character of cramps. Prolonged contractions occur when muscles fail to relax (myotonia) or when motor unit activity is continuous (Table 8-1). Prolonged, painless muscle contractions occur also

in dystonia and in other movement disorders (see Chapter 14).

Many normal children, especially preadolescent boys, complain of pain in their legs at night and sometimes during the day, especially after a period of increased activity. These pains are not true cramps. The muscle is not in spasm, the pain is diffuse and aching in quality, and the discomfort lasts for an hour or longer. Stretching the muscle does not relieve the pain. This is not a symptom of neuromuscular disease and, for want of better understanding, is usually referred to as *growing pains*. Symptoms are relieved by mild analgesics or heat.

Exercise intolerance is a relative term for an inability to maintain exercise at an expected level. The causes of exercise intolerance considered in this chapter are fatigue and muscle pain. Fatigue is a normal consequence of exercise and occurs in everyone at some level of activity. In general, weak children become fatigued more quickly than children who have normal strength. Many children with exercise intolerance and cramps, but no permanent weakness, have a defect in an enzyme needed to produce energy for muscular contraction (Table 8-2). Several such inborn errors of metabolism have been defined and others are yet to be defined. Even

■ TABLE 8–1
Diseases with Abnormal Muscle Activity

Continuous Motor Unit Activity
Neuromyotonia
Paroxysmal ataxia and myokymia (see Chapter 10)
Schwartz-Jampel syndrome
Stiff man syndrome
Thyrotoxicosis
Cramps-Fasciculation Syndrome
Myotonia
Myotonia congenita
Myotonia fluctuans
Systemic Disorders
Hypoadrenalism
Hypocalcemia (tetany)
Strychnine poisoning
Hypothryoidism
Uremia

■ TABLE 8–2
Diseases with Decreased Muscle Energy

Defects of Carbohydrate Utilization
Lactate dehydrogenase deficiency
Myophosphorylase deficiency
Phosphofructokinase deficiency
Phosphoglycerate kinase deficiency
Phosphoglycerate mutase deficiency
Defects of Fatty Acid Oxidation
Carnitine palmitoyl transferase deficiency
Very-long-chain acyl coenzyme A dehydrogenase
  deficiency
Mitochondrial (Respiratory Chain) Myopathies
Myoadenylate Deaminase Deficiency

■ TABLE 8–3
Electromyography in Muscle Stiffness

Normal Between Cramps (or may be myopathic)
Brody disease
Defects of carbohydrate metabolism
Defects of lipid metabolism
Mitochondrial myopathies
Myoadenylate deaminase deficiency
Rippling muscle disease
Tubular aggregates
Silent Cramps
Brody disease
Defects of carbohydrate metabolism
Rippling muscle disease
Tubular aggregates
Continuous Motor Activity
Neuromyotonia
Schwartz-Jampel syndrome
Stiff man syndrome
Myotonia
Myotonia congenita
Myotonic dystrophy
Schwartz-Jampel syndrome
Myopathy
Emery-Dreifuss muscular dystrophy
Rigid spine syndrome
X-linked myalgia

EMG should be the initial diagnostic test in patients with muscle stiffness that is not due to spasticity or rigidity. It usually leads to the correct diagnosis (Table 8–3).

 Abnormal Muscle Activity

CONTINUOUS MOTOR UNIT ACTIVITY

Continuous motor unit activity (CMUA) is caused by the uncontrolled release of acetylcholine (ACh) packets at the neuromuscular junction. The EMG features of CMUA are repetitive muscle action potentials in response to a single nerve stimulus; high-frequency bursts of motor unit potentials of normal morphology that start and stop abruptly; and rhythmically firing doublets, triplets, and multiplets. During long bursts the potentials decline in amplitude. This activity is difficult to distinguish from normal voluntary activity. CMUA is seen in a heterogeneous group of disorders characterized clinically by some combination of muscular pain, fasciculations, myokymia, contractures, and cramps (Table 8–4) (Auger, 1994).

Disorders with CMUA can be subdivided into

when the full spectrum of biochemical tests is available, the metabolic defect cannot be identified in some children in whom cramps develop after exercise and who have clear-cut evidence of muscle disease.

Myasthenia gravis is a disorder characterized by exercise intolerance, but it is not covered in this chapter because the usual initial symptoms are either isolated cranial nerve disturbances (see Chapter 15) or limb weakness (see Chapters 6 and 7).

Conditions that produce some combination of cramps and exercise intolerance can be divided into three groups: diseases with abnormal muscle activity, diseases with decreased energy for muscle contraction, and myopathies. As a rule, the first and third groups are symptomatic at all times, whereas the second group is symptomatic only with exercise. The first group requires EMG for diagnosis.

■ T A B L E   8 – 4
Abnormal Muscle Activity

Fasciculations: Spontaneous, random twitching of a group of muscle fibers
Fibrillation: Spontaneous contraction of a single muscle fiber, not visible through the skin
Myotonia: Disturbance in muscle relaxation following voluntary contraction or percussion
Myokymia: Repetitive fasciculations causing a quivering or undulating twitch
Neuromyotonia: Continuous muscle activity characterized by muscle rippling, muscle stiffness, and myotonia

---

syndromes in which the primary defect is believed to be within the spinal cord (stiffman syndrome) and those in which the primary defect is believed to be within the peripheral nerve (neuromyotonia). Neuromyotonia is also called *Isaac syndrome.* These disorders may be sporadic or familial in occurrence. When familial, they are usually transmitted by autosomal dominant inheritance.

Neuromyotonia

The primary abnormality in neuromyotonia is in the nerve or the nerve terminal. Most childhood cases are sporadic in occurrence, but some are transmitted by autosomal dominant inheritance.

CLINICAL FEATURES. The clinical triad includes involuntary muscle twitching (fasciculations or myokymia), muscle cramps or stiffness, and myotonia. Excessive sweating is frequently associated with the muscle stiffness. The age at onset is anytime from birth to adult life.

The initial features are muscle twitching and cramps brought on by exercise. Later these symptoms occur also at rest and even during sleep. The cramps may affect only distal muscles, causing painful posturing of the hands and feet. As a rule, the legs are affected more severely than the arms. These disorders are not progressive and do not lead to permanent disability. Attacks of cramping become less frequent and less severe with age.

In some children, cramps and fasciculations are not as prominent as stiffness, which causes abnormal limb posturing associated frequently with excessive sweating. The legs are more often affected than the arms, and the symptoms suggest dystonia (see Chapter 14). Limb posturing may begin in one foot and remain asymmetric for months. Most cases are sporadic.

Muscle mass, muscle strength, and tendon reflexes are normal. Fasciculations are sporadic and are seen only after prolonged observation.

DIAGNOSIS. Some adult-onset cases are associated with malignancy, but this is never the case in children. EMG shows CMUA, fasciculations, and sometimes myotonia. The continuous activity persists during sleep and during general and spinal anesthesia. It is progressively diminished by more distal nerve blocks, and is abolished by curare.

TREATMENT. Carbamazepine and phenytoin, at usual anticonvulsant doses, are both effective in reducing or abolishing symptoms.

Schwartz-Jampel Syndrome

The Schwartz-Jampel syndrome (osteochondromuscular dystrophy) is a hereditary disorder, probably transmitted by autosomal recessive inheritance, but possibly also by autosomal dominant inheritance (Pascuzzi et al, 1990). It is characterized by short stature, skeletal abnormalities, and persistent muscular contraction and hypertrophy.

CLINICAL FEATURES. Infants have progressive skeletal deformities, including hip dislocation, coxa vara or coxa valga, pectus carinatum, vertebral flattening, basilar impression, and dwarfism. The constellation of skeletal deformities suggests the Morquio syndrome (osteochondrodystrophy). CMUA is most prominent in the face and produces a characteristic triad that includes narrowing of the palpebral fissures (blepharophimosis), pursing of the mouth, and puckering of the chin. Blepharospasm is provoked by striking or even blowing on the eyelids (see Chapter 14). CMUA in the limbs produces stiffness of gait and exercise intolerance. Motor development during the first year is slow, but intelligence is normal.

DIAGNOSIS. EMG shows CMUA. Initial reports suggested incorrectly that the abnormal activity seen on the EMG and expressed clinically was myotonia. Myotonia may be present, but CMUA, generated in the nerve and abolished by curare, is responsible for the facial and limb symptoms. The serum concentration of creatine kinase can be mildly elevated. The muscle histologic appearance is usually normal but may show variation in fiber size and an increased number of central nuclei.

TREATMENT. Muscle stiffness is diminished by phenytoin or carbamazepine. Early treatment with relief of muscle stiffness reduces the severity of subsequent muscle deformity.

Stiffman Syndrome

Stiffman syndrome is a sporadic condition of adult life that is now considered to be immune-mediated (Grimaldi et al, 1993). It is extremely rare in children. A genetic form of stiffman syndrome, transmitted by autosomal dominant inheritance, was described in infants but is now considered to be startle disease (hyperekplexia). Startle disease is described in Chapter 1 because the main features in children and adults are paroxysmal, but the initial symptoms in newborns is stiffness. It is not the stiffman syndrome.

CLINICAL FEATURES. Following an initial period of aching and tightness in the truncal muscles, involuntary painful spasms occur without spinal deformity. Abdominal wall rigidity and contraction of thoracolumbar paraspinal muscles causes a hyperlordosis that is characteristic of the disease. The spasms are triggered by startle and by emotional upset and are relieved by sleep. Proximal limb muscles and bulbar muscles may be involved later. Tendon reflexes are active or hyperactive, and no evidence of muscle atrophy is found.

DIAGNOSIS. Individuals with stiff man syndrome and their relatives have an increased incidence of several organ-specific autoimmune disorders, especially insulin-dependent diabetes and hypothyroidism. Serum antibodies against glutamic acid decarboxylase and pancreatic islet cells are present in 60% of patients.

TREATMENT. Diazepam is the mainstay of treatment, and is useful for symptomatic relief of the spasms. Prednisone, plasma exchange, and intravenous immunoglobulin have been partially successful in treating the underlying autoimmune disease (Amato et al, 1994).

CRAMPS-FASCICULATION SYNDROME

The clinical features of the cramps-fasciculation syndrome, including the response to carbamazepine, are identical to those of neuromyotonia except that CMUA is not seen on EMG (Tahmoush et al, 1991). They are probably the same disease.

MYOTONIA CONGENITA

Myotonia congenita is a genetic disorder characterized by muscle stiffness and hypertrophy. Dystrophy does not occur, although families with features of both myotonic dystrophy and myotonia congenita have been reported. In 19% of families the trait is clearly transmitted by autosomal dominant inheritance *(Thomsen's disease)* and a smaller percentage is definitely transmitted by autosomal recessive inheritance *(Becker's disease).* Most cases are sporadic and cannot be classified genetically. In general, the autosomal recessive form has a later onset and more severe myotonia than the dominant form. However, the overlap of clinical features is considerable, and the pattern of genetic transmission cannot be determined by the clinical features alone. The abnormal gene for both the dominant and recessive forms of myotonia congenita is located on chromosome 7q23-35, at the site of the muscle chloride channel gene (Hudson et al, 1995).

CLINICAL FEATURES. Clinical features are stereotyped. After rest, muscles are stiff and difficult to move. With activity the stiffness disappears and movement may be normal. One of my patients played Little League baseball and could not sit while he was waiting to bat for fear that he would be unable to get up. The onset of the autosomal dominant type is usually dated to infancy. The myotonia causes generalized muscle hypertrophy, which gives the infant a Herculean appearance. The tongue, face, and jaw muscles are sometimes involved. Stiffness is painless and is exacerbated by exposure to cold. Percussion myotonia is present. Muscle mass, strength, and tendon reflexes are normal.

DIAGNOSIS. Diagnosis is established by EMG. Repetitive discharges at rates of 20 to 80 cycles/sec (cps) are recorded when the needle is first inserted into the muscle and again on voluntary contraction. Two types of discharges are seen: a biphasic spike potential of less than 5 ms and a positive wave of less than 50 ms. The amplitude and frequency of potentials wax and wane, producing a characteristic sound. No evidence of dystrophy is demonstrated. The serum concentration of creatine kinase is normal. Muscle biopsy specimens in patients with either the dominant or the recessive form do not contain type IIb fibers.

TREATMENT. Myotonia does not always require treatment but sometimes can be relieved by phenytoin or carbamazepine at ordinary anticonvulsant doses. Tocainide, starting at 200 mg twice a day and incrementally raised to 400 mg three times a day, is reported to improve the stiffness in children with the recessive form of the disease (Teasley et al, 1990). Acetazolamide may be beneficial in some patients.

MYOTONIA FLUCTUANS

This is the newest-described disorder of the muscle sodium channel on chromosome 17q23-25 (Hudson et al, 1995). It is transmitted by autosomal dominant inheritance and its clinical features are similar to those of myotonia congenita (Ricker et al, 1994).

CLINICAL FEATURES. The onset of stiffness is usually in the second decade and may be precipitated by general anesthesia. Myotonia affects the extraocular muscles as well as the trunk and limbs. The severity of myotonia fluctuates on a day-by-day basis, and "warming-up" relieves symptoms. A bad day may follow a day of exercise or potassium ingestion, but neither precipitant causes immediate worsening of myotonia. Cooling does not trigger or worsen myotonia.

DIAGNOSIS. EMG shows myotonia and muscle biopsy is normal. DNA analysis shows a mutation in the gene for the sodium channel α subunit.

TREATMENT. Mexilitine, a compound similar to lidocaine, prevents the myotonic stiffness in myotonia fluctuans and in paramyotonia. Acetazolamide should also be tried in this condition as well as in other sodium channel disorders.

SYSTEMIC DISORDERS

Hypoadrenalism

A small percentage of patients with Addison disease complain of cramps and pain in truncal muscles. At times, paroxysmal cramps occur in the lower torso and legs and cause the patient to double up in pain. The symptoms are relieved by hormone replacement.

Hypocalcemia and Hypomagnesemia

Tetany caused by dietary deficiency of calcium is rare in modern times, except in newborns fed cow's milk. Hypocalcemic tetany is more likely to result from hypothyroidism or hyperventilation-induced alkalosis.

The initial symptom of tetany is tingling around the mouth and in the hands and feet. With time, the tingling increases in intensity and becomes generalized. This is followed by spasms in the muscles of the face, hands, and feet. The hands assume a typical posture in which the fingers are extended, the wrist is flexed, and the thumb is abducted. Fasciculations and laryngeal spasm may be present. Percussion of the facial nerve, either just anterior to the ear or over the cheek, produces contraction of the muscles innervated by that branch of the nerve.

A similar syndrome is encountered with magnesium deficiency. In addition to the tetany, encephalopathy occurs. The cramps associated with hypocalcemia and hypomagnesemia are reversed by restoring the proper concentration of serum electrolytes.

Strychnine Poisoning

Strychnine is sometimes used as an adulterant in cocaine because it is a white odorless powder that is readily available as rat poison (Chignon, 1988). It is a competitive antagonist of glycine, a central nervous system inhibitory neurotransmitter. The clinical features of poisoning are apprehension, nausea, muscle twitching, extensor spasm, opisthotonos, and seizures. Excessive muscle contraction causes myoglobinuria and lactic acidosis. Intravenous diazepam reduces spasms and can prevent death.

Thyroid Disease

Muscle aches, cramps, and stiffness are the initial features in up to half of patients with hypothyroidism. Stiffness is worse in the morning, especially on cold days, and is probably caused by slowing of both muscular contraction and relaxation. This is different from myotonia, in which only relaxation is affected. Indeed, the stiffness of hypothyroidism is made worse by activity and may be painful, whereas myotonia is relieved by activity and is painless. The slowing of muscular contraction and relaxation is sometimes demonstrated when tendon reflexes are tested. The response tends to "hang-up."

Percussion of a muscle produces a localized knot of contraction called *myoedema*. This localized contraction lasts for up to 1 minute before slowly returning to normal.

Myokymia, CMUA of the face, tongue, and limbs, and muscle cramps develop occasionally in patients with thyrotoxicosis.

All of the neuromuscular symptoms of hypothyroidism and hyperthyroidism can be reversed by restoring the euthyroid state.

Uremia

Uremia is a known cause of polyneuropathy (see Chapter 7). However, 50% of patients complain of nocturnal leg cramps and flexion cramps of the hands even before clinical evidence of polyneuropathy is present. Excessive use of diuretics may be the triggering factor. Muscle cramps occur also in approximately one third of patients undergoing hemodialysis. Monitoring with EMG during dialysis documents a buildup of spontaneous discharges, which after several hours, usually toward the end of dialysis treatment, culminate in repetitive high-voltage discharges associated with clinical cramps. Because standard dialysis fluid is slightly hypotonic, many nephrologists have attempted to treat the cramps by administering hypertonic solutions. Either sodium chloride or glucose solutions relieve cramps in most patients. The cramps apparently result from either extracellular volume contraction or hypo-osmolarity. Similar cramps occur in children with severe diarrhea or vomiting.

 ## Decreased Muscle Energy

Three sources for replenishing adenosine triphosphate (ATP) during exercise are available: the phosphorylation of adenosine diphosphate (ADP) to ATP by phosphocreatine (PCr) within the exercising muscle; glycogen and lipids within the exercising muscles; and glucose and triglycerides brought to the exercising muscles by the blood. A fourth and less efficient source is derived from ADP via an alternate pathway using adenylate kinase and deaminase. PCr stores are the main source from which ATP is replenished during intense activity of short duration. During the first 30 seconds of intense endurance exercise, PCr is decreased by 35% and muscle glycogen stores are reduced by 25%. Exercise lasting longer than 30 seconds is associated with the mobilization of substantial amounts of carbohydrate and lipid.

The glucose required to sustain a single powerful contraction can be provided by the breakdown of muscle glycogen (glycogenolysis) and the anaerobic metabolism of glucose to pyruvate (glycolysis) (Figure 8–1). Anaerobic glycolysis is an inefficient mechanism for producing energy and is not satisfactory for endurance exercise. Endurance requires that pyruvate generated in muscle by glycolysis be metabolized aerobically in the mitochondria. Oxidative metabolism provides high levels of energy for every molecule of glucose metabolized (Figure 8–1).

The central compound of oxidative metabolism in mitochondria is acetylcoenzyme A (acetyl-CoA). Acetyl-CoA is derived from pyruvate, from fatty acids, and from amino acids. When exercise is prolonged, fatty acids become an important substrate to maintain muscular contraction. Acetyl-CoA is oxidized through the Krebs cycle and releases hydrogen ions that reduce nicotinamide adenine dinucleotide (NAD). These reduced compounds then enter a sequence of oxidation-reduction steps in the respiratory chain that liberate energy. Energy is stored as ATP. This process of liberating and storing energy is called *oxidation-phosphorylation coupling*. The production of energy for muscular contraction is therefore impaired by disorders that prevent the delivery of glucose or fatty acids, the oxidation process in the mitochondria, or the creation of ATP.

ISCHEMIC EXERCISE TEST

The ischemic exercise test is the first step in the diagnosis of muscle energy disorders and should be performed by every patient who develops cramps on exercise (Figure 8–2). Instructions for the procedure are outlined in Table 8–5. Ischemia is probably not necessary to do the test because if the work is sufficiently strenuous, the muscle is working at a level that exceeds the nourishment of nutrients delivered by the blood (Cwik and Brooke, 1996).

In most normal individuals, serum lactate concentrations are raised more than 20 mg/dl (2 mmol/L) and serum ammonia concentrations are raised more than 100 µg/dl (60 µmol/L) over baseline. If neither lactate nor ammonia concentration increases during the test, the subject did not exercise strenuously and the test should be repeated.

An abnormal increase in the concentration of serum creatine kinase, with or without failure to generate increased serum concentrations of lactate or ammonia, is an indication for muscle biopsy. Biopsy is likely to lead to the diagnosis if histochemical and biochemical techniques can be applied. Patients with a normal lactate and ammonia response and a normal creatine kinase concentration are unlikely to have an abnormal muscle biopsy result, but these patients should have an EMG. Muscle biopsy is indicated if EMG findings are abnormal or if the family has a history of cramps or muscle disease.

An elevated lactate concentration at rest suggests a mitochondrial myopathy. Failure to raise the serum lactate concentration more than 5 mg/dl (0.5 mmol/L) above baseline, coupled with a normal rise in ammonia concentration, is the basis for a diagnosis of glycogen storage disease. However, patients who lack debrancher

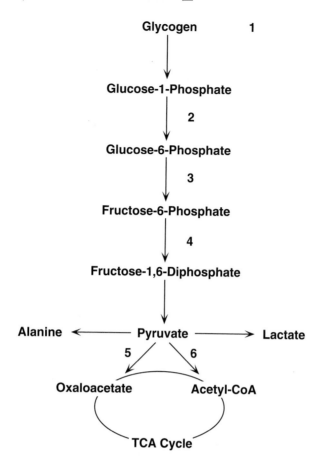

□ FIGURE 8–1 Glycogen metabolism. *1*, Myophosphorylase, initiates glycogen breakdown. *2*, Phosphoglucomutase. *3*, Phosphoglucose isomerase. *4*, Phosphofructokinase. *5*, Pyruvate carboxylase. *6*, Pyruvate dehydrogenase complex.

enzyme in both liver and muscle may have serum lactate concentrations between 5 and 10 mg/dl (0.5 to 1 mmol/L); those with only liver debrancher deficiency have a normal response.

Failure to increase ammonia concentrations more than 100 μg/dl (60 μmol/L) above baseline, coupled with a normal lactate response, suggests myoadenylate deaminase deficiency and is an indication for muscle biopsy. However, this aspect of the test produces many false-positive results.

DEFECTS OF CARBOHYDRATE UTILIZATION

Myophosphorylase Deficiency (McArdle Disease)

Myophosphorylase deficiency is transmitted by autosomal recessive inheritance. The gene defect is on chromosome 11 (Tsujino et al,

1993). Reports of autosomal dominant inheritance may represent manifesting heterozygotes. Phosphorylase activity is deficient only in muscle; the first step of glycogenolysis is prevented, and muscle glycogen is unavailable to produce glucose for energy. Liver phosphorylase concentrations are normal, and hypoglycemia does not occur.

CLINICAL FEATURES. The severity of symptoms varies with the percentage of enzyme activity. Children with only mild deficiency states have few or no symptoms until adolescence. Aching becomes increasingly prominent and then, after an episode of vigorous exercise, severe cramps are noted in the exercised muscles. Myoglobinuria is sometimes present. The pain can last for hours. Thereafter, exercise leads to repeated bouts of cramps that cause a decline in the overall level of activity. Pain begins soon after vigorous exercise is initiated, and myoglobinuria is noted several hours later. Some

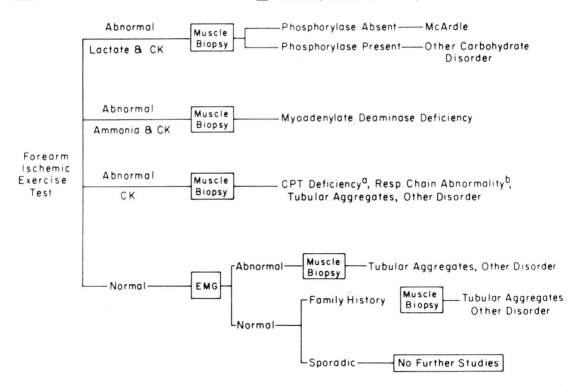

☐ FIGURE 8-2 Approach to muscle cramps and exercise intolerance. [a] Abnormal response to fasting. [b] Elevated serum lactate.

patients exercise through the pain by slowing down just before the time of fatigue. Once that point is passed, exercise may continue unimpeded. This is probably due to an increase in cardiac output, the use of blood glucose and free fatty acids as a substrate for muscle metabolism, and the recruitment of more motor units.

Examination is generally unrevealing. Muscle mass and strength and the tendon reflexes are normal. Weakness is detected only in adult patients, and even then the tendon reflexes are normal.

Myophosphorylase deficiency can also be manifested as slowly progressive proximal weakness that begins during childhood or adult life. Affected individuals may never complain of cramps on exercise or of myoglobinuria. Tendon reflexes are preserved until late in the course of disease.

DIAGNOSIS. The ischemic exercise test is the initial step to establish a defect in carbohydrate utilization. Patients with myophosphorylase deficiency develop cramps during the test and usually cannot complete the exercise, and the serum lactate concentration increases less than 5 mg/dl (0.05 mmol/L) above baseline. Normal individuals have lactate concentrations between 15 and 25 mg/dl (0.15 and 0.25 mmol/L) within

■ TABLE 8-5
Forearm Ischemic Exercise Test

1. Explain the procedure to the patient.
2. Allow the patient to rest for at least 30 minutes before the test.
3. Place the blood pressure cuff around the arm.
4. Insert the indwelling catheter in the antecubital vein and obtain blood samples for lactate, ammonia, and creatine kinase levels 10 minutes before exercise and immediately preceding it. Collect urine sample for myoglobin.
5. Inflate the cuff 20 mm Hg above systolic pressure and ask the patient to squeeze a hand dynamometer 40 times in 1 minute, and then 2 times/second for 1 minute.
6. Release the pressure in the cuff at the end of the exercise.
7. Collect blood samples for lactate, ammonia, and creatine kinase determinations at 1, 3, 5, 10, and 20 minutes following release of the cuff.
8. Collect a second urine sample for myoglobin at completion of the blood collection.

2 to 3 minutes, which rapidly decline to normal levels after 20 minutes. Cramps are not shown by EMG examination. The serum concentration of creatine kinase is elevated, and myoglobin may appear in the urine coincidentally with the cramps.

Salient features of muscle biopsy specimens are histochemical evidence of subsarcolemmal blebs containing glycogen and the absence of phosphorylase. Muscle fiber degeneration and regeneration are present immediately after an episode of cramps and myoglobinuria. Definitive diagnosis requires the biochemical demonstration of decreased myophosphorylase activity.

TREATMENT. Specific treatment is not available. Patients usually learn to live with their disorder by controlling their level of exercise.

Other Disorders of Glucose Utilization

A syndrome identical to myophosphorylase deficiency—cramps on exercise and myoglobinuria—has also been described in four other enzyme deficiencies associated with the anaerobic glycolysis of carbohydrates (see Figure 8-1). They are muscle phosphofructokinase deficiency, muscle phosphoglycerate kinase deficiency, muscle phosphoglycerate mutase deficiency, and lactate dehydrogenase deficiency. Phosphofructokinase deficiency is the most common of this group and has also been described as a cause of infantile hypotonia (see Chapter 6).

The preceding disorders are transmitted by autosomal recessive inheritance. Myophosphorylase deficiency is usually suspected because of the clinical manifestations, elevation of serum creatine kinase concentrations during attacks, and failure to produce a normal rise in venous lactate after ischemic exercise. Muscle biopsy results show subsarcolemmal collections of glycogen, but the histochemical reaction for phosphorylase is normal. These disorders are correctly identified only by biochemical analysis.

DEFECTS OF LONG-CHAIN FATTY ACID METABOLISM

Long-chain fatty acids are the principal lipid oxidized to produce acetyl-CoA.

Carnitine Palmitoyl Transferase Deficiency

Carnitine palmitoyl transferase is an essential enzyme that allows long-chain fatty acids to pass through the inner mitochondrial membrane to the inner portion of the mitochondria, where oxidation to acetyl-CoA occurs. A 50% to 75% deficiency in the activity of carnitine palmitoyl transferase produces a characteristic syndrome of exercise intolerance. The disorder is transmitted by autosomal recessive inheritance. However, the clinical expression of the deficiency varies depending on the percentage of enzyme activity and the organs involved. Carnitine palmitoyl transferase deficiency may affect several tissues other than muscle: leukocytes, platelets, fibroblasts, and liver. During periods of prolonged fasting, patients with a liver deficiency of carnitine palmitoyl transferase are slow to make ketones, and the concentration of long-chain fatty acids becomes elevated in the serum.

CLINICAL FEATURES. The features of muscle carnitine palmitoyl transferase deficiency usually begin during late childhood. No difficulty is experienced in performing even heavy exercise of short duration; energy for this activity is provided by glycogen. However, pain, tenderness, and swelling of muscles develop when sustained aerobic exercise is attempted. Severe muscle cramps, as in myophosphorylase deficiency, do not occur. Associated with the pain may be actual muscle injury characterized by increased concentrations of serum creatine kinase and the appearance of myoglobin in the urine. Muscle injury may also accompany periods of prolonged fasting, especially in patients on low-carbohydrate, high-fat diets. Prolonged exercise and prolonged fasting produce generalized muscle weakness that may lead to respiratory distress and death.

In the interval between attacks, results of muscle examination, serum concentration of creatine kinase, and EMG are usually normal, but permanent myopathy develops in some children.

DIAGNOSIS. The diagnosis is suggested by showing reduced or delayed production of ketone bodies in blood and urine when fasting. The fast should be ended by the administration of intravenous glucose at the first sign of clinical symptoms or the elevation of serum creatine kinase. Muscle biopsy may show an accumulation of lipid droplets within muscle fibers, but the results may also be normal. The definitive diagnosis requires measurement of carnitine palmitoyl transferase in platelets, fibroblasts, or muscle.

TREATMENT. Frequent carbohydrate feedings and the avoidance of prolonged aerobic activity minimize muscle destruction.

Very-Long-Chain Acyl Coenzyme A Dehydrogenase Deficiency

Four mitochondrial acyl CoA dehydrogenases are described by the chain length of their

□ F I G U R E 8 – 3 Respiratory complexes. Complex I (NADH—coenzyme Q reductase); complex II (succinate—coenzyme Q reductase); complex III (reduced coenzyme Q—cytochrome c reductase; complex IV (cytochrome c oxidase); complex V (ATP synthase).

preferred substrates: short (SCAD), medium (MCAD), long (LCAD), and very long (VLCAD). The first three are located in the mitochondrial matrix and deficiency causes recurrent coma (see Chapter 2). VLCAD is bound to the inner mitochondrial membrane and deficiency causes exercise-induced myoglobinuria (Ogilvie et al, 1994).

CLINICAL FEATURES. The only reported case is a man who developed exercise-induced muscle pain and myoglobinuria after prolonged exercise or fasting associated with aching discomfort in the legs and low back. Carbohydrate ingestion before or during exercise reduced the intensity of pain. Examination was normal.

DIAGNOSIS. Serum creatine kinase concentration is slightly elevated between attacks and increased further at the time of myoglobinuria. EMG is consistent with myopathy and muscle biopsy shows lipid storage in type I fibers. Plasma free fatty acids but not ketones increase during a 24-hour fast, suggesting impaired ketogenesis.

TREATMENT. Frequent small carbohydrate feeds are recommended.

MITOCHONDRIAL (RESPIRATORY CHAIN) MYOPATHIES

The respiratory chain, located in the inner mitochondrial membrane, consists of five protein complexes:
complex I (NADH—coenzyme Q reductase); complex II (succinate—coenzyme Q reductase); complex III (reduced coenzyme Q—cytochrome c reductase); complex IV (cytochrome c oxidase); and complex V (ATP synthase) (Figure 8-3).

Coenzyme Q is a shuttle between complexes I and II and complex III. A defect of coenzyme Q has been recorded in only one newborn, who had seizures, abnormal ocular movements, and lactic acidosis.

The clinical syndromes associated with mitochondrial disorders are continually expanding and revised (Moraes et al, 1991). The organs affected are those highly dependent on aerobic metabolism: nervous system, skeletal muscle, heart, and kidney (Table 8-6). Exercise intolerance, either alone or in combination with symptoms of other organ failure, is a common feature of mitochondrial disorders. Although several clinical syndromes have been defined, they do not correspond exactly with any one of the respiratory complexes (Table 8-7).

CLINICAL FEATURES. The age at which mitochondrial myopathies begin ranges from birth to adult life but is before 20 in 61% of patients. Half of patients have ptosis or ophthalmoplegia, one fourth have exertional complaints in the limbs, and one fourth have cerebral dysfunction. With time, considerable overlap occurs among the three groups. Seventy-five percent eventually have ophthalmoplegia and 50% have exertional complaints. Pigmentary retinopathy occurs in 33% and neuropathy in 25%.

Exercise intolerance usually develops by 10 years of age. With ordinary activity, active muscles become tight, weak, and painful, but cramps and myoglobinuria do not occur. One exception was two brothers with multiple deletions of mitochondrial DNA who had recurrent myoglobinuria and progressive weakness (Ohno et al, 1991). Nausea, headache, and breathlessness are sometimes associated features. During these episodes the serum concentration of lactate and creatine kinase may increase. Generalized weakness with ptosis and ophthalmoplegia may follow prolonged periods of activity or fasting. Such symptoms may last for several days, but recovery is usually complete.

DIAGNOSIS. A mitochondrial myopathy should be considered in all children with exer-

■ T A B L E   8 – 6
Clinical Features of Mitochondrial Disease

Nervous System
Ataxia
Central apnea
Deafness
Dementia
Hypotonia
Mental retardation
Neuropathy
Ophthalmoplegia
Optic atrophy
Retinitis pigmentosa
Heart
Cardiomyopathy
Conduction defects
Kidney
Aminoaciduria
Hyperphosphaturia
Skeletal Muscle
Exercise intolerance
Myopathy

■ T A B L E   8 – 7
Mitochondrial Disorders

Complex I (NADH—Coenzyme Q Reductase)
Congenital lactic acidosis, hypotonia, seizures, and
  apnea
Exercise intolerance and myalgia
Kearns-Sayre syndrome (see Chapter 15)
Metabolic encephalopathy, lactic acidosis, and stroke
  (see Chapter 11)
Progressive infantile poliodystrophy (see Chapter 5)
Subacute necrotizing encephalomyelopathy (see
  Chapter 5)
Complex II (Succinate—Coenzyme Q Reductase)
Encephalomyopathy (?)
**Complex III (Coenzyme QH$_2$—Cytochrome c
Reductase)**
Cardiomyopathy
Kearns-Sayre syndrome (see Chapter 15)
Myopathy and exercise intolerance with or without
  progressive external ophthalmoplegia
Complex IV (Cytochrome c Oxidase)
Fatal neonatal hypotonia (see Chapter 6)
Menkes syndrome (see Chapter 5)
Myoclonus epilepsy and ragged red fibers
Progressive infantile poliodystrophy (see Chapter 5)
Subacute necrotizing encephalomyelopathy (see
  Chapter 5)
Transitory neonatal hypotonia (see Chapter 6)
Complex V (Adenosine Triphosphate Synthase)
Congenital myopathy
Neuropathy, retinopathy, ataxia, and dementia
Retinitis pigmentosa, ataxia, neuropathy, and dementia

cise intolerance and ptosis or ophthalmoplegia. This combination of symptoms may also suggest myasthenia gravis, which can be differentiated with edrophonium chloride (Tensilon).

Some children with mitochondrial myopathies have increased concentrations of serum lactate at rest, but show lactic acidosis after exercise at 90% of predicted work rate (Nashef and Lane, 1989). Another test, easier to perform but not as sensitive as controlled exercise, is the glucose-lactate tolerance test. An ordinary oral glucose tolerance test is administered, and lactate and glucose determinations are made at the same time. In some children with mitochondrial disorders, lactic acidoses develops and glucose is slow to clear (Chi et al, 1992).

Muscle biopsy specimens show a clumping of the mitochondria, which become red when the Gomori trichrome stain is applied (Figure 8–4). These muscle cells are called *ragged-red fibers*. Only specialized laboratories can identify specific respiratory complex disturbances.

TREATMENT. Two patients with myopathy as the only feature of complex I deficiency responded to treatment with riboflavin and carnitine (Bernsen et al, 1991). Attempts to treat other patients with high doses of thiamine, menadione, or coenzyme Q have not produced encouraging results.

MYOADENYLATE DEAMINASE DEFICIENCY

The gene for the muscle form of adenosine monophosphate deaminase is encoded on chromosome 1p. Deficiency of myoadenylate deaminase is clearly a familial trait, and the mode of inheritance is probably autosomal recessive (Sinkeler et al, 1988). The deficiency state has been shown in infants with hypotonia, in children with progressive myopathies and with recurrent rhabdomyolysis (Baumeister et al, 1993), in children and adults with exercise intolerance, and in asymptomatic individuals. Establishing a cause-and-effect relationship between myoadenylate deaminase deficiency and exercise intolerance in any particular individual is often difficult because most people with the deficiency state are asymptomatic.

CLINICAL FEATURES. The typical history is one of intermittent muscle pain and weakness with exercise. The pain varies from a diffuse aching to a severe cramping type associated with muscle tenderness and swelling. Between at-

☐ F I G U R E 8 – 4 Ragged-red fibers (trichrome stain). The mitochondria are enlarged and stain intensely with hematoxylin.

tacks the children are normal. Symptoms last from 1 to 20 years, with a mean of less than 9 years.

DIAGNOSIS. During attacks the serum concentration of creatine kinase may be normal or markedly elevated. EMG and muscle histologic studies do not usually show abnormalities. The diagnosis is suggested by the ischemic exercise test (see Figure 8–2). Patients with myoadenylate deaminase deficiency fail to generate ammonia but show normal elevations of lactate. However, ammonia levels may fail to rise even in normal individuals, and enzyme analysis of muscle is required for diagnosis.

Obligate heterozygotes have reduced concentrations of myoadenylate deaminase in muscle but are capable of normal ammonia production and are asymptomatic.

TREATMENT. No treatment is available.

Myopathic Stiffness and Cramps

This section deals with several conditions that cause muscle stiffness or cramps, or both, in which the primary abnormality is thought to be in skeletal muscle.

Brody Disease

Brody disease is caused by a deficiency of calcium-activated ATPase in sarcoplasmic reticulum (Benders et al, 1994). The disorder is clearly familial but occurs only in males, suggesting X-linked inheritance.

CLINICAL FEATURES. The main clinical feature is difficulty in relaxation after contraction. Myotonia is suspected but not supported by EMG. Symptoms of exercise-induced stiffness and cramping begin in the first decade and become progressively worse with age. Unlike myotonia, stiffness becomes worse rather than better with continued exercise. Exercise can be resumed after a period of rest. Muscle strength and tendon reflexes are normal.

DIAGNOSIS. Patients with Brody disease are thought to have myotonia, but the cramps are not shown on EMG, suggesting myophosphorylase deficiency. The ischemic exercise test results are normal. Muscle biopsy results reveal type II atrophy. The diagnosis is only established by showing the biochemical defect.

TREATMENT. Dantrolene and nifedipine have been tried without success.

Cramps and Tubular Aggregates

Tubular aggregates are abnormal double-walled structures that originate from the sarcoplasmic reticulum and are located in a subsarcolemmal position (Figure 8–5). They are found in muscle biopsy specimens from patients with a variety of neuromuscular disorders but are most often present in patients with cramps or myalgia. Indeed, cramps or myalgia may be the only symptom of neuromuscular disease.

Most cases of cramps and tubular aggregates are sporadic and have a male predominance. A genetic form is transmitted by autosomal dominant inheritance.

Sporadic Cases

CLINICAL FEATURES. Onset is usually in the second or third decade. Cramps may occur at rest or be induced by exercise. Thigh and calf muscles are usually affected and become swollen, stiff, and tender. Cramping occurs more often in cold weather and may also occur at night, interfering with sleep. Myalgia is present between cramps.

Episodic stiffness of the mouth and tongue interferes with speech. Cramps are not associated with myoglobinuria. Muscle mass, strength, and tendon reflexes are normal.

DIAGNOSIS. The serum concentration of creatine kinase is normal. EMG results are normal except that in some patients the cramps are electrically silent. This suggests a disorder of

□ F I G U R E 8 – 5 Tubular aggregates (ATPase reaction). Dark material is present beneath the sarco-lemma in type I and type II fibers.

carbohydrate metabolism. An ischemic toler-ance test produces severe cramps, but lactate is generated normally with no elevation of the creatine kinase concentration.

Muscle biopsy results are the basis for a diagnosis. Light and electron microscopic ex-aminations show tubular aggregates in type II fibers. No evidence of glycogen or lipid storage is present.

TREATMENT. The cramps do not respond to medication.

Autosomal Dominant Cases

CLINICAL FEATURES. Muscle aches, cramps, and proximal weakness begin in the second de-cade (Ricker and Moxley, 1990). The cramps are exercise induced but also may occur at rest and during sleep. The legs are usually more severely affected than the arms, but the pattern of cramp-ing varies from family to family. Weakness, when it occurs, is mild and progresses slowly.

DIAGNOSIS. The serum concentration of cre-atine kinase is moderately elevated. EMG results suggest a myopathic process in some families and a neuropathic process in others. Muscle biopsy may show tubular aggregates in type I and type II fibers. Type I fiber predominance and type II hypotrophy are present in some patients.

TREATMENT. No treatment is available for either the myopathy or the cramps.

Familial X-Linked Myalgia and Cramps

Familial X-linked myalgia and cramps is a new phenotype associated with a deletion in the dystrophin gene usually associated with Duch-enne muscular dystrophy (see Chapter 7). It was described in nine males from one family (Gospe et al, 1989).

CLINICAL FEATURES. Symptoms begin in early childhood, frequently between 4 and 6 years of age. The boys first have cramps with exercise and then cramps at rest. Usually the limb muscles are affected but chest pain may occur as well. The cramping continues through-out life but is not associated with atrophy or weakness. Tendon reflexes are normal.

DIAGNOSIS. Affected family members have elevated concentrations of serum creatine ki-nase, especially after exercise. This disorder and the *McLeod phenotype* (acanthocytosis, el-evated serum concentrations of creatine kinase, and absence of the Kell antigen) are probably allelic conditions. EMG and muscle biopsy show nonspecific myopathic changes.

DNA analysis indicates a deletion in the first third of the dystrophin gene. The dystrophin molecule is smaller than normal.

TREATMENT. Phenytoin, carbamazepine, and nifedipine do not relieve the cramps. Exercise avoidance is the only way to avoid cramping.

Malignant Hyperthermia

Malignant hyperthermia is a disorder of cal-cium regulation in skeletal muscle (Heimann-Patterson, 1993). It is transmitted by autosomal dominant inheritance with variable penetrance. Attacks of muscular rigidity and necrosis in association with a rapid rise in body temperature are triggered by the administration of several inhalation anesthetics or by succinylcholine. Therefore, the syndrome is seen almost exclu-sively in the operating suite.

CLINICAL FEATURES. The first symptoms are tachycardia, tachypnea, muscle fasciculations, and increasing muscle tone. Body temperature rises dramatically, as much as 2° C per hour. All muscles become rigid, and a progressive and severe metabolic acidosis develops. Seizures and death may occur if the patient is not treated promptly.

DIAGNOSIS. The diagnosis is based on the response to anesthesia or succinylcholine. Serum concentrations of creatine kinase rise to 10 times the upper limit of normal. No reliable test for identifying susceptible individuals is available.

TREATMENT. Treatment includes termination of anesthesia, body cooling, treatment of metabolic acidosis, and intravenous injection of dantrolene, 1 to 2 mg/kg, which may be repeated every 5 to 10 minutes up to a total dose of 10 mg/kg. When malignant hyperthermia is suspected in a child, pretreatment with dantrolene before anesthetics is used.

Neuroleptic Malignant Syndrome

Neuroleptic malignant syndrome, like malignant hyperthermia, is also a disorder of the skeletal muscle calcium channel; although they have many clinical features in common, they appear to be distinct disorders (Buckley and Hutchinson, 1995).

CLINICAL FEATURES. Several neuroleptic agents may induce an idiosyncratic response characterized by muscle rigidity, hyperthermia, altered states of consciousness, and autonomic dysfunction in susceptible individuals. Phenothiazines, butyrophenones, and thioxanthenes have all been implicated. All ages have been affected, but young men predominantly. Symptoms develop over 1 to 3 days. The first symptoms are rigidity and akinesia, followed by fever, excessive sweating, urinary incontinence, and hypertension. Consciousness fluctuates, and the 20% mortality rate is due to respiratory failure.

DIAGNOSIS. The diagnosis is based primarily on clinical findings. The only helpful laboratory test results are an increased serum concentration of creatine kinase and a leukocytosis.

TREATMENT. The offending neuroleptic agent must be promptly withdrawn and general supportive care provided. Bromocriptine reverses the syndrome completely.

Rigid Spine Syndrome

Rigid spine syndrome encompasses a heterogeneous group of disorders, usually sporadic, with a male predominance. The phenotype has been associated with a vacuolar myopathy and with nemaline myopathy (Lotz and Stübgen, 1993; Topaloglu et al, 1994). Emery-Dreifuss muscular dystrophy (see Chapter 7) has similar features, but is a distinct nosologic entity.

CLINICAL FEATURES. Symptoms begin at any age, from a few months until 13 years; the average is 5 years. The first manifestation may be stiffness, weakness, or both. Exercise intolerance is common. Stiffness is characterized by marked limitation of spinal flexion, especially in the cervical and dorsolumbar portions. Scoliosis is present, and flexion contractures develop at the elbows, limiting extension. The initial symptom of weakness is usually difficulty in climbing stairs or arising from the floor. Some children are toe-walkers and may be thought to have Duchenne dystrophy.

Examination reveals a pattern of scapuloperoneal or limb-girdle weakness in addition to spinal rigidity and scoliosis. Some patients have little subcutaneous fat. Tendon reflexes are always diminished in weak muscles and sometimes in strong muscles as well.

The course is variable. In some children, weakness and rigidity progress slowly if at all. Others experience severe, progressive scoliosis that compromises respiratory effort. Contractures may form at the hip, knee, and ankle in addition to the elbow and spine. Cardiomyopathy develops in some cases, which should probably be classified as Emery-Dreifuss muscular dystrophy (see Chapter 7).

DIAGNOSIS. The serum concentration of creatine kinase is slightly elevated, and EMG is consistent with a myopathic process. Muscle biopsy usually shows fibers undergoing degeneration with fatty replacement and fibrosis. Some patients have type I predominance and others have type II predominance. Autophagic vacuoles in muscle fibers are reported in many affected children.

TREATMENT. No treatment is available for the myopathy, but scoliosis should be treated surgically to prevent respiratory distress. Patients with cardiomyopathy usually need a pacemaker.

Rippling Muscle Disease

Several families are reported under different titles in which mechanical stimulation produces electrically silent contractions. The disorder is transmitted by autosomal dominant inheritance and the responsible gene is localized to chromosome 1q in some families (Stephan et al, 1994). It is probably a disorder of skeletal muscle calcium channels that is different from the defects causing malignant hyperthermia and the neuroleptic malignant syndrome.

CLINICAL FEATURES. The onset of symptoms is usually in the second decade. Muscle pain and cramps follow exercise and persist for several hours. Stiffness occurs during rest after the patient exercises or maintains posture for long periods. Percussion of muscles causes local swelling and a peculiar rippling movement that lasts 10 to 20 seconds. Muscle hypertrophy develops. Muscle strength, tone, and coordination, as well as tendon reflexes, are normal.

DIAGNOSIS. The serum creatine kinase concentration is mildly elevated, and muscle biopsy findings are normal. EMG of the muscle swelling after percussion does not show any electrical activity.

TREATMENT. No treatment is available.

R E F E R E N C E S

Amato AA, Cornman EW, Kissel JT. Treatment of stiff-man syndrome with intravenous immunoglobulin. Neurology 1994;44:1652-1654.

Auger RG. AAEM minimonograph #44: Diseases associated with excess motor unit activity. Muscle Nerve 1994;17:1250-1263.

Baumeister FA, Gross M, Wagner DR, et al. Myoadenylate deaminase deficiency with severe rhabdomyolysis. Eur J Pediatr 1993;152:513-515.

Benders AA, Veerkamp JH, Oosternot A, et al. Ca^{2+} homostasis in Brod's disease. A study in skeletal muscle and cultured muscle cells and the effects of dantrolene and verapamil. J Clin Invest 1994;2:741-748.

Bernsen PL, Gabreels FJM, Ruitenbeek W, et al. Successful treatment of pure myopathy, associated with complex I deficiency, with riboflavin and carnitine. Arch Neurol 1991;48:334-338.

Buckley PF, Hutchinson M. Neuroleptic malignant syndrome. Neurol Neurosurg Psychiatry 1995;58:271-273.

Chi C-S, Mak S-C, Shian W-J, et al. Oral glucose lactate stimulation test in mitochondrial diseases. Pediatr Neurol 1992;8:445-449.

Cwik VA, Brooke MH. Proximal, distal, and generalized weakness. In Bradley WB, Daroff RB, Fenichel GM, et al (eds): Neurology in Clinical Practice. 2nd edition. Butterworth, Boston, 1996;359-373.

Gospe SM, Lazaro RP, Lava NS, et al. Familial x-linked myalgia and cramps: A nonprogressive myopathy associated with a deletion in the dystrophin gene. Neurology 1989;39:1277-1280.

Grimaldi LME, Martino G, Braghi S, et al. Heterogeneity of autoantibodies in stiffman syndrome. Ann Neurol 1993;34:57-64

Heiman-Patterson TD. Neuroleptic malignant syndrome and malignant hyperthermia. Med Clin North Am 1993;71:477-492.

Hudson AJ, Ebers GC, Bulman DE. The skeletal muscle sodium and chloride channel diseases. Brain 1995;118:547-563.

Lotz BP, Stübgen J-P. The rigid spine syndrome: A vacuolar variant. Muscle Nerve 1993;16:530-536.

Moraes CT, Schon EA, DiMauro S. Mitochondrial diseases: Toward a rational classification. In Appel SH, ed: Current Neurology, Vol 11. Mosby-Year Book, St Louis, 1991; 83.

Nashef L, Lane RJM. Screening for mitochondrial cytopathies: The sub-anaerobic threshold exercise test (SATET). J Neurol Neurosurg Psychiatry 1989;52:1090-1094.

Ogilvie I, Pourfarzam M, Jackson S, et al. Very long-chain acyl coenzyme A dehydrogenase deficiency presenting with exercise-induced myoglobinuria. Neurology 1994;44:467-473.

Ohno K, Tanakas M, Sahashi K, et al. Mitochondrial DNA deletions in inherited recurrent myoglobinuria. Ann Neurol 1991;29:364-369.

Pascuzzi RM, Gratianne R, Azzarelli B, et al. Schwartz-Jampel syndrome with dominant inheritance. Muscle Nerve 1990;13:1152-1163.

Ricker K, Moxley RT. Autosomal dominant cramping disease. Arch Neurol 1990;47:810-812.

Ricker K, Moxley RT, Heine R, et al. Myotonia fluctuans. A third type of muscle sodium channel disease. Arch Neurol 1994;51:1095-1102.

Shannon M. Clinical toxicity of cocaine adulterants. Ann Emerg Med 1988;17:1243-1247.

Sinkeler SP, Joosten MG, Wevers RA, et al. Myoadenylate deaminase deficiency: A clinical, genetic, and biochemical study in nine families. Muscle Nerve 1988;11:312.

Stephan DA, Buist NRM, Chittenden AB, et al. A rippling muscle disease gene is localized to 1q41: Evidence for multiple genes. Neurology 1994;44:1915-1920.

Tahmoush AJ, Alonso RJ, Tahmoush GP, et al. Cramp-fasciculation syndrome: A treatable hyperexcitable peripheral nerve disorder. Neurology 1991;41:1021-1024.

Teasley J, Garcia C, Malamut R, et al. Tocainide in pediatric patients with myotonia congenita [Abstract] Neurology 1990;40 (suppl 1):205.

Topaloglu H, Gogus S, Yalaz K, et al. Two siblings with nemaline myopathy presenting with rigid spine syndrome. Neuromusc Dis 1994;4:263-267.

Tsujino S, Shanske S, DiMauro S. Molecular genetic heterogeneity of myophosphorylase deficiency (McArdle's Disease). N Engl J Med 1993;329:241-245.

9
Sensory and Autonomic Disturbances

This chapter deals primarily with disturbed or lost sensation in the limbs and trunk. Autonomic disturbances are often associated with sensory loss but sometimes occur alone. Sensory disturbances of the face are considered in Chapter 17.

 ## Sensory Symptoms

The important symptoms of disturbed sensation are pain, dysesthesias, and loss of sensibility. Peripheral neuropathy is the most common cause of disturbed sensation at any age. As a rule, hereditary neuropathies are more likely to cause loss of sensibility without discomfort, whereas acquired neuropathies are more likely to be painful. Discomfort is more likely than numbness to bring a patient to medical attention.

Nerve root pain generally follows the course of a dermatome and is ordinarily described as deep and aching. The pain is more proximal than distal and may be constant or intermittent. When intermittent, the pain may radiate in a dermatomal distribution. The most common cause of root pain in adults is sciatica associated with lumbar disk disease. Disk disease also occurs in adolescents, usually because of trauma. In children root pain is more commonly caused by radiculitis. Examples of radiculitis are the migratory aching of a limb preceding paralysis in

the Guillain-Barré syndrome (see Chapter 7) and the radiating pain in a C5 distribution that heralds an idiopathic brachial neuritis (see Chapter 13).

Polyneuropathy involving small nerve fibers causes dysesthetic pain. This pain differs from previously experienced discomfort and is described as pins and needles, tingling, or burning. It is often compared to the abnormal sensation felt when dental anesthesia is wearing off. The discomfort is superficial, distal, and usually symmetric. Dysesthetic pain is never a feature of hereditary neuropathies in children.

Loss of sensibility is the sole initial feature in children with sensory neuropathy. Diagnosis is often delayed because clumsiness is the initial feature and strength is normal, as are tests of cerebellar function. Tendon reflexes are absent. The combination of areflexia and clumsiness should suggest a sensory neuropathy.

The pattern of sensory loss as a guide to the anatomic site of abnormality is summarized in Table 9–1.

 ## Brachial Neuritis

Three painful arm syndromes are acute idiopathic brachial neuritis (neuralgic amyotrophy), familial recurrent brachial neuritis, and reflex sympathetic dystrophy. The first two are char-

TABLE 9–1
Patterns of Sensory Loss

PATTERN	SITE
Glove-and-stocking	Peripheral nerve
One leg	Plexus or spinal cord
One arm	Plexus
Both legs	Spinal cord or peripheral nerve
Legs and trunk	Spinal cord
All limbs	Spinal cord or peripheral nerve
Unilateral arm and leg	Brain or spinal cord

acterized by some initial pain in the shoulder or arm, which then subsides and is followed by muscle atrophy. Weakness is the prominent feature, and these two syndromes are therefore discussed in Chapter 13. Although muscle atrophy also occurs in reflex sympathetic dystrophy, pain is the prominent feature and this syndrome is discussed later in this chapter.

 Congenital Insensitivity (Indifference) to Pain

Most children with congenital insensitivity to pain have a hereditary sensory neuropathy (Larner et al, 1994). Specific tests for sensory neuropathy and complete postmortem examinations were not performed in many early reports of this condition. This section is restricted to those children and families with congenital insensitivity to pain in whom sensory neuropathy was excluded and a central defect is at fault (Landrieu et al, 1990). Such children are often mentally retarded as well, and testing pain sensation is difficult. The Lesch-Nyhan syndrome is a specific disorder characterized by self-mutilation (presumably because of indifference to pain) and mental retardation without evidence of sensory neuropathy (see Chapter 5).

CLINICAL FEATURES. Children with congenital insensitivity to pain come to medical attention when they begin to crawl or walk. Their parents recognize that injuries do not cause crying and that children fail to learn the potential of injury from experience. The result is repeated bruising, fractures, ulcerations of the fingers and toes, and mutilation of the tongue. Sunburn and frostbite are common.

Examination shows absence of the corneal reflex and insensitivity to pain and temperature but relative preservation of touch and vibration sensations. Tendon reflexes are present, an important differential point from sensory neuropathy.

DIAGNOSIS. The results of electromyography (EMG), nerve conduction studies, and examination of the cerebrospinal fluid are normal.

TREATMENT. No treatment is available for the underlying insensitivity, but supportive care is needed for the repeated injuries. Life is shortened by injuries and recurrent infections.

 Foramen Magnum Tumors

Extramedullary tumors in and around the foramen magnum are known for false localizing signs and for mimicking other disorders, especially syringomyelia and multiple sclerosis. In children, neurofibroma caused by neurofibromatosis is the only tumor found in this location.

CLINICAL FEATURES. The most common initial symptom is unilateral or bilateral dysesthesias of the fingers. Half of patients experience suboccipital or neck pain. These two symptoms are often ignored early in the course. Numbness and tingling usually begin in one hand and then migrate to the other. Dysesthesias in the feet are a late occurrence. Gait disturbances, incoordination of the hands, and bladder disturbances generally follow the sensory symptoms and are so alarming that they prompt medical consultation.

Many patients have café au lait spots, but few have evidence of subcutaneous neuromas. Weakness may be confined to one arm, one side, or both legs; 25% of patients have weakness in all limbs. Atrophy of the hands is uncommon. Sensory loss may involve only one segment or may have a "cape" distribution. Pain and temperature are usually diminished, and other sensory disturbances may be present. Tendon reflexes are brisk in the arms and legs.

Patients with neurofibromatosis may have multiple neurofibromas causing segmental abnormalities in several levels of the spinal cord.

DIAGNOSIS. Magnetic resonance imaging (MRI) is the best method for showing abnormalities at the foramen magnum.

TREATMENT. Symptoms can be relieved completely by surgical excision of a neurofibroma of the C2 root.

 Hereditary Metabolic Neuropathies

ACUTE INTERMITTENT PORPHYRIA

Acute intermittent porphyria is transmitted by autosomal dominant inheritance. It is characterized by at least 50% deficiency in the activity of porphobilinogen deaminase. Individuals with similar degrees of enzyme deficiency may have considerable variation in phenotypic expression (Kauppinen and Mustajoki, 1992).

CLINICAL FEATURES. Approximately 90% of individuals with acute intermittent porphyria never have clinical symptoms. The minority who do become symptomatic have no difficulty before puberty. Symptoms are periodic and occur at irregular intervals. The attacks are triggered by alterations in hormonal levels during a normal menstrual cycle or pregnancy and by exposure to certain drugs, barbiturates especially. Most attacks begin with abdominal pain, which is often followed by nausea and vomiting. Pain in the limbs is common, and muscle weakness often develops. The weakness is a result of a motor neuropathy that causes greater weakness in proximal than distal muscles and in the arms more than the legs. Tendon reflexes are usually decreased and may be absent in weak muscles. Approximately half of patients have symptoms of cerebral dysfunction; mental changes are particularly common, and seizures can sometimes occur. Hypertension and tachycardia may accompany attacks. Chronic mental symptoms, such as depression and anxiety, sometimes continue even between attacks.

DIAGNOSIS. The risk of attacks correlates with the excretion of porphobilinogen in the urine when the patient is free of symptoms. Diagnosis is usually made by measuring porphobilinogen deaminase activity in red blood cells and urine, but erythrocyte deaminase activity is normal in some families.

TREATMENT. The most important aspect of managing symptomatic disease is to prevent acute attacks. This is done in part by avoiding known precipitating factors. During an attack, patients frequently need to be hospitalized because of severe pain. Carbohydrates are believed to reduce porphyrin synthesis and should be administered intravenously daily at a dose of 300 to 500 g as a 10% dextrose solution.

Intravenous infusions of hematin is in general use to prevent attacks and abort attacks in progress. It is given over 30 minutes or more in doses of 4 mg/kg every 12 hours during an acute attack, and 200 mg weekly to prevent attacks.

HEREDITARY TYROSINEMIA

Hereditary tyrosinemia is transmitted by autosomal recessive inheritance and is caused by deficiency of the enzyme fumarylacetoacetate hydrolase (Mitchell et al, 1990).

CLINICAL FEATURES. The major features are acute and chronic liver failure and a renal Fanconi syndrome. However, recurrent attacks of painful dysesthesias or paralysis are often the most prominent feature of the disease.

The attacks usually begin at 1 year of age, and are preceded by an infection in half of cases. Perhaps because of the child's age, the pain is poorly localized to the legs and lower abdomen. Associated with the pain is axial hypertonicity that ranges in severity from mild neck stiffness to opisthotonos. Generalized weakness occurs in 30% of attacks and may necessitate respiratory support. Less common features of attacks are seizures and self-mutilation. Between attacks, the child appears normal.

DIAGNOSIS. The diagnosis of hereditary tyrosinemia is based on showing increased blood concentrations of tyrosine and deficiency of fumarylacetoacetate hydrolase. The crises are caused in part by an acute axonal neuropathy that can be shown by EMG studies. Succinylacetone, a metabolite of tyrosine, accumulates and inhibits porphyrin metabolism. Increased urinary excretion of gamma-aminolevulinic acid is present in both acute intermittent porphyria and hereditary tyrosinemia.

TREATMENT. Children with hereditary tyrosinemia are treated with a special diet similar to the one used for phenylketonuria (see Chapter 5). During a crisis, high-carbohydrate gavage without phenylalanine or tyrosine is used to provide adequate caloric intake. Narcotics may be needed to control pain.

 ## Hereditary Sensory and Autonomic Neuropathy

The classification of hereditary sensory and autonomic neuropathy (HSAN) provided in Table 9–2 is modified from the one suggested by Dyck (1993). This classification attempts to synthesize information based on natural history, mode of inheritance, and electrophysiologic characteristics. Many of these phenotypes may be caused by several different genetic errors. In addition to the cases listed, several other disorders are described whose genetic status remains uncertain. Among these is *congenital sensory neuropathy with selective loss of small myelinated fibers,* classified as HSAN V, in which pain fibers are lost selectively.

■ TABLE 9-2
Disturbances of Sensation

Brachial Neuritis
Neuralgic amyotrophy (see Chapter 13)
Recurrent familial brachial neuropathy (see Chapter 13)
Congenital Insensitivity (Indifference) to Pain
Mental retardation
Lesch-Nyhan syndrome
With normal nervous system
Foramen Magnum Tumors
Hereditary Metabolic Neuropathies
Acute intermittent porphyria
Hereditary tyrosinemia
Hereditary Sensory and Autonomic Neuropathy (HSAN)
HSAN I (autosomal dominant)
HSAN II (autosomal recessive)
HSAN III (familial dysautonomia)
HSAN IV (with anhydrosis)
X-linked hereditary sensory neuropathy
HSAN with spastic paraplegia
Familial distal dysautonomia
Familial amyloid neuropathy
Lumbar Disk Herniation
Reflex Sympathetic Dystrophy
Syringomyelia
Thalamic Syndromes

HEREDITARY SENSORY AND AUTONOMIC NEUROPATHY TYPE I

Hereditary sensory and autonomic neuropathy type I (HSAN I) appears in the literature under several names, most commonly *hereditary sensory radiculoneuropathy*. Transmission is by autosomal dominant inheritance. As with other dominantly inherited neuropathies, variable expression is the rule. Therefore, history alone is insufficient to determine whether parents are affected; physical examination and electrophysiologic studies are required.

CLINICAL FEATURES. Symptoms begin during the second decade or later (Ouvrier et al, 1990). The major clinical features are lancinating pains in the legs and ulcerations of the feet. However, initial symptoms are usually insidious and the precise onset is often difficult to date. A callus develops on the sole of the foot, usually in the skin overlying a weight-bearing bony prominence. The callus blackens, becomes necrotic, and breaks down into an ulcer that is difficult to heal. The ulcer is preceded by sensory loss, but often it is the ulcer and not the sensory loss that first brings the patient to medical attention. Although plantar ulcers are an important fea-

ture, they are not essential for diagnosis. Most patients with HSAN I do not have ulcers. When the proband in a kindred has typical features of plantar ulcers and lancinating pain, other family members may have sensory loss in the feet, mild pes cavus or peroneal atrophy, and loss of the ankle tendon reflex.

Sensory loss in the feet is a constant feature, whereas sensory loss in the hands is variable. The hands are never affected as severely as the feet, and finger ulcers do not occur. The sensations of pain and temperature are lost before the sensations of touch and pressure. In some patients the dissociation of sensory loss is constant, whereas in others the dissociation is only a first stage before the development of global sensory loss. The ankle tendon reflex is absent, and the quadriceps tendon reflex may also be absent. Tendon reflexes in the arms are preserved.

Foot ulcers are caused by trauma to the insensitive skin of the feet. They occur more often and are more difficult to heal in boys than in girls, in individuals who wear ill-fitting shoes, and in individuals who are on their feet much of the day. Lancinating pain is a late occurrence. It comes as recurring attacks usually affecting a single arm or leg. Other limbs may be affected on subsequent days. The intensity of pain varies.

DIAGNOSIS. Autosomal dominant inheritance and sensory loss in the feet are essential for the diagnosis. The presence of plantar ulcers and lancinating pain is helpful but are not critical for the diagnosis. HSAN I can be differentiated from familial amyloid polyneuropathy on clinical grounds. Urinary incontinence, impotence, and postural hypotension are frequent features of amyloidosis but do not occur in HSAN I.

Electrophysiologic studies show slowing of sensory nerve conduction velocity and reduced amplitude of sensory action potentials. Sural nerve biopsy reveals a marked decrease or absence of myelinated fibers and a mild to moderate reduction of small myelinated fibers.

TREATMENT. No treatment is available for the neuropathy, but plantar ulcers can be prevented by good foot care. Tight shoes and activities that cause trauma to the feet should be avoided. Weight bearing must be discontinued at the first sign of a plantar ulcer. Much of the foot mutilation reported in previous years was due to secondary infection of the ulcers. This should be avoided by warm soaks, elevation, and antibiotics.

HEREDITARY SENSORY AND AUTONOMIC NEUROPATHY TYPE II

Hereditary sensory and autonomic neuropathy type II (HSAN II) probably includes several disorders transmitted by autosomal recessive inheritance. Some are relatively static and others have a progressive course (Ferriére et al, 1992). Many of the cases are sporadic, instances of parental consanguinity have been reported, and siblings are affected in some families.

CLINICAL FEATURES. Symptoms probably begin during infancy and possibly at the time of birth. Infantile hypotonia is common (see Chapter 6). Unlike HSAN I, which affects primarily the feet, HSAN II involves the arms and legs equally, as well as the trunk and forehead. The result is a diffuse loss of all sensation; touch and pressure are probably affected earlier and to a greater extent than temperature and pain. Affected infants and children are constantly hurting themselves without a painful response and are sometimes believed to have "congenital absence of pain" (Ouvrier et al, 1990). The absence of the protection that pain provides against injury results in ulcerations and infections of the fingers and toes, stress fractures, and injuries to long bones. Loss of deep sensibility causes injury and swelling of joints, and loss of touch makes simple tasks, such as tying shoes, manipulating small objects, and buttoning buttons, difficult if not impossible. Tendon reflexes are absent throughout. Sweating is diminished in all areas of decreased sensibility, but no other features of autonomic dysfunction are present.

HSAN II may be associated with impaired hearing, taste, and smell, with retinitis pigmentosa, or with the early onset of cataracts. It is not clear whether such children represent separate genetic disorders or are part of the phenotypic spectrum of a single genetic disorder.

DIAGNOSIS. The diagnosis relies primarily on the history and examination. Absence of sensory potentials confirms that the congenital absence of pain is due to peripheral neuropathy and not to a cerebral abnormality. Motor nerve conduction velocities are normal, as are the morphologic characteristics of motor unit potentials. Fibrillations are sometimes present. Sural nerve biopsy reveals an almost complete absence of myelinated fibers.

The boundary between HSAN II and HSAN IV (discussed later) is difficult to delineate. Mental retardation and anhydrosis are more prominent in HSAN IV than in HSAN II.

TREATMENT. No treatment is available for the neuropathy. However, parents must be vigilant for painless injuries. Discoloration of the skin and swelling of joints or limbs should raise the possibility of fracture. Children must be taught to avoid activities that might cause injury and to examine themselves for signs of superficial infection.

HEREDITARY SENSORY AND AUTONOMIC NEUROPATHY TYPE III

Hereditary sensory and autonomic neuropathy type III (HSAN III) is ordinarily referred to as *familial dysautonomia* or the *Riley-Day syndrome*. This disorder is present at birth. Cardinal feature are hypotonia, feeding difficulties, and poor control of autonomic function. Because neonatal hypotonia is prominent, the disorder is discussed in Chapter 6.

HEREDITARY SENSORY AND AUTONOMIC NEUROPATHY TYPE IV

Hereditary sensory and autonomic neuropathy type IV (HSAN IV) is probably a heterogeneous group of disorders transmitted by autosomal recessive inheritance. The major features are congenital insensitivity to pain, anhidrosis, and mental retardation (Rosemberg et al, 1994). All the clinical abnormalities are present at birth, and although complications of the pain-free state are a continuous problem, the underlying disease may not be progressive.

CLINICAL FEATURES. The initial symptoms are usually caused by anhidrosis rather than insensitivity to pain. Affected infants have repeated episodes of fever, sometimes associated with seizures. These episodes usually occur during the summer and are caused by the inability to sweat in response to exogenous heat. Sweat glands are present in the skin but lack sympathetic innervation. Most infants are hypotonic and areflexic. Developmental milestones are attained slowly, and by 2 or 3 years of age the child has had several self-inflicted injuries caused by pain insensitivity. Injuries may include ulcers of the fingers and toes, stress fractures, self-mutilation of the tongue, and Charcot joints.

Sensory examination shows widespread absence of pain and temperature sensation. Touch, vibration, and stereognosis are intact in some patients. Tendon reflexes are absent or hypoactive. The cranial nerves are intact and the corneal reflex and lacrimation are normal. Mild to moderate retardation is present in almost every case.

Other features, present in some children, are blond hair and fair skin, Horner syndrome, and aplasia of dental enamel.

DIAGNOSIS. Familial dysautonomia (HSAN III) and HSAN IV have many features in common and are easily confused. However, insensitivity to pain is not prominent in HSAN III and fungiform papillae of the tongue are present in HSAN IV. Anhidrotic ectodermal dysplasia is another hereditary disorder that shares many features with HSAN IV. Affected children also have unexplained fevers and abnormalities of tooth formation. However, children with ectodermal dysplasia are anhidrotic because sweat glands are absent. The nervous system is intact, and sensation to pain is present. Diagnosis of HSAN IV depends primarily on the clinical features but can be confirmed by demonstrating the absence of sensory evoked potentials, the absence of an axon reflex when histamine is injected into the skin, and the presence of sweat glands on skin biopsy specimens.

TREATMENT. No treatment is available for the underlying disease. However, constant vigilance is required to prevent injuries to the skin and bones with secondary infection.

X-LINKED HEREDITARY SENSORY NEUROPATHY

X-linked hereditary sensory neuropathy is a rare disorder described in five members of one family (Jestico et al, 1985).

CLINICAL FEATURES. Painless deformities of the feet characterized by calcaneovalgus and loss of arch are noted between the ages of 3 and 13. Repeated trauma to the feet leads to painless ulcerations. Pain and touch sensations in the feet are reduced but not absent. The ankle tendon reflex is difficult to elicit but may be obtained with reinforcement. Other tendon reflexes are present. Autonomic function is preserved.

The rate of progression varies. Ulcers tend to enlarge and lead to osteomyelitis, which may necessitate amputation. The neuropathy remains limited to the feet.

DIAGNOSIS. The only abnormality on EMG is reduction or absence of the sural nerve potential. Motor conduction velocities and motor unit potentials are normal. Sural nerve biopsy shows selective loss of the small-diameter myelinated fibers.

TREATMENT. No treatment is available, but

management requires the same concern for foot care as outlined for HSAN I.

HEREDITARY SENSORY AND AUTONOMIC NEUROPATHY WITH SPASTIC PARAPLEGIA

Most cases of hereditary sensory and autonomic neuropathy with spastic paraplegia have occurred in siblings and autosomal recessive inheritance is suspected (Thomas et al, 1994). Some patients with HSAN I or HSAN II have mild signs of corticospinal tract dysfunction, such as brisk reflexes and extensor plantar responses, but it is reasonable to consider these cases separately at the present.

CLINICAL FEATURES. The initial clinical feature may be progressive sensory neuropathy or spasticity, but eventually the sensory symptoms, affecting all modalities, cause the predominant disability. Children with early spasticity have a stiff-legged gait during infancy or early childhood and delayed motor milestones. Tendon reflexes in the legs are increased, plantar responses are extensor, and sphincter control may not be attained.

The sensory neuropathy is first noticed by the parents as a relative insensitivity to pain. This is characterized by repeated episodes of injury, ulcerations of the fingers and toes, and fractures. Pain and temperature sensations are much more severely affected than are the sensations of touch and vibration.

Intelligence is normal, and cranial nerves are unaffected. As the neuropathy becomes more profound, tendon reflexes, which initially were brisk, become depressed and are lost. When the disease begins during infancy or early childhood, the course is relentlessly progressive and may lead to early death. Disease with onset in the second decade has a slower progression.

DIAGNOSIS. A diagnosis cannot be established during early stages of the disease when spastic paraplegia is present but neuropathy is not. The development of insensitivity to pain and ulcers of the feet and fingers are essential for the diagnosis. Nerve conduction studies show prolonged sensory latencies and a reduced amplitude of action potentials. Motor conduction velocity may be normal. Sural nerve biopsy shows an axonopathy with a profound loss of myelinated fibers of all diameters and also of some unmyelinated fibers.

TREATMENT. No treatment for the underlying disease is available, but symptomatic care is needed to prevent injury to the hands and feet.

FAMILIAL DISTAL DYSAUTONOMIA

Familial distal dysautonomia is transmitted by autosomal dominant inheritance and was described in three generations of a single family (Robinson et al, 1989).

CLINICAL FEATURES. Symptoms begin during childhood. Vasodilation is not induced by exercise, and burning pain occurs in the digits because of ischemia. Running causes swelling and reddening of the feet. The skin of the hands and feet is dry and cracks easily. Pedal pulses, tendon reflexes, and sensation are normal. The disorder does not shorten life expectancy.

DIAGNOSIS. Warming of the hands or feet does not produce sweating. Motor and sensory nerve conduction is normal.

TREATMENT. Vasodilatory agents and sympathetic nerve block are not helpful. Symptoms are best managed by alterations in lifestyle.

FAMILIAL AMYLOID POLYNEUROPATHY

Familial amyloid polyneuropathy is a heterogenous group of disorders, all transmitted by autosomal dominant inheritance, in which amyloid is deposited in the peripheral somatic and autonomic nervous systems. The abnormality is caused by a mutation in the gene for prealbumin located on chromosome 18 (Benson, 1995). Other organs may be affected. The disorder has been described in several different nationalities and in each one a different subunit protein is affected.

CLINICAL FEATURES. Symptoms begin between the second and seventh decades, most often between the ages of 25 and 35. Dysesthesias are an early feature. Pain and temperature sensations are lost first, followed by touch, pressure, and vibration sensations. Lancinating pains and foot ulcers may be present, suggesting the diagnosis of HSAN I. However, autonomic dysfunction is much more profound and occurs earlier in the course of amyloid neuropathy than in HSAN I. Symptoms of autonomic dysfunction include impotence, constipation, diarrhea, fecal or urinary incontinence, and anhidrosis. Cardiac involvement is relatively common, as evidenced by bundle branch block, left ventricular hypertrophy, and atrioventricular dissociation. Postural hypotension occurs in approximately 10% of patients.

Motor involvement is a late feature; weakness and atrophy occur in both the hands and the feet. Tendon reflexes are depressed or absent in all limbs. Symptoms of other organ involvement tend to be mild. Vitreous opacities and perivascular amyloid deposition in retinal vessels are common. Some patients have proteinuria, but renal insufficiency is rare.

The course of disease is a steady progression, leading to cachexia and death within 15 years. Postmortem studies show amyloid deposition predominantly in peripheral nerves and blood vessels and to a lesser degree in cardiac muscle, smooth muscle, spleen, and kidneys.

DIAGNOSIS. Clinical symptoms of a hereditary mixed motor sensory neuropathy with prominent autonomic dysfunction should suggest the diagnosis of familial amyloid polyneuropathy. Electrophysiologic findings are consistent with a mixed motor sensory neuropathy of the axonal type. Examination shows amyloid deposition around the sural nerve causing compression within the endoneurium and in the walls of the vasa nervorum.

TREATMENT. No treatment is available for the underlying disease. Cardiac arrhythmias may necessitate a permanent cardiac pacemaker. Treatment of autonomic dysfunction is symptomatic.

 Lumbar Disk Herniation

Lumbar disk herniation in children is usually caused by trauma. Almost all cases occur after age 10; they are more common in boys than in girls and are frequently sports related. Because lumbar disk herniation is unusual in children, diagnosis may be delayed for months or years.

CLINICAL FEATURES. Sciatica or back pain or both are the initial features. Twenty percent of patients never have back pain, but all have sciatica at some time in the course. Almost half of patients report bilateral sciatica.

Physical findings may include diminished lumbar lordosis, vertebral muscle spasm, and scoliosis. The patient tries to hold the lumbar spine rigid. Point tenderness may be present over the involved disk space. Straight leg raising usually provokes sciatica. Sensation to pinprick may be diminished in the distribution of the L5-S1 dermatome, and the ankle tendon reflex is diminished or absent in more than half of patients.

DIAGNOSIS. Radiographs of the lumbosacral spine reveal minor congenital anomalies (hemivertebrae, sacralization of the lumbar spine) in an unusually large number of cases. The diagnosis is confirmed by computed tomography of the spine or by myelography.

TREATMENT. Bed rest provides immediate relief in the majority of patients, but surgery is sometimes required for permanent relief of symptoms.

 Reflex Sympathetic Dystrophy

In the medical literature, reflex sympathetic dystrophy has several names, including *causalgia, algodystrophy, neurovascular reflex dystrophy, post-traumatic sympathetic dystrophy,* and *Sudeck atrophy.* The essential feature is sustained burning pain in a limb, combined with vasomotor and pseudomotor dysfunction, leading to atrophic changes in skin, muscle, and bone following trauma. The inciting trauma, which may be accidental or surgical, injures the nerves in a limb or the cervical spinal cord. The mechanism of reflex sympathetic dystrophy remains a debated issue, and several different central and peripheral mechanisms probably produce the same result (Bhatia et al, 1993).

CLINICAL FEATURES. The mean age at onset in children is 11 years, and girls are affected more often than boys (Wilder et al, 1992). Reflex sympathetic dystrophy frequently follows trauma to one limb with or without fracture. The trauma may be relatively minor, and the clinical syndrome is so unusual that many affected individuals are first labeled "hysterical" or "malingering." Time until onset after injury is usually within 1 or 2 months, but the average interval from injury to diagnosis is 1 year.

The first symptom is pain at the site of injury, which progresses either proximally or distally without regard for dermatomal distribution or anatomic landmarks. Generalized swelling and vasomotor disturbances of the limb follow in 80% of children. Pain is intense, described as burning or aching, and is out of proportion to the injury. It may be maximally severe at onset or may become progressively worse for 3 to 6 months. Pain is exacerbated by movement or dependence, causing the arm to be held in a position of abduction and internal rotation as if it were swaddled to the body. The hand becomes swollen and hyperesthetic and feels warmer.

Children with reflex sympathetic dystrophy do better than adults. Reported outcomes vary widely, probably based on the standard of diagnosis. In my own experience, most begin recovering within 6 to 12 months. Long-term pain is unusual, as are the trophic changes of the skin and bones that often occur in adults. Recovery is usually complete and recurrence is unusual.

DIAGNOSIS. The diagnosis is based on the clinical features and cannot be confirmed by laboratory tests. Because the syndrome follows accidental or surgical trauma, litigation is commonplace, and careful documentation of the examination is needed. One simple test is to immerse the affected limb in warm water. Wrinkling of the skin of the fingers or toes requires an intact sympathetic innervation. The absence of wrinkling is evidence of a lesion in either the central or the peripheral sympathetic pathway. The other unaffected limb is used as a control.

TREATMENT. I have been satisfactorily treating children with range of motion exercises and over-the-counter analgesics. Treatment of more severe syndromes, as occur in adults, includes the oral administration of guanethidine, 20 to 30 mg/day, prednisone with or without stellate ganglion blockade, and sympathectomy.

 Syringomyelia

Syringomyelia is a generic term for a fluid-filled cavity within the substance of the spinal cord (Gower et al, 1994). The cavity varies in length and may extend into the brainstem. Such a cephalic extension is termed *syringobulbia.* The cavity, or *syrinx,* is centrally placed in the gray matter and may enlarge in all directions. The cervicothoracic region is a favorite site, but thoracolumbar syrinx also occurs, and occasionally a syrinx extends from the brainstem to the conus medullaris.

The mechanism of syrinx formation has been debated. Cavitation of the spinal cord sometimes follows trauma and infarction, but these are not important mechanisms of syringomyelia in children. In childhood, primary syringomyelia is generally regarded as either a congenital malformation or a cystic astrocytoma. In the past, a congenital cyst could be distinguished from astrocytoma only by postmortem examination. Astrocytomas of the spinal cord, like those of the cerebellum, may have large cysts with only a nubbin of solid tumor. The development of MRI has greatly enhanced antemortem diagnosis of cystic astrocytoma by showing small areas of increased signal intensity in one or more portions of the cyst. Cystic astrocytoma is more likely to produce symptoms during the first decade, whereas congenital syringomyelia becomes symptomatic in the second decade or later and is usually associated with the Chiari anomaly. Cystic astrocytoma of the spinal cord is considered further in Chapters 12 and 13; this section deals primarily with congenital syringomyelia.

CLINICAL FEATURES. The initial symptoms of syringomyelia depend on the cyst location. Because the cavity is near the central canal, crossing fibers subserving pain and temperature are often affected first. When the syrinx is in the cervical area, pain and temperature are typically lost in a "cape" or "vest" distribution. However, early involvement is often unilateral or at least asymmetric and sometimes involves the fingers before the shoulders. Touch and pressure are ordinarily preserved until the cyst enlarges into the posterior columns or the dorsal root entry zone. Loss of pain sensibility in the hands often leads to injury, ulceration, and infection, as seen in hereditary sensory and autonomic neuropathies. Pain is not ordinarily a feature of syringomyelia, but lancinating limb pain is occasionally reported.

Scoliosis is common and torticollis may be an initial sign in children with cervical cavities. As the cavity enlarges into the ventral horn, weakness and atrophy develop in the hands and may be associated with fasciculations; pressure on the lateral columns causes hyperreflexia and spasticity in the legs. Very long cavities may produce lower motor neuron signs in all four limbs. Sphincter control is sometimes impaired. The posterior columns are generally the last to be affected, so that vibration sense and touch are preserved until relatively late in the course. The progress of symptoms is extremely slow and insidious. The spinal cord accommodates well to the slowly developing pressure within. Thus, at the time a physician is consulted, a long history of minor neurologic handicap such as clumsiness or difficulty running may be elicited.

Bulbar signs are relatively uncommon and usually asymmetric. They include hemiatrophy of the tongue with deviation on protrusion, facial weakness, dysphasia, and dysarthria. The descending pathway of the trigeminal nerve is frequently affected, causing loss of pain and temperature sensations on the same side of the face as the facial weakness and tongue hemiatrophy.

□ F I G U R E 9 – 1 Cervical syringomyelia. MRI demonstrates a long cavity, beginning *(arrow)* just below the foramen magnum.

DIAGNOSIS. MRI is the diagnostic test of choice. It not only shows the cavity (Figure 9–1) and the Chiari malformation, but also shows the presence of small foci of glioma.

TREATMENT. An approach to surgical management has been developed based on MRI criteria (Milhorat et al, 1992). Syrinxes occurring with hydrocephalus and communicating with the fourth ventricle do well following ventriculoperitoneal shunt. Syrinxes associated with Chiari I malformations collapse after shunting from the syrinx to the cerebellopontine angle, and noncommunicating syrinxes often collapse after excision of an extramedullary obstruction.

 Thalamic Pain

The thalamic pain syndrome of Dejerine and Roussy occurs almost exclusively in adults following infarction of the thalamus or of the white matter of the parietal lobe. Similar symptoms sometimes occur in patients with thalamic glioma. Such tumors more often produce hemiparesis than thalamic pain.

CLINICAL FEATURES. Touching the affected limb or part of the body produces intense discomfort described as "sharp," "crushing," or "burning." Suffering is considerable, and the quality of pain is unfamiliar to the patient. Several different modes of stimulation, such as changes in ambient temperature, auditory stimulation, and even changes in emotional state, can accentuate the pain. Despite the severity of these dysesthesias, the affected limb is otherwise anesthetic to ordinary sensory testing.

DIAGNOSIS. The presence of thalamic pain should prompt imaging studies to determine the presence of tumor, infarction, or demyelinating disease.

TREATMENT. The combination of levodopa and a peripheral decarboxylase inhibitor may be helpful for relieving pain. If this does not prove satisfactory, some combination of analgesic and tranquilizing medication should be administered.

REFERENCES

Benson MD. Amyloidosis. In Scriver CR, Beaudet AL, Sly WS, et al, eds. The Metabolic Basis of Inherited Disease, 7th edition. McGraw-Hill, New York, 1995;4157-4194.

Bhatia KP, Bhatt MH, Marsden CD. The causalgia-dystonia syndrome. Brain 1993;116:843-851.

Dyck PJ. Neuronal atrophy and degeneration predominantly affecting peripheral sensory and autonomic neurons. In Dyck PJ, Thomas PK, Griffin JW, et al, eds. Peripheral Neuropathy. WB Saunders, Philadelphia, 1993;1065-1093

Ferriére G, Guzzetta F, Kulakowski S, et al. Nonprogressive type II hereditary sensory autonomic neuropathy: A homogeneous clinicopathologic entity. J Child Neurol 1992;7:364-370.

Gower DJ, Pollay M, Leech R. Pediatric syringomyelia. J Child Neurol 1994;9:14-21.

Jestico JV, Urry PA, Efphimiou J. An hereditary sensory and autonomic neuropathy transmitted as an X-linked recessive trait. J Neurol Neurosurg Psychiatry 1985;48:1259-1264.

Kauppinen R, Mustajoki P. Prognosis of acute porphyria: Occurrence of acute attacks, precipitating factors, and associated diseases. Medicine 1992;71:1-13.

Landrieu P, Said G, Allaire C. Dominantly transmitted congenital indifference to pain. Ann Neurol 1990;27:574-578.

Larner AJ, Moss J, Rossi ML, et al. Congenital insensitivity to pain: A 20 year follow up. J Neurol Neurosurg Psychiatry 1994;57:973-974.

Milhorat TH, Johnson WD, Miller JI, et al. Surgical treatment of syringomyelia based on magnetic resonance imaging criteria. Neurosurgery 1992;31:231-234.

Mitchell G, Larochelle J, Lambert M, et al. Neurologic crises in hereditary tyrosinemia. N Engl J Med 1990;322:432-437.

Ouvrier R, McLeod JG, Pollard J. Sensory neuropathies. In Peripheral Neuropathy in Childhood. International Review of Child Neurology Series. Raven Press, New York, 1990;127-138.

Robinson B, Johnson R, Abernathy D, et al. Familial distal dysautonomia. J Neurol Neurosurg Psychiatry 1989;52:1281-1285.

Rosemberg S, Marie SKN, Kliemann S. Congenital insensitivity to pain with anhidrosis (hereditary sensory and autonomic neuropathy type IV). Pediatr Neurol 1994;11:50-56.

Thomas PK, Misra VP, King RHM, et al. Autosomal recessive hereditary sensory neuropathy with spastic paraplegia. Brain 1994;117:651-659.

Wilder RT, Berde CB, Wolohan M, et al. Reflex sympathetic dystrophy in children: Clinical characteristics and follow-up of seventy patients. J Bone Joint Surg 1992;74A:910-919.

10
Ataxia

The term *ataxia* is used to denote disturbances in the fine control of posture and movement that are normally controlled by the cerebellum and its major input systems from the frontal lobes and the posterior columns of the spinal cord. The initial and most prominent feature is usually an abnormal gait. The ataxic gait is wide based, lurching, and staggering, and in the observer it provokes disquiet for fear that the patient is in danger of falling. The same gait is seen in people who are attempting to walk in a vehicle that has several directions of movement at once, such as a railroad train.

When an abnormality occurs in the vermis of the cerebellum, the child cannot sit still but constantly moves the body to-and-fro and bobs the head (*titubation*). In contrast, disturbances of the cerebellar hemispheres cause a tendency to veer in the direction of the affected hemisphere, with dysmetria and hypotonia in the ipsilateral limbs. Bifrontal lobe disease may produce symptoms and signs that are indistinguishable from cerebellar disease.

Loss of sensory input to the cerebellum, because of peripheral nerve or posterior column disease, necessitates constant looking at the feet to know their location in space. The gait is also wide based but is not so much lurching as careful. The foot is raised high with each step and slaps down heavily on the ground. Station and gait are considerably worse with the eyes closed and the patient may actually fall to the floor (positive Romberg sign). Sensory ataxia is more likely to cause difficulty with fine finger movements than with reaching for objects.

Other features of cerebellar disease are a characteristic speech which varies in volume and has an increased separation of syllables (*scanning speech*), hypotonia, limb and ocular dysmetria, and tremor.

The differential diagnosis of a child with acute ataxia or recurrent attacks of ataxia (Table 10-1) is quite different from that of a child with chronic static or progressive ataxia (Table 10-2). Therefore, these two presentations are discussed separately in the text. However, a slowly progressive ataxia may be noticed "acutely," and children with recurrent ataxia may never return to baseline after each attack and have a progressive ataxia superimposed on the acute attacks.

Acute or Recurrent Ataxia

The two most common causes of ataxia among children who were previously healthy and then suddenly have an ataxic gait are drug ingestion and acute postinfectious cerebellitis (Gieron-Korthals et al, 1994). Migraine, brainstem encephalitis, and an underlying neuroblastoma are the next considerations (Table 10-1). Recurrent ataxia is uncommon and is usually caused by hereditary disorders; migraine is the most common cause, and disorders of pyruvate metabolism are second.

BRAIN TUMOR

Primary brain tumors ordinarily cause chronic progressive ataxia and are discussed later in this chapter. However, acute ataxia may be the initial

■ TABLE 10-1
Acute or Recurrent Ataxia

Brain Tumor
Conversion Reaction
Drug Ingestion
Encephalitis (Brainstem)
Genetic Disorders
Dominant recurrent ataxia
Episodic ataxia type 1
Episodic ataxia type 2
Hartnup disease
Maple syrup urine disease
Pyruvate dehydrogenase deficiency
Migraine
Basilar
Benign paroxysmal vertigo
Postinfectious-Immune
Acute postinfectious cerebellitis
Miller Fisher syndrome
Multiple sclerosis
Myoclonic encephalopathy and neuroblastoma
Pseudoataxia (Epileptic)
Trauma
Hematoma (see Chapter 2)
Postconcussion
Vertebrobasilar occlusion
Vascular Disorders
Cerebellar hemorrhage
Kawasaki disease

■ TABLE 10-2
Chronic or Progressive Ataxia

Brain Tumors
Cerebellar astrocytoma
Cerebellar hemangioblastoma (Von Hippel-Lindau
  disease)
Ependymoma
Medulloblastoma
Supratentorial tumors (see Chapter 4)
Congenital Malformations
Basilar impression
Cerebellar aplasias
Cerebellar hemisphere aplasia
Dandy-Walker malformation (see Chapter 18)
Vermal aplasia
Chiari malformation
Hereditary Ataxias
Autosomal dominant inheritance
  Dentatorubropallidoluysian atrophy
  Machado-Joseph disease
  Olivopontocerebellar degeneration
Autosomal recessive inheritance
  Abetalipoproteinemia
  Ataxia-ocular motor apraxia
  Ataxia-telangiectasia
  Ataxia with diffuse central nervous system
    hypomyelination
  Ataxia with episodic dystonia
  Friedreich ataxia
  Hartnup disease
  Hypobetalipoproteinemia
  Juvenile GM_2 gangliosidosis
  Juvenile sulfatide lipidoses
  Maple syrup urine disease
  Marinesco-Sjögren syndrome
  Pyruvate dehydrogenase deficiency
  Ramsay-Hunt syndrome
  Refsum disease (HSMN IV) (see Chapter 7)
  Respiratory chain disorders (see Chapter 8)
  Sea-blue histiocytosis
X-linked inheritance
  Adrenoleukodystrophy (see Chapter 5)
  Leber optic neuropathy (see Chapter 16)
  With deafness
  With deafness and loss of vision
  With adult-onset dementia

feature of brain tumors because of bleeding, sudden shifts in position that cause hydrocephalus, or growth. In addition, early clumsiness may be overlooked until it becomes severe enough to cause an obvious gait disturbance. For this reason, brain imaging is recommended for most children with acute cerebellar ataxia (Fig. 10-1).

CONVERSION REACTION

CLINICAL FEATURES. Hysterical gait disturbances are common in children, especially girls between 10 and 15 years of age. Hysteria is involuntary, usually provides a secondary gain such as attention, and should be distinguished from malingering, which is a voluntary act. Hysterical gait disturbances are often extreme and if so are termed *astasia-abasia.* The child appears to sit without difficulty but when brought to standing immediately begins to sway from the waist. A wide-based stance is not used to increase stability. Instead the child lurches, staggers, and otherwise travels across the room from object to object. The lurching maneuvers are often complex and require extraordinary balance. Strength, tone, sensation, and tendon reflexes are normal.

DIAGNOSIS. Hysterical gait disturbances are usually diagnosed by observation; laboratory tests are not ordinarily required to exclude other possibilities.

TREATMENT. Determination of the precipitating stress is important. Conversion may represent a true call for help in a desperate situation such as child abuse. Such cases require referral to a multispecialty team able to deal with the whole family.

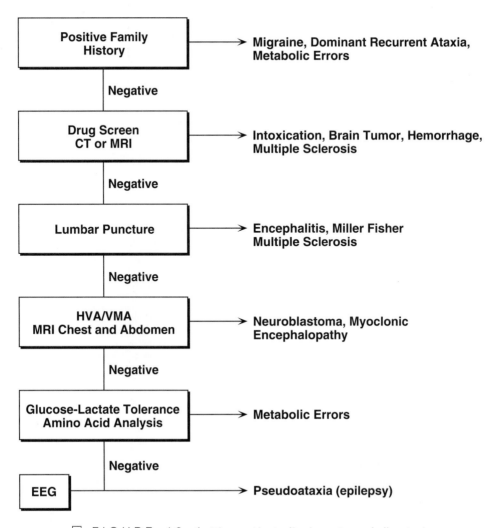

☐ FIGURE 10 – 1 Diagnostic studies in acute cerebellar ataxia.

Most children with hysterical gait disturbances are responding to a more immediate and less serious life-stress. Symptoms can usually be treated by the use of suggestion and do not require psychiatric referral except when conversion is used repeatedly to handle stress.

DRUG INGESTION

The incidence of accidental drug ingestion is highest between 1 and 4 years of age.

CLINICAL FEATURES. An overdosage of most psychoactive drugs causes ataxia, disturbances in personality or sensorium, and sometimes seizures. Toxic doses of anticonvulsant drugs, especially phenytoin, may cause marked nystagmus and ataxia without an equivalent alteration in sensorium. Excessive use of antihistamines in the treatment of an infant or young child with allergy or an upper respiratory tract infection may cause ataxia. This is especially true in children with otitis media, who may have underlying unsteadiness because of middle-ear infection.

DIAGNOSIS. The parents or care providers of every child with acute ataxia should be carefully questioned concerning drugs intentionally administered to the child and other drugs accessible in the home. Specific inquiry should be made concerning the use of anticonvulsant or psychoactive drugs by family members. Urine should be screened for drug metabolites, and blood should be sent for analysis when a specific drug is suspected.

TREATMENT. Treatment depends on the specific drug ingested and its blood concentration. In most cases of ataxia caused by drug ingestion, the drug can be safely eliminated spontaneously if vital function is not compromised, if acid-base balance is not disturbed, and if liver and kidney function is normal. In life-threatening situations, dialysis may be necessary while vital function is supported in an intensive care unit.

ENCEPHALITIS (BRAINSTEM)

Ataxia may be the initial feature of viral encephalitis affecting primarily the structures of the posterior fossa. Echoviruses, coxsackieviruses, and adenoviruses have been implicated as etiologic agents.

CLINICAL FEATURES. Cranial nerve dysfunction is often associated with the ataxia. A more diffuse encephalitis characterized by declining consciousness and seizures may develop later. Meningismus is sometimes present. The course is variable, and although most children recover completely, some are left with considerable neurologic impairment. Those who have only ataxia and cranial nerve palsies, with no disturbance of neocortical function, tend to recover best. Such cases cannot be distinguished from the Miller Fisher syndrome on clinical grounds alone.

DIAGNOSIS. Diagnosis requires showing a cellular response, primarily mononuclear leukocytes, in the cerebrospinal fluid, with or without some elevation of the protein content. Prolonged interpeak latencies of the brainstem auditory evoked response are evidence of an abnormality within the brainstem parenchyma and not the peripheral sensory input system. The electroencephalogram (EEG) is usually normal in children with brainstem encephalitis who have a normal sensorium.

TREATMENT. No specific treatment is available for the viral infection.

GENETIC DISORDERS

Dominant Recurrent Ataxias

Several families have been reported in whom episodic ataxia and vertigo are transmitted by autosomal dominant inheritance. At least two distinct genetic defects are recognized; Episodic ataxia type 1 (EA-1) and episodic ataxia type 2 (EA-2) (Griggs and Nutt, 1995).

Episodic Ataxia Type 1 (Paroxysmal Ataxia and Myokymia)

EA-1 is caused by a mutation of the potassium channel gene on chromosome 12p. It is probably related to the syndrome of paroxysmal choreoathetosis (see Chapter 1) (Lubbers et al, 1995). The additional feature of continuous motor unit activity (see Chapter 8) suggests a defect in membrane stability affecting the central and peripheral nervous system.

CLINICAL FEATURES. The onset of attacks is usually between 5 and 7 years of age. The child has sudden awareness that an attack is to begin by the sensation of spreading limpness or stiffness lasting a few seconds. Incoordination, trembling of the head or limbs, and blurry vision often follows. Some children feel warm and perspire. Some can continue standing or walking, but most sit down. Attacks usually last less than 10 minutes, but can be as long as 6 hours. They may begin spontaneously but are usually brought on by sudden and unexpected movement (kinesiogenic). Startle and anxiety increase the potential for attacks. Myokymia of the hands is observed even between attacks.

DIAGNOSIS. The clinical diagnosis is based on the history of typical attacks and the family history. Electromyography confirms the diagnosis by showing continuous motor unit activity, most often in the hands but also in the proximal arm muscles and sometimes the face.

TREATMENT. Acetazolamide reduces the frequency of attacks or completely stops them in about half of patients. The effect is noted within a few days. Some patients respond to phenytoin.

Episodic Ataxia Type 2 (Acetazolamide-Responsive Ataxia)

The gene for EA-2 maps to chromosome 19p at a site that may be allelic with the gene for familial hemiplegic migraine (see Chapter 11).

CLINICAL FEATURES. The onset of attacks is generally during school-age or adolescence. In EA-2, the child first becomes unsteady and is then unable to maintain posture because of vertigo and ataxia. Vomiting is frequent and severe. Jerk nystagmus, sometimes with a rotary component, is seen during attacks. One to three attacks may occur each month with symptoms lasting from 1 hour to 1 day. Attacks become milder and less frequent with age. Slowly progressive truncal ataxia and nystagmus may persist between attacks. In some patients, ataxia is the only symptom, others have only vertigo, and still others have only nystagmus. Most affected individuals are normal between attacks, but some have nystagmus and are clumsy.

DIAGNOSIS. Diagnosis is based on the clinical features and a family history of the disorder. Magnetic resonance imaging (MRI) may show selective atrophy of the cerebellar vermis. Basilar artery migraine and benign paroxysmal vertigo can be distinguished from dominant recurrent ataxia because in these conditions, older family members have migraine but do not have recurrent ataxia. Further, attacks of benign paroxysmal vertigo rarely last more than a few minutes.

None of the other hereditary recurrent ataxias, other than migraine, are transmitted by autosomal dominant inheritance. Nevertheless, disorders of pyruvate metabolism, many of which cause intermittent ataxia, must be excluded.

TREATMENT. Daily oral acetazolamide prevents recurrence of attacks in almost every case. Its mechanism of action is unknown. The dose is generally 125 mg twice a day in young children, and 250 mg twice a day in older children. Flunarizine, 5 to 10 mg/day, may serve as an alternative therapy when acetazolamide is not tolerated. Anticonvulsant and antimigraine medications are without value.

Hartnup Disease

Hartnup disease is a rare disorder transmitted by autosomal recessive inheritance (Levy, 1995). The basic error is a defect of amino acid transport in cells of the proximal renal tubules and small intestine. The result is massive aminoaciduria and the retention of amino acids in the small intestine, where they are converted by bacteria into useless or toxic products that may be absorbed. Tryptophan is converted to nonessential indole products instead of nicotinamide.

CLINICAL FEATURES. Affected children are normal at birth but may be slow in attaining developmental milestones. Most achieve only borderline intelligence; others are normal. Affected individuals are photosensitive and have a severe, pellagra-like skin rash after exposure to sunlight. The rash is attributed to nicotinamide deficiency. Many patients have episodes of limb ataxia, sometimes associated with nystagmus. Mental changes, ranging from emotional instability to delirium, or states of decreased consciousness may occur. Tone is decreased, and the tendon reflexes are normal or exaggerated. The neurologic disturbances are triggered by stress or intercurrent infection and may be due to the intestinal absorption of toxic amino acid breakdown products.

Most patients have both rash and neurologic disturbances, but each can occur without the other. Neurologic symptoms progress over several days and last from a week to a month before recovery occurs.

DIAGNOSIS. The constant features of Hartnup disease is massive aminoaciduria involving neutral monoaminomonocarboxylic amino acids. These include alanine, serine, threonine, asparagine, glutamine, valine, leucine, isoleucine, phenylalanine, tyrosine, tryptophan, histidine, and citrulline.

TREATMENT. The rash can be prevented by daily oral administration of nicotinamide, 50 to 300 mg. Whether nicotinamide has a beneficial effect on the neurologic symptoms is not known. A high-protein diet is also recommended to make up for the amino acid loss.

Maple Syrup Urine Disease (Intermittent)

Maple syrup urine disease is a disorder of branched-chain amino acid metabolism caused by deficiency of the enzyme branched-chain ketoacid dehydrogenase. The defect is transmitted by autosomal recessive inheritance. Three phenotypes are associated with this enzyme deficiency. The *classic* form begins as seizures in the newborn (see Chapter 1), the *intermediate* form causes progressive mental retardation (see Chapter 5), and the *intermittent* form causes recurrent attacks of ataxia and encephalopathy (Chuang and Shih, 1995).

CLINICAL FEATURES. Affected individuals are normal at birth. Between 5 months and 2 years, episodes of ataxia, irritability, and progressive lethargy are provoked by minor infections, surgery, or a diet that is rich in protein. The length of an attack is variable; most children recover spontaneously, but some die of severe metabolic acidosis. Psychomotor development remains normal in survivors.

DIAGNOSIS. The urine has a maple syrup odor during the attack, and the blood and urine have elevated concentrations of branched-chain amino acids and ketoacids. Between attacks the concentrations of branched-chain amino acids and ketoacids are normal in both blood and urine. The diagnosis is established by showing the enzyme deficiency in cultured fibroblasts.

TREATMENT. Children with intermittent maple syrup disease need a protein-restricted diet. Some have a thiamine-responsive enzyme defect and should be tried on 1 g of thiamine a day for the acute attack. If this is successful, a maintenance dose of 100 mg/day is recommended. The main objective during an acute attack is to reverse ketoacidosis. Protein should not be given. Peritoneal dialysis may be helpful in life-threatening situations.

Pyruvate Dehydrogenase Deficiency

The pyruvate dehydrogenase (PDH) complex is responsible for the oxidative decarboxylation of pyruvate to carbon dioxide and acetyl-coenzyme A (CoA) (Fujii et al, 1994). Disorders of the complex are associated with several neurologic conditions, including subacute necrotizing encephalomyelopathy (Leigh syndrome), mitochondrial myopathies, and lactic acidosis. The complex contains three main components that are termed E1, E2 and E3. E1 consists of two alpha subunits encoded on the X chromosome and two beta subunits. An X-linked form of PDH-E1 deficiency is characterized by episodes of intermittent ataxia and lactic acidosis.

CLINICAL FEATURES. Most patients show mild developmental delay during early childhood. Episodes of ataxia, dysarthria, and sometimes lethargy usually begin after 3 years of age. In more severely affected patients, episodes may begin during infancy and are associated with generalized weakness and states of decreased consciousness. Some attacks are spontaneous, but others are provoked by intercurrent infection, stress, or a high-carbohydrate meal. Attacks recur at irregular intervals and may last from 1 day to several weeks.

The severity of neurologic dysfunction in any individual probably reflects the level of residual enzyme activity. Those with generalized weakness are also areflexic and have nystagmus or other disturbances in ocular motility. Ataxia is the predominant symptom. Intention tremor and dysarthria may be present. Hyperventilation is common and may be caused by metabolic acidosis.

Patients with almost complete PDH deficiency die of lactic acidosis and central hypoventilation during infancy.

DIAGNOSIS. Many patients have mild elevation in the concentration of blood lactate between attacks; all have elevated concentrations of blood lactate and pyruvate during attacks. Some have hyperalaninemia as well. The diagnosis of a pyruvate dysmetabolism state may be further verified by an oral glucose tolerance test. When oral glucose is administered, hyperglycemia is prolonged and blood concentrations of lactate are elevated. The test may provoke clinical symptoms. The diagnosis is established by analysis of enzyme activity in cultured fibroblasts, leukocytes, or muscle.

TREATMENT. Patients are usually treated with thiamine (100 to 600 mg/day) and a high-fat (>55%), low-carbohydrate diet. Unfortunately, current treatments do not prevent disease progression in most patients. In addition, daily oral acetazolamide, 125 mg twice a day in small children and 250 mg twice a day in older children, may significantly abort the attacks. Biotin and thiamine supplements have been used in several patients, but the value of vitamin supplementation has not been established.

MIGRAINE

Basilar Migraine

The term *basilar (artery) migraine* is used to characterize recurrent attacks of brainstem or cerebellar dysfunction that occur as symptoms of a migraine attack. Girls are affected more often than boys. The peak incidence is during adolescence, but attacks may occur at any age. Infant-onset cases are more likely to be manifested as benign paroxysmal vertigo.

CLINICAL FEATURES. Gait ataxia occurs in approximately 50% of patients. Other symptoms include visual loss, vertigo, tinnitus, alternating hemiparesis, and paresthesias of the fingers, toes, and corners of the mouth. An abrupt loss of consciousness, usually lasting for only a few minutes, may be reported. Cardiac arrhythmia and brainstem stroke are rare life-threatening complications. Neurologic disturbances are usually followed by a severe, throbbing, occipital headache. Nausea and vomiting occur in less than one third of cases.

Children may have repeated basilar migraine attacks, but with time the episodes evolve into a pattern of classic migraine. Even during attacks of classic migraine, the patient may continue to complain of vertigo and even ataxia.

DIAGNOSIS. Several authors have stressed the association of seizures and occipital lobe spike discharges with attacks of basilar migraine (De

Romanis, et al, 1993). I believe that such cases should be considered examples of benign occipital epilepsy and not migraine (see Chapter 1). In basilar migraine the EEG shows occipital intermittent delta activity during and just after an attack. However, the boundary between basilar artery migraine and benign occipital epilepsy remains ill-defined.

TREATMENT. I treat basilar artery migraine as I would other forms of migraine (see Chapter 3) and do not use anticonvulsant drugs, as suggested by others, unless I believe that I am treating benign occipital epilepsy.

Benign Paroxysmal Vertigo

Benign paroxysmal vertigo is primarily a disorder of infants and preschool children but may occur in older children.

CLINICAL FEATURES. Episodes are characterized by the sudden onset of vertigo. True cerebellar ataxia is not present, but vertigo is so profound that posture cannot be maintained. The child either lies motionless on the floor or indicates the need to be held by a parent. Consciousness is not altered, and headache is not reported. The predominant symptoms are pallor, nystagmus, and fright. Episodes last only minutes and may recur at irregular intervals. With time, attacks of paroxysmal vertigo are replaced by episodes of headache and vomiting that are more readily recognized as migraine.

DIAGNOSIS. The diagnosis is primarily clinical and laboratory tests are useful only to exclude other possibilities. A family history of migraine, though not necessarily paroxysmal vertigo, can be obtained in almost every case. Some parents indicate that they experience vertigo with their attacks of migraine. Only in rare cases does a parent have a history of benign paroxysmal vertigo.

TREATMENT. The attacks are so brief and harmless that treatment is seldom indicated. Standard migraine therapy can be used when the child grows older and vertiginous episodes are replaced by headache and vomiting.

POSTINFECTIOUS/IMMUNE DISORDERS

In many of the conditions discussed in this section, an altered immune state is blamed for cerebellar dysfunction and sometimes for other neurologic deficits. Preceding viral infections are usually incriminated but are documented in only half of cases. Considering that children have an average of four to six viral infections a year, it is not surprising that 50% of any group of children have a history of a viral illness during the preceding 30 days. The only vaccine that has been linked to acute cerebellar ataxia is that for varicella.

Acute Cerebellar Ataxia

Acute cerebellar ataxia usually affects children between 2 and 7 years of age, but it may occur as late as 16 years (Connolly et al, 1994). Males and females are affected equally and the incidence among family members is not increased.

A preceding illness is identified in 80% of cases; 25% have had varicella, 50% have had a presumed "viral" illness, and the other 5% are attributed to vaccination or Epstein-Barr virus.

CLINICAL FEATURES. The onset is explosive. A previously healthy child awakens from a nap and cannot stand. *Ataxia is maximal at onset.* Some worsening may occur during the first hours, but a longer progression, or a waxing and waning course, makes the diagnosis unlikely. Ataxia varies from mild unsteadiness while walking to complete inability to stand or walk. Even when ataxia is severe, sensorium is clear and the child is otherwise normal. Tendon reflexes may be present or absent; their absence suggests Miller Fisher syndrome. Nystagmus, when present, is usually mild. Chaotic movements of the eyes (opsoclonus) should suggest the myoclonic encephalopathy-neuroblastoma syndrome.

Symptoms may begin to remit after a few days, but recovery of normal gait takes 3 weeks to 5 months. Patients with pure ataxia of the trunk or limbs and only mild nystagmus are likely to recover completely. Marked nystagmus or opsoclonus (see "Myoclonic Encephalopathy"), tremors of the head and trunk, or moderate irritability is likely to be followed by persistent neurologic sequelae.

DIAGNOSIS. The diagnosis of acute postinfectious cerebellitis is one of exclusion. Every child should have drug screening and most will have a brain imaging study. The necessity of imaging the brain in typical cases, especially those with varicella infection, is debatable. Lumbar puncture is indicated when encephalitis is suspected.

TREATMENT. Acute postinfectious cerebellitis is a self-limited disease. Treatment is not required.

Miller Fisher Syndrome

The Miller Fisher syndrome is characterized by ataxia, ophthalmoplegia, and areflexia. A similar disorder with ataxia and areflexia but without ophthalmoplegia is called *acute ataxic neuropathy* (Taly et al, 1991). Some believe that the Miller Fisher syndrome is a variant of the Guillain-Barré syndrome, others believe that it is a form of brainstem encephalitis (Najim et al, 1994). In support of the hypothesis of a Guillain-Barré-like immune-mediated hypothesis is the finding that *Campylobacter jejuni* is a causative agent in both the Miller Fisher syndrome and the Guillain-Barré syndrome (Jacobs et al, 1995).

CLINICAL FEATURES. A viral illness precedes the neurologic symptoms by 5 to 10 days in 50% of cases. Either ophthalmoparesis or ataxia may be the initial feature. Both are present early in the course. The initial ocular motor disturbance is paralysis of upgaze, followed by loss of lateral gaze, and then downgaze. Recovery takes place in the reverse order. The Bell phenomenon may be preserved despite paralysis of voluntary upward gaze, suggesting the possibility of a supranuclear palsy. Ptosis occurs but is less severe than the vertical gaze palsy.

Ataxia is more prominent in the limbs than in the trunk and like the areflexia is probably caused by decreased peripheral sensory input. Weakness of the limbs may be noted. Unilateral or bilateral facial weakness occurs in a significant minority of children. Recovery generally begins within 2 to 4 weeks after symptoms become maximal and is complete within 6 months.

DIAGNOSIS. The clinical distinction between the Miller Fisher syndrome and brainstem encephalitis can be difficult. Disturbances of sensorium, multiple cranial nerve palsies, an abnormal EEG, or prolongation of the interpeak latencies of the brainstem auditory evoked response should suggest a brainstem encephalitis. The cerebrospinal fluid profile in the Miller Fisher syndrome parallels that of the Guillain-Barré syndrome. A cellular response is noted early in the course and protein elevation occurs later.

TREATMENT. Corticosteroids, adrenocorticotropic hormone (ACTH), and plasmapheresis are not beneficial. The outcome in untreated children is excellent.

Multiple Sclerosis

Multiple sclerosis is usually a disease of young adults, but may occur in children as young as 24 months. Whether the childhood forms of multiple sclerosis are etiologically distinct from the adult types is not established.

CLINICAL FEATURES. The female-to-male ratio varies from 2:1 to 4:1. Ataxia, concurrent with a febrile episode, is the most common initial feature in children, followed by encephalopathy, hemiparesis, or seizures. Intranuclear ophthalmoplegia, unilateral or bilateral, develops in one third of patients (see Chapter 15).

The clinical features that occur in multiple sclerosis are so variable that a single prototype cannot be provided. The essential feature is repeated episodes of demyelination in noncontiguous areas of the central nervous system. Each episode is characterized by the rapid development of focal neurologic deficits that persist for weeks and months; afterward the child has partial or complete recovery. Recurrences are separated by months or years and are frequently associated with febrile illnesses. Lethargy, nausea, and vomiting sometimes accompany the attacks in children, but rarely in adults.

The child is usually irritable and shows truncal and limb ataxia. Tendon reflexes are generally brisk throughout. Long-term outcome is unpredictable.

DIAGNOSIS. Multiple sclerosis may be suspected at the time of the first attack, but definitive diagnosis requires recurrence to establish a polyphasic course. Examination of the cerebrospinal fluid at the time of exacerbation shows less than 25 lymphocytes/mm^3, a normal or mildly elevated protein content, and sometimes the presence of oligoclonal bands.

MRI is the best technique to show demyelination (Figure 10-2), but the extent and severity of lesions may not correlate with the clinical syndrome (Osborn et al, 1990). Visual evoked responses are useful to document prior or concurrent optic neuritis, and peroneal somatosensory evoked responses can be used to document myelitis.

TREATMENT. A course of ACTH or corticosteroids is recommended at the time of acute exacerbations. Prednisone is generally administered orally at a dosage of 2 mg/kg/day for 1 week and is then rapidly tapered and discontinued at the end of a month. Some believe that ACTH is superior to corticosteroids in adults with multiple sclerosis. Aqueous ACTH, 80 units, is given intravenously over 8 hours in 5% dextrose and water each day for 3 days. Forty units of ACTH gel is then given intramuscularly every 12 hours for 7 days. Each injection is reduced by 5 units every 3 days. Improvement, when it occurs, is expected during the first 2 weeks.

☐ FIGURE 10–2 MRI in multiple sclerosis. Two areas of increased signal intensity are present in the cerebellum.

Interferon beta (betaseron) is a newly approved agent for managing the relapsing type of multiple sclerosis. It reduces the frequency of relapse but is not recommended for progressive disease (Arnason, 1994).

Myoclonic Encephalopathy/ Neuroblastoma Syndrome

Myoclonic encephalopathy is a syndrome characterized by chaotic eye movements (dancing eyes opsoclonus), myoclonic ataxia, and encephalopathy. It may occur as an idiopathic syndrome or be caused by an occult neuroblastoma. The common pathophysiologic mechanism is an altered immune state. The clinical presentation and the neurologic outcome are the same regardless of whether neuroblastoma is present.

CLINICAL FEATURES. The mean age at onset is 19 months, with a range from 6 months to 6 years. Unlike acute postinfectious cerebellitis and the Miller Fisher syndrome, in which neurologic symptoms are fully expressed within 1 to 2 days, the evolution of symptoms in myoclonic encephalopathy may take a week or longer.

Either ataxia or chaotic eye movements may bring the child to medical attention. Almost half

of affected children show personality change or irritability, suggesting the presence of a more diffuse encephalopathy. Some are described as having a cerebellar ataxia, whereas others are said to be incoordinated because of myoclonus, constant rapid muscular contractions that have an irregular occurrence and a widespread distribution (see Chapter 14). Opsoclonus is a disorder of ocular muscles that is similar to myoclonus. It is characterized by spontaneous, conjugate, irregular jerking of the eyes in all directions. The movements are most prominent with attempts to change fixation and are then associated with blinking or eyelid flutter. Opsoclonus persists even in sleep and becomes more severe with agitation.

DIAGNOSIS. The myoclonic encephalopathy syndrome can be diagnosed on clinical grounds, but laboratory investigation is required to determine the underlying cause. The presence of an occult neuroblastoma should be suspected in all children with recurrent ataxia or the myoclonic encephalopathy syndrome. Acute ataxia that progresses over several days or waxes and wanes is more likely to be caused by neuroblastoma than by postinfectious acute cerebellar ataxia.

In children with myoclonic encephalopathy caused by occult neuroblastoma, the tumor is equally likely to be in the chest or the abdomen. In contrast, only 10% to 15% of neuroblastomas are in the chest when myoclonic encephalopathy is absent. The usual studies to detect neuroblastoma are MRI of the chest and abdomen (Figure 10–3), and measurement of the urinary excretion of homovanillic acid (HVA) and vanillylmandelic acid (VMA). However, radioisotope studies using metaiodobenzylguanidine (MIBG) and other specific isotopes may become the studies of choice (Parisi et al, 1993).

TREATMENT. Partial or complete remission of the neurologic syndrome may occur regardless of whether neuroblastoma is present. In most patients the course is prolonged, with waxing and waning of neurologic dysfunction. Either ACTH or oral corticosteroids provide partial or complete relief of symptoms in 80% of patients, including those with neuroblastoma. Marked improvement usually occurs 1 to 4 weeks after initiation of therapy. Relapses occur when therapy is discontinued but may also occur while treatment is in progress.

Neuroblastoma, when present, must be removed. However, the long-term neurologic outcome is the same whether or not neuroblastoma is present (Koh et al, 1994). Approximately half of affected children will have impaired motor ability, and one third will have some disturbance in intellectual function.

Pseudoataxia (Epileptic)

CLINICAL FEATURES. Ataxia and other gait disturbances can be the only clinical features of seizure activity. Both limb and gait ataxia may be present, and the child's epilepsy may not have been previously recognized. If the child is already taking anticonvulsant drugs, the gait disturbance may be blamed on overdose. During the ataxic episode the child may appear inattentive or confused. Like other seizure manifestations, ataxia is sudden in onset and episodic.

DIAGNOSIS. The absence of nystagmus should suggest that ataxia is a seizure manifestation and is not caused by drug toxicity. The usual EEG findings concurrent with ataxia are prolonged, generalized, 2- to 3-Hz spike-wave complexes that have a frontal predominance. This is the typical EEG finding in the Lennox-Gastaut syndrome (see Chapter 1). Such discharges are ordinarily associated with myoclonic jerks or akinetic seizures. Either one occurring momentarily, but repeatedly, could interrupt smooth movement and produce ataxia.

TREATMENT. Pseudoataxia usually responds to anticonvulsant drugs. Clonazepam and valproate are most often used for slow spike-wave discharges (see Chapter 1).

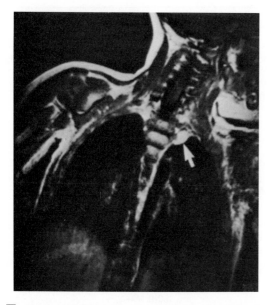

☐ F I G U R E   1 0 – 3 Apical neuroblastoma *(arrow)* demonstrated by MRI in a child with normal radiographs and CT scans of the chest.

TRAUMA

Mild head injuries are common in children, and are an almost daily occurrence in toddlers. Recovery is always complete despite considerable parental concern. More serious head injuries, associated with loss of consciousness, seizures, and cerebral contusion, are less common but still account for several thousand deaths in children annually. Ataxia may follow head injuries, even mild injuries. In most of these cases the ataxia is part of the so-called postconcussion syndrome, in which no structural derangement of the nervous system can be shown by imaging studies. In others a cerebellar contusion or posterior fossa hematoma may be present (see Chapter 2).

Ataxia may also follow cervical injuries, especially during sports. These are usually caused by trauma to the vertebrobasilar artery.

Postconcussion Syndrome

CLINICAL FEATURES. Many adults complain of headache, dizziness, and mental changes following even a mild head injury. Some of these symptoms also occur after head injury in children and probably represent a transitory derangement of cerebral function caused by the trauma. Even mild head trauma can cause a cerebral axonopathy, which may explain the persistence of symptoms.

In infants and small children the most prominent postconcussive symptom is ataxia. This is not necessarily a typical cerebellar ataxia but may be only an unsteady gait. No limb dysmetria is present, and other neurologic functions are normal.

In older children with postconcussive syndromes, headache and dizziness are as common as ataxia. The headache is usually described as low grade and constant, sometimes made worse by movements of the head. Gait is less disturbed, possibly because an older child better compensates for dizziness, but the sensation of unsteadiness is still described.

DIAGNOSIS. The diagnosis is based on the clinical syndrome. Cranial CT at the time of injury to exclude intracranial hemorrhage is abnormal but MRI may show foci of high signal intensity on T_2-weighted images, indicating axonal injury (Mittl et al, 1994).

TREATMENT. Ataxia usually clears completely within 1 month and always within 6 months. Decreased activity during this time is recommended. Usually no further treatment is required.

Vertebrobasilar Occlusion

Trauma to the vertebrobasilar arteries may occur with chiropractic manipulation and sports injuries. The vertebral arteries are encased in bony canals from C2 to the foramen magnum. Sudden stretching of the arteries by hyperextension or hyperflexion of the neck causes endothelial injury and thrombosis.

CLINICAL FEATURES. Symptoms are noted within minutes or hours of injury. Vertigo, nausea, and vomiting are the initial symptoms of brainstem ischemia. Occipital headache may be present as well. Ataxia is due to incoordination of the limbs on one side. It may be maximal at onset or progress over several days.

Examination shows some combination of unilateral brainstem disturbances (diplopia, facial weakness) and ipsilateral cerebellar dysfunction.

DIAGNOSIS. CT or MRI shows a unilateral infarction in the cerebellar hemisphere. The lateral medulla may also be infarcted. The location of arterial thrombosis is visualized by arteriography.

TREATMENT. Many children recover completely in the months that follow injury. The value of anticoagulation has not been established.

VASCULAR DISORDERS

Cerebellar Hemorrhage

Spontaneous cerebellar hemorrhage in children, in the absence of a coagulopathy, is due to arteriovenous malformation, even though less than 10% of intracranial arteriovenous malformations in children are in the cerebellum. The two major features of cerebellar hemorrhage are ataxia and headache.

Kawasaki Disease

Kawasaki disease is a systemic vasculitis that occurs predominantly in infants and children.

CLINICAL FEATURES. Five of the following six criteria are required for diagnosis: fever, conjunctival congestion, reddening of the oropharynx and lips, indurative edema of the limbs, polymorphic exanthems, and lymphadenopathy. Arthralgia, carditis, and aseptic meningitis may be associated features. The disease is thought to be identical to childhood polyarteritis nodosa.

Multiple infarcts may occur in the brain. Acute ataxia, facial palsy, ocular motor palsies, and hemiplegia may occur. Prognosis is guarded, partly because of the neurologic complications but mainly because of coronary artery disease.

DIAGNOSIS. Clinical features of multisystem disease are essential for diagnosis. Abnormal laboratory findings include an increased sedimentation rate, a positive test for C-reactive protein, and increased serum complement and globulin levels. Typical changes of arteritis are demonstrated by skin biopsy.

TREATMENT. No effective method of treatment has been established. Aspirin is usually recommended. Corticosteroids are thought to increase coronary artery disease. Some studies suggest that intravenous high-dose gammaglobulin may be useful.

 Chronic or Progressive Ataxia

Brain tumor is always an initial concern when progressive ataxia develops in previously normal children, especially if headache is present as well (Table 10-3). Congenital abnormalities that cause ataxia are often associated with some degree of mental deficiency. The onset of symptoms may occur during infancy or be delayed until adult life. Friedreich ataxia is the

■ T A B L E 1 0 – 3
Metabolic Screening in Progressive Ataxias

DISEASE	ABNORMALITY
BLOOD	
Adrenoleukodystrophy	Very-long-chain fatty acids
Ataxia-telangiectasia	IgA, IgE, alpha-fetoprotein
Abetalipoproteinemia	Lipoproteins, cholesterol
Hypobetalipoproteinemia	Lipoproteins, cholesterol
Mitochondrial disorders	Lactate, glucose-lactate tolerance
Sulfatide lipidoses	Arylsulfatase A
URINE	
Hartnup disease	Amino acids
Maple syrup urine disease	Amino acids
FIBROBLASTS	
GM$_2$ gangliosidosis	Hexosaminidase
Refsum disease	Phytanic acid
Carnitine acetyltransferase deficiency	Carnitine acetyltransferase
BONE MARROW	
Neurovisceral storage	Sea-blue histiocytes

most common hereditary form of progressive ataxia. The causes of chronic or progressive ataxia are usually easy to diagnose and many are treatable. Failure to establish a diagnosis can have unfortunate consequences for the child.

BRAIN TUMORS

Neuroectodermal tumors are the second most common malignancy of childhood and the most common solid tumor. Posterior fossa tumors are more common than supratentorial tumors between the ages of 1 and 8 years and account for approximately 50% of brain tumors in children of all ages. The four major tumors of the posterior fossa are cerebellar astrocytoma, brainstem glioma, ependymoma, and medulloblastoma. The initial feature of brainstem glioma is cranial nerve dysfunction and not ataxia (see Chapter 15). Although this discussion is limited to tumors of the posterior fossa, it is important to remember that supratentorial brain tumors may also cause ataxia. Approximately one quarter of children with supratentorial brain tumors have gait disturbances at the time of their first hospitalization, and many of these have signs of "cerebellar dysfunction." Gait disturbances occur with equal frequency whether supratentorial tumors are in the midline or the hemispheres, whereas cerebellar signs are more common with midline tumors.

Cerebellar Astrocytoma

Cerebellar astrocytomas comprise 12% of brain tumors in children. The tumor usually grows slowly in the cerebellar hemisphere, and consists of a large cyst with a mural nodule. It may be in the hemisphere, in the vermis, in both the hemisphere and vermis, or may occupy the fourth ventricle. Midline tumors are likely to be solid (Abdollahzadeh et al, 1994).

CLINICAL FEATURES. Both sexes are affected equally. The peak incidence is at 5 to 9 years of age, but may be as early as infancy. Headache is the most common initial complaint in school-age children, whereas unsteadiness of gait and vomiting are the initial symptoms in preschool children. Headache can be insidious and intermittent; only rarely is there typical morning headache and vomiting. The first complaints of headache and nausea are usually attributed to a flulike illness. Only when symptoms persist is the possibility of increased intracranial pressure

considered. In infants and small children, symptoms of increased intracranial pressure are often relieved by the separation of cranial sutures. For this reason gait disturbances without headache or vomiting are the common initial sign of cerebellar astrocytoma in infants.

Papilledema is present in most affected children at initial examination but is often absent in infants with separation of cranial sutures. Ataxia is present in three quarters, dysmetria in half, and nystagmus in only a quarter. Ataxia varies in severity from a wide-based lurching gait to a subtle alteration of gait observed only with tandem walking or quick turning. It is caused in part by the cerebellar location of the tumor and in part by hydrocephalus. When the tumor is in the cerebellar hemisphere, ipsilateral or bilateral dysmetria may be present. Other neurologic signs sometimes present in children with cerebellar astrocytoma are abducens palsy, multiple cranial nerve palsies, stiff neck, and head tilt.

DIAGNOSIS. CT or MRI is suitable for diagnosis.

TREATMENT. Children with life-threatening hydrocephalus should undergo a shunting procedure as the first step in treatment. The shunt relieves many of the symptoms and signs, including ataxia. Corticosteroids are sufficient to relieve pressure in many children with less severe hydrocephalus.

The 5-year survival after surgical removal approaches 95%. The mural nodule must be located and removed at surgery or the tumor may recur. The totality of tumor resection is difficult to determine at the time of resection and the surgeon's estimate can be improved by postoperative enhanced CT (Schneider et al, 1992). The need for adjuvant radiotherapy is not established.

Deeper tumors that involve the floor of the fourth ventricle are rarely removed in toto. Local recurrence is common after partial resection. Repeat surgery may be curative in some cases, but postoperative radiation therapy appears to offer a better prognosis following partial resection. In one series, the overall disease-free survival rates following either surgery alone or surgery and radiotherapy were 92% at 5 years and 88% at 25 years (Garcia et al, 1989). Chemotherapy is not currently recommended for low-grade cerebellar astrocytomas regardless of the degree of surgical resection.

High-grade cerebellar astrocytoma (glioblastoma) has rarely been reported in children. More than 30% of childhood patients have dissemination of tumor through the neuraxis (spinal cord drop metastases). Examination of cerebrospinal fluid for cytologic features and complete myelography are recommended following surgical resection in all patients with glioblastoma. If either result is abnormal, whole-axis radiation therapy is indicated.

Cerebellar Hemangioblastoma (Von Hippel-Lindau Disease)

Von Hippel-Lindau disease is a multisystem disorder transmitted by autosomal dominant inheritance. The most prominent feature is hemangioblastomas of the cerebellum and retina (Maher et al, 1990). All children with cerebellar hemangioblastomas have von Hippel-Lindau disease. Among adults, 60% have isolated tumors and do not have the genetic defect. The expression of von Hippel-Lindau disease is variable even within the same kindred. The most common features are cerebellar and retinal hemangioblastoma (59%), renal carcinoma (28%), and pheochromocytoma (7%).

CLINICAL FEATURES. Mean age at onset of cerebellar hemangioblastoma in von Hippel-Lindau disease is 32 years; onset before 15 is unusual. The initial features are headache and ataxia. Retinal hemangioblastomas occur at a younger age and may cause visual impairment resulting from hemorrhage as early as the first decade. They may be multiple and bilateral and appear on ophthalmoscopic examination as a dilated artery leading from the disk to a peripheral tumor with an engorged vein.

DIAGNOSIS. The gene locus for von Hippel-Lindau has been mapped to chromosome 3p35 by positional cloning. Identification of the gene locus allows the identification of asymptomatic, affected family members who need annual examinations to look for treatable abnormalities. Such examinations should include indirect ophthalmoscopy and renal ultrasound, and gadolinium-enhanced MRI of the brain every 3 years.

The clinical diagnosis of von Hippel-Lindau disease is based on the presence of any of the following: more than one hemangioblastoma of the central nervous system, an isolated hemangioblastoma associated with a visceral cyst or renal carcinoma, or any known manifestation with a family history of disease.

TREATMENT. Cryotherapy or photocoagulation of smaller retinal lesions can lead to complete tumor regression without visual loss. Cerebellar hemangioblastoma should be treated surgically and can often be totally extirpated.

Ependymoma

Posterior fossa ependymoma is derived from the cells that line the roof and floor of the fourth ventricle. These tumors can extend into both lateral recesses and grow out to the cerebellopontine angle. They account for 10% of primary brain tumors in children.

CLINICAL FEATURES. The peak incidence in children is from birth to 4 years. Both sexes are affected equally. The clinical features evolve slowly and are often present for several months before medical consultation is sought. Symptoms of increased intracranial pressure are the first feature in 90% of children. Disturbances of gait and coordination, neck pain, or cranial nerve dysfunction is the initial feature in the remainder. Half of affected children have ataxia, usually of the vermal type, and one third have nystagmus. Head tilt or neck stiffness is present in one third of children and indicates extension of tumor into the cervical canal.

Although steady deterioration is expected, some children have an intermittent course. Episodes of headache and vomiting, ataxia, and even nuchal rigidity lasting for days or weeks are followed by periods of well-being. These intermittent symptoms are caused by transitory obstruction of the fourth ventricle or aqueduct by the tumor acting in a ball-valve fashion.

DIAGNOSIS. CT and MRI are equally useful for diagnosis. The ventricular system is almost always markedly dilated. MRI is better at showing the tumor's location in the fourth ventricle and its extraventricular extensions.

TREATMENT. The goals of surgical therapy are to relieve the hydrocephalus and to remove as much tumor as possible without damaging the fourth ventricle. Postoperative irradiation to the posterior fossa, but not the neuraxis, is indicated (Rousseau et al, 1994). With surgery alone, the 5-year survival rate is 15% for supratentorial ependymomas and 35% for infratentorial tumors. A postoperative mortality rate of approximately 30% is noted in several series. Survival in children correlates with the primary location and the regional and distant tumor spread. Subarachnoid seeding occurs most frequently in high-grade tumors and tumors in the posterior fossa. High-grade ependymomas and ependymoblastomas are likely to seed the spinal subarachnoid space and require whole-neuraxis radiation.

Medulloblastoma

Medulloblastoma is a primitive neuroectodermal tumor with the capacity to differentiate into neuronal and glial tissue. Most tumors are in the vermis or fourth ventricle with or without extension into the cerebellar hemispheres. Approximately 10% are in the hemisphere alone.

CLINICAL FEATURES. Most series indicate a male-to-female ratio of 3:2. Ninety percent of cases have their onset during the first decade, and the remainder during the second decade. Medulloblastoma is the most common primary brain tumor, with onset of symptoms during infancy.

The tumor grows rapidly, and the interval between onset of symptoms and medical consultation is generally brief; 2 weeks in 25% of cases and less than a month in 50%. Vomiting is an initial symptom in 58% of children, headache in 40%, an unsteady gait in 20%, and torticollis or stiff neck in 10%. The predominance of vomiting with or without headache as an early symptom is probably caused when the tumor irritates the floor of the fourth ventricle. Gait disturbances are more common in young children and are characterized by refusal to stand or walk rather than by ataxia.

Two thirds of children have papilledema at the time of initial examination. Truncal ataxia and limb ataxia are equally common, and both may be present. Only 22% of children have nystagmus. Tendon reflexes are hyperactive when hydrocephalus is present and hypoactive when the tumor is causing primarily cerebellar dysfunction.

DIAGNOSIS. Medulloblastoma is readily diagnosed with CT or MRI (Figure 10–4). The tumors are highly vascular and become enhanced when contrast medium is used.

TREATMENT. The prognosis for children with medulloblastoma is greatly improved by the combined use of surgical extirpation, radiation therapy, and chemotherapy. The role of surgery is to provide histologic identification, debulk the tumor, and relieve obstruction of the fourth ventricle. Ventriculoperitoneal shunting may be needed to reduce intracranial pressure, even before decompressive resection.

The overall 5-year survival is approximately 40%. Survival is better in children who have gross total tumor resection as compared with partial resection or biopsy. Craniospinal radiation increases survival better than local field radiation. Survival is significantly improved by the use of adjuvant chemotherapy (Packer et al, 1994).

☐ F I G U R E   1 0 – 4 MRI of medulloblastoma. The tumor is seen as a mass in the vermis of the cerebellum.

CONGENITAL MALFORMATIONS

Basilar Impression

Basilar impression is a disorder of the craniovertebral junction in which the odontoid process is displaced posteriorly and compresses the spinal cord or brainstem.

CLINICAL FEATURES. The first symptoms are often head tilt, neck stiffness, and headache. The onset of symptoms is frequently precipitated by minor trauma to the head or neck. Examination shows ataxia, nystagmus, and hyperreflexia.

DIAGNOSIS. MRI is the best method to visualize the cervicomedullary junction and may also be useful to delineate an associated Chiari malformation or syringobulbia (Figure 10–5) Johnson and Smoker, 1994).

TREATMENT. Surgical decompression of the foramen magnum usually relieves symptoms.

Cerebellar Malformations

Cerebellar Hemisphere Hypoplasia

Congenital hypoplasia of the cerebellum occurs in humans as an autosomal recessive disease and can be experimentally induced in immature animals by cytotoxic drugs, irradiation, or viral infection. The common histologic feature is the absence of granular cells with a relative preservation of Purkinje cells. In the human hereditary form, granular cell degeneration may continue postnatally and cause progressive cerebellar dysfunction during infancy. Most cases of human cerebellar hypoplasia are sporadic, and although the causes are diverse, the clinical features are relatively constant (Sarnat, 1992).

CLINICAL FEATURES. Developmental delay and hypotonia are the first features suggesting a cerebral abnormality in the infant. Titubation of the head is a constant feature and some combination of ataxia, dysmetria, and intention tremor is also noted. A jerky coarse nystagmus is usually present. Tendon reflexes may be increased or diminished. Those with hyperactive reflexes probably have congenital abnormalities of the corticospinal tract in addition to cerebellar hypoplasia. Seizures occur in some hereditary and some sporadic cases. Other neurologic signs and symptoms may be present, depending on associated malformations. Mental retardation is a constant feature but varies from mild to severe.

DIAGNOSIS. MRI is the study of choice (Figure 10-5). It not only shows the extent of cerebellar hypoplasia but also associated anomalies. The folial pattern of the cerebellum is prominent, and there is compensatory enlargement of the fourth ventricle, cisterna magna, and vallecula.

TREATMENT. No treatment is available.

Vermal Aplasia

Aplasia of the vermis is relatively common and often associated with other cerebral malforma-

tions. All or part of the vermis may be missing, and when the vermis is incomplete, the caudal portion is usually lacking (Al Shahwan et al, 1995).

CLINICAL FEATURES. Partial agenesis of the cerebellar vermis may be asymptomatic. Four families with dominantly inherited aplasia of the anterior vermis have been reported; whether the pattern is autosomal or X-linked dominant is unknown (Rivier and Echenne, 1992). Symptoms are nonprogressive and vary from only mild gait ataxia and upbeating nystagmus to severe ataxia.

Complete agenesis causes titubation of the head and truncal ataxia. Vermal agenesis is frequently associated with other cerebral malformations, producing a constellation of symptoms and signs referable to neurologic dysfunction. Two such examples are the Dandy-Walker malformation (see Chapter 18) and the *Joubert syndrome*.

Cerebellar vermal agenesis is a constant feature of the Joubert syndrome, but several other cerebral malformations are usually present as well. More than one sibling in a family may be involved, but the parents are normal. The typical clinical features in newborns and infants is periods of hyperpnea, usually about 120 breaths/min and lasting for up to 16 seconds, alternating with episodes of apnea lasting up to 12 seconds. Abnormal, conjugate jerking eye movements are seen in half of infants. Most infants are hypotonic. Tendon reflexes may be normal or exaggerated. All patients are mentally retarded, and some are microcephalic. Several affected children have died unexpectedly, possibly from respiratory failure.

DIAGNOSIS. MRI shows agenesis of the vermis of the cerebellum with enlargement of the cisterna magna. Other cerebral malformations, such as agenesis of the corpus callosum, may be observed as well.

TREATMENT. No treatment is available.

Chiari Malformation Type I

The type I Chiari malformation is a displacement of the cerebellar tonsils and posterior vermis of the cerebellum through the foramen magnum, compressing the spinomedullary junction. The type II Chiari malformation has an additional downward displacement of a dysplastic lower medulla and a lumbosacral meningomyelocele (see Chapter 12).

CLINICAL FEATURES. The onset of symptoms is frequently delayed until adolescence or adult life. Major clinical features are headache, head tilt, pain in the neck and shoulders, ataxia, and lower cranial nerve dysfunction. Physical signs vary among patients. Features found in approximately half of cases include: weakness of the arms, hyperactive tendon reflexes in the legs, nystagmus, and ataxia.

DIAGNOSIS. MRI provides the best visualization of posterior fossa structures. The distortion of the cerebellum and the hindbrain is precisely identified (Figure 10–6).

TREATMENT. Surgical decompression of the foramen magnum to at least the C3 vertebra is recommended. More than half of patients are significantly improved by surgery.

HEREDITARY ATAXIA

Autosomal Dominant Inheritance

Eight autosomal dominant cerebellar ataxia have been identified by genotype (Rosenberg, 1995). Only three have onset during childhood and all are caused by an expanding trinucleotide repeats. The dominantly inherited ataxias are difficult to differentiate on clinical grounds because considerable phenotypic variability exists even within a kindred.

Dentatorubropallidoluysian Atrophy (DRPLA)

DRPLA is a progressive atrophy of the globus pallidus and subthalamic nucleus associated with an unstable trinucleotide repeat on the short are of chromosome 12 (Warner et al, 1995).

CLINICAL FEATURES. The onset of symptoms may be in childhood or adult life. The clinical syndromes vary widely within a kindred depending on the size of the trinucleotide repeat. Patients with childhood onset usually have a progressive myoclonic epilepsy syndrome (see Chapter 1), whereas those with an adult onset have ataxia, dementia, and chorea as initial features. Dementia, dysarthria, and ataxia of gait and limbs eventually occur in all cases.

DIAGNOSIS. DRPLA is easily differentiated from sporadic cases by family history and the diagnosis is established by showing the unstable trinucleotide repeat.

TREATMENT. Myoclonus and seizures should be treated with valproate (see Chapter 1).

Machado-Joseph Disease

Machado-Joseph disease is genetically homogeneous. The genetic abnormality is a trinucleotide repeat at 14q24.32 (Rosenberg, 1995). It originated in Portuguese-Azorean populations and was transmitted worldwide by Portuguese sailors during the age of exploration. The age at onset appears to be earlier with each generation

□ F I G U R E 1 0 – 6 Chiari malformation. MRI demonstrates displacement of the cerebellar tonsils *(arrow)* into the foramen magnum.

(anticipation) and onset during adolescence is relatively common.

CLINICAL FEATURES. Machado-Joseph disease is characterized by a degeneration of all motor systems: cerebellar, extrapyramidal, pyramidal, and motor unit. The initial symptom is usually ataxia. Unsteadiness of gait is followed by dysmetria of the hands. Nystagmus is often present and tendon reflexes may be diminished or brisk if the corticospinal tracts are involved.

Within a family some members have predominantly a dystonic disorder, others have ataxia and pyramidal signs, and still others show amyotrophy. Dystonia is somewhat more common than ataxia as the initial feature in children. Bulging eyes are a characteristic, but not constant, early feature of the disorder. Multimotor system degeneration eventually develops in all cases, with death occurring in middle to late adult life.

DIAGNOSIS. Diagnosis depends on the clinical features and a family history of the disease. Neurodiagnostic studies do not add to the physical examination. In families with several affected members, individuals recognize the disease in themselves and may not seek medical attention.

TREATMENT. Treatment is not available for the underlying genetic defect, but Parkinson-like symptoms may be reversed by levodopa and dystonia may respond to trihexyphenidyl.

Olivopontocerebellar Atrophy (OPCA) Type I

The olivopontocerebellar degenerations have their onset from adolescence to 65 years of age. They are divided into three genotypes. Spinocerebellar atrophy (SCA) type 1, type 2, and type 3. SCA1 is the only type that may have onset before age 20. The genotype is a trinucleotide repeat at 6p22-23. Paternal transmission is associated with larger repeat size and earlier onset of symptoms (Dubourg et al, 1995).

SCA2 and SCA3 have adult onset and are not discussed here. The abnormal gene sites are on chromosomes 12 and 14, respectively.

SCA3 is now recognized as an expression of Machado-Joseph disease and is associated with trinucleotide repeats (Junck and Fink, 1996).

CLINICAL FEATURES. Cerebellar ataxia is invariably present and is usually the initial feature. Gait ataxia, dysmetria, dysdiadochokinesia, finger-nose ataxia, and decomposition of movement are present. Patients with childhood onset

often have mental retardation and seizures. Tendon reflexes are exaggerated, and the plantar response is usually extensor. Optic nerve atrophy is a constant finding in some families. Other variable features include nystagmus, dysarthria, decreased pupillary response, ptosis, and impaired position sense.

DIAGNOSIS. Diagnosis depends on the clinical features and a family history.

TREATMENT. No treatment is available.

Autosomal Recessive Inheritance

Abetalipoproteinemia

Abetalipoproteinemia is a disorder of lipid metabolism transmitted by autosomal recessive inheritance. Other terms for the disorder are *acanthocytosis* and the *Bassen-Kornzweig syndrome*. Apolipoprotein B, which is essential for the synthesis and structural integrity of low-density and very-low-density lipoproteins, is missing from the serum. The results are fat malabsorption and a progressive deficiency of vitamins A, E, and K.

CLINICAL FEATURES. Fat malabsorption is present from birth, and most newborns come to medical attention because of failure to thrive, vomiting, and large volumes of loose stool. The correct diagnosis may be made at that time.

Psychomotor development during infancy is delayed. A cerebellar ataxia develops in one third of children during the first decade and in almost every child by the end of the second decade. The progression of symptoms may suggest Friedreich ataxia. Tendon reflexes are usually lost by 5 years of age. Progressive limb ataxia is characterized by gait disturbances, dysmetria, and difficulty with performing rapid alternating movements. Ataxia progresses until the third decade and then becomes stationary. Proprioceptive sensation is lost in the hands and feet, and pinprick and temperature sensations are mildly reduced. Sensory loss results from demyelination in the posterior columns of the spinal cord and the peripheral nerves.

Retinitis pigmentosa is an almost constant feature of abetalipoproteinemia. The age at onset is variable but is usually during the first decade. The initial symptom is night blindness. Nystagmus is common and may be caused either by the cerebellar disturbance or by loss of central vision.

DIAGNOSIS. The acanthocyte is the hallmark of abetalipoproteinemia and other lipoprotein deficiencies. It is an abnormal erythrocyte characterized by thorny projections from the cell surface that prevent normal rouleau formation and cause a very low erythrocyte sedimentation rate. Between 50% and 70% of peripheral erythrocytes undergo transformation to acanthocytes. Acanthocytes are also seen in association with other neurologic disorders in which lipoproteins are normal (see discussions of McLeod syndrome and neuroacanthocytosis).

Severe anemia, with hemoglobin levels less than 8 g/dl (5 mmol/L), is common in young children, but not in adults. The anemia may result from malabsorption and can be corrected with parenteral supplementation of iron or folate. Plasma cholesterol levels are less than 100 mg/dl (2.5 mmol/L), and triglyceride levels are less than 30 mg/dl (0.3 mmol/L). The diagnosis is confirmed by the absence of apolipoprotein B in plasma. Parents should be screened for apolipoprotein B as well. In abetalipoproteinemia the heterozygote is normal; if partial deficiency of apolipoprotein B is present, the diagnosis of familial hypobetalipoproteinemia is more likely.

TREATMENT. It is not clear how much of the neurologic abnormality is a direct effect of lipoprotein deficiency and how much is caused by deficiency of fat-soluble vitamins. Steatorrhea in newborns responds to a restricted intake of triglycerides containing long-chain fatty acids. In addition to maintaining a low-fat diet, for the rest of their lives, patients should take daily doses of vitamin E, 200 to 300 IU/kg, and vitamin A, 200 to 400 IU/kg. Evidence supports that vitamin supplementation not only prevents or retards the development of neurologic sequelae, but also may reverse a neuropathy or myopathy already present.

Ataxia-Ocular Motor Apraxia

Ataxia-ocular motor apraxia is transmitted as an autosomal recessive trait (Gascon et al, 1995). The defect may be allelic with ataxia-telangiectasia, with which it shares the neurologic features but not the disorder of immunity.

CLINICAL FEATURES. Development is normal during the first year. Sometime between age 1 and 7, the child develops ataxia of gait followed by ataxia of the trunk and arms. The progression of neurologic deterioration is slow and eventually stabilizes. All patients have choreic movements, and some have tremor as well. Abnormal movements of the head caused by ocular motor apraxia develop between the ages of 6 and 12

years (see Chapter 15). Oculomotor apraxia is a disturbance of voluntary gaze with intact following responses. Consequently, the head turns first and the eyes follow after. The apraxia of gaze is both vertical and horizontal. Tendon reflexes are normal in the arms but diminished or absent in the legs. Intellectual function is normal or decreased.

DIAGNOSIS. Ataxia-ocular motor apraxia is distinguished from ataxia-telangiectasia because the onset of ataxia is after the first year and because only the nervous system is involved. MRI shows cerebellar atrophy.

TREATMENT. No treatment is available.

Ataxia-Telangiectasia

Ataxia-telangiectasia is a multisystem disorder affecting primarily the nervous and immune systems. It is transmitted by autosomal recessive inheritance, and the genetic abnormality is on the long arm of chromosome 11. Ataxia telangiectasia has worldwide distribution, occurs in all races, and occurs in 1 in 40,000 births (Gatti et al, 1991).

CLINICAL FEATURES. The principal feature is a progressive truncal ataxia that begins during the first year. In infants, choreoathetosis develops instead of, or in addition to, ataxia. The ataxia begins as clumsiness and progresses so slowly that cerebral palsy is often the erroneous diagnosis. Oculomotor apraxia is present in 90% of patients but may be mild at first and overlooked (see Chapter 15). Many children are said to have a dull or expressionless face. Intellectual development is normal at first but often lags with time. One third of children ultimately function in the mildly retarded range.

Telangiectasia usually develops after 2 years of age and sometimes as late as age 10. It first appears on the bulbar conjunctivae, giving the eyes a bloodshot appearance. Similar telangiectasia appears on the upper half of the ears, on the flexor surfaces of the limbs, and in a butterfly distribution on the face. Telangiectasia may be exacerbated by exposure to sun or by irritation or friction.

Recurrent sinopulmonary infection is one of the more serious features of the disease and reflects an underlying immunodeficiency. The synthesis of antibodies and certain immunoglobulin subclasses is disturbed because of disorders of B cell and helper T-cell function. Serum and salivary IgA is absent in 70% to 80% of children and IgE is absent or diminished in 80% to 90%.

The IgM concentration may be elevated in compensation for the IgA deficiency. The thymus has an embryonic appearance, and alpha-fetoprotein concentrations are elevated in the majority of patients.

Taken together, the many features of this disease suggest a generalized disorder of tissue differentiation and cellular repair. The result is an increased incidence of neoplasia, especially lymphoma and lymphocytic leukemia. Two thirds of patients are dead by 20 years of age. Infection is the most common cause of death and neoplasia is second.

DIAGNOSIS. The diagnosis should be suspected in infants who have a combination of ataxia, chronic sinopulmonary infections, and oculomotor apraxia. As the child gets older, the addition of telangiectasia to the other clinical features makes the diagnosis a certainty. Complete studies of immunocompetence should be performed. Elevated concentrations of alpha-fetoprotein and carcinoembryonic antigen are the most constant laboratory markers. Ataxia-ocular motor apraxia without telangiectasia or abnormal immunity occurs as a genetic trait that is probably different from ataxia-telangiectasia.

TREATMENT. All infections must be treated vigorously. Intravenous antibiotics are sometimes required for what would otherwise be a trivial sinusitis in a normal child. Patients with ataxia telangiectasia are exquisitely sensitive to radiation, which produces cellular and chromosomal damage. Radiation may be a precipitant in the development of neoplasia. Therefore, despite the frequency of sinopulmonary infections, radiologic studies must be minimized.

Ataxia with Diffuse Central Nervous System Hypomyelination

This disorder is apparently transmitted by an autosomal recessive trait because it occurs in male and female siblings (Schiffman et al, 1994).

CLINICAL FEATURES. Development is normal during the first year. Some clumsiness may be noted during the second year but the onset of progressive ataxia and diplegia is usually after age 2. Dysarthria and seizures may occur but cognitive function and ocular motility are preserved. Optic atrophy may occur late in the course. Muscle tone is depressed but tendon reflexes are exaggerated and the plantar response is extensor. Long-term outcome is not established.

DIAGNOSIS. MRI shows diffuse homogeneous hypodensity of the white matter and lysosomal and peroxisomal enzyme concentrations are normal. No biochemical defect is identified.

TREATMENT. No treatment is available.

Ataxia with Episodic Dystonia

The combination of ataxia, brisk tendon reflexes, and episodic dystonia is transmitted as an autosomal recessive trait. No underlying metabolic disturbance has been identified. The syndrome begins in the first decade with the onset of progressive ataxia, which is followed by episodes of dystonia that may be unilateral. The dystonia responds to anticonvulsant drugs. The syndrome shares many features with the syndrome of familial paroxysmal choreoathetosis, except for the pattern of inheritance and the progressive nature of the ataxia (see Chapter 1).

Friedreich Ataxia

The term *Friedreich ataxia* has been used in a generic sense to describe all spinocerebellar degenerations. This usage was never helpful and has been discarded. Strict clinical criteria for Friedreich ataxia define a more homogeneous group of patients who have a predictable course and genetic linkage to chromosome 9q (Hanauer et al, 1990).

CLINICAL FEATURES. The strict criteria for diagnosis include autosomal recessive inheritance, onset of ataxia or scoliosis before 20 years of age, rapid early progression, and absence of ophthalmoplegia and dementia. Heterozygotes are asymptomatic, and the presence of abnormal signs, such as pes cavus or scoliosis, in parents should suggest a dominantly inherited ataxia or Charcot-Marie-Tooth disease.

The onset is usually between 2 and 16 years of age, but symptoms may begin earlier or later. The initial feature is ataxia or clumsiness of gait in 95% of cases and scoliosis in 5%. The course is one of steady deterioration; most patients are confined to a wheelchair within 20 years of onset. Dysarthria always develops. Disturbances of ocular motility occurs in 32% of patients, deafness in 8%, and titubation of the head in 4%. Symptoms of cerebellar dysfunction are more severe and more common in the arms than in the legs. Finger-nose ataxia and difficulty in performing rapid alternating movements develop in almost every patient. Only 28% of patients show the same symptoms in the legs, but spastic weakness is often present and may hide the cerebellar signs.

All tendon reflexes are absent in 75% of children. Absent tendon reflexes in the legs was thought to be an essential feature for diagnosis. It is now recognized that the abnormal gene location in children with Freidreich ataxia and retained reflexes maps to the same 9q location (Palau et al, 1995). Extensor plantar responses are present in 89%. Joint position sense and vibration sense are absent in the feet in 90% and in the hands in 27%. Light touch and pain sensations are impaired in less than 10% of patients.

Scoliosis develops in 79% and pes cavus in 55% of patients. The severity of the skeletal deformities varies and is usually mild. A cardiomyopathy characterized by dyspnea on exertion, palpitations, and angina develops in 40% of patients. Systolic ejection murmurs, heard best over the apex or left sternal edge, are relatively common.

Diabetes is present in 10% of patients and has its onset during the third decade. It tends to be severe, may be difficult to control with insulin, and significantly contributes to death from the disease.

DIAGNOSIS. The diagnosis relies primarily on the clinical features. Motor nerve conduction velocities in the arms and legs are slightly slower than normal. In contrast, sensory action potentials are either absent or markedly reduced in amplitude. Spinal somatosensory evoked responses are usually absent.

Common changes on the electrocardiogram (ECG) are a reduced amplitude of T waves and left- or right-ventricular hypertrophy. Arrhythmias and conduction defects are uncommon.

TREATMENT. The underlying disturbance is not curable, but symptomatic treatment is available. Severe scoliosis should be prevented by surgical stabilization. The development of cardiomyopathy must be monitored by regular ECG and chest radiographs to determine heart size. Chest pain on exertion responds to propranolol, and congestive heart failure responds to digitalis. Patients should be checked for diabetes and should be given insulin when necessary.

Hypobetalipoproteinemia

CLINICAL FEATURES. Several different disorders are associated with hypocholesterolemia and reduced, but not absent, concentrations of apolipoprotein B and apolipoprotein A. Some patients with this lipid profile have no neurologic symptoms; others have severe ataxia beginning in infancy. Malabsorption does not occur, but the infant fails to thrive and has progressive fatty cirrhosis of the liver. Severe hypotonia and

absence of tendon reflexes are noted in the first months. The course is characterized by inanition, slow development, and recurrent infection. Death occurs in the second year.

DIAGNOSIS. Total serum lipid content is normal, and the concentration of triglycerides is increased. Total high- and low-density lipoprotein cholesterol concentrations are reduced, as are levels apolipoprotein B and apoprotein A^1.

TREATMENT. No treatment is available.

Juvenile GM_2 Gangliosidosis

All juvenile forms of both alpha- and beta-hexosaminidase-A deficiency are transmitted by autosomal recessive inheritance. Some, like Tay-Sachs disease, are restricted to Ashkenazi Jews, whereas others occur in individuals of non-Jewish descent (see Chapter 5). In all of these conditions, GM_2 gangliosides are stored within the central nervous system (Gravel et al, 1995).

CLINICAL FEATURES. Several different syndromes have been described; some resemble the Ramsay Hunt syndrome, and others mimic Friedreich ataxia or other spinocerebellar degenerations. Clumsiness of gait and ataxia are the usual early features. Onset is usually after age 2 years of age, but can be as late as adult life. Intention tremor is frequently an associated feature. Affected children may be considered clumsy for several years before neurologic deterioration is evident. Although ataxia is a constant feature, other neurologic findings and the rate of progression vary from family to family but are relatively constant within a kindred. Associated neurologic disturbances may include spasticity, dysarthria, optic atrophy, athetoid posturing of the hands, and dementia. Many patients eventually enter a vegetative state.

Other findings in some families include pes cavus, scoliosis, and visceromegaly.

DIAGNOSIS. Any child with an apparent "spinocerebellar degeneration" may have juvenile GM_2 gangliosidosis. Diagnosis requires the measurement of alpha- and beta-hexosaminidase activity in fibroblasts or the demonstration of neuronal ganglioside storage by rectal biopsy.

TREATMENT. No treatment is available.

Juvenile Sulfatide Lipidosis

Sulfatide lipidosis (metachromatic leukodystrophy) is a disorder of central and peripheral myelin metabolism caused by deficient activity of the enzyme arylsulfatase A. The defective gene is on chromosome 22q and is transmitted by autosomal recessive inheritance. The late infantile form is discussed in Chapters 5 and 7 (Kolodny and Fluharty, 1995).

CLINICAL FEATURES. Onset is usually between 4 and 12 years but may be as early as infancy or as late as adult life. When onset is in infancy, the initial symptoms are developmental delay and clumsiness. School-age children have spasticity, progressive ataxia of the trunk and limbs, and generalized tonic-clonic convulsions. Mental deterioration follows. Peripheral neuropathy is not a prominent clinical feature, but motor conduction velocities are usually prolonged late in the course. Protein concentration in the cerebrospinal fluid may be normal or only slightly elevated.

Once symptoms start, progression is relatively rapid. Most children deteriorate into a vegetative state and die within 10 years. The time from onset to death ranges from 3 to 17 years and cannot be predicted by age at onset.

DIAGNOSIS. Among the many causes of progressive ataxia, this is the only one that demonstrates rapid and severe degeneration of multiple neurologic systems. It should be especially considered when the family has a history of similar illness. Nevertheless, many such families have gone for years without diagnosis. Physicians are frequently misled by normal motor conduction velocities early in the course. MRI shows widespread demyelination of the cerebral hemispheres. Patients with late-onset disease are often thought to have multiple sclerosis. Diagnosis requires the demonstration of markedly reduced or absent arylsulfatase A in peripheral leukocytes.

TREATMENT. Treatment is not available.

Marinesco-Sjögren Syndrome

The Marinesco-Sjögren syndrome, characterized by cerebellar ataxia, congenital cataracts, and mental retardation, is transmitted by autosomal recessive inheritance. It is probably a mitochondrial disorder because ragged-red fibers are seen on muscle biopsy and exercise induces a hyperlactemia (Torbergsen et al, 1991).

CLINICAL FEATURES. A constant feature is cataracts, which may be congenital or develop during infancy. The type of cataract varies and is not specific. Cerebellar dysfunction during infancy is characterized by dysarthria, nystagmus, and ataxia of trunk and limbs. Strabismus and hypotonia are frequently present in childhood.

Developmental delay is a constant feature but varies from mild to severe. Other features include short stature, delayed sexual development, pes valgus, and scoliosis.

Although the onset of symptoms is in infancy, the progress is slow or stationary. Ataxia leads to confinement in a wheelchair by the third or fourth decade, and the life span is significantly shortened.

DIAGNOSIS. Diagnosis of the Marinesco-Sjögren syndrome relies primarily on the triad of bilateral cataracts, progressive cerebellar ataxia, and mental retardation. The underlying biochemical defect is unknown, and laboratory tests are not helpful.

TREATMENT. No treatment is available.

Ramsay Hunt Syndrome

Ramsay Hunt syndrome, also termed *dyssynergia cerebellaris myoclonica,* is a progressive degeneration of the dentate nucleus and superior cerebellar peduncle characterized by myoclonus, cerebellar ataxia, and infrequent seizures in the absence of dementia (Marsden et al, 1990). Many patients will prove to have mitochondrial encephalomyopathies (see Chapter 5). Sporadic occurrence is common, and autosomal recessive inheritance is only presumed.

CLINICAL FEATURES. Sporadic cases are not homogeneous, but a general clinical picture can be delineated. The initial symptom is clumsiness, usually noted during the first decade, which evolves into progressive ataxia. Intention tremor and dysarthria may follow. Myoclonus usually begins in the second decade. It is present at rest, but is made worse by attempted movement. Myoclonus may be so severe as to throw the patient to the floor. The combination of ataxia and myoclonus is severely disabling. Generalized tonic-clonic convulsions develop late in the course and are not a constant feature. Tendon reflexes are depressed and scoliosis may be present.

DIAGNOSIS. The diagnosis of Ramsay Hunt syndrome is based on the combination of cerebellar ataxia and myoclonus. However, diagnosing the syndrome does not diagnose a disease. Variants with autosomal dominant inheritance, as well as other syndromes causing myoclonic epilepsy, must be considered (see Chapter 1). MRI may show atrophy of the pons, cerebellar peduncles, and cerebellum. EEG frequently shows epileptiform activity of the slow spike-wave type.

TREATMENT. Seizures usually respond to ordinary anticonvulsant drugs. Valproate is specifically useful in reducing the severity and frequency of myoclonus.

Sea-Blue Histiocytoses

Sea-blue histiocytoses are a heterogeneous group of neurovisceral storage diseases that includes Niemann-Pick disease. In many, the enzymatic error has not been established. Sea-blue histiocytes are large macrophages 20 to 60 μm in diameter with a single eccentric nucleus and a prominent nucleolus. Wright-Giemsa staining reveals blue or blue-green granules in the cytoplasm that contain ceroid, lipofuscin, and sphingomyelin. The histiocytes are present in the bone marrow, liver, and lymph glands.

CLINICAL FEATURES. The initial features may be hepatosplenomegaly or neurologic deterioration. Onset of symptoms can be as early as 2 months of age, but more commonly occurs after 1 year and sometimes after 10 years of age. Ataxia and spasticity are prominent features. The initial progress of neurologic dysfunction is so slow that the child is thought to have cerebral palsy. Involuntary movements and tremor may be present.

Neurologic deterioration accelerates as the child gets older. Later symptoms include dementia, seizures, speech disturbances, and supranuclear ophthalmoplegia. Severe bulbar palsy leads to aspiration and death.

DIAGNOSIS. Sea-blue histiocytosis is a diagnosis of exclusion. When sea-blue histiocytes are present in the bone marrow or liver, an extensive search for a lysosomal enzyme defect must be made. Niemann-Pick disease type C should be especially suspect (see Chapter 5).

TREATMENT. No treatment is available. Liver transplantation was tried in one patient without success.

Other Metabolic Disorders

Hartnup disease and maple syrup urine disease were both described in the section on acute or recurrent ataxia. After an acute attack of these diseases, some patients never return to baseline but instead have chronic progressive ataxia. Such patients should be screened for metabolic disorders (Table 10–3). Refsum disease is an inborn error of phytanic acid metabolism and is transmitted by autosomal recessive inheritance. The cardinal features are retinitis pigmentosa,

chronic or recurrent polyneuropathy, and cerebellar ataxia. Affected individuals usually have either night blindness or neuropathy (see Chapter 7).

Disorders of pyruvate metabolism and the respiratory chain enzymes produce widespread disturbances in the nervous system and are described in Chapters 5, 7, and 8. The common features among the several disorders of mitochondrial metabolism include lactic acidosis, ataxia, hypotonia, ophthalmoplegia, mental retardation, and peripheral neuropathy. These disorders are suggested by a raised concentration of blood lactate or the production of lactic acidosis by administration of a standard glucose tolerance test. A deficiency of pyruvate dehydrogenase may produce acute, recurrent, or chronic ataxias and is discussed in the section on acute or recurrent ataxia. Respiratory chain disorders produce a combination of ataxia, dementia, myoclonus, and seizures.

X-Linked Inheritance

Ataxia may be the initial feature of the infantile form of adrenoleukodystrophy (see Chapter 5). The clinical features of adrenoleukodystrophy can mimic a spinocerebellar degeneration and should be considered in any family with only males affected. An X-linked ataxia associated with hypotonia, deafness, and loss of vision in early childhood is described in several generations of a Dutch family (Arts et al, 1993). Other families have only ataxia and deafness. The abnormal gene site and gene product has not been established and it is not possible to know if these are allelic or different disorders.

Ataxia with Dementia

CLINICAL FEATURES. Age at onset of ataxia with dementia is 2 to 3 years. The initial features are delayed developmental milestones, clumsiness, and intention tremor. Early school performance is acceptable. Progressive ataxia and spasticity develop in affected males during the second decade. Incoordination becomes progressively severe, leading to loss of ambulation. Progressive dementia begins in the third and fourth decades. Death usually occurs in the seventh decade.

Cerebellar, corticospinal, and intellectual function are abnormal. Other neurologic systems are intact.

DIAGNOSIS. CT or MRI shows cerebellar atrophy. No biochemical defect has been identified. Adrenoleukodystrophy is a major consideration, and plasma concentrations of very-long-chain fatty acids should be determined.

TREATMENT. No treatment is available.

REFERENCES

Abdollahzadeh M, Hoffman HJ, Blazer SI. Benighn cerebellar astrocytoma in childhood: Experience at the Hospital for Sick Children 1980-1992. Child Nerv Syst 1994;10:380-383.

Al Shahwan SA, Bruyn GW, Al Deeb SM. Non-progressive familial congenital cerebellar hypoplasia. J Neurol Sci 1995;128:71-77.

Arnason BGW. Interferon beta in multiple sclerosis. Neurology 1993;43;641-643.

Arts WFM, Loonen MCB, Sengers RCA, et al. X-linked ataxia, weakness, deafness, and loss of vision in early childhood with a fatal course. Ann Neurol 1993;33:535-539.

Chuang DT, Shih VE. Disorders of branched chain amino acid and keto acid metabolism. In Scriver CR, Beaudet AL, Sly WS, et al, eds: The Metabolic and Molecular Basis of Inherited Disease, 7th edition. McGraw-Hill, New York, 1995;1239-1278.

Connolly AM, Dodson WE, Prensky AL, et al. Course and outcome of acute cerebellar ataxia. Ann Neurol 1994;35: 673-679.

De Romanis F, Buzzi MG, Assenza S, et al. Basilar migraine with electrophysiologic findings of occipital spike-wave complexes; a long-term study in seven children. Cephalgia 1993;13;192-196.

Dubourg O, Dürr A, Cancel MS, et al. Analysis of the SCA1 CAG repeat in a large number of families with dominant ataxia: Clinical and molecular correlations. Ann Neurol 1995;37:176-180.

Fujii T, Van Coster RN, Old SE, et al. Pyruvate dehydrogenase deficiency: Molecular basis for intrafamilial heterogeneity. Ann Neurol 1994;36:83-89.

Garcia DM, Latifi HR, Simpson JR, et al. Astrocytomas of the cerebellum in children. J Neurosurg 1989;71:661-664.

Gascon GG, Abdo N, Sigut D, et al. Ataxia-oculomotor apraxia syndrome. J Child Neurol 1995;10:118-122.

Gatti RA, Boder E, Vinters HV, et al. Ataxia-telangiectasia: An interdisciplinary approach to pathogenesis. Medicine 1991; 70:99-117.

Gieron-Korthals MA, Westberry KR, Emmanuel PJ. Acute childhood ataxia: 10 year experience. J Child Neurol 1994;9:381-384.

Gravel RA, Clarke JTR, Kaback MM, et al. The G_{M2} gangliosidoses. In Scriver CR, Beaudet AL, Sly WS, et al, eds: The Metabolic and Molecular Basis of Inherited Disease, 7th edition. McGraw-Hill, New York, 1995;2839-2882.

Griggs RC, Nutt JG. Episodic ataxias as channelopathies. Ann Neurol 1995;37:285-286.

Jacobs BC, Endtz H, van der Meche FG, et al. Serum anti-GQ1b IgG antibodies recognize surface epitopes on *Campylobacter jejuni* from patients with Miller Fisher syndrome. Ann Neurol 1995;37:260-264.

Johnson MH, Smoker WR. Lesions of the craniovertebral junction. Neuroimaging Clin North Am 1994;4:599-617.

Koh PS, Raffensperger JG, Berry S, et al. Long-term outcome in children with opsiclonus-myoclonus and ataxia and coincident neuroblastoma. J Pediatr 1994;125:712-716.

Kolodny EH, Fluharty AL. Metachromatic leukodystrophy and multiple sulfatase deficiency. In Scriver CR, Beaudet AL, Sly WS, et al, eds: The Metabolic and Molecular Basis of Inherited Disease, 7th edition. McGraw-Hill, New York, 1995;2693.

Levy HL. Hartnup disorder. In Scriver CR, Beaudet AL, Sly WS, et al, eds: The Metabolic and Molecular Basis of Inherited Disease, 7th edition. McGraw-Hill, New York, 1995; 3629.

Lubbers WJ, Brunt ERP, Scheffer H, et al. Hereditary myokymia and paroxysmal ataxia linked to chromosome 12 is responsive to acetazolamide. J Neurol Neurosug Psychiatry 1995;59:400-405.

Maher ER, Yates JRW, Harries R, et al. Clinical features and natural history of von Hippel-Lindau disease. Q J Med 1990;77:1151-1163.

Marsden CD, Harding AE, Obeso JA. Progressive myoclonic ataxia (the Ramsay Hunt Syndrome). Arch Neurol 1990;47: 1121-1125.

Mittl RL, Grossman RI, Hiehle RW, et al. Prevalence of MR evidence of diffuse axonal injury in patients with mild head injury and normal head CT findings. Am J Neuroradiol 1994;15:1583-1589.

Najim A-DS, Anderson M, Eeg-Olofsson O, et al. Neuro-ophthalamic manifestations of the syndrome of ophthalmoplegia, ataxia, and areflexia: a review. Acta Neurol Scand 1994;89:157-163.

Osborn AG, Harnsberger HR, Smoker WRK, et al. Multiple sclerosis in adolescents: CT and MR findings. AJNR 1990; 11:489-494.

Packer RJ, Sutton LN, Elterman R, et al. Outcome for children with medulloblastoma treated with radiation and cisplatin, CCNU, and vincristine chemotherapy. J Neurosurg 1994;81:690-698.

Palau F, Michele GD, Vilchez JJ, et al. Early-onset ataxia with cardiomyopathy and retained tendon reflexes maps to the Freidreich's ataxia locus on chromosome 9q. Ann Neurol 1995;37:359-362.

Parisi MT, Hattner RS, Matthay KK, et al. Optimized diagnostic strategy for neuroblastoma in opsiclonus-myoclonus. J Nuclear Med 1993;34:1922-1926.

Rivier F, Echenne B. Dominantly inherited hypoplasia of the vermis. Neuropediatrics 1992;23:206-208.

Rosenberg RN. Autosomal dominant cerebellar phenotypes: The genotype has settled the issue. Neurology 1995;45:1-5.

Rousseau P, Habrand JL, Sarrazin D, et al. Treatment of intracranial ependymomas of children: Review of a 15-year experience. Int J Radiat Oncol Biol Phys 1994;15:381-386.

Sarnat HB: Cerebral Dysgenesis. Embryology and Clinical Expression. New York: Oxford University Press, 1992.

Schiffmann R, Moller JR, Trapp BD, et al. Childhood ataxia with diffuse central nervous system hypomyelination. Ann Neurol 1994;35:331-340.

Schneider JH, Raffel C, McComb JG. Benign cerebellar astrocytomas of childhood. Neurosurgery 1992;30:58-62.

Taly AB, Prasad A, Vasanth A, et al. Acute ataxic neuropathy: A clinical, electrophysiological, and morphological study. Acta Neurol Scand 1991;84:398-402.

Torbergsen T, Aasly J, Borud U, et al. Mitochondrial myopathy in Marinesco-Sjögren syndrome. J Ment Defic Res 1991;35:154-159.

Warner TT, Williams LD, Walker RWH, et al. 1995;37:452-459. A clinical and molecular genetic study of dentatorubropallidoluysian atrophy in four European families. Ann Neurol 1995;37:452-459.

11
Hemiplegia

The approach to children with hemiplegia must distinguish between acute hemiplegia, in which weakness develops within a few hours, and chronic progressive hemiplegia, in which weakness evolves over days, weeks, or months. The distinction between an acute and an insidious onset should be easy but can be problematic. In children with a slowly evolving hemiplegia, early weakness may be missed until an obvious level of functional disability is reached; then the hemiplegia seems new and acute.

An additional presentation of hemiplegia is found in infants who come to medical attention because they are slow in meeting motor milestones or are not using one hand. They have a static structural problem from birth (hemiplegic cerebral palsy), but the clinical features are not apparent until the child is old enough to use the affected limbs.

Magnetic resonance imaging (MRI) has become the diagnostic modality of choice for investigating all forms of hemiplegia, and is especially informative in hemiplegic cerebral palsy to show migrational defects that are also causing seizures. Magnetic resonance arteriography (MRA) is a developing technique that will obviate the need for arteriography in many children (Wiznitzer and Masaryk, 1991).

Hemiplegic Cerebral Palsy

The term *hemiplegic cerebral palsy* comprises several pathologic entities that result in limb weakness on one side of the body. In premature infants the most common cause is periventricular hemorrhagic infarction (see Chapter 4). In full-term infants the underlying causes are more often cerebral malformations (Figure 11-1), cerebral infarction, and intracerebral hemorrhage. Imaging studies of the brain are useful to provide the family with a definitive diagnosis (Steinlin et al, 1993). This often relieves guilt and prevents litigation against the obstetrician.

Infants with hemiplegia from birth are often brought to evaluation because crawling or walking is delayed and attention is directed at the legs. An associated but seldom recognized feature is that hand dominance was established during the first year; this is *not* normal. Unilateral facial weakness is never associated, probably because bilateral cortiobulbar innervation of the lower face persists until birth.

Infants with injury to the dominant hemisphere can develop normal speech in the nondominant hemisphere, but it is at the expense of visuoperceptual and spatial skills (Vargha-Khadem et al, 1992). Infants with hemiplegia and early-onset seizures are an exception; they show cognitive disturbances of verbal and nonverbal skills.

NEONATAL INFARCTION

Cerebral infarction from arterial occlusion occurs more often in full-term newborns than in premature newborns. Three patterns of infarction are seen with MRI (Smith and Baumann, 1991): (1) arterial border zone infarction is

□ FIGURE 11-1 Schizencephaly. The rim of gray matter around the defect in the left hemisphere indicates that the abnormity is a schizencephaly rather than an infarction. The child's main abnormality was hemiplegia.

usually associated with resuscitation and probably is caused by hypotension; (2) multiartery infarction is less often associated with perinatal distress and may be caused by congenital heart disease, disseminated intravascular coagulation, and polycythemia; and (3) single-artery infarction can be caused by injury to the cervical portion of the carotid artery during a difficult delivery owing to either misapplication of obstetric forceps or hyperextension and rotation of the neck with stretching of the artery over the lateral portion of the upper cervical vertebrae. However, trauma is a rare associated event and the cause of most single-artery infarctions, especially large infarctions in the frontal or parietal lobes, cannot be determined.

CLINICAL FEATURES. Newborns with large single-artery infarcts appear normal at birth, but develop repetitive, focal, or generalized seizures during the first 4 days postpartum. Some recover fully, but most are left with a hemiparesis that spares the face.

DIAGNOSIS. MRI is necessary to show small infarcts, but large infarcts in the complete distribution of the middle cerebral artery can be detected by ultrasound. Follow-up imaging studies may show either unilateral enlargement of the lateral ventricle or porencephaly in the distribution of the middle cerebral artery con-

tralateral to the hemiparesis. Hemiatrophy of the pons contralateral to the abnormal hemisphere may be an associated feature.

Maternal use of cocaine during pregnancy can cause cerebral infarction and hemorrhage in the fetus. Cocaine can be detected in the newborn's urine during the first week postpartum.

TREATMENT. Anticonvulsant drugs are usually effective for seizure control (see Chapter 1). Hemispherectomy or commissurotomy should be considered in children with intractable focal seizures (see "Epilepsy Surgery" in Chapter 1).

NEONATAL HEMORRHAGE

Small unilateral parietal or temporal hemorrhages occur almost exclusively in full-term newborns and are not associated with either trauma or asphyxia. Larger hemorrhages into the temporal lobe sometimes result when excessive force is applied with obstetric forceps, but more often they are idiopathic. Intraventricular hemorrhage may be an associated feature.

CLINICAL FEATURES. Newborns with small hemorrhages are normal at birth and seem well until seizures begin, anytime during the first week. The symptoms of larger hemorrhages may be apneic spells or seizures, or both. Seizures may be focal or generalized, and hemiplegia or hypotonia is present on examination. Some infants recover completely, whereas others are left with hemiplegia and mental retardation.

DIAGNOSIS. Seizures and apneic spells usually prompt lumbar puncture to exclude the possibility of sepsis. The cerebrospinal fluid is grossly bloody. Computed tomography (CT) shows hemorrhage (Figure 11-2) and follow-up studies show focal encephalomalacia.

TREATMENT. Treatment is available for seizures, but not for hemorrhage.

⇨ Acute Hemiplegia

The sudden onset of an acute, focal neurologic deficit suggests either a vascular or an epileptic mechanism (Table 11-1). Infants and children who have acute hemiplegia can be divided almost equally into two groups according to whether or not the hemiplegia was preceded by epilepsia partialis continua. Both groups may have seizures on the paretic side after hemiplegia is established. Cerebral infarction, usually in the distribution of the middle cerebral artery, accounts for one quarter of cases in which seizures precede the hemiplegia and more than half of cases in which hemiplegia is the initial feature. Whatever the cause, the probability of a permanent motor deficit is almost 100% when the initial feature is epilepsia partialis continua and about 50% when it is not.

ALTERNATING HEMIPLEGIA

This is a rare and poorly understood clinical syndrome with hemiplegia as a cardinal feature. Its nosologic identity has been linked to migraine, epilepsy, and familial paroxysmal choreoathetosis. All cases are sporadic, with the exception of one family in whom chromosomal analysis showed a balanced reciprocal translocation [46,XY,t(3;9)(p26;q34)] in the patient, in all

☐ FIGURE 11–2 Moyamoya disease. Arteriography demonstrates occlusion of the carotid artery at the siphon and new anastomotic vessel formation (arrow).

■ TABLE 11–1
Differential Diagnosis of Acute Hemiplegia

Alternating hemiplegia
Asthmatic amyotrophy (see Chapter 13)
Cerebrovascular disease
Diabetes mellitus
Epilepsy
Hypoglycemia (see Chapter 2)
Kawasaki disease (see Chapter 10)
Migraine
Trauma
Tumor

the affected living relatives, and in one unaffected sibling (Mikati et al, 1992). In this family, the onset of attacks was before 18 months in all affected children except one child whose first attack was at age 3 years.

CLINICAL FEATURES. Affected infants are developmentally normal before the attacks begin, which usually occurs before 18 months of age (Bourgeois et al, 1993). The initial attacks may be hemiplegia, dystonia, or both. As a rule, young infants have more dystonic features and older children are more likely to have flaccid hemiplegia. Brief episodes of monocular or binocular nystagmus, lasting 1 to 3 minutes, are often associated with both dystonic and hemiplegic attacks. Because the attacks have an abrupt onset, dystonia is often thought to be a seizure, and hemiplegia a stroke. Most reports of epileptic seizures during infancy are probably dystonic attacks.

The duration of hemiplegia varies from minutes to days and intensity waxes and wanes during a single episode. During long attacks, hemiplegia may shift from side to side or both sides may be affected. The arm is usually affected more than the leg and walking may not be impaired. Hemiplegia disappears during sleep and reappears on awakening, but not immediately.

Dystonic episodes may primarily affect the limbs on one side, causing hemidystonia, or affect the trunk, causing opisthotonic posturing. Some children scream during attacks as if in pain. Headache is sometimes reported at the onset of attack but not afterward. Writhing movements that suggest choreoathetosis may be associated.

Mental retardation is recognized early in the course and mental regression occurs with time. Stepwise neurologic impairment occurs as well, as if recovery from individual attacks is incomplete.

DIAGNOSIS. Results of electroencephalography (EEG), cerebral arteriography, and MRI are normal. The diagnosis relies entirely on the clinical features.

TREATMENT. Anticonvulsant and antimigraine medications have consistently failed to prevent attacks or prevent progression. Flunarizine, a calcium channel blocking agent, is recommended to reduce the frequency of attacks, but its efficacy is not established.

Alternating hemiplegia and dopa-responsive dystonia (see Chapter 14) share the feature of episodic dystonia with diurnal variation, and levodopa-carbidopa should be tried in infants with attacks of dystonia.

CEREBROVASCULAR DISEASE

The annual incidence of cerebral infarction in children after the newborn period is 1.2 per 100,000, and the combined incidence of non-traumatic intracerebral and subarachnoid hemorrhage is 1.5 per 100,000 (Broderick et al, 1993). The incidence rate is slightly higher in black than in white children. Approximately 66% of strokes in children are associated with a known risk factor (Table 11–2) (Kerr et al, 1993).

Stroke is usually considered when a previously healthy child suddenly becomes hemiparetic or develops any focal neurologic disturbance. The diagnosis of stroke is then confirmed by cranial CT or MRI. Clinical features vary with the age of the child and the location of the stroke. Hemiplegia, either immediately or as a late sequela, is one of the more common features.

Infarction is identified on CT as an area of increased lucency that becomes enhanced with contrast material. As a rule, the lucency cannot be visualized in the first 24 hours after stroke. Cerebral infarction is often superficial, affecting both gray and white matter, and is in the distribution of a single artery. Multiple infarcts suggest either embolism or vasculitis. Small, deep lesions of the internal capsule are rare, but can occur in infants.

The evaluation of a child with cerebral infarction is summarized in Table 11–3. The usual line of investigation includes tests for coagulopathies, vaculitis, and vasculopathies, a search for cardiac sources of emboli, and cerebral arteriography.

Intracerebral hemorrhage is readily identified as an area of increased density on a non-contrast-enhanced CT. It is frequently surrounded by edema and may produce a mass effect with shift of midline structures.

Arteriovenous Malformations

Supratentorial malformations may cause acute or chronic, progressive hemiplegia. Acute hemiplegia is usually caused by intraparenchymal hemorrhage. The major clinical features of hemorrhage into a hemisphere are loss of consciousness, seizures, and hemiplegia. Large hematomas shift midline structures and increase intracranial pressure. Arteriovenous malformations are discussed fully in Chapter 4.

Brain Tumors

Acute hemiplegia from brain tumor is usually caused by hemorrhage into or around the tumor. The underlying tumor may be hidden by the hemorrhage on CT and is better appreciated on MRI (see Chapter 4).

Carotid and Vertebral Artery Disorders

Cervical Infections

Unilateral and bilateral occlusions of the cervical portion of the internal carotid arteries may occur in children with a history of chronic tonsillitis and cervical lymphadenopathy. Whether

■ TABLE 11–2
Causes of Stroke

Cerebrovascular Malformations
Arteriovenous malformation
Fibromuscular dysplasia
Hereditary hemorrhagic telangiectasia
Sturge-Weber syndrome

Coagulopathies/Hemoglobinopathies
Antiphospholipid antibodies/lupus anticoagulant
Congenital coagulation defects
Disseminated intravascular coagulation
Drug-induced thrombosis
Malignancy
Sickle cell anemia/disease
Thrombocytopenic purpura

Heart Disease
Arrhythmia
Atrial myxoma
Bacterial endocarditis
Cardiac catheterization
Cardiomyopathy
Cyanotic congenital defects
Mitral valve prolapse
Prosthetic heart valve
Rhabdomyoma
Rheumatic heart disease

Trauma
Arterial dissection
Blunt trauma to neck
Intraoral trauma
Vertebral manipulation

Vasculitis
Carotid infection
Drug abuse (amphetamines and cocaine)
Hemolytic-uremic syndrome (see Chapter 2)
Hypersensitivity vasculitis
Isolated angiitis
Kawasaki disease (see Chapter 10)
Meningitis (see Chapter 4)
Mixed connective tissue disease
Systemic lupus erythematosus
Takayasu arteritis

Vasculopathies
Homocystinuria (see Chapter 5)
Mitochondrial encephalopathy, lactic acidosis, and stroke (MELAS)
Moyamoya disease

■ TABLE 11-3
TABLE 11-3
Evaluation of Cerebral Infarction

Blood

Antiphospholipid anti- bodies, antiDNA anti- bodies, complete blood count, culture, erythrocyte sedimentation rate, lactic acid, lipid profile	Bacterial endocarditis Hypercoaguable state Hyperlipidemia Leukemia Lupus erythematosis MELAS Polycythemia Sickle cell anemia Vasculitis

Urine

Cocaine, nitroprusside reaction, urinalysis	Cocaine abuse Homocystinuria Nephritis Nephrosis

Heart

Echocardiography, electrocardiography	Bacterial endocarditis Congenital heart disease Mitral valve prolapse Rheumatic heart disease

Brain

Arteriography, magnetic resonance imaging	Arterial dissection Arterial thrombosis Arteriovenous malfor- mation Fibromuscular hypoplasia Moyamoya disease Vasculitis

this is cause and effect or coincidence is uncertain. It is speculated that tonsillitis produces carotid arteritis.

Unilateral cerebral infarction may occur in the course of cat-scratch disease (see Chapter 2) and mycoplasmal pneumonia. In both diseases, the presence of submandibular lymph node involvement is associated with arteritis of the adjacent carotid artery.

Necrotizing fasciitis is a serious cause of inflammatory arteritis with subsequent occlusion of one or both carotid arteries. The source of parapharyngeal space infection is usually chronic dental infection. Mixed aerobic and anaerobic organisms are isolated on culture.

CLINICAL FEATURES. The usual sequence in cervical arteritis is fever and neck tenderness followed by sudden hemiplegia. Bilateral hemiplegia may occur when both sides are infected.

DIAGNOSIS. The offending organism or organisms must be identified by culture of the throat or lymph nodes specimens. Carotid occlusion is identified by arteriography.

TREATMENT. Aggressive therapy with antibiotics, especially for necrotizing fasciitis, is indi-

cated. The outcome is variable, and recovery may be partial or complete.

Fibromuscular Dysplasia

Fibromuscular dysplasia is an idiopathic segmental nonatheromatous disorder of the internal carotid artery. The cervical portion of the artery is most often affected.

CLINICAL FEATURES. Transitory ischemic attacks and stroke are the only clinical features. Fibromuscular dysplasia is primarily a disease of women over 50 years of age but can occur in children.

DIAGNOSIS. Arteriography shows an irregular contour of the internal carotid artery in the neck, resembling a string of beads. Concomitant fibromuscular dysplasia of the renal arteries should be suspected if hypertension is present.

TREATMENT. The occlusion may be treated by operative transluminal balloon angioplasty or by carotid endarterectomy. The long-term prognosis in children is unknown.

Trauma to the Carotid Artery

Children may experience carotid thrombosis and dissection from seemingly trivial injuries sustained in child abuse (grabbing and shaking the neck) or during exercise and sports. The carotid artery also may be injured in the tonsillar fossa during a tonsillectomy or when a child falls with a blunt object (i.e., pencil, lollipop) in the mouth.

CLINICAL FEATURES. The onset of symptoms is usually delayed for several hours and sometimes days. The delay probably represents the time needed for thrombus to form within the artery. Clinical features usually include hemiparesis, hemianesthesia, hemianopia, and aphasia when the dominant hemisphere is affected. Deficits may be transitory or permanent, but some recovery always occurs. Seizures are uncommon.

DIAGNOSIS. Carotid occlusions in the neck can be seen using ultrasonic imaging, MRA, and arteriography.

TREATMENT. Neither anticoagulation nor surgical repair has proved useful in reversing hemiplegia.

Trauma to Vertebral Artery

Vertebral artery thrombosis or dissection may follow minor neck trauma, especially rapid neck rotation. The site of occlusion is usually at the C1-C2 level (Garg et al, 1993).

CLINICAL FEATURES. The usual features of vertebral artery injury are headache and brainstem dysfunction. Repeated episodes of hemiparesis associated with bitemporal throbbing headache and vomiting may occur and are readily misdiagnosed as basilar artery migraine. The outcome is relatively good, survival is the rule, and chronic neurologic disability is unusual.

DIAGNOSIS. The clue to diagnosis is the presence of one or more areas of infarction on CT or MRI. This should raise the possibility of stroke and lead to arteriography. Occlusion of the basilar artery is then visualized.

TREATMENT. No treatment is proven to be effective, but aspirin prophylaxis is often recommended.

Cocaine Use

Cocaine is a potent vasoconstrictor that causes infarction in several organs. Stroke occurs mainly in young adults and may follow any route of administration but takes place more often when "crack" is smoked (Levine et al, 1991). The interval from administration to stroke is unknown in most cases but may be minutes to hours. Intracerebral and subarachnoid hemorrhage are more common than cerebral infarction and often occur in people with underlying aneurysms or arteriovenous malformations. Infarction is probably caused by vasospasm or vasculitis.

Heart Disease

Congenital Heart Disease

Cerebrovascular complications of congenital heart disease are most likely in children with cyanotic disorders. The usual complications are venous sinus thrombosis in infants and embolic arterial occlusion in children. Emboli may occur from valvular vegetations or bacterial endocarditis. In either case the development of cerebral abscess is a major concern. Cerebral abscess of embolic origin is exceedingly uncommon in children younger than 2 years of age with congenital heart disease and occurs only as a complication of meningitis or surgery.

CLINICAL FEATURES. Venous thrombosis occurs most often in infants with cyanotic heart disease who are dehydrated and polycythemic. One or more sinuses may become occluded. Failure of venous drainage always increases intracranial pressure. Hemiparesis is a major clinical feature and may occur on first one side and then the other when the sagittal sinus is obstructed. Seizures and decreased consciousness are almost always associated features. The mortality rate is high in infants with thrombosis of major venous sinuses, and most survivors have neurologic morbidity.

Children with cyanotic heart disease are at risk for arterial embolism when vegetations are present within the heart or if a right-to-left shunt allows peripheral emboli to bypass the lungs and reach the brain. This can occur spontaneously or at the time of cardiac surgery. The potential for cerebral abscess formation increases in children with right-to-left shunt because decreased arterial oxygen saturation lowers cerebral resistance to infection.

The initial feature is sudden onset of hemiparesis associated with headache, seizures, and loss of consciousness. Seizures may at first be focal and recurrent but then become generalized.

DIAGNOSIS. MRI is the preferred procedure for the detection of venous thrombosis and emboli. A pattern of hemorrhagic infarction is seen adjacent to the site of venous thrombosis, and multiple areas of infarction are associated with embolization.

The CT appearance may be normal during the first 12 to 24 hours following embolization. By the next day a low-intensity lesion can be observed with contrast enhancement. Although the sequence is consistent with a sterile embolus, the possibility of subsequent abscess formation must be considered. Enhanced CT or MRI should be repeated within 1 week to search for ring enhancement as a sign of abscess development.

TREATMENT. Treatment for venous thrombosis is primarily supportive and directed toward correcting dehydration and controlling increased intracranial pressure. Dexamethasone can be used to decrease cerebral volume, but osmotic diuretics are contraindicated and may cause further thrombosis. The infarction is usually hemorrhagic, and anticoagulants are contraindicated. Distinguishing a septic from a sterile thrombosis is impossible and all infants should be treated with antibiotics.

Children with arterial emboli, but without evidence of hemorrhagic infarction, should undergo anticoagulation to prevent further embolization. If the infarction is associated with cerebral edema and a mass effect, dexamethasone should be administered as well. All such children should begin antibiotic therapy to prevent cerebral abscess formation. If an abscess does not form, antibiotics can be stopped after 1 week. If an abscess forms, therapy must be continued for 6 to 8 weeks.

Mitral Valve Prolapse

Mitral valve prolapse is a familial disorder present in 5% of children. It is almost always asymptomatic but is estimated to cause recurrent attacks of cerebral ischemia in 1 in every 6,000 cases each year (Cheng, 1989). The attacks are attributed to sterile emboli from thrombus originating either from the prolapsing leaflet or at its junction with the atrial wall.

CLINICAL FEATURES. The initial feature is usually a transitory ischemic attack in the distribution of the carotid circulation producing partial or complete hemiparesis. Weakness usually clears within 24 hours, but recurrent episodes, not necessarily in the same arterial distribution, are the rule. Basilar insufficiency is less common and usually results in visual field defects. The interval between recurrences varies from weeks to years. Fewer than 20% of individuals are left with permanent neurologic deficits.

DIAGNOSIS. Only 25% of patients have late systolic murmurs or a midsystolic click. In the remainder, a cardiac examination shows no abnormalities. Two-dimensional echocardiography is required to establish the diagnosis.

TREATMENT. No treatment is needed for asymptomatic children with auscultatory or electrocardiographic abnormalities, nor is specific treatment available for a transient ischemic attack. However, once a child has suffered a transitory attack of ischemia, aspirin should be administered daily to reduce the likelihood of further thrombus formation in the heart.

Rheumatic Heart Disease

The frequency and severity of rheumatic fever and rheumatic heart disease in North America had been decreasing for several decades. Unfortunately, the incidence of acute rheumatic fever is now increasing. Rheumatic heart disease involves the mitral valve in 85% of patients, the aortic valve in 54%, and the tricuspid and pulmonary valves in less than 5%.

CLINICAL FEATURES. The main features of mitral valve disease are cardiac failure and arrhythmia. Aortic valve disease is often asymptomatic. Neurologic complications are always

due to bacterial endocarditis or embolism from a valvular vegetation during surgery. Symptoms are much the same as in congenital heart disease, except that cerebral abscess is less common.

DIAGNOSIS. Children are known to have rheumatic heart disease long before their first stroke. The onset of neurologic abnormalities, except in the period following cardiac surgery, should suggest bacterial endocarditis as the underlying cause. Embolization is a more likely explanation in the postoperative period. Multiple blood cultures may be needed to identify the organism and select the best drug for intravenous antibiotic therapy.

TREATMENT. Bacterial endocarditis must be treated vigorously with intravenous antibiotics.

Hypercoagulable States

Venous thrombosis in children is usually due to a hypercoagulable state, polycythemia, or dehydration. Congenital heart disease and cancer, two of the leading causes, are discussed in previous sections. Congenital deficiency or defect of an anticoagulant or fibrinolytic protein, such as antithrombin III, causes repeated venous thromboses in children (Whitlock et al, 1989). Partial thrombosis of the sagittal sinus may also occur in young women taking oral contraceptives and during pregnancy.

The *lupus anticoagulant* and the *anticardiolipin antibody* are antiphospholipid antibodies associated with several syndromes that include arterial or venous thrombosis (Angelini et al, 1994).

CLINICAL FEATURES. The typical features of venous thrombosis is headache and obtundation caused by increased intracranial pressure, seizures, and successive hemiplegia on each side. An inherited hypercoaguable state should be suspected in children with recurrent venous thromboses, a family history of venous thrombosis, or thrombosis at an unusual site.

Arterial thromboses usually cause ischemic stroke in the distribution of a single cerebral artery.

DIAGNOSIS. Venous thrombosis should be suspected when hemiplegia and increased intracranial pressure suddenly develop. The diagnosis of sagittal sinus thromboses is suggested when parasagittal hemorrhage or infarction is associated with a flow void in the sagittal sinus on MRI. Cerebral arteriography is the more definitive procedure.

The initial laboratory studies on a child with venous thrombosis include screening hematologic and coagulations studies. Detailed studies of anticoagulant or fibrinolytic proteins should be done when a hypercoaguable state is suspected.

TREATMENT. Symptomatic treatment is directed at decreasing intracranial pressure and rehydrating the patient without increasing cerebral edema. Anticoagulant therapy is often required.

Idiopathic Infarction

Capsular Stroke

Small, deep infarcts involving the internal capsule are usually seen in adults with hypertensive angiopathy. They also occur, but very rarely, in infants and young children. The onset of weakness is sudden and may occur during sleep or wakefulness.

CLINICAL FEATURES. The face and limbs are involved and a typical hemiplegic posture and gait develop. Hypalgesia and decreased position sense are difficult to show in infants, but can be seen in older children. Larger infarcts affecting the striatum and the internal capsule of the dominant hemisphere cause speech disturbances. At the onset of hemiplegia, the child is mute and lethargic. As speech returns, evidence of dysarthria and aphasia develops. Eventually speech becomes normal. Hemiplegia may clear completely in the following year, but some children have residual weakness of the hand.

DIAGNOSIS. Capsular infarcts are demonstrated by MRI. A cause is rarely determined despite extensive study (see Table 11–3).

TREATMENT. No treatment is available.

Cerebral Artery Infarction

Acute infantile hemiplegia may result from infarction in the distribution of the middle cerebral artery or one of its branches, the posterior cerebral artery, or the anterior cerebral artery.

CLINICAL FEATURES. Sudden hemiplegia is the typical initial feature. Hemianesthesia, hemianopia, and aphasia (with dominant hemisphere infarction) are present as well. Some children are lethargic at the onset of symptoms, but consciousness is seldom lost completely.

In approximately one third of cases, epilepsia partialis continua precedes the hemiplegia. In such cases, permanent hemiplegia is a constant feature and epilepsy is common. When hemiplegia occurs without seizures, half of patients recover completely and the remainder are left with partial paralysis.

DIAGNOSIS. Complete occlusion of the middle cerebral artery produces a large area of lucency on CT involving the cortex, underlying white matter, basal ganglia, and internal capsule. Occlusion of superficial branches of the middle cerebral artery produces a wedge-shaped area of lucency extending from the cortex into the subjacent white matter.

TREATMENT. Seizures should be treated with anticonvulsant drugs (see Chapter 1). When seizures are intractable, hemispherectomy or commissurotomy should be considered (see "Epilepsy Surgery" in Chapter 1).

Lipoprotein Disorders

Familial lipid and lipoprotein abnormalities may cause premature cerebrovascular disease in infants and children. These disorders are transmitted by autosomal dominant inheritance.

CLINICAL FEATURES. Ischemic episodes cause transitory or permanent hemiplegia, sometimes associated with hemianopia, hemianesthesia, and aphasia. The family has a history of cerebrovascular and coronary artery disease developing at an early age.

DIAGNOSIS. Most children have low plasma concentrations of high-density lipoprotein (HDL) cholesterol, others have high plasma concentrations of triglycerides, and some have both. The mechanism of arteriosclerosis is lipoprotein-mediated endothelial damage with secondary thrombus formation.

TREATMENT. Dietary treatment and daily aspirin administration are indicated.

Mitochondrial Encephalopathy, Lactic Acidosis, and Stroke

Mitochondrial encephalopathy, lactic acidosis, and stroke (MELAS) is usually associated with a point mutation in mitochondrial DNA causing a biochemical defect in complex I (NADH coenzyme Q reductase) (Koo et al, 1993).

CLINICAL FEATURES. Affected children are usually normal at birth (Hirano and Pavlakis, 1994). Onset during infancy is characterized by failure to thrive, growth retardation, and progressive deafness. The main neurologic features in later-onset cases are recurrent attacks of prolonged migraine-like headaches and vomiting, seizures (myoclonic, focal, generalized) that often progress to status epilepticus, the sudden onset of focal neurologic defects (hemiplegia, hemianopia, aphasia), and encephalopathy. Mental deterioration, when present, occurs anytime during childhood. Neurologic abnormalities are initially intermittent and then become progressive, leading to coma and death.

DIAGNOSIS. MRI shows multifocal infarctions that do not conform to definitive vascular territories. The initial infarctions are often in the occipital lobes; progressive disease affects the cerebral and cerebellar cortices, the basal ganglia, and the thalamus. The concentration of lactate in the blood and cerebrospinal fluid is elevated. Ragged-red fibers are noted on muscle biopsy (see Chapter 7).

TREATMENT. No treatment is available.

Moyamoya Disease

Moyamoya disease is a slowly progressive, bilateral occlusion of the internal carotid arteries starting at the carotid siphon. The basilar artery is sometimes occluded as well. Because the occlusion is slowly progressive, multiple anastomoses have time to form between the internal and external carotid arteries. The result is a new vascular network at the base of the brain composed of collaterals from the anterior or posterior choroidal arteries, the basilar artery, and the meningeal arteries. On angiography, these telangiectasias produce a hazy appearance, like a puff of smoke, from which the Japanese word *moyamoya* is derived (Figure 11-2). The disorder is worldwide in distribution, with a female-to-male bias of 3:2. The underlying cause or causes have not been identified, but an arteritis is suspected.

CLINICAL FEATURES. The initial symptoms vary from recurrent headache to abrupt hemiparesis. Infants and young children tend to have an explosive onset characterized by the sudden development of complete hemiplegia affecting face and limbs. The child is at least lethargic and sometimes comatose. When the child is sufficiently alert to be examined, hemianopia, hemianesthesia, and aphasia may be found. Some children have chorea of the face and all limbs that may be worse on one side. Recovery follows, but before it is complete, new episodes of focal neurologic dysfunction occur on either the same or the opposite side. These episodes include hemiparesis, hemianesthesia, or aphasia, alone or in combination. The outcome is generally poor. Most children are left with chronic weakness of one or both sides, epilepsy, and mental retardation. Some have died.

Recurrent transient ischemic attacks are an alternative manifestation. These are characterized by episodic hemiparesis and dysesthesias lasting minutes or hours. Consciousness is retained. Attacks are frequently triggered by hyperpnea or excitement and may recur daily. After 4 or 5 years, the attacks cease but the child may be left with residual deficits.

Repeated episodes of monoparesis or symptoms of subarachnoid hemorrhage are other possible features of moyamoya disease. Monoparesis generally occurs after infancy, and subarachnoid hemorrhage after 16 years of age.

DIAGNOSIS. CT or MRI usually shows a large cerebral infarction caused by stenosis in the internal carotid artery. Definitive diagnosis requires arteriographic demonstration of bilateral stenosis in the distal internal carotid arteries and the development of collaterals in the basal ganglia and meninges.

Antiphospholipid antibody was associated with one child with moyamoya disease and the ischemic episodes stopped after administration of intravenous immunoglobulin (Schoning et al, 1994).

TREATMENT. Intravenous verapamil was reported to be effective early in the course to provide return of function and radiographic evidence of increased perfusion. Temporal muscle graft, in which temporal muscle is placed over the arachnoid, has been attempted and found useful in providing better circulation to the superficial cortex. However, this approach seems unlikely to add substantially to the natural development of arterial anastomoses.

Sickle Cell Anemia

Sickle cell anemia is a genetic disorder of black children that is transmitted by autosomal recessive inheritance. Neurologic complications occur in up to 25% of homozygotes and may occur at times of stress, such as surgery, in heterozygotes. The abnormal erythrocytes clog large and small vessels, decreasing total, hemispheric, or regional blood flow. Cerebral infarction usually occurs in the region of arterial border zones.

CLINICAL FEATURES. The major systemic features are jaundice, pallor, weakness, and fatigability from chronic hemolytic anemia. Half of homozygotes show symptoms by 1 year and all have symptoms by 5 years of age.

Strokes occur at the time of a thrombotic, vaso-occlusive crisis. Such crises are frequently precipitated by dehydration or anoxia and are characterized by fever and pain in the abdomen and chest. Focal or generalized seizures are the initial neurologic feature in 70% of patients. After the seizures have ended, hemiplegia and other focal neurologic deficits are noted. Some recovery follows, but there is a tendency for recurrent strokes, epilepsy, and mental retardation. Strokes affecting both hemispheres produce a pseudobulbar palsy with brainstem dysfunction.

The worst case is a child who is in a coma and has meningismus. Such a case is usually caused by a diffuse decrease in cerebral blood flow associated with subarachnoid or intracerebral hemorrhage. The mortality rate is high.

DIAGNOSIS. The abnormal hemoglobin can be diagnosed at birth with acid agar gel electrophoresis or microcolumn chromatography. In most affected children sickle cell anemia is diagnosed long before their first stroke. The extent of cerebral infarction and hemorrhage during a cerebral vaso-occlusive crisis can be documented by CT or MRI. After several such crises, cortical atrophy may be present.

Cerebral arteriography should be avoided, because it offers little additional information and carries the risk of increasing ischemia.

TREATMENT. A vaso-occlusive crisis requires prompt hydration, oxygen administration, and transfusions of packed red blood cells. Hydration should not reach the point of increasing cerebral edema. Recurrent strokes may be prevented by a regimen of regular transfusions designed to keep the level of hemoglobin A above 60%.

Vasculopathies

Hypersensitivity Vasculitis

The term *hypersensitivity vasculitis* covers several disorders that have a known underlying cause (drugs, infection) and are characterized by purpura of the legs and venulitis. Neurologic complications occur only in *Henoch-Schönlein purpura,* for which the cause is not established but is thought to be an antecedent infection.

CLINICAL FEATURES. The systemic features of Henoch-Schönlein purpura are fever, a purpuric rash on the extensor surfaces of the limbs, and abdominal pain with nausea and vomiting. Joint and renal disturbances may be present. Almost half of affected children have headache and abnormalities on EEG (Ostergaard and Storm, 1991). Focal neurologic deficits occur in one third of patients, with hemiplegia accounting for half of these cases. Hemiplegia may be preceded by a seizure, and may be associated with hemianesthesia, hemianopia, and aphasia. These deficits may be permanent.

DIAGNOSIS. Infarction or hemorrhage, or both, may be demonstrated by CT or MRI.

TREATMENT. Corticosteroids are used to treat the underlying disease.

Isolated Angiitis of the Central Nervous System

Isolated angiitis of the central nervous system is an inflammation of small cerebral vessels. It is rare in children (Barron et al, 1993). The clinical features are recurrent headache, sometimes of a migrainous type, encephalopathy, and stroke. Arteriography shows multiple areas of irregular narrowing of the cerebral vessels. Corticosteroid therapy may be beneficial, but additional treatment with pulse cyclophosphamide is often required.

Systemic Lupus Erythematosus

Several collagen vascular disorders can cause neurologic disturbances in adults, but systemic lupus erythematosus is the main cause in children. *Mixed connective tissue disease* is a rare cause of either large vessel occlusion or hemorrhage secondary to fibrinoid necrosis (Graf et al, 1993).

CLINICAL FEATURES. The clinical features of lupus in children is similar to those in adults except for a higher incidence of hepatosplenomegaly, chorea (see Chapter 14), nephritis, and avascular necrosis (White, 1994). Most children have fever, arthralgia, and skin rash at the time of diagnosis. Neurologic features are present in one quarter of children at the time of diagnosis. Unlike systemic complaints, neurologic disturbances are likely to progress or develop anew even after treatment is initiated. Neurologic dysfunction develops in about one third of children sometime during the course of disease. Headache, seizures, cranial neuropathies, and mental disorders are common features. Hemiplegia usually follows a seizure and may be caused by cerebral infarction or hemorrhage.

Neurologic episodes during treatment are often complications of immunosuppression, such as fungal meningitis, rather than primary complications of the underlying disease (Wong et al, 1991).

DIAGNOSIS. The diagnosis of lupus requires a compatible clinical syndrome and the detection of an abnormal titer of antinuclear antibody or anti-DNA antibody to native DNA. The presence of anticardiolipin antibodies is associated with hemolytic anemia and thrombotic events (Seaman et al, 1995). CT or MRI of the head is useful to determine the presence of hemorrhage or infarction. Results of cerebral arteriography may be normal.

TREATMENT. Large doses of corticosteroids are the mainstay of therapy, but the mortality is higher in children than in adults.

Takayasu Arteritis

Takayasu arteritis, a disorder of unknown cause, involves the aorta and its major branches.

CLINICAL FEATURES. Onset usually occurs between 15 and 20 years of age, but may occur as early as infancy. Ninety percent of patients are female. The most common features are hypertension, absent pulses, and vascular bruits. Stroke occurs in only 5% to 10% of patients and is usually characterized by focal seizures and sudden hemiplegia.

DIAGNOSIS. CT reveals a focal hypodense area, indicating infarction. Arteriography shows involvement of the ascending aorta and its major branches. Cardiac catheterization is necessary to define the full extent of arteritis. Some vessels have a beaded appearance; others terminate abruptly and have prestenotic dilatation.

TREATMENT. Aggressive immunosuppressive therapy with prednisone, 2 mg/kg/day, and azathioprine, 1 mg/kg/day, is indicated. If the disease is left untreated, the mortality rate is 75%. Early diagnosis and treatment can lead to full recovery.

DIABETES MELLITUS

Acute but transitory attacks of hemiparesis occur in children with insulin-dependent diabetes mellitus. Complicated migraine is a suggested mechanism, but the pathophysiology remains unknown.

CLINICAL FEATURES. Attacks frequently occur during sleep in a child with a respiratory illness. Hemiparesis is present on awakening; the face and arm are more affected than the leg. Sensation is intact, but aphasia is present if the dominant hemisphere is affected. Tendon reflexes may be depressed or brisk in the affected arm and an extensor plantar response can usually be elicited.

Headache is a constant feature and may be unilateral or generalized. Some patients are nauseated. The family does not have a history of migraine.

Attacks last for 3 to 24 hours, and recovery is complete. Recurrences are common.

DIAGNOSIS. Stroke is not a complication of juvenile insulin-dependent diabetes, except during episodes of ketoacidosis (see Chapter 2). Head CT in children with transitory hemiplegia does not show infarction. EEG shows a focus of polymorphic delta activity that returns to normal after several days.

TREATMENT. Although some children have further attacks, no way of preventing recurrences has been established. Prophylactic phenobarbital was useful in one child.

EPILEPSY

Absence Status

Absence attacks in children are characterized by brief episodes of staring or eye blinking associated with 3-Hz generalized spike-wave complexes on the EEG (see Chapter 1). Prolonged absence attacks are characterized by confusion and automatisms similar to complex partial seizures. In addition, a variant form of absence status exists with hemiparesis as the primary feature.

CLINICAL FEATURES. Some patients have a history of generalized tonic-clonic seizures but are not known to have a prior history of absence. The patient seems confused, has poor motor performance, and is unable to carry on a conversation. Transitory hemiparesis or face-hand weakness is noted, and aphasia may be present. The attack ends spontaneously or with the intravenous administration of diazepam.

DIAGNOSIS. EEG is essential for diagnosis. Several different epileptiform patterns may be seen. The most common pattern is 3-Hz spike-wave complexes from the frontal region during an attack. These complexes are often generalized but always have a unilateral predominance.

TREATMENT. Standard anticonvulsant drugs provide seizure control. However, the appropriate class of drugs to use in any individual is difficult to determine. Some respond to phenytoin or carbamazepine, whereas others respond to ethosuximide, valproate, or clonazepam.

Hemiparetic Seizures

Todd paralysis is a term used to describe hemiparesis that lasts minutes or days and follows a focal or generalized seizure. It most often occurs when seizures are prolonged or caused by an underlying structural abnormality. An ischemic mechanism has been suggested.

Hemiparesis may be a seizure manifestation as well as a postictal event. The seizures are called *hemiparetic* or *focal inhibitory* seizures. Todd paralysis may be difficult to distinguish from hemiparetic seizures, because it is not always clear whether a seizure preceded the hemiparesis or whether the hemiparesis is ictal or postictal.

CLINICAL FEATURES. The initial feature may be a brief focal seizure followed by flaccid hemiparesis or the abrupt onset of flaccid monoparesis or hemiparesis. Consciousness is not impaired, and the child seems well otherwise. The severity and distribution of weakness fluctuate, affecting one limb more than the other, and sometimes the face. Tendon reflexes are normal in the hemiparetic limbs, but the plantar response may be extensor.

DIAGNOSIS. EEG shows recurrent spike-and-slow-wave discharges in the contralateral hemisphere. A radioisotope scan shows increased focal uptake in the affected hemisphere. Results of MRI, CT, and cerebral arteriography are normal.

TREATMENT. Seizures respond to standard anticonvulsant drugs (see Chapter 1).

INFECTIONS

Hemiplegia occurs during the course of bacterial meningitis, resulting from vasculitis or venous thromboses, and during the course of viral encephalitis, especially herpes simplex, resulting from parenchymal necrosis. In both bacterial and viral infections, hemiplegia is usually preceded by prolonged or repetitive focal seizures.

Brain abscess may cause hemiplegia, but its evolution is usually slowly progressive rather than acute.

MIGRAINE

Migraine is a hereditary disorder associated with paroxysmal alterations in cerebral blood flow. Transitory neurologic abnormalities may accompany the attack but these are believed to be caused by a primary neuronal disturbance rather than cerebral ischemia. However, cerebral infarction may occur in adolescents during a prolonged attack of classic migraine.

The occurrence of focal motor deficits, usually hemiplegia or ophthalmoplegia (see Chapter 15), during an occasional migraine attack is called *complicated migraine*. In some families, hemiplegic migraine is a familial trait. This condition is called *familial hemiplegic migraine*.

Complicated Migraine

CLINICAL FEATURES. The family has a history of migraine, but other family members have not experienced hemiplegia during an attack. The evolution of symptoms is variable but usually includes scintillating or simple scotomas, unilateral dysesthesias of the hand and mouth, and unilateral weakness of the arm and face. The leg is usually spared. Occurring concurrently with hemiparesis is a throbbing frontotemporal headache contralateral to the affected hemisphere. Nausea and vomiting follow. The patient falls asleep and has usually recovered on awakening. Hemiparesis lasts less than 24 hours.

DIAGNOSIS. Migraine is a clinical diagnosis that relies heavily on a positive family history of the disorder. During an attack of hemiplegic migraine, an EEG focus of polymorphic delta activity is present in the hemisphere contralateral to weakness. Arteriography is contraindicated and may prolong the attack.

TREATMENT. The management of migraine is summarized in Chapter 3.

Familial Hemiplegic Migraine

Familial hemiplegic migraine differs from complicated migraine because other family members with migraine have had at least one hemiplegic attack. The trait is transmitted by autosomal dominant inheritance and the gene location is on chromosome 19p, possibly allelic with the gene for hereditary paroxysmal cerebellar ataxia (Joutel et al, 1995).

CLINICAL FEATURES. Attacks are stereotyped, occur primarily in childhood or adolescence, are precipitated by trivial head trauma, and rarely occur more often than once a year. The hemiplegia, although usually more severe in the face and arm, affects the leg too, and always outlasts the headache (Marchioni et al, 1995). Hemianesthesia of the hemiplegic side is a prominent feature. Aphasia occurs when the dominant hemisphere is affected. Confusion, stupor, or psychosis may be present during an attack. The psychosis includes both auditory and visual hallucinations, as well as delusions. Occasionally, patients have fever and a stiff neck.

Symptoms last for 2 or 3 days. When the attack is over, the neurologic deficits usually resolve completely, but permanent sequelae are possible. A gaze-evoked nystagmus may persist between attacks (Elliott et al, 1996). Recurrent hemiplegic attacks may occur on either the same or the opposite side.

DIAGNOSIS. A family history of hemiplegic migraine is essential for diagnosis. MRI may show atrophy of the cerebellar vermis that worsens with age.

TREATMENT. Because familial hemiplegic migraine and acetazolamide-responsive episodic ataxia are allelic conditions, a trial of acetazolamide is indicated.

TRAUMA

Trauma accounts for half of all deaths in children. Approximately 10% of traumatic injuries in children are not accidental. Head injury is the leading cause of death from child abuse, and half of survivors are left with permanent neurologic handicaps.

Epidural hematoma, subdural hematoma, cerebral laceration, and intracerebral hemorrhage can produce focal signs such as hemiplegia. However, brain swelling is such a prominent feature of even trivial head injury in children that diminished consciousness and seizures are the typical clinical features (see Chapter 2).

TUMORS

The initial clinical feature of primary tumors of the cerebral hemispheres is more likely to be chronic progressive hemiplegia than acute hemiplegia. However, tumors may cause acute hemiplegia when they bleed or provoke seizures and must be considered in the evaluation of acute hemiplegia.

 Chronic Progressive Hemiplegia

The important causes of chronic progressive hemiplegia are brain tumor, brain abscess, and arteriovenous malformations. The initial features of all three are often those of increased intracranial pressure; they are discussed in Chapter 4. Progressive hemiplegia is sometimes an initial feature of demyelinating diseases, which are discussed in Chapters 5 and 10 (Table 11–4).

■ T A B L E 1 1 – 4
Progressive Hemiplegia

Arteriovenous malformation (see Chapter 4)
Brain abscess (see Chapter 4)
Cerebral hemisphere tumor (see Chapter 4)
Demyelinating diseases
  Adrenoleukodystrophy (see Chapter 5)
  Late-onset globoid leukodystrophy (see Chapter 5)
  Multiple sclerosis (see Chapter 10)
Sturge-Weber syndrome

Sturge-Weber Syndrome

The Sturge-Weber syndrome is a sporadic neurocutaneous disorder characterized by the association of a venous angioma of the pia mater with a port-wine stain of the face (Pascual-Castroviejo et al, 1993).

CLINICAL FEATURES. The cutaneous angioma is flat and variable in size but usually involves the upper lid. It is unilateral in 70% of children and ipsilateral to the venous angioma of the pia. Even when the facial nevus is bilateral, the pial angioma is usually unilateral. The size of the cutaneous angioma does not predict the size of the intracranial angioma.

Seizures occur in 80% of children with Sturge-Weber syndrome. Onset is generally within the first year and the seizure type is usually focal motor, sometimes leading to partial or generalized status epilepticus (see Chapter 1). Eighty percent of children with Sturge-Weber who have seizures in the first year will show developmental delay and mental retardation (Sujansky and Conradi, 1995).

Hemiplegia, contralateral to the facial angioma, occurs in up to 50% of children. It is often noted initially after a focal-onset seizure and progresses in severity after subsequent seizures. Transitory episodes of hemiplegia that cannot be related to clinical or EEG evidence of seizure activity may occur. Some episodes are associated with migraine-like headache and others occur in the absence of other symptoms, and may be caused by transitory ischemia.

DIAGNOSIS. The association of neurologic abnormalities and a port-wine stain of the face should suggest the Sturge-Weber syndrome. The eyelid and the skin above the eye should be examined for angioma in any child with focal motor seizures. The pial angioma is best visualized by a contrast-enhanced MRI and only rarely by angiography.

TREATMENT. The seizures are often difficult to control with anticonvulsant medications.

Surgery is recommended when seizures are refractory and disabling (Roach et al, 1994). Hemispherectomy is often required but local resection is satisfactory for patients with localized lesions.

REFERENCES

Angelini L, Ravelli A, Caporali R, et al. High prevalence of antiphospholipid antibodies in children with idiopathic cerebral ischemia. Pediatrics 1994;94:500-503.

Barron TE, Ostrov BE, Zimmerman RA, et al. Isolated angiitis of CNS: Treatment with pulse cyclophosphamide. Pediatr Neurol 1993;9:73-75.

Bourgeois M, Acardi J, Goutiéres F. Alternating hemiplegia of childhood. J Pediatr 1993;122:673-679.

Broderick J, Talbot T, Prenger E, et al. Stroke in children within a major metropolitan area: The surprising importance of intracerebral hemorrhage. J Child Neurol 1993;8: 250-255.

Cheng TO. Mitral valve prolapse. Annu Rev Med 1989;40: 201-211.

Elliot MA, Peroutka SJ, Welch S, et al. Familial hemiplegic migraine, nystagmus, and cerebellar atrophy. Ann Neurol 1996;39:100-106.

Garg BP, Ottinger CJ, Smith RR, et al. Strokes in children due to vertebral artery trauma. Neurology 1993;43:2555-2558.

Graf WD, Milstein JM, Sherry DD. Stroke and mixed connective tissue disease. J Child Neurol 1993;8:256-259.

Hirano M, Pavlakis SG. Mitochondrial myopathy, encephalopathy, lactic acidosis, and strokelike episodes (MELAS): Current concepts. J Child Neurol 1994;9:4-13.

Joutel A, Ducros A, Vahedi K, et al. Genetic heterogeneity of familial hemiplegic migraine. Am J Hum Genet 1995;55: 1166-1172.

Kerr LM, Anderson DM, Thompson JA, et al. Ischemic stroke in the young: Evaluation and comparison of patients six months to thirty-nine years. J Child Neurol 1993;8:266-270.

Koo B, Becker LE, Chuang S, et al. Mitochondrial encephalomyopathy, lactic acidosis, stroke-like episodes (MELAS): Clinical, radiological, pathological, and genetic observations. Ann Neurol 1993;34:25-32.

Levine SR, Brust JCM, Futrell N, et al. A comparative study of the cerebrovascular complications of cocaine: Alkaloidal versus hydrochloride—a review. Neurology 1991;41:1173-1177.

Marchioni E, Galimberta CA, Soragna D, et al. Familial hemiplegic migraine versus migraine with prolonged aura: An uncertain diagnosis in a family report. Neurology 1995;45:33-37.

Mikati MA, Maguire H, Barlow CE, et al. A syndrome of autosomal dominant alternating hemiplegia: Clinical presentation mimicking intractable epilepsy; and physiologic investigations. Neurology 1992;42:2251-2257.

Ostergaard JR, Storm K. Neurologic manifestations of Schönlein-Henoch purpura. Acta Paediatr Scand 1991;80: 339-342.

Pascual-Casroviejo I, Diaz-Gonzalez C, Garcia-Melian RM, et al. Sturge-Weber syndrome: Study of 40 patients. Pediatr Neurol 1993;9:283-288.

Roach ES, Riela AR, Chugani HT, et al. Sturge-Weber syndrome: Recommendations for surgery. J Child Neurol 1994;9:190-192.

Schöning M, Klein R, Krägeloh-Mann I, et al. Antiphospholipid antibodies in cerebrovascular ischemia and stroke in childhood. Neuropediatrics 1994;25:8-14.

Seaman DE, Londino AV Jr, Kwoh CK, et al. Antiphospholipid antibodies in pediatric systemic lupus erythematosus. Pediatrics 1995;96:1040-1045.

Smith CD, Baumann RJ. Clinical features and magnetic resonance imaging in congenital and childhood stroke. J Child Neurol 1991;6:263-272.

Steinlin M, Good M, Martin E, et al. Congenital hemiplegia: Morphology of cerebral lesions and pathogenetic aspects from MRI. Neuropediatrics 1993;24:224-229.

Sujansky E, Conradi S. Sturge-Weber syndrome: Age of onset of seizures and glaucoma and the prognosis for affected children. J Child Neurol 1995;10:49-58.

Vargha-Kadem F, Isaacs E, Van Der Werf S, et al. Development of intelligence and memory in children with hemiplegic cerebral palsy: The deleterious consequences of early seizures. Brain 1992;115:315-329.

Whitlock JA, Janco RL, Phillips JA III. Inherited hypercoagulable states in children. Am J Pediatr Hematol Oncol 1989;11:170-173.

White PH. Pediatric systemic lupus erythematosus and neonatal lupus. Rheum Dis Clin North Am 1994;20:119-127.

Wiznitzer M, Masaryk TJ. Cerebrovascular abnormalities in pediatric stroke: Assessment using parenchymal and angiographic magnetic resonance imaging. Ann Neurol 1991;29: 585-589.

Wong KL, Woo EKW, Yu YL, et al. Neurological manifestations of systemic lupus erythematosus: A prospective study. Q J Med 1991;81:857-860.

12

Paraplegia and Quadriplegia

The term *paraplegia* is used in this text to denote the partial or complete weakness of both legs, therefore obviating need for the term *paraparesis*. Many conditions described fully in this chapter are abnormalities of the spinal cord. The same spinal abnormality can cause paraplegia or quadriplegia, depending on the location of injury. Therefore, the two are discussed together in this chapter. The term *quadriplegia* is used to denote partial or complete weakness of all limbs, and the term *quadriparesis* is not used.

Approach to Paraplegia

Weakness of both legs, without any involvement of the arms, suggests an abnormality of either the spinal cord or the peripheral nerves. Ordinarily, peripheral neuropathies are readily identified by the pattern of distal weakness and sensory loss, atrophy, and loss of tendon reflexes (see Chapters 7 and 9). In contrast, spinal paraplegia causes spasticity, exaggerated tendon reflexes, and a dermatomal level of sensory loss. Disturbances in the conus medullaris and cauda equina, especially congenital malformation, may produce a complex of signs in which spinal cord or peripheral nerve localization is difficult. Indeed, both may be involved. Spinal paraplegia may be asymmetric at first, and then the initial feature is monoplegia (see Chapter 13). When anatomic localization between the spinal cord and peripheral nerves is difficult, electromyogra-

phy (EMG) and nerve conduction studies are useful in making the distinction.

Paraplegia is sometimes caused by cerebral abnormalities. In such a case, the child's arms as well as the legs are usually weak. However, leg weakness is so much greater than arm weakness that paraplegia is the chief complaint. It is important to remember that both the brain and the spinal cord may be abnormal and that the abnormalities can be in continuity (syringomyelia) or separated (Chiari malformation and myelomeningocele).

Spinal Paraplegia and Quadriplegia

The conditions that cause acute, chronic, or progressive spinal paraplegia are listed in Table 12-1. In the absence of trauma, the acute onset or rapid progression of paraplegia is caused by either spinal cord compression or myelitis. Spinal cord compression from any cause is a medical emergency requiring rapid diagnosis and therapy to avoid permanent paraplegia. Corticosteroids have the same dehydrating effect on the spinal cord as on the brain and provide transitory decompression before surgery.

Several techniques are available to visualize the spinal cord. Each has its place, and sometimes more than one technique must be used to achieve a comprehensive picture of the disease process. However, as resolution is increased and scan time decreased by newer magnetic reso-

■ TABLE 12–1
Spinal Paraplegia

Adrenomyeloneuropathy (Adrenoleukodystrophy)
Congenital Malformations
Arachnoid cyst
Arteriovenous malformations
Atlantoaxial dislocation
Caudal regression syndrome
Dysraphic states
   Chiari malformation
   Myelomeningocele
   Tethered spinal cord
Syringomyelia (see Chapter 9)
Familial Spastic Paraplegia
Autosomal dominant
Autosomal recessive
X-linked recessive
Infections
Asthmatic amyotrophy (see Chapter 13)
Diskitis
Epidural abscess
Herpes zoster myelitis
Polyradiculoneuropathy (see Chapter 7)
Tuberculous osteomyelitis
Lupus Myelopathy
Neonatal Cord Infarction
Transverse Myelitis
Devic disease
Encephalomyelitis
Idiopathic
Trauma
Concussion
Epidural hematoma
Fracture dislocation
Neonatal cord trauma (see Chapter 6)
Tumors
Astrocytoma
Ependymoma
Neuroblastoma
Other

nance imaging (MRI) instruments, MRI is becoming the procedure of choice.

SYMPTOMS AND SIGNS

Clumsiness of gait, refusal to stand or walk, and loss of bladder or bowel control are the common complaints of spinal paraplegia. Clumsiness of gait is the usual feature of slowly progressive disorders. The decline in function can be sufficiently insidious to be overlooked for years. Refusal to stand or walk is a symptom of an acute process. When a young child refuses to support weight, the underlying cause may be weakness or pain. Sometimes both are present.

Scoliosis is a feature of many spinal cord disorders. It is seen with neural tube defects, spinal cord tumors, and several degenerative disorders. The presence of scoliosis, in females before puberty and in males of all ages, should strongly suggest either a spinal cord disorder or a neuromuscular disease (see Chapters 6 and 7).

Abnormalities in the skin overlying the spine, such as an abnormal tuft of hair, pigmentation, a sinus opening, or a mass, may indicate an underlying dysraphic state. Spina bifida is almost always an associated feature.

Foot deformities and especially stunted growth of a limb are malevolent signs of lower spinal cord dysfunction. The usual deformity is foreshortening of the foot, *pes cavus*. In such cases disturbances of bladder control are often an associated feature.

Spinal myoclonus is often misdiagnosed as seizure activity or fasciculations. It is characterized by brief, irregular contractions of small groups of muscles and persists in sleep. Myoclonus is caused by irritation to pools of motor neurons and interneurons, usually by an intramedullary tumor or syrinx. The dermatomal distribution of the myoclonus localizes the site of irritation within the spinal cord.

ADRENOMYELONEUROPATHY

Adrenomyeloneuropathy is one phenotype of adrenoleukodystrophy, an X-linked disorder caused by impaired ability to oxidize very-long-chain fatty acids (see Chapter 5). Paraparesis begins after age 20 and slowly progresses throughout adult life. Intellect is not usually impaired and prolonged survival is the rule (Moser et al, 1992).

CONGENITAL MALFORMATIONS

Some congenital malformations, such as caudal regression syndrome and myelomeningocele, are obvious at birth. Many others do not cause symptoms until the teens or later. Congenital malformations must always be considered when progressive paraplegia appears in childhood.

Arachnoid Cysts

Arachnoid cysts of the spinal cord, like those of the brain (see Chapter 4), are usually asymptomatic and discovered incidentally on imaging studies. Familial cases should suggest neurofibromatosis type 2 (see Chapter 5).

CLINICAL FEATURES. Arachnoid cysts may be single or multiple and are usually thoracic. Symptomatic arachnoid cysts are unusual in children and are most often encountered in adolescents and young adults. The features are back or radicular pain and paraplegia. Symptoms are intensified when the child is standing and intermittent when the child changes position. They have a tendency to become more severe with time.

DIAGNOSIS. MRI is the diagnostic modality of choice. The cyst has the same MRI characteristics as cerebrospinal fluid.

TREATMENT. Shunting of the cyst is curative but should not be undertaken unless the cyst is known to be symptomatic. It is a common mistake to blame a subarachnoid cyst for symptoms that have another cause.

Arteriovenous Malformations

Arteriovenous malformations of the spinal cord are uncommon in childhood. The youngest patient reported was 1 year old, and only 14% of childhood cases begin before age 5.

CLINICAL FEATURES. The progression of symptoms is usually insidious, and the time from onset to diagnosis may be several years. Subacute or chronic pain is the initial feature in one third of patients, and subarachnoid hemorrhage in one quarter. Paraplegia is an early feature in only one third, but monoplegia or paraplegia is present in almost all children at the time of diagnosis. Most children have a slowly progressive spastic paraplegia and loss of bladder control.

When subarachnoid hemorrhage is the initial manifestation, the malformation is more likely to be in the cervical portion of the spinal cord. Blunt trauma to the spine may be a precipitating factor. The onset of paraplegia or quadriplegia is then acute and associated with back pain.

Back pain and episodic weakness that improve completely or in part may be initial features in some children, but impairment is progressive. This type of presentation is misleading and diagnosis may be delayed for several years.

DIAGNOSIS. MRI has replaced myelography as the first step in diagnosis. It distinguishes intramedullary from dural and extramedullary locations of the malformation and even allows recognition of thrombus formation. Arteriography is still necessary to demonstrate the intramedullary extent of the malformation and all of the feeding vessels.

TREATMENT. The potential approaches to therapy for intraspinal and intracranial malformations are similar (see Chapter 4).

Atlantoaxial Dislocation

The odontoid process is the major factor preventing dislocation of C1 onto C2. Aplasia of the odontoid process can occur alone or as part of Morquio syndrome, other mucopolysaccharidoses, Klippel-Feil syndrome, several types of genetic chondrodysplasia, and some chromosomal abnormalities (Crockard and Stevens, 1995). Asymptomatic atlantoaxial subluxation is thought to occur in 20% of children with Down syndrome as a result of congenital hypoplasia of the articulation of C1 and C2; symptomatic dislocation is much less common.

CLINICAL FEATURES. Congenital atlantoaxial dislocation produces an acute or slowly progressive quadriplegia that may begin anytime from the neonatal period to adult life. When the onset is in a newborn, the clinical features resemble an acute infantile spinal muscular atrophy (see Chapter 6). The infant has generalized hypotonia with preservation of facial expression and extraocular movement. The tendon reflexes are absent at first but then become hyperactive.

Dislocations during childhood frequently follow a fall or head injury. In such cases symptoms may begin suddenly and include not only those of myelopathy but also those related to vertebral artery occlusion (Bhatnagar et al, 1991).

Morquio syndrome is primarily a disease of the skeleton with only secondary abnormalities of the spinal cord. Beginning in the second year or thereafter, affected children have development of prominent ribs and sternum, knock-knees, progressive shortening of the neck, and dwarfism. The odontoid process is aplastic or absent. Acute, subacute, or chronic cervical myelopathy develops, sometimes precipitated by a fall. An insidious onset is characterized by loss of endurance, fainting attacks, and a "pins and needles" sensation in the arms.

The essential feature of the *Klippel-Feil syndrome* is a reduced number and abnormal fusion of cervical vertebrae. As in Morquio syndrome, the head appears to rest directly on the shoulders, the posterior hairline is low, and movement in all directions is limited. Elevation of the scapulae and deformity of the ribs (Sprengel deformity) are frequently present. Weakness and atrophy of the arm muscles and mirror movements of the hands are associated with the paraplegia. Associated abnormalities may be present in several different organ systems.

Symptomatic atlantoaxial dislocation in children with Down syndrome may occur anytime from infancy to the twenties. Females are affected more often than males. Symptoms include neck pain, torticollis, and an abnormal gait. Spinal cord compression is progressive and leads to quadriplegia and urinary incontinence.

DIAGNOSIS. Lateral radiographs of the cervical portion of the spine in extension and flexion may show atlantoaxial instability, but computed tomography (CT) of the cervical vertebrae provides better documentation of the instability and of the spinal cord compression. When Morquio syndrome is suspected, the urine should be checked for keratan sulfate.

TREATMENT. Surgical stabilization of the atlantoaxial junction must be considered in any child with evidence of spinal cord compression. The choice of surgical procedure depends on the mechanism of compression.

Caudal Regression Syndrome

The term *caudal regression syndrome* covers several malformations of the caudal spine that range from sacral agenesis to sirenomelia, in which only one leg is present (Towfighi and Housman, 1991). The mechanism of caudal regression is poorly understood. Although the name implies that the cord was formed properly and then regressed, defects in neural tube closure and prosencephalization are often associated features (Martìnez-Frìas et al, 1994). The risk of caudal regression is greater among infants of diabetic mothers.

The clinical spectrum varies from absence of the lumbosacral spinal cord, resulting in small paralyzed legs, to a single malformed leg associated with malformations of the rectum and genitourinary tract.

Chiari Malformation

The type I Chiari malformation is elongation of the cerebellar vermis with herniation of its caudal end through the foramen magnum. The type II malformation combines the cerebellar herniation with distortion and dysplasia of the medulla and occurs in more than 50% of children with lumbar myelomeningocele (Azimullah et al, 1991). The herniated portion may become ischemic and necrotic and can cause compression of the brainstem and upper cervical spinal cord.

CLINICAL FEATURES. The initial features of the type I malformation are often insidious. Headache and neck pain are the first features in 38% of children, and weakness in 56%. Eighty percent show motor deficits on examination, usually atrophy and hyporeflexia in the arms and spasticity and hyperreflexia in the legs. Sensory loss and scoliosis are each present in half of cases.

The type II malformation should be suspected in every child with myelomeningocele. In most the cerebellar displacement is asymptomatic. Hydrocephalus may be caused by aqueductal stenosis or by an obstruction of the outflow of cerebrospinal fluid from the fourth ventricle from herniation. Respiratory distress is the most important feature of the Chiari malformation and the usual cause of death. Rapid respirations, episodes of apnea, and Cheyne-Stokes respirations may occur. Other evidence of brainstem compression are poor feeding, vomiting, dysphagia, and paralysis of the tongue. Sudden cardiorespiratory failure is the usual cause of death.

DIAGNOSIS. The malformation is best visualized by MRI of the posterior fossa and cervical cord, but recognition of bony abnormalities of the cervical cord may require CT or plain radiographs.

TREATMENT. Newborns with myelomeningocele and respiratory distress caused by the Chiari malformation are often treated with posterior fossa decompression. Unfortunately, the results are not encouraging. Posterior fossa decompression is usually successful in relieving symptoms of cord compression in older children without myelomeningocele. Ventriculoperitoneal shunt may be required as well.

Myelomeningocele

Dysraphia comprises all defects in the closure of the neural tube and its coverings. Closure occurs during the third and fourth weeks of gestation. The mesoderm surrounding the neural tube gives rise to dura, skull, and vertebrae, but not to the skin. Therefore, defects in the final closure of the neural tube and its mesodermal case do not preclude the presence of a dermal covering.

Despite extensive epidemiologic studies, the cause of myelomeningocele remains unknown. Causes are likely to be multifactorial, including both genetic and environmental factors (Chatkupt et al, 1994). Because women who have previously had a child with dysraphia have an approximate 2% risk of recurrence, prenatal diagnosis can be offered to prevent repetition.

Alpha-fetoprotein is the principal plasma protein of the fetus and is present in amniotic fluid. When the fetus has a defect of the skin that allows the exudation of plasma proteins, the concentration of alpha-fetoprotein in the amniotic fluid increases. Prenatal diagnosis is possible in every case by the combination of measuring the maternal serum concentration of alpha-fetoprotein and performing an ultrasound examination of the fetus (Nadel et al, 1990).

The incidence of dysraphic defects has been declining in the United States and the United Kingdom. This decline cannot be explained by antenatal screening alone and may be caused in part by changes in critical environmental factors.

Because the ingestion of folic acid supplements during early pregnancy reduces the incidence of neural tube defects, all women of child-bearing age are advised to consume 0.4 mg of folic acid daily (Centers for Disease Control, 1992). Supplements of 4 mg/day of folic acid are suggested for women with a prior history of delivering a child with a neural tube defect from at least 4 weeks before the conception through the first 3 months of pregnancy.

CLINICAL FEATURES. *Spina bifida cystica,* the protrusion of a cystic mass through the defect, is an obvious deformity of the newborn's spine. More than 90% are thoracolumbar. Among newborns with spina bifida cystica the protruding sac is a meningocele without neural elements in 10% to 20% and is a myelomeningocele in the rest. Meningoceles tend to have a partial dermal covering and are often pedunculated, with a narrow base connecting the sac to the underlying spinal cord. Myelomeningoceles usually have a broad base, are poorly epithelialized, and ooze a combination of cerebrospinal fluid and serum. Remnants of the spinal cord are fused to the exposed portion of the dome.

In newborns with spina bifida cystica, it is important to determine the extent of neurologic dysfunction caused by the myelopathy, the potential for the development of hydrocephalus, and the presence of other malformations in the nervous system and in other organs. When myelomeningocele is the only deformity, the newborn is alert and responsive and has no difficulty in feeding. Diminished consciousness or responsiveness and difficulty in feeding should suggest perinatal asphyxia or cerebral malformations such as hydrocephalus. Cyanosis, pallor, or dyspnea may be caused by associated malformations in the cardiovascular system. Multiple major defects are present in 27% of cases.

Location of the myelomeningocele with reference to the ribs and iliac crest provides reasonably accurate information concerning the spinal segments involved. Several patterns of motor dysfunction may be observed depending on the cyst's location. Motor dysfunction results from interruption of the corticospinal tracts and from dysgenesis of the segmental innervation. At birth the legs are flaccid and the hips are dislocated. Spastic paraplegia, a spastic bladder, and a level of sensory loss develop in infants with a thoracic lesion. Segmental withdrawal reflexes below the level of the lesion, which indicate the presence of an intact but isolated spinal cord segment below the cyst, are present in half of patients. Infants with deformities of the conus medullaris maintain a flaccid paraplegia, have lumbosacral sensory loss, lack a withdrawal response in the legs, and have a distended bladder with overflow incontinence.

Only 15% of newborns with myelomeningocele have clinical evidence of hydrocephalus at birth, but hydrocephalus can be detected in 60% of affected newborns by ultrasound. Hydrocephalus eventually develops in 80%. The first clinical features of hydrocephalus often follow the repair of the myelomeningocele, but the two are not related. Aqueductal stenosis is the cause of hydrocephalus in three quarters of infants with myelomeningocele.

DIAGNOSIS. The diagnosis of spina bifida cystica is made by examination alone. EMG may be useful to clarify the distribution of segmental dysfunction. Cranial ultrasound should be performed on every newborn to look for hydrocephalus. CT and MRI are useful to define malformations of the brain, especially the Chiari malformation (see Figure 10-7). This information may be needed in making therapeutic decisions. Even when hydrocephalus is not present at birth, ultrasound should be repeated in 2 to 4 weeks to evaluate ventricular size.

TREATMENT. The chance of surviving the first year is poor unless the back is closed. However, closure is not a "surgical emergency" and can be delayed for a week or longer without influencing the survival rate. Other factors associated with an increased mortality are a high spinal location of the defect and clinical hydrocephalus at birth. The long-term outcome depends on the degree of mental retardation and the neurologic deficit from the spinal defect.

Tethered Spinal Cord

The conus medullaris is sometimes anchored to the base of the vertebrae by a thickened filum terminale, a lipoma, a dermal sinus, or a diastematomyelia. Spina bifida occulta is usually an associated feature, and for this reason these anomalies are considered part of the spectrum of dysraphia. As the child grows, the tether causes the spinal cord to stretch and the lumbosacral segments to become ischemic. The mitochondrial oxidative metabolism of neurons is impaired, and neurologic dysfunction follows.

Dermal sinus is a midline opening of the skin usually marked by a tuft of hair or port-wine stain. It is caused by an abnormal invagination of ectoderm into the posterior closure site of the neural tube. Most sinuses terminate subcutaneously as a blind pouch or dermoid cyst. Others extend through a spina bifida to the developing neuraxis, at which point they attach to the dura or the spinal cord as a fibrous band or dermoid cyst. Such sinuses tether the spinal cord and may also serve as a route for bacteria from the skin to reach the subarachnoid space and cause meningitis.

Diastematomyelia consists of a bifid spinal cord (also diplomyelia) that is normal in the cervical and upper thoracic regions and then divides into lateral halves (Figure 12-1). Two types of diastematomyelia occur with equal frequency. In one type each half of the cord is surrounded by its own dural sheath and the two halves are separated by a fibrous or bony septum. Once the cord separates, it never rejoins. In the other type the two halves are surrounded by a single dural sheath, no septum is present, and the two halves rejoin after one or two segments. Therefore, splitting of the spinal cord is not caused by the presence of a septum,

but is instead a primary disturbance in the formation of luminal borders caused by faulty closure of the neural tube. It is usually associated with other dysraphic disturbances such as spina bifida occulta or cystica.

CLINICAL FEATURES. The initial features of a tethered spinal cord occur at any age, from infancy to young adulthood. The clinical features vary with age. External signs of spinal dysraphism (tuft of hair, subcutaneous lipoma, dermal sinus) are present in more than half of patients, and spina bifida occulta or sacral deformity is present in almost 90%.

Infants and young children are most likely to show clumsiness of gait, stunted growth or deformity of one foot or leg, and disturbances in bladder function. These may occur alone or in combination. Consequently, the first specialist consulted may be an orthopedic surgeon, a urologist, a neurologist, or a neurosurgeon. The progression of symptoms and signs is insidious, and at first most children are believed to have a static problem. Children with only a clumsy gait or disturbances in urinary control tend to have normal or exaggerated tendon reflexes and an extensor plantar response. In some children, the ankle tendon reflex is diminished or absent on one or both sides. Children with foot deformity usually have pes cavus and stunted growth of the entire leg. The other leg may appear normal or have a milder deformity without a growth disturbance. The tendon reflexes in the deformed foot are more likely to be diminished than increased.

The initial feature of tethered spinal cord in older children and adolescents is either clumsiness of gait or scoliosis. Bilateral, but mild, foot deformities are sometimes present and urinary incontinence and constipation may be reported. Tendon reflexes in the legs are usually exagger-

□ F I G U R E   1 2 – 1   Diplomyelia. MRI shows two cords with two central canals. An enlarged segment with a cystic center is seen on longitudinal section.

ated at the knees and ankles, and the plantar response is usually extensor.

DIAGNOSIS. MRI is the appropriate diagnostic test and is particularly useful in the detection of lumbosacral lipoma (Brophy et al, 1989). The essential feature of a tethered spinal cord is a low-lying conus medullaris. At 28 weeks' gestational age, the tip of the conus is at the L3 vertebral level. It generally rises one level by 40 weeks' gestation. A conus tip below the L2 to L3 interspace in children 5 years and older is always abnormal.

TREATMENT. Surgical relief of the tethering prevents further deterioration of neurologic function. However, improvement of pre-existing deficits occurs in only 25% of patients with lipoma and in 50% of patients with a thickened filum terminale.

FAMILIAL SPASTIC PARAPLEGIA

Familial spastic paraplegia is a heterogeneous group of genetic disorders in which the prominent clinical feature is progressive spastic paraplegia. Degeneration occurs in the lateral and posterior columns of the spinal cord, and for this reason these disorders are classified in the broader category of spinocerebellar degenerations. Some families have pure spastic paraplegia without clinical evidence of degeneration in the posterior columns or cerebellar pathways. Familial spastic paraplegia is transmitted by autosomal dominant inheritance in 70% of cases and by autosomal recessive inheritance in the remainder. Genetic heterogeneity exists even within the dominant and recessive forms. An X-linked form has been reported in less than 20 families. Linkage studies have mapped the abnormal gene to the long arm of the X chromosome (Cambi et al, 1995).

Autosomal Dominant Inheritance

CLINICAL FEATURES. Children with dominantly inherited spastic diplegia do not have prominent disturbances of other neurologic systems. The age at onset ranges from 1 to 68 years, with the mean at 29 years (Dürr et al, 1994). Early and late onset occurs among members of the same family. Motor milestones are normal in affected infants except for toe-walking. Their condition is frequently misdiagnosed as cerebral palsy, especially if the affected parent is asymptomatic or has only a mildly stiff gait. Increased tone is more prominent than

weakness. Tone increases slowly for 10 years and then stabilizes. At this point the child may have minimal stiffness of gait or be unable to stand or walk.

Tendon reflexes are usually increased in the legs and arms, and ankle clonus may be present. Occasionally, tendon reflexes at the ankle are diminished or absent. This may be caused by an associated axonal neuropathy. Increased reflexes are usually the only sign of involvement of the arms. Vibratory and position sense is diminished in half of patients. One third have urinary symptoms, usually in the form of frequency and urgency, and one third have a pes cavus deformity.

DIAGNOSIS. Familial spastic paraplegia is difficult to diagnose in the absence of a family history of the defect. It should be suspected in any child with very slowly progressive spastic paraplegia. Laboratory studies are not helpful except to exclude other conditions such as spinal cord compression and adrenoleukodystrophy.

TREATMENT. No treatment is available.

Autosomal Recessive Inheritance

Autosomal recessive inheritance of hereditary spastic paraplegia is characterized by involvement of other neurologic systems (Appleton et al, 1991). The associated features vary from family to family, suggesting genetic heterogeneity.

CLINICAL FEATURES. Spastic paraplegia may begin during infancy but can be delayed until until the teens. Involvement of other neurologic systems follows the establishment of spastic paraplegia. The common associated features are cerebellar dysfunction, pseudobulbar palsy, sensory neuropathy, and pes cavus. These features may be present in any combination.

Children with sensory neuropathy lose the tendon reflexes in the legs that had once been hyperactive. Some have delayed development and never achieve bladder control. When sensory loss is progressive, the symptoms resemble those of familial sensory neuropathies, described in Chapter 9. The outcome varies from mild disability to wheelchair confinement.

DIAGNOSIS. The onset of paraplegia is in infancy. In the absence of a family history, the course of disease suggests cerebral palsy until the progressive nature of the spasticity is recognized. Sensory neuropathy with mutilation of digits may lead to the erroneous diagnosis of syringomyelia. Laboratory tests are useful only to exclude other diagnoses.

TREATMENT. No treatment is available for the underlying defect, but supportive care for the sensory neuropathy is needed (see Chapter 9).

INFECTIONS

Primary myelitis from acquired immune deficiency syndrome (AIDS) is uncommon in children and is not discussed in this section.

DISKITIS

Diskitis is a relatively common disorder of childhood in which one disk space is inflamed; adjacent vertebral bodies may be affected as well. The cause is uncertain, but bacterial infection, viral infection, and trauma have been suspected. *Staphylococcus aureus* is the organism most often grown on culture of disk material removed by needle biopsy and is probably the major cause. The same organism is sometimes isolated from cultures of the blood.

CLINICAL FEATURES. The initial feature is either difficulty walking or pain. Difficulty walking occurs almost exclusively in children less than 3 years of age. The typical child has a low-grade fever, is observed to be limping, and then refuses to stand or walk. This symptom complex evolves over 24 to 48 hours. Affected children prefer to lie on their sides rather than to rest supine, resist being brought to standing, and then seem uncomfortable and walk with a shuffling gait. Examination shows loss of lumbar lordosis. The hips or back is sometimes tender.

Pain as an initial feature occurs more often after 3 years of age. The pain may be abdominal or vertebral. When abdominal, the pain gradually increases in intensity and may radiate from the epigastrium to the umbilicus or pelvis. Abdominal pain in association with low-grade fever and an elevated peripheral white blood cell count invariably suggests the possibility of appendicitis or other intra-abdominal disease. Fortunately, abdominal pain is the least common presenting feature.

Back pain is the most common complaint. Older children may indicate a specific area of pain and tenderness. Younger children may have only an abnormal posture intended to splint the painful area. Back pain usually leads to prompt diagnosis because attention is immediately directed to the spine. Examination reveals point tenderness, loss of lumbar lordosis, and decreased movement of the spine.

□ FIGURE 12-2 Diskitis. MRI reveals collapse of the disk space *(arrow)* and demineralization of the adjoining vertebral bodies.

DIAGNOSIS. Diskitis should be considered in all children who have a sudden back pain or refuse to walk and in whom neurologic findings are normal. Strength, tone, and tendon reflexes in the legs are normal. Radiographs of the spine reveal narrowing of the affected intervertebral space, most often in the lumbar region but sometimes as high as the C5 to C6 positions. The inflammation within the disk is best demonstrated by MRI, which shows osteomyelitis of the surrounding vertebrae as well as of the disk space (Figure 12-2).

TREATMENT. Whether antibiotics are effective is a matter of controversy. However, a course of treatment directed at *S. aureus* seems reasonable, even if the organism cannot be grown on culture. Immobilization is important, as much to reduce pain as to encourage healing. Bed rest is sufficient immobilization for most children.

Epidural Abscess

Most epidural abscesses result from hematogenous spread of bacteria, most often hemolytic *S. aureus,* rather than direct extension from vertebral osteomyelitis. The abscess is usually located on the dorsal surface of the midthoracic or lower lumbar spine, at which point the epidural space is large. The source of infection may be cutaneous or intra-abdominal, and often no source can be identified. Despite occasional reports of epidural abscess in infancy, it rarely occurs in children less than 10 years of age.

CLINICAL FEATURES. A bacterial infection or trauma to the back is described as an antecedent event in some children. The initial feature is usually back pain, which increases in severity and localizes at the site of the abscess. An effort is made to splint the trunk in extension; flexion and coughing intensify the pain. Fever is often present at the onset of pain but may be delayed for days. Headache, vomiting, and stiff neck often develop and suggest the diagnosis of meningitis. At this stage, examination reveals a rigid spine with tenderness to percussion over the involved area.

Symptoms of root irritation and spinal cord compression develop 3 to 6 days after localized back pain begins. Because the abscess is usually thoracic, root irritation is characterized by radiating pain around the chest or into the groin. Spinal cord compression is characterized by progressive paraplegia and bladder dysfunction. Back pain intensifies and is more severe than the pain associated with spinal cord compression by tumor. Fever also suggests abscess.

Epidural abscess in the thoracic region may cause flaccid or spastic paraplegia with hyperreflexia in the legs, while abscess in the lumbar region causes flaccid paraplegia and diminished tendon reflexes.

DIAGNOSIS. Most children with spinal epidural abscess undergo lumbar puncture because meningitis is suspected. If the abscess is lumbar and is pierced by the spinal needle, meningitis will follow. The cerebrospinal fluid is usually sterile, with an increased concentration of protein and a mixed pleocytosis in which lymphocytes predominate. The concentration of glucose is normal. Definitive diagnosis requires MRI of the painful area.

TREATMENT. Intravenous antibiotics directed against *S. aureus* should be started immediately when spinal epidural abscess is suspected. As with other causes of spinal cord compression, early surgical decompression is essential. The likelihood of recovery is diminished with each day that paraplegia is allowed to persist.

Herpes Zoster Myelitis

Immunosuppressed individuals may experience reactivation of the varicella-zoster virus that had been latent in sensory ganglia following primary chicken-pox infection (Devinsky et al, 1991).

CLINICAL FEATURES. The spinal cord becomes involved within 3 weeks after a truncal rash appears. The myelopathy usually progresses for 3 weeks, but progression may last long as 6 months in people with AIDS. Cord involvement is bilateral in 80% of cases.

DIAGNOSIS. Diagnosis depends on recognition of the characteristic herpetic rash at the dermatomal level of the myelitis. The spine should be imaged to exclude other causes. The cerebrospinal fluid shows a pleocytosis and protein elevation that is greatest at the time of maximal neurologic deficit.

TREATMENT. Corticosteroids and acyclovir are recommended for treatment, although their benefit is uncertain.

Tuberculous Osteomyelitis

Vertebral infection is caused by hematogenous dissemination. Any level of the vertebral column may be affected. The infection usually begins in one vertebral body and then spreads to adjacent vertebrae and the surrounding soft tissue. Less than 20% of patients with tuberculous osteomyelitis have symptoms of spinal cord dysfunction. The pathophysiologic mechanisms include epidural abscess, arteritis, and vertebral collapse. In addition, tuberculous granuloma of the spine may occur in the absence of vertebral disease.

CLINICAL FEATURES. Tuberculosis of the vertebrae and spine is primarily a disease of children and young adults. Young children with vertebral osteomyelitis not extending to the spinal cord may refuse to walk because of pain, and their symptoms may mimic paraplegia. The prominent features are fever, anorexia, and back pain. In children less than 10 years of age, infection is generally diffuse, affecting several vertebrae and adjacent tissues. Older children tend to have localized infection, but with a higher incidence of spinal cord compression.

The symptoms and signs of spinal cord compression from tuberculosis are similar to those described for epidural abscess, except that progression is slower.

DIAGNOSIS. The cerebrospinal fluid is usually under pressure and shows a pleocytosis with polymorphonuclear leukocytes predominating early in the course and lymphocytes predominating in the later stages. The total cell count rarely exceeds 500 cells/mm^3. Protein concentrations are elevated, and glucose concentrations are depressed. Acid-fast organisms can be seen on stained smear and can be isolated on cultures of the cerebrospinal fluid.

Early stages of vertebral osteomyelitis can be shown by technetium bone scan or plain radiographs. As the disease progresses, radiographs reveal collapse of adjacent vertebrae and gibbus formation.

TREATMENT. Tuberculous osteomyelitis and meningitis should be treated in a similar fashion. The recommended drug combinations are oral isoniazid, 20 mg/kg/day (up to 500 mg/day); intramuscular streptomycin, 20 mg/kg/day (up to 1 g/day); and oral rifampin, 15 mg/kg/day (up to 15 mg/kg). Streptomycin and rifampin are continued for 8 weeks following clinical improvement, and isoniazid is continued for 2 years.

LUPUS MYELOPATHY

Transverse myelopathy is a rare complication of systemic lupus erythematosus (Provenzale and Bouldin, 1992). The usual features are back pain, rapidly progressive paraplegia, and bowel and bladder dysfunction. Sensory loss is not a constant feature. The protein concentration of the cerebrospinal fluid is elevated. Recovery is poor and mortality is high.

NEONATAL CORD INFARCTION

Infarction of the spinal cord is a hazard in newborns undergoing umbilical artery catheterization. The artery of Adamkiewicz arises from the aorta at the level of T10 to T12 and is the major segmental artery to the thoracolumbar spinal cord. Embolization of the artery may occur if the catheter tip is placed between levels T8 and T11. The result is acute and sometimes irreversible paraplegia. A similar syndrome can occur in premature or small-for-dates newborns who have not been catheterized (Singer et al, 1991). The mechanism is not established but may be caused by hypotension.

TRANSVERSE MYELITIS

Transverse myelitis is an acute demyelinating disorder of the spinal cord that evolves in hours or days. It may occur alone or in combination with demyelination in other portions of the nervous system. The association of transverse myelitis and optic neuritis is called *Devic disease;* acute demyelination throughout the neuraxis is called *diffuse encephalomyelitis.* These terms are descriptive and do not suggest an underlying cause.

Multiple sclerosis is usually suspected in adults with transverse myelitis, although only 20% eventually have other demyelinating lesions (Jeffery et al, 1993). Multiple sclerosis is uncommon in childhood, and the initial feature is more likely to be cerebellar or extraocular dysfunction than myelitis (see Chapter 10).

Transverse myelitis, and especially encephalomyelitis, in children is frequently attributed to a preceding viral infection or immunization. No evidence supports such a notion. School-age children average four to six "viral" episodes annually. Therefore, half of children with any illness may give a history of a viral infection within the preceding 30 days. Similarly, despite several case reports, a cause-and-effect relationship has not been established between licensed vaccines and demyelinating disorders of the central nervous system (Institute of Medicine, 1994).

CLINICAL FEATURES. Mean age at onset is 9 years. Symptoms progress rapidly, and maximal deficit is attained within 2 days (Adams and Armstrong, 1990). The level of myelitis is usually thoracic and demarcated by the sensory loss. Asymmetric leg weakness is common. The bladder fills and does not empty voluntarily. Tendon reflexes may be increased or reduced. Recovery begins after 6 days but may be incomplete. Fifty percent of patients make a full recovery, 10% have no recovery, and 40% recover incompletely. Most resume walking, but many continue to have sensory disturbances.

Several children are reported with *relapsing myelitis* (Tippett et al, 1991), and I am seeing an adolescent boy who has had three attacks over 10 years, each time recovering completely. None have developed multiple sclerosis or more disseminated disease.

DIAGNOSIS. MRI of the spine should be performed to exclude acute cord compression, and it sometimes shows swelling at the level of myelitis. Cranial MRI is indicated to exclude more widespread disease. Vision should be checked daily because of the possibility of Devic disease.

TREATMENT. Corticosteroids are generally used despite the absence of controlled studies. High-dose intravenous therapy followed by tapering doses of prednisone is recommended.

Devic Disease (Neuromyelitis Optica)

I believe that Devic disease is a distinct disorder that occurs mainly in children and is not part of the spectrum of multiple sclerosis. This view is not shared by many authorities in the field. No cause can be determined in most children with Devic disease.

A temporal association between pulmonary tuberculosis and Devic disease is seen in adolescents and adults (Silber et al, 1990). In these cases the neurologic disease appears to be an immune reaction to tuberculosis and not caused by antituberculous therapy.

CLINICAL FEATURES. A history of anorexia or a flulike syndrome a few days or a week before the first neurologic symptoms is common. The anorexia may be part of the acute demyelinating illness rather than a viral infection. Myelitis precedes optic neuritis in 13% of patients, and follows it in 76%; myelitis and neuritis occur simultaneously in 10%. Optic neuritis and transverse myelitis generally occur within 1 week of each other. The child remains irritable while the neurologic symptoms are evolving.

Bilateral optic neuritis occurs in 80% of patients (see Chapter 16). Both eyes may be affected at onset, or one eye may become affected before the other. Loss of vision is acute and accompanied by pain. Blindness is often complete within hours. The initial ophthalmoscopic examination may have normal results but more often shows swelling of the disk. The pupils are dilated, and response to light is sluggish.

Myelitis is heralded by back pain and discomfort in the legs. The legs become weak, and the patient has difficulty standing and walking. Paraplegia becomes complete; it is first flaccid and then becomes spastic. Tendon reflexes may be diminished at first but later become exaggerated and are associated with extensor plantar responses. The bladder is spastic, and the patient has overflow incontinence. In some patients, a sensory level may be detected, but more often the sensory deficit is patchy and difficult to delineate in an irritable child.

The course of Devic disease varies. Some evolve into an encephalomyelitis (see "Diffuse Encephalomyelitis"), some have permanent paraplegia, and most recover but not always completely.

DIAGNOSIS. Acute transverse myelitis may be caused by spinal cord compression syndrome, and a space-occupying mass must be excluded by MRI. If MRI shows the area of demyelination,

☐ FIGURE 12-3 Demyelination of the spinal cord in an adolescent girl with multiple sclerosis.

then MRI of the head is indicated to look for other lesions (Figure 12-3).

The cerebrospinal fluid in children with Devic disease is usually abnormal. The protein content is mild to moderately elevated, and a mixed pleocytosis of neutrophils and mononuclear cells is present.

TREATMENT. A course of corticosteroids is usually suggested for children with Devic disease. Although the value of corticosteroids is not established, most physicians believe they are beneficial. The regimen is the same as for diffuse encephalomyelitis. Bladder care with intermittent catheterization is imperative, as are measures to prevent bed sores and infection. The family and the child often need psychological counseling.

Diffuse Encephalomyelitis

Diffuse encephalomyelitis is discussed in the section on Devic syndrome and in Chapter 2. The major clinical difference from Devic disease is that the cerebral hemispheres are affected as well as the spinal cord. Cerebral demyelination may precede, follow, or occur concurrently with the myelitis.

CLINICAL FEATURES. In addition to the myelitis, an encephalopathy characterized by decreased consciousness, irritability, and spastic quadriplegia occurs. If the brainstem is affected, dysphagia, fever, cranial nerve palsies, and irregular respiration are present.

DIAGNOSIS. The full extent of demyelination can be appreciated only with MRI. Multiple white matter lesions that become confluent are noted in the cerebral hemispheres (see Figure 2–2), cerebellum, and brainstem. Adrenoleukodystrophy must be excluded by measuring very-long-chain fatty acids.

TREATMENT. Most authorities agree that corticosteroids should be administered. Prednisone, 2 mg/kg/day (not to exceed 100 mg), or its equivalent in a parenteral form is the initial dose, which is then tapered over a 4-week period depending on the response. The benefit of such a course of therapy is not established, but some patients become corticosteroid dependent and have a relapse when prednisone is discontinued. Such children require long-term alternate-day therapy.

TRAUMA

Spinal cord injuries are relatively rare, especially before adolescence. The major cause is motor vehicle accidents, followed by sports-related injuries. The injuries affect the cervical spinal cord in 65% of cases before 15 years of age and 71% of cases before 9 years of age. Fifteen percent of patients have injuries at multiple levels. Neurologic function that is intact immediately after the injury remains intact afterward. Even those with incomplete function are likely to recover completely. Evidence of complete transection on initial examination indicates that paralysis is permanent.

Spinal Cord Concussion

A direct blow on the back may produce a transitory disturbance in spinal cord function (Zwimpfer and Bernstein, 1990). The dysfunction is caused by edema (spinal shock); the spinal cord is intact.

CLINICAL FEATURES. Most injuries occur at the level of the cervical cord or the thoracolumbar juncture. The major clinical features are flaccid paraplegia or quadriplegia, a sensory level at the site of injury, loss of tendon reflexes, and urinary retention. Recovery begins within a few hours and is complete within a week.

DIAGNOSIS. At the onset of weakness, a spinal cord compression syndrome such as epidural hematoma cannot be excluded, and an imaging study of the spine is necessary.

TREATMENT. Children with spinal cord concussion should be treated with methylprednisolone as outlined in the section on spinal cord transection.

Compressed Vertebral Body Fractures

CLINICAL FEATURES. Compression fractures of the thoracolumbar region occur when a child jumps or falls from a height greater than 10 feet and lands in a standing or sitting position. The spinal cord itself is not transected, but spinal cord concussion may cause paraplegia. Back pain at the fracture site is immediate and intense. Nerve roots are compressed, causing pain that radiates into the groin and legs.

DIAGNOSIS. Thoracolumbar radiographs reveal the fracture, but when paraplegia is present, a spinal cord imaging study is usually performed as well, and the results prove to be normal.

TREATMENT. Immobilization relieves the back pain and promotes healing of the fracture.

Fracture Dislocation and Spinal Cord Transection

Transection of the spinal cord from fracture dislocation of the vertebral column injury is usually caused by a motor vehicle accident. A forceful flexion of the spine fractures the articular facets and allows the vertebral body to move forward or laterally, with consequent contusion or transection of the spinal cord. The common sites of traumatic transection are the levels C1 to C2, C5 to C7, and T12 to L2.

CLINICAL FEATURES. Neurologic deficits at and below the level of spinal cord contusion or transection are immediate and profound. Many children with fracture dislocations sustained head injuries at the time of trauma and are unconscious.

Immediately after the injury the child has flaccid weakness of the limbs below the level of the lesion associated with loss of tendon and cutaneous reflexes (spinal shock). In high cervical spinal cord lesions, the knee and ankle tendon reflexes, anal reflex, and plantar response may be elicited during the initial period of spinal shock. Spinal shock lasts for approximately 1 week in infants and young children and up to 6 weeks in adolescents.

First the superficial reflexes return, then the plantar response becomes one of extension, and finally massive withdrawal reflexes (mass reflex)

□ FIGURE 12–4 Fracture dislocation. C4 is dislocated on C5, causing compression *(arrow)* of the cord.

appear. The mass reflex is triggered by trivial stimulation of the foot or leg, usually in a specific zone unique to the patient. The response at first is dorsiflexion of the foot, flexion at the knees, and flexion and adduction at the thighs. Later, there are also contraction of the abdomen, sweating, piloerection, and emptying of the bladder and bowel. During this time of heightened reflex activity the tendon reflexes return and become exaggerated.

Below the level of injury, sensation is lost to a variable degree, depending on the completeness of the transection. When the injury is incomplete, sensation begins to return within weeks and may continue to improve for up to 2 years. Patients with partial or complete transections may complain of pain and tingling below the level of injury.

In addition to the development of a small, spastic bladder, autonomic dysfunction includes constipation, lack of sweating, orthostatic hypotension, and disturbed temperature regulation.

DIAGNOSIS. Fracture dislocation is readily identified by radiographs of the vertebrae. Imaging of the spinal cord produces further information on the presence of compressive hematomas and the structural integrity of the spinal cord (Figure 12–4). The presence of a complete block on myelography indicates a poor prognosis for return of function.

TREATMENT. The immediate treatment of fracture dislocation is to reduce the dislocation

and prevent further damage to the cord. This is accomplished by corticosteroids, surgery, and immobilization. An intravenous infusion of methylprednisolone, 30 mg/kg within the first 8 hours after injury, and followed by 4 mg/kg/hr for 23 hours, significantly reduces neurologic morbidity (Bracken et al, 1992). Long-term management of spinal cord injuries is beyond the scope of this text but is best accomplished at specialized centers.

Spinal Epidural Hematoma

Spinal epidural hematoma usually results from direct vertebral trauma and is especially common in children with an underlying bleeding tendency. The hematoma causes symptoms by progressive compression of the cord and is manifested like any other extradural mass lesion. Diagnosis is usually based on MRI. Treatment is surgical evacuation.

TUMORS OF THE SPINAL CORD

Astrocytoma, ependymoma, and neuroblastoma are the common spinal cord tumors of childhood. Sarcomas are next in frequency, followed by neurofibroma and then by several different secondary tumors such as teratoma, dermoid tumor, and chondroma. Motor deficits, usually paraplegia, are an early feature in 86% of spinal cord tumors, and back pain in 63%.

Astrocytoma

The problem of differentiating cystic astrocytoma of the spinal cord from syringomyelia is discussed in Chapter 9 (see "Syringomyelia").

CLINICAL FEATURES. Astrocytomas are usually long and may extend from the lower brainstem to the conus medullaris. The initial features of multiple-segment spinal astrocytomas may be seen in the arms or legs. One syndrome is characterized primarily by weakness of one arm. Pain in the neck may be associated, but bowel and bladder function are normal. Examination shows mild spastic weakness of the legs. The solid portion of the tumor is in the neck and its caudal extension is cystic.

A second syndrome is characterized by progressive spastic paraplegia, sometimes associated with thoracic pain. Scoliosis may be present. In these patients, the solid portion of the tumor is in the thoracic or lumbar region. When solid tumor extends into the conus medullaris, tendon reflexes in the legs may be diminished or absent and bowel and bladder function are impaired. Intra-axial tumors of the cervicomedullary junction are often low grade and have an indolent course (Robertson et al, 1994). They may cause cranial nerve dysfunction or spinal cord compression. Cranial nerve dysfunction is manifested by difficulty in swallowing and nasal speech (see Chapter 17).

DIAGNOSIS. MRI is the definitive diagnostic procedure. It allows visualization of both the solid and cystic portions of the tumor (Figure 12–5).

TREATMENT. Complete resection should be attempted whenever possible. A laminectomy is performed over the solid portion of the tumor. With microsurgical technique, the solid portion is removed and the cystic portion is aspirated. MRI should be repeated 1, 6, and 12 months after surgery. The benefits of radiation therapy, either after resection or at the time of recurrence, are not established (Rossitch et al, 1990).

□ FIGURE 12–5 Astrocytoma of the cervical cord. The tumor demonstrates an intense signal *(arrow)* on T$_2$-weighted images.

Ependymoma

Ependymomas are composed primarily of ependymal cells and arise from the lining of the ventricular system or central canal. They are more often intracranial than intraspinal in children. When intraspinal, they tend to be located in the lumbar region or in the cauda equina but may occur anywhere along the neuraxis.

CLINICAL FEATURES. Clinical features vary with the location of the tumor. The initial feature may be scoliosis, pain in the legs or back, paresthesia, or weakness in one or both legs. Diagnosis may be delayed for years when scoliosis is the only sign. Eventually, all children have difficulty walking, and this is the symptom that usually leads to appropriate diagnostic testing.

Cervical ependymoma is manifested by stiff neck and cervical pain that is worse at night. Tumors of the cauda equina may sometimes rupture and produce meningismus, fever, and pleocytosis mimicking bacterial meningitis.

Spastic paraplegia is the usual finding on examination. Cervical tumors cause weakness of one arm as well. Tumors of the cauda equina produce flaccid weakness and atrophy of leg muscles associated with loss of tendon reflexes.

DIAGNOSIS. MRI is the primary modality for imaging tumors of the spinal cord. Lumbar puncture is rarely indicated but shows an elevated protein content of the cerebrospinal fluid.

TREATMENT. Microsurgical techniques make possible the complete removal of intramedullary ependymoma. The role of postoperative local radiation therapy in treating benign tumors is uncertain. Malignant ependymomas of the spinal cord are unusual in children, but require total neuraxis irradiation when present.

Neuroblastoma

Neuroblastoma is the most common extracranial solid tumor of infancy and childhood. It produces neurologic dysfunction by direct invasion, by metastasis, and by distant "humoral" effects (see Chapter 10). Half of cases occur before 2 years of age and 60% occur before 1 year. Neuroblastoma is derived from cells of the sympathetic chain and cranial ganglia. Tumors in a paraspinal location may extend through a neural foramen and compress the spinal cord.

CLINICAL FEATURES. Paraplegia is the initial manifestation of neuroblastoma extending into the epidural space from a paravertebral origin. Because most affected children are infants, the first symptom is usually refusal to stand or walk. Mild weakness may progress to complete paraplegia within hours or days. Examination generally reveals a flaccid paraplegia, a distended bladder, and exaggerated tendon reflexes in the legs. Sensation may be difficult to test.

DIAGNOSIS. Radiographs of the chest usually show the extravertebral portion of the tumor, and the extent of spinal compression is delineated with MRI.

TREATMENT. In children with an acute spinal cord compression, some relief can be provided by high-dose corticosteroids before surgical extirpation and radiation therapy. The survival rate in infants with neuroblastoma confined to a single organ is greater than 60%.

Other Tumors

Other spinal cord tumors of infancy and childhood include sarcoma, neurofibroma, dermoid tumor, teratoma, and epidermoid tumor. Meningioma almost never occurs before the third decade.

The clinical features of the various spinal cord tumors are much alike. Paraplegia and back pain are prominent. Sensory deficits and sphincter disturbances are less common and depend on tumor location. MRI usually leads to the diagnosis, and excision of the tumor is ordinarily the first step in treatment.

Cerebral Paraplegia and Quadriplegia

Almost all progressive disorders of the brain that result in quadriplegia also have dementia as an initial or prominent feature (see Chapter 5). Pure paraplegia of cerebral origin is unusual. At the very least, the patient has impairment of fine finger movements and increased tendon reflex activity in the arms. Pure paraplegia should always direct attention to the spinal cord.

Cerebral Palsy

Cerebral palsy is a chronic motor disability of cerebral origin, appearing early in life, and not caused by a progressive disease. The prevalence of moderately severe cases is approximately 2 per 1,000 live births; the prevalence of cerebral palsy has increased among very small premature infants as more have survived (Kuban and Leviton, 1994).

■ T A B L E   1 2 – 2
Slowly Progressive Disorders Sometimes Misdiagnosed as Cerebral Palsy

CONDITION	CHAPTER
Polyneuropathy	
GM$_1$ gangliosidosis type II	5
Hereditary motor and sensory neuropathies	7
Infantile neuroaxonal dystrophy	5
Metachromatic leukodystrophy	5
Ataxia	
Abetalipoproteinemia	10
Ataxia-telangiectasia	10
Friedreich ataxia	10
Spasticity-Chorea	
Familial spastic paraplegia	12
Glutaric aciduria type I	14
Lesch-Nyhan syndrome	5
Niemann-Pick disease type C	5
Pelizaeus-Merzbacher disease	5
Rett syndrome	5

Many slowly progressive disorders are mistakenly diagnosed as cerebral palsy (Table 12-2). Perinatal asphyxia is a known cause of cerebral palsy but accounts for only a minority of cases. Most cerebral palsy is due to prenatal factors that are difficult to identify with precision in an individual patient.

Cerebral palsy is not always a permanent condition. Many infants with only mild motor impairments improve and achieve normal motor function in childhood. Unfortunately, up to 25% of such children will be retarded or will have some behavioral or cognitive disturbance.

Traditionally, the cerebral palsies have been classified by the pattern of motor impairment. The spastic types are paraplegia or diplegia, quadriplegia, and hemiplegia (see Chapter 11). The hypotonic types are ataxic (see Chapter 10) and athetoid (see Chapter 14).

Spastic Diplegia (Paraplegia)

Diplegia means that all four limbs are affected but that the legs are affected more severely than the arms. The motor impairment in the arms may be limited to increased responses of tendon reflexes; such children are classified as paraplegic. Spastic diplegia is usually caused by periventricular leukomalacia in children born prematurely. Cystic lesions in the white matter are often unilateral, or at least asymmetric, causing a hemiplegia superimposed on spastic diplegia (Rogers et al, 1994).

CLINICAL FEATURES. Many children with spastic diplegia have normal tone, or even hypotonia, during the first 4 months. The onset of spasticity in the legs is insidious and slowly progressive during the first year. Four-point creeping is impossible because of leg extension, and early ambulation is usually achieved by either rolling or crawling on the floor with the belly on the ground, using the arms to pull the body forward.

Sitting up alone is delayed or never achieved. From the supine position, the infant pulls to standing rather than to sitting. Sitting is later made possible by bending forward at the waist, to compensate for the lack of flexion at the hip and knee, and placing one hand on the floor for balance. Most children with spastic diplegia stand on their toes, with flexion at the knees and an increased lumbar lordosis. Walking is difficult because of the stiffness in the legs and can be accomplished only by throwing the body forward or side to side to transfer weight.

Examination shows spasticity of the legs and lesser spasticity of the arms. The tendon reflexes are exaggerated in all limbs. Reflex sensitivity and responsiveness are increased; percussion at the knee causes a crossed adductor response. Ankle clonus and an extensor plantar response are usually present. When the infant is suspended vertically, strong contractions of the adductor muscles cause the legs to cross at the thigh (*scissoring*).

Subluxation or dislocation of the hips is relatively common in children with severe spasticity; this is caused in part by the constant adduction of the thighs and also by insufficient development of the hip joint resulting from delayed standing or inability to stand.

DIAGNOSIS. Spastic diplegia is a clinical diagnosis. Abnormalities in the deep white matter secondary to periventricular leukomalacia are easily identified by MRI, but children with a known history of perinatal distress secondary to prematurity do not require follow-up imaging studies. The important consideration is not to mistake cerebral palsy for a progressive disease of the brain or cervical portion of the spine. Features that suggest a progressive disease are a family history of "cerebral palsy," deterioration of mental function, loss of motor skills previously obtained, atrophy of muscles, and sensory loss.

TREATMENT. There are probably as many "methods" to manage spastic diplegia and quadriplegia as there are children with cerebral palsy. In general, a multidisciplinary approach, including infant stimulation, physical therapy, and occupational therapy, is used to help the child achieve an adequate functional status. Controlled clinical trials are rarely accomplished and one such trial concluded that physical therapy offered no short-term advantage (Palmer et al, 1988). Most drugs to relieve spasticity have marginal benefit and often cause unacceptable sedation.

Selective posterior rhizotomy has emerged as a useful procedure for the treatment of spasticity (Park and Owen, 1992). The best results are obtained in children younger than 8 years of age. Surgery is also useful to relieve contractures but should be carefully planned so that it is performed only once. Surgery is followed by a program of physical therapy that maintains the desired range of motion.

Spastic Quadriplegia

All limbs are affected, often the legs worse than the arms. If the arms are worse than the legs, the condition is sometimes called *double hemiplegia*. Most spastic quadriplegia is caused by intrauterine disease, usually malformations. Hypoxic-ischemic encephalopathy of the term newborn accounts for a minority of cases.

CLINICAL FEATURES. Developmental delay is profound, and the infant is quickly identified as neurologically abnormal. Failure to meet motor milestones, abnormal posturing of the head and limbs, and seizures are the common reasons for neurologic evaluation.

In severely affected children, the supine posture is characteristic. The head and neck are retracted, the arms are flexed at the elbows with the hands clenched, and the legs are held in extension. Infantile reflexes (Moro and tonic-neck) are obligatory and stereotyped and persist after 6 months of age. Microcephaly is frequently an associated feature.

Because both hemispheres are damaged, supranuclear bulbar palsy (dysphagia and dysarthria) is common. Disturbances in vision and ocular motility are frequently associated features and seizures occur in 50% of affected children.

DIAGNOSIS. Diagnosis is based on clinical findings. Laboratory studies are useful when the underlying cause is not obvious or the possibility of a genetically transmitted defect exists. MRI of the brain is especially useful to show malformations.

TREATMENT. Treatment is the same as described in the section on spastic diplegia (paraplegia).

REFERENCES

Adams C, Armstrong D. Acute transverse myelopathy in children. Can J Neurol Sci 1990;17:40-45.

Appleton RE, Farrell K, Dunn HG. "Pure" and complicated forms of hereditary spastic paraplegia presenting in childhood. Dev Med Child Neurol 1991;33:304-312.

Azimullah PC, Smit LME, Rietveld-Knol E, et al. Malformations of the spinal cord in 53 patients with spina bifida studied by magnetic resonance imaging. Child Nerv Syst 1991;7:63-66.

Bhatnagar M, Sponseller PD, Carroll C IV, et al. Pediatric atlantoaxial instability presenting as cerebral and cerebellar infarcts. J Pediatr Orthop 1991;11:103-107.

Bracken MB, Shepard MJ, Collins WF, et al. Methylprednisolone or naloxone treatment after acute spinal-cord injury: 1-year follow-up data. Results of the second National Acute Spinal Cord Injury Study. J Neurosurg 1992;76:23-31.

Brophy JD, Sutton LN, Zimmerman RA, et al. Magnetic resonance imaging of lipomyelomeningocele and tethered cord. Neurosurgery 1989;25:336-340.

Cambi F, Tartaglino L, Lublin F, et al. X-linked pure familial spastic paraparesis: Characterization of a large kindred with magnetic resonance imaging studies. Arch Neurol 1995;52:665-669.

Centers for Disease Control. Recommendations for the use of folic acid to reduce the number cases of spina bifida and other neural tube defects. MMWR 41(No. RR-14):1, 1992.

Chatkupt S, Skurnick JH, Jaggi BS, et al. Study of genetics, epidemiology, and vitamin usage in familial spina bifida in the United States in the 1990s. Neurology 1994;44:65-70.

Crockard HA, Stevens JM. Craniovertebral junction anomalies in inherited disorders: Part of the syndrome or caused by the disorder. Eur J Pediatr 1995;154:504-512.

Devinsky O, Eun-Sook C, Petito CK, et al. Herpes zoster myelitis. Brain 1991;114:1181-1196.

Dürr A, Brice A, Serdaru M, et al. The phenotype of "pure" autosomal dominant spastic paraplegia. Neurology 1994;44:1274-1277.

Institute of Medicine. Adverse Events Associated with Childhood Vaccines: Evidence Bearing on Causality. National Academy Press, Washington D.C., 1994; 84-86.

Jeffery DR, Mandler RN, Davis LE. Transverse myelitis: Retrospective analysis of 33 cases, with differentiation of cases associated with multiple sclerosis and parainfectious events. Arch Neurol 1993;50:532-535.

Kuban KCK, Leviton A. Cerebral palsy. N Engl J Med 1994; 330:188-195.

Martinez-Frìas ML, Bermejo E, Garcia A, et al. Holoprosencephaly associated with caudal dysgenesis: A clinical-epidemiological analysis. Am J Med Genet 1994;53:46-51.

Moser HW, Moser AB, Smith KD, et al. Adrenoleukodystrophy: Phenotypic variability and implications for therapy. J Inher Metab Dis 1992;15:645-664.

Nadel AS, Green JK, Holmes LB, et al. Absence of need for amniocentesis in patients with elevated levels of maternal serum alpha-fetoprotein in normal ultrasonographic examinations. N Engl J Med 1990;323:557-561.

Palmer FB, Shapiro BK, Wachtel RC, et al. The effects of physical therapy on cerebral palsy. A controlled trial in spastic diplegia. N Engl J Med 1988;318:803-808.

Park TS, Owen JH. Surgical management of spastic diplegia in cerebral palsy. N Engl J Med 1992;326:745-749.

Provenzale J, Bouldin TW. Lupus-related myelopathy: Report of three cases and review of the literature. J Neurol Neurosurg Psychiatry 1992;55:830-835.

Robertson PL, Allen JC, Abbott IR, et al. Cervicomedullary tumors in children: A distinct subset of brainstem gliomas. Neurology 1994;44:1798-1803.

Rogers B, Msall M, Owens T, et al. Cystic periventricular leukomalacia and types of cerebral palsy in preterm infants. J Pediatr 1994;125:S1-S8.

Rossitch E Jr, Zeidman SM, Burger PC, et al. Clinical and pathological analysis of spinal cord astrocytomas in children. Neurosurgery 1990;27:193-196.

Silber MH, Willcox PA, Bowen RM, et al. Neuromyelitis optica (Devic's syndrome) and pulmonary tuberculosis. Neurology 1990;40:934-938.

Singer R, Joseph K, Gilai AN, et al. Nontraumatic, acute neonatal paraplegia. J Pediatr Orthop 1991;11:588-593.

Tippett DS, Fishman PS, Panitch HS. Relapsing transverse myelitis. Neurology 1991;41:703-706.

Towfighi J, Housman C. Spinal cord abnormalities in caudal regression syndrome. Acta Neuropathol 1991;81:458-466.

Zwimpfer TJ, Bernstein M. Spinal cord concussion. J Neurosurg 1990;72:894-900.

13
Monoplegia

Flaccid weakness of one limb is usually caused by abnormalities of the spine or the proximal portion of nerves. Many conditions that cause paraplegia or quadriplegia begin as monoplegia. Therefore the differential diagnosis of spinal paraplegia provided in Table 12-1 must also be consulted for monoplegia. In addition, several cerebral disorders that cause hemiplegia may begin as a monoplegia, so the tables in Chapter 11 should be consulted as well.

 ## Approach to Monoplegia

Refusal to use a limb may be caused by either pain or weakness. Painful limbs are usually caused by injury, but they may also be caused by arthritis, infection, or tumor. A trivial pull of the arm may dislocate the radial head in some infants and cause an apparent monoplegia. Pain and weakness together are a feature of plexitis.

The differential diagnosis of acute monoplegia is summarized in Table 13-1. Plexopathies and neuropathies are the leading causes of pure monoplegia. Stroke often affects one limb more than the other, usually the arm more than the leg. The presentation suggests monoplegia, but careful examination often reveals increased tendon reflexes and an extensor plantar response in the seemingly unaffected leg. Any suggestion of hemiplegia, rather than monoplegia, or increased tendon reflexes in the paretic limb should focus attention on the brain and cervical cord as the pathologic site.

Chronic progressive brachial monoplegia is uncommon. When it occurs, syringomyelia and

tumors of the cervical cord or brachial plexus should be suspected. Chronic progressive weakness of one leg suggests a congenital malformation or tumor of the spinal cord.

A monomelic form of spinal muscular atrophy, affecting only one leg or one arm, is reported repeatedly from Asia but is less common in Europe and the United States. However, childhood-onset spinal muscular atrophies may be asymmetric at onset and first appear as a monoplegia.

 ## Plexopathies
ACUTE IDIOPATHIC PLEXITIS

Acute plexitis is a demyelinating disorder of the brachial or lumbar plexus thought to be immune mediated. Brachial plexitis is far more common than lumbar plexitis.

Brachial Plexitis

Brachial plexitis (brachial neuritis, neuralgic amyotrophy) occurs from infancy to adult life. An antecedent infectious disease is recorded in 25% of patients; this is not a significant association, but a 10% to 20% rate of prior immunization with tetanus toxoid may be significant (Institute of Medicine, 1994). The site of immunization does not correlate with the arm involved.

CLINICAL FEATURES. The onset of symptoms is usually explosive. Pain, the initial feature in 95% of patients, is frequently localized to the shoulder but may be more diffuse or limited to the lower arm. It is severe, may awaken the

■ TABLE 13-1
Differential Diagnosis of Acute Monoplegia

Complicated Migraine (see Chapter 11)
Dislocation of the Radial Head
"Hemiparetic" Seizures (see Chapter 11)
Plexopathy and Neuropathy
Acute neuritis
    Asthmatic plexitis
    Idiopathic plexitis
    Osteomyelitis plexitis
    Poliomyelitis (see Chapter 7)
    Tetanus toxoid plexitis
Hereditary
    Hereditary brachial neuritis
    Hereditary neuropathy with liability to pressure palsy
Injury
    Lacerations
    Pressure injuries
    Traction injuries
Stroke (see Table 11–2)

patient, and is described as sharp, stabbing, throbbing, or aching. The duration of pain, which is frequently constant, varies from several hours to 3 weeks. As the pain subsides, weakness appears. Weakness is in the distribution of the upper plexus alone in half of patients, and the entire plexus in most of the rest. Lower plexitis alone is unusual. Although the initial pain has abated, paresthesias may accompany the weakness.

Two thirds of patients report improved strength during the month after onset. Upper plexus palsies improve faster than do lower plexus palsies. Among all patients, one third recover within 1 year, three quarters by 2 years, and 90% by 3 years. After 3 years, further improvement may occur but permanent residua should be expected. Recurrences are unusual and less severe than the initial episode.

DIAGNOSIS. Pain and weakness in one arm are also symptoms of spinal cord compression, and an imaging study of the spinal cord is often needed. However, when the onset is characteristic of brachial plexus neuritis, the diagnosis can be established by the clinical features and diagnostic tests can be deferred.

The cerebrospinal fluid is usually normal. A slight lymphocytosis and mild elevation in protein content are sometimes noted. Electromyography (EMG) and nerve conduction studies are helpful in showing the extent of plexopathy. Electrical evidence of bilateral involvement is often present in patients with unilateral symptoms.

TREATMENT. Corticosteroids have not been shown to affect outcome. Range of motion exercises are recommended.

Lumbar Plexitis

Lumbar plexitis occurs at all ages and is similar to brachial plexitis, except that the leg is affected instead of the arm. An immune mechanism is suspected, but no association with antecedent viral infection or immunization has been established.

CLINICAL FEATURES. Fever is often the first symptom and is followed, after 3 to 8 days, by pain in one or both legs (Awerbuch et al, 1989). The pain has an abrupt onset and may occur in a femoral or sciatic distribution. Sciatica, when present, suggests disk disease. Young children refuse to stand or walk, and older children begin to limp.

Weakness may develop concurrently with pain or may be delayed for as long as 3 weeks. The onset of weakness is insidious and often difficult to date, but usually it begins 8 days after the onset of pain. Weakness progresses for a week and then stabilizes. Tendon reflexes are absent in the affected leg but are present in other limbs.

Recovery is characterized first by abatement of pain and then by increasing strength. The average time from onset of pain to maximal recovery is 18 weeks, with a range of 8 weeks to several years. Functional recovery is almost universal, but mild weakness may persist.

DIAGNOSIS. The sudden onset of pain and weakness of one leg suggests spinal cord or disk disease. Magnetic resonance imaging (MRI) of the spine is a means of excluding other disorders; the results are invariably normal in lumbar plexitis. The cerebrospinal fluid is normal except for a mild elevation of protein concentration. EMG performed 3 weeks after onset shows patchy denervation.

TREATMENT. Corticosteroids do not affect outcome. Range of motion exercises are recommended.

OSTEOMYELITIS-NEURITIS

Apparent limb weakness caused by pain is a well-recognized phenomenon. However, a true brachial neuritis may occur in response to osteomyelitis of the shoulder. The mechanism is thought to be ischemic nerve damage caused by vasculitis.

CLINICAL FEATURES. Osteomyelitis-neuritis occurs predominantly during infancy. The initial feature is a flaccid arm without pain or tenderness. Body temperature may be normal at first but soon becomes elevated. Pain develops on movement of the shoulder, and tenderness to palpation follows. No swelling is present. The biceps and triceps reflexes may be depressed or absent.

DIAGNOSIS. Osteomyelitis of the proximal humerus should be suspected when brachial plexitis develops during infancy. Radiographs of the humerus become abnormal at the end of the first week, when they show destruction of the lateral margin of the humerus, but a focal area of uptake in the proximal humerus, the scapula, or both are seen shortly after onset using radioisotope bone scan. After 3 weeks EMG shows patchy denervation in the muscles innervated by the upper plexus. These results support the idea that this is a true plexitis and not just a painful limb.

The organism can be identified in aspirate from the shoulder joint or by blood cultures. Group B *Streptococcus* is often isolated in specimens from young infants, and other species of bacteria are found in older children.

TREATMENT. Intravenous antibiotics, usually penicillin, must be administered for 3 to 4 weeks. Recovery of arm strength may be incomplete.

ASTHMATIC AMYOTROPHY (HOPKINS SYNDROME)

Sudden flaccid paralysis of one or more limbs, resembling poliomyelitis, may occur during recovery from an asthmatic attack (Liedholm et al, 1994). All affected children had been immunized against poliomyelitis. The syndrome is believed to be caused by anterior horn cell infection by a neurotropic virus other than poliovirus (Shahar et al, 1991). Adenovirus, echovirus, and coxsackievirus have been isolated from stool, throat, or cerebrospinal fluid in some cases.

CLINICAL FEATURES. Age at onset is from 1 to 11 years and the male-to-female ratio is 7:4. The interval between the asthmatic attack and the paralysis is 1 to 11 days, with an average of 5 days. Among reported cases, monoplegia occurred in 90%; the arm was involved twice as often as the leg. The remainder have had hemiplegia or diplegia. Meningeal irritation is not present. Sensation is intact, but the paralyzed limb is painful in half of cases. Recovery is incomplete, and all affected children have some degree of permanent paralysis.

DIAGNOSIS. Asthmatic amyotrophy is primarily a clinical diagnosis based on the sequence of events. It must be distinguished from paralytic poliomyelitis and idiopathic brachial neuritis. The distinction from paralytic poliomyelitis is based on the normal cerebrospinal fluid in asthmatic amyotrophy. A few white blood cells may be present in the cerebrospinal fluid but never to the extent encountered in poliomyelitis, and the protein concentration is normal.

EMG during the acute phase shows active denervation of the paralyzed limb, but the pattern of denervation does not follow the radicular distribution expected in a brachial neuritis.

TREATMENT. Treatment is directed to the symptoms and includes analgesics for pain and physical therapy.

HEREDITARY BRACHIAL PLEXOPATHY

Focal familial recurrent neuropathy has two major phenotypes: hereditary brachial plexopathy and hereditary neuropathy with liability to pressure palsies (see "Mononeuropathies," later in this chapter). The phenotypes are genetically distinct but can be confused because isolated nerve palsies may occur in hereditary brachial plexopathy and brachial plexopathy is reported in patients with hereditary neuropathy with liability to pressure palsies (Gouider et al, 1994). Both disorders are transmitted by autosomal dominant inheritance.

CLINICAL FEATURES. Hereditary brachial plexopathy may be difficult to distinguish from idiopathic brachial plexitis in the absence of a family history or a patient's history of similar episodes. Events that may trigger an attack in genetically predisposed individuals include infection, emotional stress, strenuous use of the affected limb, and childbirth. Immunization has not been implicated.

The initial attack usually occurs during the second or third decade but may appear in childhood. When brachial plexus palsy is present at birth, it is usually misinterpreted as traumatic even when the family history is known. Weakness resolves completely, only to recur later in childhood.

Attacks are characterized by severe arm pain that may be exacerbated by movement. Weakness follows in days to weeks; it is usually maximal within a few days and always by 1 month. The entire plexus may be involved, but most often the upper trunk is affected alone or most severely. Examination shows proximal arm weakness and sometimes distal weakness. Tendon reflexes cannot be elicited from affected muscles. Weakness persists for weeks to months, during which time atrophy and fasciculations are observed. Pain, which is frequently the only sensory finding, subsides after the first week.

Recovery begins weeks to months after maximal weakness is attained. Return of function is usually complete, although some residual weakness may persist after repeated attacks. The frequency of attacks is variable; several attacks may occur within a single year, but two or three attacks per decade is more usual.

Occasional patients have an episode of lumbar plexopathy, which is characterized by pain in the thigh and by proximal weakness. Brachial and lumbar plexopathies are never concurrent, although bilateral brachial plexopathy is a relatively common event. Isolated cranial nerve palsies are reported in families with hereditary brachial plexopathy. The vagus nerve is most often affected, causing hoarseness and difficulty in swallowing. Transitory facial palsies and unilateral hearing loss are reported as well.

DIAGNOSIS. The family history, early age at onset, unique triggering events, recurrences, and involvement of other nerves differentiate hereditary brachial plexopathy from idiopathic brachial neuritis. EMG shows a diffuse axonopathy in the affected arm and some evidence of denervation in the asymptomatic arm. Asymptomatic legs are electrically normal.

TREATMENT. Corticosteroid use is not beneficial. Analgesics may be needed at the onset of an attack. Range of motion exercises are recommended.

NEONATAL BRACHIAL NEUROPATHY

The incidence of neonatal brachial plexus birth injuries is approximately 1/1,000 live births (Laurent and Lee, 1994). They are caused by excessive traction. The upper plexus is injured when the head is suddenly pulled away from the arm. This occurs in vertex position when the head is forcefully pulled to deliver the aftercoming shoulder or when the head and neck are forced downward by normal contractions while the shoulder is caught by the pelvis. Injuries in breech position occur when the arm is pulled downward to free the aftercoming head or when the head is rotated to occipitoanterior, but the shoulder is fixed. Complete (upper and lower) plexus injuries occur during vertex deliveries when traction is exerted on a prolapsed arm and in breech deliveries when the trunk is pulled downward but an aftercoming arm is fixed.

CLINICAL FEATURES. Most neonatal brachial plexus injuries occur in large full-term newborns of primiparous mothers, especially when the fetus is malpositioned and the delivery is long and difficult. Although brachial plexus injuries are traditionally divided into those involving the upper roots (named for Erb and Duchenne) and those involving the lower roots (named for Klumpke), solitary lower-root injuries are unusual (Laurent et al, 1993). Only the C5 through C7 roots are affected in 70%, only the C8 and the T1 roots in 8%, and the complete plexus in 22%. Bilateral, but not necessarily symmetric, involvement occurs in 8% of cases.

Because the upper plexus (C5 to C7) is almost always involved, the posture of the arm is typical and reflects weakness of the proximal muscles. The arm is abducted and internally rotated at the shoulder and is extended and pronated at the elbow, so that the partially flexed fingers face backward. Extensions of the wrist is lost and the fingers are fisted. The biceps and triceps reflexes are absent. Injuries that extend higher than the C4 segment result in ipsilateral diaphragmatic paralysis.

Newborns with a complete brachial plexus palsy have a flaccid, dry limb with neither proximal nor distal movement. A Horner syndrome is sometimes associated. Sensory loss to pinprick is pinprick is present with partial or complete palsies but may not conform to the segmental pattern of weakness.

DIAGNOSIS. Brachial plexus palsy is easily recognized by the typical posture of the arm and by failure of movement when the Moro reflex is tested. Because the injury often takes place during a long and difficult delivery, asphyxia may be present as well. In such cases focal arm weakness may be missed because of generalized hypotonia. Approximately 10% of newborns with brachial plexus injuries have facial nerve palsy and fractures of the clavicle or humerus.

TREATMENT. Spontaneous recovery rates of 70% or more are reported, and one goal of therapy is to prevent the development of contractures. This is accomplished by range of motion exercises; splinting or other forms of immobilization should be avoided. Significant recovery occurs throughout the first year, but infants who show no improvement in strength at the end of 4 months are unlikely to show functional improvement later. Surgical reconstruction of the plexus (nerve grafts, neuroma excision, etc.) should be considered in infants with no evidence of spontaneous recovery at 4 months (Laurent and Lee, 1994).

POSTNATAL INJURIES

Brachial Plexus

Traction and pressure injuries of the brachial plexus are relatively common because of its superficial position. Motor vehicle and sports accidents account for the majority of severe injuries. However, mild injuries can occur when an adult suddenly yanks a child's arm, either protectively or to force movement; by a blow to the shoulder, such as in a football scrimmage or from the recoil of a rifle; because of prolonged wearing of a heavy knapsack; when the arm is kept hyperextended during surgery; and by pressure in the axilla from poorly positioned crutches.

CLINICAL FEATURES. Mild injuries do not affect all portions of the plexus equally. Diffuse weakness is uncommon. Pain may be an important initial feature, and sensory loss is uncommon. Recovery begins within days or weeks and is complete. Atrophy does not occur.

More severe injuries are usually associated with fractures of the clavicle and scapula and dislocation of the humerus. The upper plexus is generally affected more severely than is the lower plexus, but complete paralysis may be present at the onset. Sensory loss is less marked than weakness, and the two may not correspond in distribution. Pain is common, not only from the plexopathy but also from the bone and soft tissue injuries. The most painful injuries are those associated with root avulsion.

Tendon reflexes are absent, and atrophy develops in denervated muscle. Recovery progresses proximal to distal and can be plotted by the Tinel sign: tingling in the distal part of a limb caused by tapping over the regenerating segment of a nerve. Complete reinnervation, when it occurs, may take several months or years. The completeness of recovery depends on the severity and nature of the injury. Pressure and traction injuries in which anatomic integrity is not disturbed recover best, whereas injuries that tear the nerve or avulse the root do not recover at all.

DIAGNOSIS. EMG is useful in identifying the pattern of nerve injury and in providing information on prognosis. Even with mild traction injuries the amplitude of motor and sensory action potentials is attenuated and motor and sensory conduction is slowed.

TREATMENT. Mild injuries do not require treatment other than range of motion exercises. For more severe traction injuries, resting the limb for the first month is usually necessary. During that time, analgesia is needed for pain and the muscles can be stimulated electrically, away from the site of injury, to maintain tone. Range of motion exercises should be started after the pain subsides.

Fractures and dislocations causing pressure on the brachial plexus must be corrected promptly. Where nerves have been lacerated, anatomic integrity must be restored surgically.

Lumbar Plexus

The lumbar plexus is much less likely to be injured than is the brachial plexus because the former is surrounded by the pelvis and the very heavy muscles of the proximal leg.

CLINICAL FEATURES. Lumbar plexus injuries are almost always associated with fracture-dislocation of the pelvis. Motor vehicle accidents or falls from considerable height are required to produce sufficient force to fracture the pelvis. Therefore the patient usually has multiple injuries and the lumbar plexus injury may not be identified early.

Lumbar plexus injuries produce a patchy weakness that is difficult to differentiate from mononeuritis multiplex.

DIAGNOSIS. EMG is very helpful in making the distinction between plexus injuries and nerve injuries.

TREATMENT. Fracture-dislocations must be treated to relieve pressure on the plexus. As with brachial plexus injuries, the completeness of recovery depends on the anatomic integrity of the nerves.

PLEXUS TUMORS

Brachial plexus tumors in childhood are rare; when they do occur they are likely to be malignant. The important primary tumor is a malignant schwannoma, and the important secondary tumors are neuroblastoma and other primitive neuroectodermal tumors arising in the chest.

➡ Mononeuropathies

RADIAL NEUROPATHY

The radial nerve is most often injured in the spinal groove of the humerus, just below the takeoff of the motor branch to the triceps muscle. Injury may occur with fractures of the humerus or by external pressure. Such pressure usually results when a sleeping or sedated patient is in a position that compresses the nerve between the humerus and a hard surface, such as an operating room table or chair.

CLINICAL FEATURES. Radial nerve injuries in the spiral groove are characterized by wristdrop and fingerdrop. The brachioradialis muscle may be weak and its tendon reflex lost. Sensory disturbances are restricted to the back of the hand near the base of the thumb. With the wrist dropped, a fist is mechanically difficult to make but the finger flexors are not weak.

DIAGNOSIS. Electrophysiologic studies are useful for locating the site of injury and assessing the anatomic integrity of the nerve and the prognosis for recovery.

TREATMENT. Pressure injuries recover completely in 6 to 8 weeks. During that time a splint is useful for placing the wrist in extension so that the patient can flex the fingers.

ULNAR NEUROPATHY

The most common site of ulnar injury is the elbow. This type of injury can result from external pressure, recurrent dislocation of the nerve from its groove, and fracture of the distal humerus.

CLINICAL FEATURES. Paresthesias are experienced on the ulnar side of the hand, the little finger, and the ring finger. Tapping the ulnar groove increases the discomfort. Hand strength is lost and the intrinsic muscles become wasted. Sensation over the little finger and the adjacent side of the ring finger is diminished or absent.

DIAGNOSIS. The injury's precise localization along the course of the nerve is readily determined by electrophysiologic techniques.

TREATMENT. Minor pressure injuries do not require treatment, and recovery is complete within a few weeks. Surgical repair is often needed for injuries to the elbow that cause fracture or nerve dislocation.

MEDIAN NEUROPATHY

Nontraumatic median neuropathies are caused by compression of the nerve in the carpal tunnel; traumatic injuries occur at the elbow (Deymeer and Jones, 1994). Compression at the carpal tunnel in children may be caused by a storage disease such as mucolipidosis, but idiopathic cases occur as well. Fracture at the elbow is the usual cause of traumatic median neuropathy.

CLINICAL FEATURES. The most common feature is numbness and pain in the hand. Nontraumatic median neuropathy is often bilateral. Weakness and atrophy are more likely to occur in traumatic injuries of the nerve than in carpal tunnel entrapment.

DIAGNOSIS. EMG is very useful to localize the lesion, especially when surgical decompression is an option.

TREATMENT. Surgical decompression may be beneficial for both nontraumatic and traumatic injuries.

PERONEAL NEUROPATHY

The peroneal nerve lies in a superficial position adjacent to the fibula and is readily compressed against the bone by external force. This most often occurs in children who have undergone significant weight loss or trauma to the nerve (Jones et al, 1993). The prenatal onset of a peroneal palsy, presumably caused by pressure, was documented by EMG in one newborn (Jones et al, 1996).

CLINICAL FEATURES. The prominent feature is an acute painless footdrop. Both dorsiflexion and eversion of the foot are weak. Sensation is usually intact, but sometimes there is numbness over the lower lateral leg and dorsum of the foot. When only the deep branch of the peroneal nerve is involved, sensory loss is restricted to a small triangle between the first two toes.

Complete or significant spontaneous recovery is the rule except when the palsy was caused by considerable trauma.

DIAGNOSIS. Electrodiagnosis is useful in discriminating peroneal nerve lesions from disturbances of the fifth lumbar root.

TREATMENT. A footdrop brace is a useful aid to walking until recovery is complete.

HEREDITARY NEUROPATHY WITH LIABILITY TO PRESSURE PALSY

Hereditary neuropathy with liability to pressure palsy is characterized by the development of a mononeuropathy following trivial trauma (Gabreëls-Festen et al, 1992). In some cases, the brachial plexus is affected. The disorder is transmitted as an autosomal dominant trait and most families have a deletion in chromosome 17p (Mariman et al, 1994).

CLINICAL FEATURES. The first episode usually occurs during the second or third decade. Typical precipitating factors include sleeping on a limb, body contact in sports, constrictive clothing, or positioning during surgery. Individuals quickly learn to avoid activities that provoke episodes. Superficial nerves (radial, ulnar, median, peroneal) are the ones most commonly affected. The resulting mononeuropathy is painless and affects both motor and sensory fibers. Tendon reflexes are lost. Recovery is complete within days to weeks.

DIAGNOSIS. Except for the family history, the first episode might suggest an ordinary pressure palsy, although the trivial nature of the trauma should alert the physician to the underlying neuropathy.

Electrophysiologic studies show slow conduction time, not only in the affected limb but in all limbs. Generalized slowing of conduction can be shown in other family members between attacks.

TREATMENT. No treatment is available for the underlying neuropathy. Lifestyle may need to be altered to avoid pressure palsies. Acute episodes should be treated with physical therapy. Some patients eventually develop a generalized motor and sensory neuropathy.

IDIOPATHIC PROGRESSIVE NEUROPATHIES

An insidiously progressive axonal neuropathy involving only a single nerve of one leg is described in children and young adults (Engstrom et al, 1993). All patients had weakness and some had sensory loss as well. The cause is unknown and entrapment excluded. I have personally seen an adolescent male with insidiously progressive motor and sensory neuropathy of the entire brachial plexus of one arm. Extensive evaluation and observation over several years failed to show an underlying cause in the reported cases of mononeuropathy and my own case of brachial plexus palsy.

Monomelic Spinal Muscular Atrophy

Spinal muscular atrophies are genetic disorders characterized by progressive degeneration of anterior horn cells (see Chapter 7). Focal and generalized forms are worldwide in distribution, but most monomelic forms are reported from Japan and India (Donofrio, 1994).

CLINICAL FEATURES. Monomelic spinal muscular atrophy is usually sporadic in occurrence and has a male bias of 10:1. A single report describes a segmental spinal muscular atrophy affecting one hand and then the other in male identical twins (Tandan et al, 1990).

Age at onset is between 10 and 25 years but generally after 15 years. The progression of weakness and wasting is insidious. The arm is affected more often than the leg, and the distribution of weakness may be only proximal, be only distal, or involve the entire limb. The initial weakness and wasting are often unilateral and involve muscles innervated by C7, C8, and T1. Bilateral weakness is usually present within 2 years. Tremor of one or both hands is often associated with the wasting. Fasciculations are then noted in the proximal muscles and their appearance heralds weakness and wasting. Progression is slow, and spontaneous arrest within 5 years is the rule. However, another limb may become affected after a gap of 15 years.

DIAGNOSIS. Monomelic spinal muscular atrophy is a rare disorder, and other causes of monoplegia must be excluded. Fasciculations are present in the affected muscles. EMG and muscle biopsy findings are consistent with denervation, but nerve conduction velocities are normal. MRI of the spinal cord shows no abnormalities.

TREATMENT. Treatment is supportive and includes physical and occupational therapy.

REFERENCES

Awerbuch GI, Nigro MA, Dabrowski E, et al. Childhood lumbosacral plexus neuropathy. Pediatr Neurol 1989;5: 314-316.

Deymeer F, Jones HR Jr. Pediatric median mononeuropathies: A clinical and electromyographic study. Muscle Nerve 1994;17:755-762.

Donofrio PD. AAEM Case report 328: Monomelic amyotrophy. Muscle Nerve 1994;17:1129-1134.

Engstrom JW, Layzer RB, Olney RK, et al. Idiopathic, progressive mononeuropathy in young people. Arch Neurol 1993;50:20-23.

Gabreëls-Festen AAWM, Gabreëls FJM, Joosten EMG, et al. Hereditary neuropathy with liability to pressure palsies in childhood. Neuropediatrics 1992;23:138-143.

Gouider R, LeGuern E, Emile J, et al. Hereditary neuralgic amyotrophy and hereditary neuropathy with liability to pressure palsies: Two distinct clinical, electrophysiologic, and genetic entities. Neurology 1994;44:2250-2252.

Institute of Medicine. Adverse Events Associated With Childhood Vaccines: Evidence Bearing On Causality. National Academy Press, Washington D.C., 1994.

Jones Jr HR, Felice KJ, Gross PT. Pediatric peroneal mononeuropathy: A clinical and electromyographic study. Muscle Nerve 1993;16:1167-1173.

Jones Jr HR, Herbison GJ, Jacobs SR, et al. Intrauterine onset of a mononeuropathy: Peroneal neuropathy in a newborn with electromyographic findings at age one day compatible with prenatal onset. Muscle Nerve 1996;19:88-91.

Laurent JP, Lee R, Shenaq S, et al. Neurosurgical correction of upper brachial plexus birth injuries. J Neurosurg 1993;79:197-203.

Laurent JP, Lee RT. Birth-related upper brachial plexus injuries in infants: Operative and nonoperative approaches. J Child Neurol 1994;9:111-117.

Liedholm JLA, EEG-Olofsson O, Ekenberg BEK, et al. Acute postasthmatic amyotrophy (Hopkins syndrome). Muscle Nerve 1994;17:769-772.

Mariman ECM, Gabreëls-Festen AAWM, van Beersum SEC, et al. Prevalence of the 1.5-Mb 17p deletion in families with hereditary neuropathy with liability to pressure palsies. Ann Neurol 1994;36:650-655.

Shahar EM, Hwang PA, Niesen CE, et al. Poliomyelitis-like paralysis during recovery from acute bronchial asthma: Possible etiology and risk factors. Pediatrics 1991;88:276-279.

Tandan R, Sharma KR, Bradley WG, et al. Chronic segmental spinal muscular atrophy of upper extremities in identical twins. Neurology 1990;40:236-239.

14
Movement Disorders

Involuntary movements are usually associated with abnormalities of the basal ganglia and their connections and may occur in several different neurologic disorders. Abnormal movements can be the main or initial feature of disease, or they can occur as a late manifestation. The former type is discussed in this chapter, and the latter is discussed in other chapters.

 ## Approach to the Patient

Movement disorders cannot be adequately described; they must be seen. If abnormal movements are not present at the time of examination, the parents should be instructed to videotape the movements at home. Some relatively common movements are recognizable by description, but the rich variety of abnormal movements and postures that may occur defies classification. The most experienced observer will at times mistake one movement for another or will have difficulty conceptualizing the nature of an abnormal movement.

Many abnormal movements are paroxysmal or at least intermittent. Some are induced by movement, startle, emotional upset, or sleep. The physician should ask what makes the movement worse, and if they are action induced, the child should be asked to perform the action during the examination. Paroxysmal movements raise the question of epilepsy. Indeed, many neurologic disorders of childhood are characterized by the concurrent presence of seizures and involuntary movements. All cases of nocturnal paroxysmal dystonia are now believed to be frontal lobe seizures (see Chapter 1). The clinical and conceptual distinction between spinal myoclonus and spinal seizures remains a gray area. No absolute rules distinguish involuntary movements from seizures, but in general the following guidelines apply: (1) involuntary movements, with the exception of spinal myoclonus, abate or disappear during sleep and seizures persist or may worsen; (2) involuntary movements usually have a more stereotyped appearance and, with the exception of acute drug reactions, are more persistent than seizures; (3) seizures are often characterized by loss of consciousness or awareness, and involuntary movements are not; and (4) seizures are usually accompanied by epileptiform activity on electroencephalography (EEG) and involuntary movements are not.

Involuntary contraction of a muscle that does not move a joint may be a fasciculation, a focal seizure, or myoclonus. Low-amplitude jerking movements that move a joint or muscles may be focal seizures, chorea, myoclonus, tics, or hemifacial spasms. High-amplitude jerking movements that move a limb or limbs may be seizures, ballismus, or myoclonus. Slow, writhing movements and abnormal posturing may be due to athetosis, dystonia, continuous motor unit activity (see Chapter 8), or seizures. Rhythmic movements may be caused by tremors, seizures, or myoclonus.

 Chorea and Athetosis

Chorea is a rapid jerk affecting any part of the body and may be incorporated into a voluntary movement to hide the jerk. The movements are repetitive but neither rhythmic nor stereotyped, and they migrate from side to side and limb to limb. Because the involuntary movement flows into a voluntary movement, it gives the appearance of constant movement *(restlessness)*. Restlessness is also caused by *akasthisia,* an inward compulsion to move (discussed later). Depending on the condition, chorea may be unilateral or bilateral and may affect the face and trunk as well as the limbs.

Chorea is more readily observed when separated from the superimposed voluntary movement that follows. This is achieved by asking the child to raise both hands upward beside the head with palms facing each other. Low-amplitude jerking movements occur that turn the arm into pronation. When the child is asked to grip the examiner's fingers lightly, the grip alternately tightens and loosens, as if the patient is "milking" the examiner's hands. Hypotonia is common in many conditions causing chorea. Tendon reflexes may be normoreactive, but at times a choreic jerk occurs during the patellar response, producing an extra kick.

Athetosis is a slow, writhing movement of the limbs that may occur alone but is often associated with chorea (choreoathetosis). Athetosis without chorea is almost always due to perinatal brain injury. Kernicterus was the major cause, but perinatal asphyxia is now predominant. Many children with athetosis have atonic cerebral palsy, and others have spastic diplegia.

Ballismus is a high-amplitude, violent flinging of a limb from the shoulder or pelvis. It is considered an extreme form of chorea. In adults it may occur in limbs contralateral to a vascular lesion in the subthalamic nucleus; in children it is almost always associated with chorea and is seen in Sydenham chorea and lupus erythematosus.

Tardive dyskinesia is a complex syndrome characterized by buccolingual masticatory movements that include tongue protrusion, lip smacking, puckering, and chewing. It is decidedly uncommon in children. Psychotropic drugs are the usual cause of tardive dyskinesia. It may be considered a subtype of chorea, or at least a

■ TABLE 14–1
Differential Diagnosis of Chorea as an Initial or Prominent Symptom

Cardiopulmonary Bypass Surgery
Genetic Disorders
Abetalipoproteinemia (see Chapter 10)
Ataxia-telangiectasia (see Chapter 10)
Benign familial chorea
Fahr disease
Familial paroxysmal choreoathetosis (see Chapter 1)
Glutaric aciduria
Hallervorden-Spatz disease
Hepatolenticular degeneration (Wilson disease)
Huntington disease (see Chapter 5)
Lesch-Nyhan syndrome (see Chapter 5)
Machado-Joseph disease (see Chapter 5)
Neuroacanthocytosis
Drug-Induced Movement Disorders
Anticonvulsants
Antiemetics
Oral contraceptives
Psychotropic agents
Stimulants
Theophylline
Systemic Conditions
Hyperthyroidism
Lupus erythematosus
Pregnancy (chorea gravidarum)
Sydenham (rheumatic) chorea
Tumors of Cerebral Hemisphere (see Chapter 4)

related disorder, and is sometimes associated with choreic movements of the limbs.

The differential diagnosis of chorea and choreoathetosis is summarized in Tables 14-1 and 14-2. Chorea is a cardinal feature of the conditions listed in Table 14-1. Nevertheless, many are detailed elsewhere in the text because concurrent features are more prominent. Although abnormal movements are the only manifestation, familial paroxysmal choreoathetosis is described in Chapter 1 because it is more likely to be confused with epilepsy than with other causes of chorea.

Table 14-2 contains a partial list of conditions in which chorea and choreoathetosis may occur, but in which they are either late features or at least not prominent early in the course. Movement disorders are relatively common in many progressive cerebral degenerations. In contrast, chorea may be misinterpreted as seizures when it develops during an acute illness such as bacterial meningitis, metabolic encephalopathies, or encephalitis. At times the movement disorder is due to the underlying brain disorder and at times to drugs used in treatment.

■ TABLE 14-2
Conditions That May Include Choreoathetosis

Alternating Hemiplegia (see Chapter 11)
Bilateral Striatal Necrosis (see "Dystonia")
Cerebral Palsy
Congenital malformations (see Chapters 5 and 18)
Intrauterine disease (see Chapter 1)
Perinatal asphyxia (see Chapter 1)
Unknown causes
Genetic Disorders
Ceroid lipofuscinosis (see Chapter 5)
Idiopathic torsion dystonia
Incontinentia pigmenti (see Chapter 1)
Pelizaeus-Merzbacher disease (see Chapter 5)
Phenylketonuria (see Chapter 5)
Porphyria (see Chapter 7)
Infectious Diseases
Bacterial meningoencephalitis (see Chapter 4)
Viral encephalitis (see Chapter 2)
Metabolic Encephalopathies (see Chapter 2)
Addison disease
Burn encephalopathy
Hypernatremia
Hypocalcemia
Hypoparathyroidism
Vitamin B_{12} deficiency
Rett Syndrome (see Chapter 5)
Vascular
Moyamoya disease (see Chapter 11)
Poststroke (see Chapter 11)

CARDIOPULMONARY BYPASS SURGERY

Severe choreoathetosis is seen in 1% to 10% of children with congenital heart disease following cardiopulmonary bypass surgery and profound hypothermia (Medlock et al, 1993). Deep hypothermia and circulatory arrest are not essential factors in the pathophysiology but are often associated. The mechanism of basal ganglia injury is unknown.

CLINICAL FEATURES. Most affected children are more than 1 year of age and have cyanotic heart disease with systemic to pulmonary collaterals. Choreoathetosis begins within 2 weeks postoperatively and may be associated with oral-facial dyskinesias, hypotonia, affective changes, and pseudobulbar signs. Some children have only mild chorea that resolves spontaneously within 2 months. Others have severe exhausting chorea, unresponsive to treatment, that results in either death or severe neurologic morbidity. Some cognitive disturbance is expected in all survivors.

DIAGNOSIS. The diagnosis is made on the clinical features alone. Magnetic resonance imaging (MRI) results are normal during the acute illness.

TREATMENT. Sedation is needed to prevent exhaustion in severely affected children. The choreoathetosis is refractory to drug therapy.

DRUG-INDUCED CHOREA

Choreiform movements and akathisia or dystonic posturing may occur as effects of drugs, especially dopamine antagonists. Chorea and akathisia are more likely to be dose-related effects, whereas dystonia is usually an idiosyncratic reaction (see "Dystonia"). Phenytoin and ethosuximide may induce chorea as a toxic or idiosyncratic manifestation. Phenothiazines and haloperidol are associated with idiosyncratic dystonic reactions and tardive dyskinesia, and stimulant drugs (dextroamphetamine and methylphenidate) are associated with chorea, akathisia, and tic (see "Tic and Tourette Syndrome").

Tardive Dyskinesia

The term *tardive dyskinesia* denotes drug-induced choreiform movements. These movements are often limited to the lingual facial and buccal muscles and appear late ("tardive") in the course of drug therapy. Drug-induced buccolingual dyskinesia is unusual in children.

Tardive dyskinesias are most often associated with drugs used to modify behavior (neuroleptics), such as phenothiazines or haloperidol, and antiemetics, such as metoclopramide and prochlorperazine; they also occur in children with asthma treated with theophylline (Pranzatelli et al, 1991). The incidence of tardive dyskinesia in children taking neuroleptic drugs is estimated at 1%. I suspect that such children were taking very large dosages to treat major behavioral disorders.

CLINICAL FEATURES. Tardive dyskinesia is a complex of stereotyped movements. It usually affects the mouth and face, resembles chewing, and includes tongue protrusion and lip smacking; the trunk may be involved in rocking movements and the fingers in alternating flexion and extension resembling piano playing. Limb chorea, dystonia, myoclonus, tics, and facial grimacing may be associated features. These movements are exacerbated by stress and relieved by sleep.

Symptoms appear from months to years after starting therapy and are not related to changes in dosage. In children the movements usually cease when the drug is discontinued, but they may remain unchanged in adults.

DIAGNOSIS. Drug-induced dyskinesia should be suspected in any child who shows abnormal movements of the face or limbs while taking neuroleptic drugs. It is important to distinguish tardive dyskinesia from facial tics in children with Tourette syndrome and from facial mannerisms in children with schizophrenia.

TREATMENT. All neuroleptic drugs should be discontinued as quickly as possible after symptoms of dyskinesia develop. This may not be possible when drugs are needed to treat psychosis. In such circumstances the movements sometimes respond to diazepam.

Emergent Withdrawal Syndrome

Chorea and myoclonus may appear for the first time after neuroleptic drugs are abruptly discontinued or greatly reduced in dosage. Lingual-facial-buccal dyskinesia may be present as well. The symptoms are self-limited and cease in weeks to months.

GENETIC DISORDERS

The initial feature of abetalipoproteinemia and ataxia-telangiectasia is usually a cerebellar ataxia. Chorea may occur in both conditions, but only in ataxia-telangiectasia does chorea occur without ataxia. Huntington disease is an important cause of chorea and dystonia and is described in most texts as a movement disorder. However, because the initial features of the childhood form of Huntington disease is usually declining school performance, it is discussed in Chapter 5.

Benign Familial (Hereditary) Chorea

Benign familial chorea is a rare disorder transmitted by autosomal dominant inheritance (Wheeler et al, 1993). Benign familial chorea and familial paroxysmal choreoathetosis (see Chapter 1) may be genetically related disorders.

CLINICAL FEATURES. The onset of chorea is usually in early childhood, often when the child is beginning to walk. Motor development is sometimes delayed. Other possible features are intention tremor, dysarthria, hypotonia, and athetosis. Intelligence is normal. Most children

■ TABLE 14-3
Generic and Brand Names of Drugs

GENERIC NAME	BRAND NAME (MANUFACTURER)
Benztropine	Cogentin (Merck, Sharp & Dohme)
Carbamazepine	Tegretol (Geigy)
Clomipramine	Anafranil (Basel)
Clonazepam	Klonipin (Roche)
Clonidine	Catapres (Boehringer Ingelheim)
Dextroamphet-amine	Dexedrine (Smith, Kline & French)
Diazepam	Valium (Roche)
Fluoxetine	Prozac (Dista)
Haloperidol	Haldol (McNeil)
Methylphenidate	Ritalin (CIBA)
Metoclopramide	Reglan (Robins)
Phenothiazines	
Chlorpromazine	Thorazine (Smith, Kline, Beecham)
Fluphenazine	Permitil (Schering); Prolixin (Squibb)
Thioridazine	Mellaril (Sandoz)
Pimozide	Orap (McNeil)
Primidone	Mysoline (Ayerst)
Tetrabenazine	Nitoman (Roche)*
Trihexyphenidyl	Artane (Lederle)
Valproate	Depakene (Abbott)

*Not available in the United States.

have only chorea, which becomes less pronounced by adolescence. Adults may be asymptomatic or may have mild hypotonia and ataxia.

DIAGNOSIS. Benign familial chorea may be difficult to distinguish from other causes of chorea in children, especially familial paroxysmal chorea. A family history of the disorder is critical to diagnosis but can be overlooked because of incomplete expression in parents. Chorea is continuous and not episodic or paroxysmal. Computed tomography (CT) and EEG results are normal.

TREATMENT. Chlorpromazine or haloperidol is beneficial in some individuals (Table 14-3).

Fahr Disease

The combination of encephalopathy and progressive calcification of the basal ganglia is called *Fahr disease.* It may be familial or sporadic. Familial cases are transmitted by autosomal recessive or autosomal dominant inheritance. Those with dominant inheritance are usually associated with hypoparathyroidism or pseudohypoparathyroidism. Some sporadic cases probably represent autosomal recessive inheritance and others are caused by systemic disease. The common mechanism of diseases with basal ganglia calcification are thought to be defective iron transport and free-radical production (Beall et al, 1989).

CLINICAL FEATURES. Onset may be anytime from childhood to adult life but is consistent within a family. Disorders occurring before 10 years of age are likely to be different from those that occur in adults. Affected children may have a Cockayne syndrome phenotype (see Chapter 16): dwarfism, senile appearance, and retinitis pigmentosa. Mental deterioration and choreoathetosis are constant features. Ataxia, dysarthria, spasticity, and seizures are variable. Progressive neurologic deterioration results in early disability and death.

DIAGNOSIS. Plain radiographs of the skull show bilateral calcifications in the region of the basal ganglia that are localized more precisely by CT (Manyam et al, 1992). Calcifications appear first in the dentate nuclei and pons, then in the basal ganglia, and finally in the corpus callosum.

Parathyroid function must be assessed in every child with basal ganglia calcification to exclude the possibility of either hyperparathyroidism or pseudohypoparathyroidism.

TREATMENT. No treatment is available for the underlying condition except in cases of parathyroid dysfunction. The symptoms can be treated symptomatically.

Hallervorden-Spatz Disease

Hallervorden-Spatz disease is a rare hereditary disorder of iron metabolism. Transmission by autosomal recessive inheritance is presumed (Swaiman, 1991).

CLINICAL FEATURES. The disorder becomes symptomatic between 2 and 10 years of age in more than half of patients but may appear as late as the third decade. The prominent features are choreoathetosis, dystonia, rigidity, and dysarthria. Dystonia may be more prominent than chorea. Retinitis pigmentosa and seizures each occur in 20% to 25% of cases. Mental deterioration and spasticity follow, with progression to spastic immobility and death within 5 to 10 years.

DIAGNOSIS. Antemortem diagnosis is based primarily on the clinical presentation and is difficult to establish in the absence of a family history of the disorder. T_2-weighted MRI shows low-intensity signal images from the globus pallidus with a central area of increased signal intensity, known as the *eye-of-the-tiger* sign, which is believed to be characteristic of the disease (Schaffert et al, 1989).

Postmortem examination shows degeneration of the pallidum and substantia nigra with deposition of iron-containing material.

TREATMENT. Levodopa reduces symptoms in some patients but not in others. Benztropine, 2 mg twice daily, may also be beneficial. Agents that chelate iron have not proved effective.

Neuroacanthocytosis

Familial and nonfamilial cases of a progressive neurologic disorder are described in which the main features are chorea and acanthocytosis with normal lipoprotein levels (Hardie et al, 1991). The acanthocyte is an abnormal erythrocyte that has thorny projections from the cell surface. Erythrocyte deformity is enhanced by incubating the cells in saline solution for 5 minutes (Feinberg et al, 1991).

CLINICAL FEATURES. Onset is usually in adult life but may occur as early as the first decade. Chorea or dystonia of the limbs and face occurs in all cases. Tics, oromandibular dyskinesia and dystonia, and self-mutilation of the lips may be associated features. Phenotypic variability is considerable and may include axonal neuropathy, loss of tendon reflexes, dementia, seizures, and neurosis.

DIAGNOSIS. The association of acanthocytes or echinocytes (cells with rounded projections) and neurologic disease in the absence of lipoprotein abnormality is required for diagnosis. McLeod syndrome is excluded by testing for the Kell antigen (see Chapter 8).

TREATMENT. Only the symptoms can be treated. Death occurs 10 to 20 years after onset.

PAROXYSMAL CHOREOATHETOSIS

Paroxysmal choreoathetosis occurs in children who are otherwise normal and in children with an obvious underlying static encephalopathy. The normal children have a genetic disease, *familial paroxysmal choreoathetosis* (see Chapter 1), and the abnormal children may have one of several nongenetic disorders. The mechanism of paroxysmal choreoathetosis of all causes is unknown.

Acquired paroxysmal choreoathetosis occurs most often in children with cerebral palsy. Either hemiplegia or diplegia may be present, and the involuntary movements affect only the paretic limbs. The onset of the movement disorder often occurs 10 or more years after the acute encephalopathy. One patient had paroxysmal choreoathetosis precipitated by sound and light that was attributed to an arteriovenous malformation of the parietal lobe (Shintani et al, 1991).

SYSTEMIC DISORDERS

Hyperthyroidism

The ocular manifestations of thyrotoxicosis are discussed in Chapter 15. Tremor is the most common associated movement disorder. Chorea is unusual, but when present it may affect the face, limbs, and trunk. The movements cease when the child becomes euthyroid.

Lupus Erythematosus

CLINICAL FEATURES. Lupus-associated chorea is uncommon but may be the initial feature of the disease, beginning 7 years before to 3 years after the appearance of systemic features. It is indistinguishable from Sydenham chorea in appearance. Average duration is 12 weeks, but one fourth of patients have recurrences. Additional neurologic features of lupus (ataxia, psychosis, seizures) are common in children who have chorea but occur only after the appearance of systemic symptoms. Therefore, chorea may be a solitary manifestation of disease.

DIAGNOSIS. The diagnosis is clear in children with known lupus erythematosus. When chorea is the initial feature of lupus, it must be differentiated from Sydenham chorea. The erythrocyte sedimentation rate may be elevated in both conditions and is not a distinguishing feature. The presence of elevated concentrations of antinuclear antibodies is critical to diagnosis.

TREATMENT. Children with neurologic manifestations of lupus erythematosus should be treated with high doses of corticosteroids. The overall outcome is poor.

Pregnancy (Chorea Gravidarum)

Chorea should not be accepted as a complication of pregnancy. More likely, pregnancy has added one more stress to an underlying condition. The major considerations are an initial attack or recurrence of Sydenham chorea and lupus erythematosus.

Sydenham (Rheumatic) Chorea

Sydenham chorea is the most common cause of acquired chorea in children. It is a cardinal feature of rheumatic fever and is sufficient alone to make the diagnosis. It occurs primarily in populations with untreated streptococcal infections. One hypothesis is that when genetically predisposed children are exposed to group A beta-hemolytic streptococcus infection, antibodies mistakenly attack cells in the basal ganglia and cause inflammation (Swedo, 1995).

CLINICAL FEATURES. The onset is frequently insidious, and diagnosis is often delayed. Chorea, hypotonia, dysarthria, and emotional lability are cardinal features. Difficulty in school may bring the child to medical attention. Chorea causes the child to be restless, and discipline by the teacher results in emotional excess. Obsessive-compulsive behavior may be present (Swedo et al, 1993). The behavioral change is often thought to be a sign of mental illness.

Examination reveals a fidgeting child with migratory chorea of limbs and face. The limbs of only one side may be affected initially, but the chorea eventually becomes generalized in most patients. Efforts to conceal chorea with voluntary movement only add to the appearance of restlessness.

Gradual improvement occurs over several months. Most patients recover completely. Rheumatic valvular heart disease develops in one third of untreated patients.

DIAGNOSIS. The diagnosis is established by the clinical features and cannot be confirmed by laboratory tests. The differential diagnosis is mainly between Sydenham chorea, lupus-associated chorea, and drug-induced chorea. Blood should be examined for lupus antinuclear antibodies and for thyroid function. The onset of Sydenham chorea is usually 4 months after the provocative streptococcal infection, and by that time the antistreptolysin O titer is back to normal or only slightly increased.

During the time of illness, T_2-weighted MRI may show increased signal intensity in the putamen and globus pallidus that resolves when the child has recovered (Traill et al, 1995).

TREATMENT. Pimozide usually controls the acute neurologic symptoms without producing sedation (Shannon and Fenichel, 1990). If pimozide does not relieve the symptoms, benzodiazepines, phenothiazines, or haloperidol should be tried. All children with Sydenham chorea must be treated as if they had acute rheumatic fever: penicillin in high doses for 10 days to eradicate active streptococcal infection, and prophylactic penicillin therapy until age 21.

 Dystonia

Dystonia is a disturbance of posture caused by simultaneous contracture of agonist and antagonist muscles. The posturing is initiated by

■ TABLE 14–4
Differential Diagnosis of Abnormal Posturing

Dystonia
Hysteria
Muscular dystrophy
Myotonia
Neuromyotonia
Rigidity
Spasticity
Stiffman syndrome

■ TABLE 14–5
Differential Diagnosis of Dystonia in Childhood

Focal Dystonia
Blepharospasm
Drug-induced dystonia
Generalized dystonia beginning as focal dystonia
HARP syndrome
Torticollis
Writer's cramp
Generalized Genetic Dystonias
Ataxia with episodic dystonia (see Chapter 10)
Ceroid lipofuscinosis (see Chapter 5)
Cytochrome b deficiency
Dopa-responsive dystonia
Familial paroxysmal choreoathetosis (see Chapter 1)
Glutaric acidemia type I
Hallervorden-Spatz disease (see "Chorea")
Hepatolenticular degeneration (Wilson disease)
Huntington disease (see Chapter 5)
Idiopathic torsion dystonia
Infantile bilateral striatal necrosis
Leber disease (see Chapter 16)
Machado-Joseph disease (see Chapter 10)
Transient paroxysmal dystonia of infancy (see Chapter 1)
Generalized Symptomatic Dystonias
Perinatal cerebral injury (see Chapter 1)
Postinfectious
Poststroke
Post-traumatic
Toxin-induced
Tumor-induced
Hemidystonia
Alternating hemiplegia (see Chapter 11)
Antiphospholipid syndrome (see Chapter 11)
Basal ganglia tumors
Neuronal storage disorders

■ TABLE 14–6
Differential Diagnosis of Blepharospasm in Childhood

Continuous motor unit activity
Drug-induced
Encephalitis
Hemifacial spasm
Hepatolenticular degeneration (Wilson disease)
Huntington disease
Hysteria
Myokymia
Myotonia
Schwartz-Jampel syndrome
Seizures

involuntary movement in the limbs, face, or trunk; the movement has a writhing quality. The overall appearance is not of an involuntary movement disorder, but rather of an abnormal posture of the limbs or trunk and grimacing of the face. Involvement may be of a single body part (*focal dystonia*), two or more contiguous body parts (*segmental dystonia*), the arm and leg on one side of the body (*hemidystonia*), or of one or both legs and the contiguous trunk and any other body part (*generalized dystonia*).

The differential diagnosis of abnormal posturing is summarized in Table 14–4. Continuous motor unit activity (see Chapter 8) may be difficult to distinguish from dystonia by clinical inspection alone, especially when only one or two limbs are affected. The two disorders are differentiated by electromyography, which is recommended in most cases.

Persistent focal dystonias are relatively common in adults but are unusual in children except when drug induced. Most dystonias in children that begin focally eventually become generalized. Children with focal, stereotyped movements of the eyelids, face, or neck are much more likely to have a tic than focal dystonia. Only childhood forms of focal dystonia are listed in Table 14–5.

Generalized dystonia usually begins in one limb. The patient has difficulty performing an act rather than a movement, so that the foot becomes dystonic when walking forward but may not be dystonic when sitting, standing, or running.

FOCAL DYSTONIAS

Blepharospasm

Blepharospasm is an involuntary spasmodic closure of the eyes. The differential diagnosis for children is summarized in Table 14–6. Essential blepharospasm, an incapacitating condition, is a disorder of middle or late adult life and never begins in childhood. Tics account for almost all cases of involuntary eye closure in children. Eye fluttering occurs during absence seizures (see

Chapter 1) but is not confused with dystonia. Focal dystonia involving eye closure in children is almost always drug induced.

Blepharospasm and orofacial dystonia in adults may be helped by treatment with baclofen, clonazepam, trihexyphenidyl, tetrabenazine with lithium, and subcutaneous injections of botulinum A toxin (Jankovic and Brin, 1991).

Drug-Induced Dystonia

Acute Reactions

Focal or generalized dystonia may occur as an acute idiosyncratic reaction following a first dose of phenothiazine or haloperidol. Possible reactions include trismus, opisthotonos, torticollis, and oculogyric crisis. Difficulty with swallowing and speaking may occur. Metoclopramide, a nonphenothiazine antiemetic that blocks postsynaptic dopamine receptors, may produce acute and delayed (tardive) dystonia. The acute reactions are usually self-limited or respond to treatment with benztropine, but they may be prolonged and resistant to therapy.

Tardive Dystonia

The onset of dystonia is usually 3 to 11 days after treatment with neuroleptic drugs is initiated. The dystonia is usually generalized in children but may be focal in adults. Spontaneous remissions are unusual. Tetrabenazine is helpful in most patients, and anticholinergics offer relief in others.

HARP SYNDROME

HARP is an acronym for hypoprebetalipoproteinemia, acanthocytosis, retinitis pigmentosa, and pallidal degeneration. The disorder shares many features with Hallevorden-Spatz disease, neuroacanthocytosis (see "Chorea"), and abetalipoproteinemia (see Chapter 10). These genetic disorders, all transmitted by autosomal recessive inheritance, may represent variable clinical features of a contiguous gene defect (Orrell et al, 1995).

CLINICAL FEATURES. The early features are night blindness from retinitis pigmentosa and mild mental subnormality. Dystonic dysarthria develops during adolescence and causes difficulty in speech and swallowing. Facial expression is decreased and the jaw and facial reflexes

■ TABLE 14–7

Differential Diagnosis of Torticollis and Head Tilt

Benign paroxysmal torticollis
Cervical cord syringomyelia (see Chapter 12)
Cervical cord tumors (see Chapter 12)
Cervicomedullary malformations (see Chapters 10 and 18)
Diplopia (see Chapter 15)
Dystonia
Familial paroxysmal choreoathetosis (see Chapter 1)
Juvenile rheumatoid arthritis
Posterior fossa tumors (see Chapter 10)
Sandifer syndrome
Spasmus nutans (see Chapter 15)
Sternocleidomastoid injuries
Tic and Tourette syndrome

are lost. Eye movements are normal and generalized dystonia does not follow. Mental deterioration and seizures are not part of the syndrome.

DIAGNOSIS. MRI shows the eye-of-the-tiger appearance of the pallidum that is usually considered diagnostic of Hallevorden-Spatz disease. Acanthocytes and echinocytes are seen in preparations of washed erythrocytes. Quantitation of lipoprotein fractions shows that very-low-density lipoprotein cholesterol and intermediate-density lipoprotein cholesterol and intermediate-density lipoprotein cholesterol levels are only 10% of normal.

TREATMENT. Treatment for the underlying defect is not available.

Torticollis

The differential diagnoses of torticollis and head tilt are summarized in Table 14–7. The first step in diagnosis is to distinguish fixed from nonfixed torticollis. In fixed torticollis the neck cannot be readily moved back to the neutral position. This may be caused by structural disturbance of the cervical vertebrae, or because movement causes pain and is therefore resisted.

Evidence of concurrent dystonia in the face or limbs indicates the need for further evaluation directed at underlying causes of dystonia. Torticollis associated with hyperactive tendon reflexes, ankle clonus, or extensor plantar responses suggests a cervical spinal cord disturbance and is an indication for MRI of the cervical portion of the spine (see Figure 10–7). Symptoms of increased intracranial pressure indicate a posterior fossa tumor with early herniation. When torticollis is the only abnormal feature, the underlying causes are focal dystonia, injuries to the neck muscles, and juvenile rheumatoid arthritis.

Nonfixed torticollis that occurs in attacks suggests benign paroxysmal torticollis or familial paroxysmal choreoathetosis. The combination of head tilt and nystagmus is termed *spasmus nutans* (see Chapter 15). Tic produces head turning but is so spasmodic that it should not be confused with torticollis.

Benign Paroxysmal Torticollis

The cause of benign paroxysmal torticollis is not fully understood (Cohen et al, 1993). It is believed to be a migraine variant closely related to benign paroxysmal vertigo (see Chapter 10) in some infants, but not in others.

CLINICAL FEATURES. Onset is always in the first year and is characterized by episodes in which the head is tilted to one side (not always the same side) and may be slightly rotated. The child may resist efforts to return the head to a neutral position, but this can be overcome. Some children have no other symptoms, whereas others have pallor, irritability, malaise, and vomiting. Most attacks last for 1 to 3 days, end spontaneously, and tend to recur three to six times a year. Children who are old enough to stand and walk become ataxic during attacks.

With time the attacks may evolve into episodes characteristic of benign paroxysmal vertigo or classic migraine, or may simply cease without further symptoms. The disorder has been described in siblings, but more often the family history is only of migraine.

DIAGNOSIS. The disorder should be suspected in any infant with attacks of torticollis that remit spontaneously. A family history of migraine should be sought. Familial paroxysmal choreoathetosis and familial paroxysmal dystonia do not begin during early infancy. *Sandifer syndrome,* intermittent torticollis associated with hiatal hernia, is an alternative consideration.

TREATMENT. No treatment is available or needed for the acute attacks.

Writer's Cramp

Writer's cramp is a focal dystonia that may occur only when writing, when performing other specific manual tasks such as typing or playing the piano (*occupational cramp*), or with nonspecific use of the hands. The cramp is more often isolated, but may be associated with other focal dystonias, such as torticollis, or with generalized dystonia.

CLINICAL FEATURES. Onset is almost always after 20 years of age, but may be in the second decade. Initial features are any of the following: aching in the hand when writing, loss of handwriting neatness or speed, and difficulty in holding a writing implement. All three symptoms are eventually present. Dystonic postures occur when the patient attempts to write. The hand and arm lift from the paper and the fingers may flex or extend. Writing with the affected hand becomes impossible and the patient learns to write with the nondominant hand, which may also become dystonic.

Symptoms are at first intermittent and are especially severe when others observe the writing. Later the cramp occurs with each attempt at writing. Some patients have lifelong difficulty with using the dominant hand for writing and may have difficulty with other manual tasks as well. Others experience remissions and exacerbations, and a minority of patients develop generalized dystonia.

DIAGNOSIS. Unfortunately, most people with writer's or occupational cramp are thought to have psychiatric illness despite the lack of associated psychopathologic features. Early diagnosis can save considerable expense and concern. Isolated focal dystonia must be distinguished from generalized dystonia with focal onset. Family history should be explored thoroughly and examination repeated to determine the presence of dystonia in other body parts.

TREATMENT. The same medications used to treat generalized dystonia should be used in patients with focal dystonia (see "Idiopathic Torsion Dystonia").

GENERALIZED GENETIC DYSTONIAS

Cytochrome b Deficiency

Mitochondrial disorders cause widespread dysfunction of the central and peripheral nervous system (see Chapters 5, 8, and 11). Partial cytochrome b deficiency was identified in an 18-year-old girl in whom clinical features of idiopathic torsion dystonia developed at age 2 (Nigro et al, 1990). The possibility of mitochondrial dysfunction was suggested by an increased concentration of lactate and pyruvate in venous blood, and by CT evidence of bilateral hypodensities in the putamen. A muscle biopsy specimen showed ragged-red fibers (see Chapter 8) and deficiency of cytochrome b.

Dopa-Responsive Dystonia

Dopa-responsive dystonia is also called the *dystonia-parkinsonism syndrome, dystonia with diurnal variation,* and *Segawa disease* (Calne, 1994). Dopa-responsive dystonia is inherited as an autosomal dominant trait with a 31% penetrance rate. The abnormal gene is located on the short arm of chromosome 14 and is responsible for the production of tetrahydrobiopterin, an essential cofactor in converting tyrosine to dopamine (Tanaka et al, 1995). Most reported cases of "juvenile parkinsonism" are probably variants of dopa-responsive dystonia (Nygaard et al, 1991).

CLINICAL FEATURES. Age at onset is usually between 4 and 8 years but may be as early as infancy. Early-onset cases are often misdiagnosed as cerebral palsy. The initial feature is nearly always a gait disturbance caused by leg dystonia. Flexion at the hip and knee and plantar flexion of the foot cause toe-walking. Both flexor and extensor posturing of the arms develops, and finally parkinsonian features appear: cogwheel rigidity, masklike facies, and bradykinesia. The disease reaches a plateau in adolescence. Postural or intention tremor occurs in almost half of patients, but typical parkinsonian tremor is unusual.

Diurnal fluctuation in symptoms occurs in more than half of patients. Symptoms are considerably improved on awakening and become worse later in the day. Movement and exercise exacerbate dystonia in some patients, and other disorders with exercise-induced dystonia as the main or only clinical features may be expressions of the same genetic error.

DIAGNOSIS. Dopa-responsive dystonia may be difficult to differentiate from other genetic disorders with dystonia because of phenotypic variation among family members (see also "Rapid-Onset Dystonia-Parkinsonism"). Diagnosis by mutation analysis will be commercially available. Important clues to diagnosis are features of parkinsonism without other neurologic signs, diurnal variation in severity of symptoms, exacerbation of symptoms with exercise, and response to levodopa.

TREATMENT. A small dose of levodopa usually provides immediate and complete relief in most patients, even when treatment is initiated long after symptoms begin. No other

dystonia responds so well. Carbidopa-levodopa should be started at the lowest possible dose and slowly increased until a response is established. Long-term therapy is beneficial and required; symptoms return when the drug is discontinued.

Trihexyphenidyl, in doses lower than ordinarily needed to treat idiopathic torsion dystonia, and bromocriptine are also effective.

Glutaric Acidemia Type I

Glutaric acidemia type I is a rare inborn error in the catabolism of lysine, hydroxylysine, and tryptophan. It is transmitted by autosomal recessive inheritance and is caused by deficiency of glutaryl-coenzyme A dehydrogenase (Kyllerman et al, 1994).

CLINICAL FEATURES. Megalencephaly is usually present at birth. Neurologic findings may be otherwise normal. Two patterns have been described in affected infants. The initial feature in two thirds of infants is an acute encephalitis-like illness characterized by somnolence, irritability, and excessive sweating. Seizures sometimes occur. The prognosis in such cases is poor. Afterward, development regresses and progressive choreoathetosis and dystonia occur. The other pattern is more insidious and the prognosis is better. Affected infants are at first hypotonic, and later have mild developmental delay and dyskinesias. Many are often misdiagnosed as "cerebral palsy" (see Chapter 12).

DIAGNOSIS. Metabolic acidosis may be present. Abnormal amounts of glutaric, 3-hydroxyglutaric, 3-hydroxybutyric, and acetoacetic acids are found in the urine. The diagnosis is established by showing the enzyme deficiency in cultured fibroblasts. CT often shows diffuse attenuation of cerebral white matter and cerebral atrophy, most marked in the frontal and temporal lobes.

TREATMENT. The course of disease may be improved by protein restriction and riboflavin supplementation.

Hepatolenticular Degeneration (Wilson Disease)

Hepatolenticular degeneration is transmitted by autosomal recessive inheritance (Petrukhin and Gilliam, 1994). The disorder may be caused by a disturbance in the biliary excretion of copper and its incorporation into ceruloplasmin. The defective gene is located on chromosome 13. Symptoms result from the accumulation of copper in the liver, brain, and cornea.

CLINICAL FEATURES. Hepatic failure is the prominent clinical feature in children less than 10 years of age, usually without neurologic symptoms or signs. Neurologic manifestations with only minimal symptoms of liver disease are more likely when the onset of symptoms is in the second decade. A single symptom, such as a disturbance of gait or speech, is often the initial feature and may remain unchanged for years. Eventually the initial symptom worsens and new features develop: dysarthria (97%), dystonia (65%), dysdiadochokinesia (58%), rigidity (52%) gait and postural abnormalities (42%), tremor (32%), and drooling (23%).

Dystonia of bulbar muscles is responsible for three prominent features of the disease: dysarthria, a fixed pseudosmile (risus sardonicus), and a high-pitched whining noise on inspiration.

Psychiatric disturbances precede the neurologic abnormalities in 20% of cases. They range from behavioral disturbances to paranoid psychoses. Dementia is not an early feature of disease.

The Kayser-Fleischer ring, a yellow-brown granular deposit at the limbus of the cornea, is a certain indicator of the disease. It is caused by copper deposition in the Descemet membrane and is present in all patients with neurologic manifestations, although it may be absent in children with liver disease alone.

DIAGNOSIS. Hepatolenticular degeneration should be considered in any child with dysarthria and dystonia. The further association of chronic liver disease increases the probability of hepatolenticular degeneration. The diagnosis is established by showing an increased copper content by liver biopsy or by the demonstration of a Kayser-Fleischer ring by slit-lamp examination. Ninety-six percent of patients will have a serum ceruloplasmin concentration of less than 20 mg/dl, corresponding to less than 56 μg/dl of ceruloplasmin copper.

MRI shows increased signal intensity and decreased size of the caudate, putamen, subcortical white matter, midbrain, and pons. MRI findings do not correlate well with clinical features (Prayer et al, 1990).

TREATMENT. The treatment of choice is the oral administration of D-penicillamine, 250 mg four times a day for children more than 10 years of age and half as much for children less than 10. Penicillamine must always be given on an empty stomach together with a daily dose of 25 mg pyridoxine. Twenty-four-hour urinary copper

secretion is then monitored and the dose is adjusted to produce urinary excretion of copper at a rate of 2 mg/day during the first year. Later, an excretion of 1 mg/day is considered satisfactory. Improvement is slow, and neurologic improvement frequently takes several months. Worsening may occur during the first months of therapy, but this should not be a cause for alarm. When treatment is started early, the results are quite satisfactory, without excess morbidity and mortality.

Discontinuation of penicillamine results in rapid clinical deterioration, which may prove fatal. The replacement of penicillamine with trientine, a chelating agent, prevents the adverse course associated with penicillamine withdrawal.

Siblings of patients with Wilson disease should be carefully screened for disease and treated as early as possible.

Idiopathic Torsion Dystonia

Idiopathic torsion dystonia probably encompasses several genetic disorders characterized by generalized dystonia without other symptoms of neurologic deterioration. Most forms are transmitted by autosomal dominant inheritance. *Dystonia musculorum deformans* is an older name for the same disorders. The frequency of idiopathic torsion dystonia in Ashkenazi Jews is 5 to 10 times greater than in other groups, and the abnormal gene maps to chromosome 9 at the q32-34 site (Bressman et al, 1994). Nonfamilial cases probably represent autosomal dominant inheritance with incomplete penetrance. The penetrance rate is 40% and the expression is highly variable (Fletcher et al, 1990).

CLINICAL FEATURES. Age at onset has a bimodal distribution; for early onset the mode is 9 years, and for late onset the mode is 45 years. The early onset cases are more genetically homogeneous. The limbs are usually affected before the trunk. The initial features may be in the arms, legs, or larynx. Early leg involvement is more common in children than adults. Despite the focal features at onset, dystonia always becomes generalized in children, affecting the limbs and trunk. Spontaneous stabilization is the rule, but remission is unusual. The eventual outcome varies from complete disability to functional independence.

Other clinical features include dysarthria, orofacial movements, dysphagia, postural tremor, and blepharospasm. Mental deterioration does not occur, but as a group, patients with familial disease have a lower IQ than those with sporadic cases.

DIAGNOSIS. Diagnosis depends on the clinical features of dystonic movements and postures, normal perinatal history, no exposure to drugs, no evidence of intellectual or corticospinal deterioration, and no demonstrable biochemical disorder.

A syndrome of *rapid-onset dystonia-parkinsonism* may be a variant of idiopathic torsion dystonia (Dobyns et al, 1993). The disorder is characterized by the acute (hours) or subacute (days to weeks) development of generalized dystonia and parkinsonism that responds poorly to treatment with levodopa. Age at onset is 14 to 45 years. The disorder is transmitted as an autosomal dominant trait and is linked to the site for idiopathic torsion dystonia on chromosome 9.

TREATMENT. A trial of levodopa is reasonable in any child with new-onset dystonia even though it is not effective in idiopathic torsion dystonia. If dopa fails, then trihexyphenidyl is the drug of choice and is usually effective. High dosages are required, usually 30 mg/day in three divided doses. Dosages as high as 80 mg/day are sometimes necessary. Such high dosages can be tolerated in children if built up slowly, but are rarely tolerated by adults. The response cannot be predicted from measurement of plasma concentrations.

If trihexyphenidyl is not effective, baclofen should be added (Greene and Fahn, 1992). The initial dosage is 5 to 10 mg/day, increased 10 mg weekly until benefit is attained or adverse reactions occur. Diazepam is an alternate to baclofen and should also be added at low dosages and slowly increased as tolerated. If a patient does not respond to this combination, tetrabenazine or some combination of carbamazepine, benztropine, pimozide, or bromocriptine can be tried.

Infantile Bilateral Striatal Necrosis

Bilateral striatal necrosis occurs in several clinical disorders, many genetic, that share pathologic features of bilateral, symmetric, spongy degeneration of the corpus striatum with variable degeneration of the globus pallidus. These disorders may appear in infancy or early childhood.

CLINICAL FEATURES. Two clinical syndromes are associated with infantile bilateral striatal necrosis. One is characterized by an insidious onset during infancy or childhood and with a long clinical course that includes dystonia, cognitive impairment, seizures, and death. Most of these cases are probably mitochondrial disorders; a point mutation in the mitochondrial ATPase 6 gene was shown in one child (Meirleir et al, 1995). A clinical and pathologic overlap exists between progressive infantile bilateral striatal necrosis and subacute necrotizing encephalomyelopathy (see Chapter 5) and Leber hereditary optic neuropathy (see Chapter 16) (Leuzzi et al, 1992).

The other syndrome begins as an acute encephalopathy, usually following a febrile illness with nausea and vomiting (Rosemberg et al, 1993). The major features are dystonia and tremor. The severity of symptoms may fluctuate at the time of intercurrent illness. Some children recover spontaneously; others are permanently impaired. One child with a progressive neurologic disorder experienced an acute encephalopathy and then developed MRI evidence of bilateral striatal necrosis (Mizuguchi et al, 1994).

DIAGNOSIS. Diagnosis is suggested by showing static or progressive striatal necrosis on serial MRI examinations (Roig et al, 1993). Postmortem examination shows diffuse but patchy neuronal loss and marked gliosis in the striatum and globus pallidus.

TREATMENT. No treatment is available.

SYMPTOMATIC GENERALIZED DYSTONIA

Dystonia may be caused by an underlying tumor, an active encephalopathy (hypoxic, infectious, or metabolic), or prior brain damage caused by encephalopathy, trauma, or stroke.

CLINICAL FEATURES. The onset of dystonia may be at the time of an acute encephalopathy, after the acute phase is over, or several years later when the encephalopathy is thought to be static. Delayed-onset chorea and dystonia in children with perinatal disturbances such as asphyxia or kernicterus usually begin by 2 to 3 years of age, but may be delayed for 17 years (Saint Hilaire et al, 1991). After involuntary movements appear, they tend to become progressively more severe, but intellectual decline is not an associated feature. Delayed-onset dystonia is usually generalized.

Hemidystonia most often occurs after stroke or head injury but may be a symptom of neuronal storage diseases or tumors of the basal ganglia, alternating hemiplegia, and the antiphospholipid antibody syndrome (see Chapter 11). The dystonic limbs are contralateral to the damaged basal ganglia.

DIAGNOSIS. Children with a known cause for the development of dystonia or chorea need not be studied extensively. The new symptoms are discouraging for patients and families, who have adjusted to a fixed neurologic deficit. They may be assured that this is not evidence of new degeneration in the brain, but only the appearance of new symptoms from old lesions. This sequence is most likely when injury is perinatal and brain maturation is required to manifest involuntary movements.

The appearance of hemidystonia, even when the predisposing event is known, necessitates MRI to look for localized changes that may require treatment, such as an expanding cyst. The possibility of tumor must be considered in children who had been neurologically intact before hemidystonia appeared.

TREATMENT. The drugs used to treat symptomatic dystonia are no different from those used for genetic dystonia, but the results may not be as favorable.

 ## Hemifacial Spasm

Hemifacial spasm is characterized by involuntary, irregular contraction of the muscles innervated by one facial nerve. It is very rare in children. The spasms may develop because of aberrant regeneration following facial nerve injury, as a result of posterior fossa tumor, or without apparent cause.

CLINICAL FEATURES. Spasms are embarrassing and disturbing but not painful. The orbicularis oculi muscles are affected first and most commonly, causing forced closure of the eye. As facial muscles on one side become affected, the mouth is pulled to one side. Spasms may occur several times a minute, especially during times of stress. The subsequent course depends on the underlying cause.

DIAGNOSIS. Hemifacial spasm in children may be mistaken for a focal siezure. The stereotyped appearance of the spasm and a concurrent normal EEG are distinguishing features. Posterior fossa tumor must be suspected in every child with hemifacial spasm. MRI is indicated unless symptoms can be explained by a known history of facial nerve injury.

TREATMENT. Some patients respond to treatment with carbamazepine at anticonvulsant doses (see Chapter 1), but most have no response to medical therapy. Injection of botu-

linum toxin into the muscles in spasm is the treatment of choice. Surgical procedures to relieve pressure on the facial nerve from adjacent vessels are of questionable value.

 ## Mirror Movements

Mirror movements are defined as involuntary movements of one side of the body, usually the hands, that occur as mirror reversals of an intended movement on the other side of the body (Cohen et al, 1991). They are normal during infancy and tend to disappear before 10 years of age, coincident with myelination of the corpus callosum. Persistence of mirror movements may be a familial trait caused by ipsilateral and contralateral organziation of the corticospinal pathways (Rasmussen, 1993). Obligatory mirror movements are abnormal even in infants and suggest a congenital abnormality at the cervicomedullary junction.

 ## Myoclonus

The term *myoclonus* encompasses several involuntary movements characterized by rapid muscle jerks. They are less frequent and severe during sleep but may not disappear. Myoclonus may be rhythmic or nonrhythmic; focal, multifocal, or generalized; or spontaneous or activated by movement (action myoclonus) or sensory stimulation (reflex myoclonus).

Nonepileptic myoclonus must be distinguished from tic, chorea, tremor, and seizures. Tics are usually more complex and stereotyped movements than myoclonus and can be briefly suppressed by voluntary effort; myoclonus cannot be suppressed. Chorea is more random than myoclonus and tends to be incorporated into voluntary movement; myoclonus is never part of a larger movement. Rhythmic myoclonus and tremor look alike and are distinguished with certainty only by special studies. Tremor is a continuous to-and-fro movement, whereas rhythmic myoclonus has a pause between movements.

An etiologic classification of myoclonus is summarized in Table 14–8. *Physiologic myoclonus* occurs in normal people when falling asleep, during sleep (nocturnal myoclonus), when waking up, and during times of anxiety. Nocturnal myoclonus is a rhythmic jerking of the legs during sleep that is common in children. It

■ TABLE 14-8
Etiologic Classification of Myoclonus

Physiologic
Anxiety-induced
Exercise-induced
Sleep jerks and nocturnal myoclonus
Essential
Epileptic (see Chapter 1)
Symptomatic
Post-central nervous system injury
  Hypoxia (see Chapter 2)
  Trauma (see Chapter 2)
  Stroke (see Chapter 11)
Basal ganglia degenerations
  Idiopathic torsion dystonia
  Hallervorden-Spatz disease
  Hepatolenticular degeneration (Wilson disease)
  Huntington disease (see Chapter 5)
Drug-induced
  Carbamazepine
  Levodopa
  Tricyclic antidepressants
Lysosomal storage diseases (see Chapter 5)
Metabolic encephalopathies (see Chapter 2)
  Dialysis syndromes
  Disorders of osmolality
  Hepatic failure
  Renal failure
Myoclonic encephalopathy (see Chapter 10)
  Idiopathic
  Neuroblastoma
Spinal cord tumor (see Chapter 12)
Spinocerebellar degenerations (see Chapter 10)
Toxic encephalopathies (see Chapter 2)
Viral encephalitis

should be distinguished from the *restless legs syndrome,* a genetic disorder transmitted by autosomal dominant inheritance (Walters et al, 1994). The syndrome is characterized by leg discomfort at rest that is relieved by movement. It is often attributed to "growing pains." Periodic limb movements mainly occur during sleep but also during wakefulness.

Epileptic myoclonus is associated with epileptiform activity on the EEG (see Chapter 1). *Symptomatic myoclonus* is caused by drugs or follows a cerebral injury, or is part of a generalized and usually progressive encephalopathy.

ESSENTIAL MYOCLONUS

Essential myoclonus is a chronic condition of focal, segmental, or generalized jerking that is aggravated by action or stress. Affected people are otherwise normal. It's occurrence is usually sporadic, but when familial, it is transmitted by autosomal dominant inheritance.

CLINICIAL FEATURES. Onset is in the first or second decade. Males and females are affected equally. The movements are predominantly in the face, trunk, and proximal muscles. They are usually generalized but may be restricted to one side of the body. No other neurologic disturbances develop, and life span is not affected. Essential tremor may be present in the same family.

DIAGNOSIS. The diagnosis is established by the clinical features and a family history when available. Symptomatic and epileptic myoclonus must be eliminated by careful neurologic examination, EEG, and brain imaging study. Even then, a period of observation and repeat laboratory investigations may be necessary to eliminate other causes.

TREATMENT. Mild essential myoclonus does not require treatment. Clonazepam is the drug of choice. Carbamazepine, tetrabenazine, and valproate have been found useful in symptomatic myoclonus and may be beneficial in generalized myoclonus as well.

SYMPTOMATIC MYOCLONUS

Myoclonus is often a symptom of an underlying neurologic disease. It tends to be generalized when caused by diffuse, progressive encephalopathies (such as lysosomal storage diseases) and segmental when there is a focal lesion of the brainstem or spinal cord. Multifocal myoclonus may occur as a non-dose-dependent side effect of carbamazepine therapy in children (Dhuna et al, 1991).

Posthypoxic Myoclonus (Lance-Adams Syndrome)

Posthypoxic myoclonus is a form of action myoclonus in patients who have suffered an episode of hypoxia. It does not follow hypoxic-ischemic encephalopathy of the newborn. Single or repetitive myoclonic jerks occur when voluntary movement is attempted. Facial and pharyngeal muscles may be affected, interfering with speech and swallowing. Cerebellar disturbances are usually associated findings.

Myoclonus usually begins during recovery from anoxic encephalopathy and is lifelong. It may respond to valproate, 5-hydroxytryptophan, or clonazepam.

Segmental (Focal) Myoclonus

Segmental myoclonus is an involuntary contraction of contiguous muscles innervated by the brainstem or spinal cord. It may be rhythmic or nonrhythmic. Rhythmic segmental myoclonus looks like a focal seizure. The underlying causes in children are limited mainly to demyelinating diseases and intrinsic tumors. Cystic astrocytoma of the spinal cord is the major cause of spinal myoclonus and may be the initial feature (see Chapter 12).

Palatal myoclonus is the most common segmental myoclonus of brainstem origin. It is a unilateral or bilateral rhythmic contraction of the palate (80 to 180/min) that usually persists during sleep. It may be associated with rhythmic contractions of the eyes, larynx, neck, diaphragm, trunk, and limbs. Palatal myoclonus is caused by lesions in the central tegmental tract or dentato-olivary pathways. The median interval between the precipitating cause and the onset of palatal myoclonus is 10 to 11 months.

Clonazepam and tetrabenazine are the most useful drugs in the treatment of segmental myoclonus.

➡ Tic and Tourette Syndrome

Tics or *habit spasms* are complex, stereotyped movements (motor tic) or utterances (verbal tic) that are sudden, brief, and purposeless. They may be confused with chorea but can be readily distinguished by their stereotyped appearance. A tic can be accurately described and reproduced by an observer, chorea can not. Tics can be suppressed for short periods of time, with some discomfort, and are never incorporated into a voluntary movement. Chorea is harder to suppress and is usually elaborated into a voluntary movement. Tic and chorea are both exacerbated by stress and disappear during sleep.

Tourette syndrome is any combination of verbal and motor tics. It should not be considered a separate disease, but rather part of a phenotypic spectrum that includes simple motor tic, attention-deficit disorder, and obsessive-compulsive behavior. The syndrome is believed to be transmitted as a highly penetrant, autosomal dominant trait in which tics and attention-deficit disorder are more commonly expressed in males and obsessive-compulsive disease in females (Kurlan et al, 1994). Bilineal transmission

is common and may correlate with the severity of disease.

CLINICAL FEATURES. Affected children are not mentally disturbed before symptoms begin. Although the frequency of behavioral disturbances is increased in children with Tourette syndrome, the movement disorder and the behavioral disturbances should each be considered an expression of the same underlying genetic defect; one does not cause the other.

Onset is anytime from 2 to 15 years of age, with the mean between 6 and 7 years. Neck muscles are often affected first, causing a head movement in which the child appears to be tossing hair back from the face. A haircut is frequently the first unsuccessful intervention. New motor tics develop either in place of, or in addition to, existing tics. They usually affect the head, eyes, or face. Common tics include eye blinking, grimacing, lip smacking, and shrugging of one or both shoulders.

The initial verbal tics are usually a clearing of the throat, a snorting or sniffing noise, and a coughlike noise. Many children who make sniffing or coughing noises will undergo an extensive evaluation for allergy and are found to be allergic to something (isn't everyone?). Desensitization is then the next unsuccessful intervention. Grunting and hissing are other verbal tics. Coprolalia is a rare symptom in children (Goldenberg et al, 1994). The profanity is quickly suppressed and replaced by barking or coughing noises.

Symptoms wax and wane spontaneously and in response to stress. Tics usually become less frequent when children are out of school. Most children outgrow their tics, but some have lifelong difficulty and others have prolonged remissions with recurrence in middle age or later.

Half of children with tics have an attention-deficit disorder and a third have an obsessive-compulsive disorder. Attention-deficit disorder is characterized by hyperactivity, short attention span, restlessness, poor concentration, and impaired impulse control. This syndrome is often treated with methylphenidate, a drug that has the potential to accentuate tics in genetically predisposed children.

Obsessive-compulsive disease is characterized by ritualistic actions and thoughts, which may include touching things repeatedly, placing objects in a certain place, washing and rewashing hands, obsessive thoughts about sex or violence, and counting objects. A history of obsessive-compulsive disorder in family members, especially mothers, can be elicited with the following questions. Do you routinely go back and check the door and lights after you leave the house? Do you have routines in the way that you clean the house or fold clothes that must be followed every time? The diagnosis of obsessive-compulsive disorder is assured if the mother responds that these habits are driving her family crazy.

DIAGNOSIS. The diagnosis is established by history and observation. Laboratory tests are not helpful and need not be done in obvious cases. EEG, MRI, and psychological test results are normal.

Tics do not ordinarily occur in degenerative diseases of the nervous system or as an adverse reaction to drugs. Drug-induced tics should be considered the potentiation of Tourette syndrome in a genetically predisposed child. Carbamazepine, as well as amphetamine and methylphenidate, may trigger the symptoms. Withdrawal of the potentiating drug does not always stop the tics.

TREATMENT. Most children with tics and Tourette syndrome do not require drug treatment. The decision to prescribe medication depends on whether the tics bother the child. Drugs should not be used if the tics bother the parents but do not disturb the child's life. The parents must be told that tics are not a sign of progressive neurologic or mental illness, are made worse by stress, and will diminish in frequency if ignored.

Drug treatment is often difficult to evaluate because the disorder's natural history is one of exacerbation and remission. The most useful drugs to control tic are pimozide, fluphenazine, and haloperidol (Singer and Walkup, 1991). They are probably equally effective but I use pimozide first, then fluphenazine, on the basis of a lower incidence of adverse effects. The dosage of pimozide is initially 2 mg/day in two divided doses and is increased 2 mg each week as needed. The maintenance dosage is 0.2 mg/kg/day or 10 mg/day, whichever is less. Fluphenazine is started at 1 mg/day and increased 1 mg each week. The usual maintenance dosage is 2 to 6 mg/day, and should not exceed 10 mg. Haloperidol is started as a single dose of 0.5 mg at night and is slowly increased by 0.5 mg each week until tics are reasonably controlled or adverse reactions are noted. The usual maintenance dosage is 1 to 3 mg/day in two divided doses. The major toxic effects of all three drugs are sedation, irritability, and depression of appe-

tite. Dystonia and akathisia are idiosyncratic reactions. Clonidine is recommended by many neurologists and should be tried when the response to other drugs is unsatisfactory.

Any of these drugs may lose their efficacy after prolonged use, but effectiveness may return after an interval of withholding the drug. Interrupted therapy with one drug or alternating between two drugs is reasonable.

Obsessive-compulsive disorder, when it occurs as part of the Tourette phenotype, is best treated with fluoxetine, a modest dose of 10 to 20 mg each morning may be effective. Fluoxetine is also useful for treating tics in conjunction with pimozide. It may work by reducing stress.

 Tremor

Tremor is an involuntary oscillating movement with a fixed frequency. The product of tremor frequency and amplitude are constant; because frequency decreases with age, amplitude increases. Shuddering, cerebellar ataxia or dysmetria, and asterixis are not tremors because they lack rhythm. Myoclonus may be rhythmic but is interrupted between oscillations.

All normal people have a low-amplitude *physiologic tremor* inherent to movement that is not ordinarily observed without instrumentation. Physiologic tremor may be enhanced to a clinically detectable level by situations (anxiety, excitement, exercise, fatigue, stress) and drugs (adrenergic agonists, nicotine, prednisone, thyroid hormone, xanthines). Hyperthyroidism is routinely associated with enhanced physiologic tremor.

Parkinsonism is a common cause of pathologic tremors in adults, but it does not occur in children except when drug induced or as part of a complex degenerative disorder. Typical parkinsonian tremor is seldom present in these situations. Essential (familial) tremor is the major cause of tremor in children.

ESSENTIAL (FAMILIAL) TREMOR

Essential (familial) tremor is a monosymptomatic condition probably transmitted as an autosomal dominant trait (Bain et al, 1994). Penetrance is eventually complete but the age at onset may be delayed until 65 years. Essential tremor that begins during childhood is not associated with other neurologic disturbances. Adult-onset tremor is sometimes associated with dystonia or Parkinsonism, and such cases are usually sporadic in occurrance (Koller et al, 1994).

Shuddering attacks in young children may be a form of essential tremor and occur in families where other members have essential tremor (Barron and Younkin, 1992).

CLINICAL FEATURES. Essential tremor occurs only in a limb being used. The head, face, and neck are sometimes affected. Neck tremor gives the appearance of torticollis. The frequency of essential tremor is typically between 4 and 8 Hz.

Childhood-onset tremor usually appears in the second decade but can begin as early as 2 years of age. Essential tremor may impair function, especially schoolwork, and therefore disturbs the patient. In young children, the tremor has the appearance of restlessness or clumsiness. Later, its nature as an action tremor is appreciated.

Tremor is enhanced by greater precision of movement and therefore appears first and most prominently in the hands. It is further enhanced by anxiety, concentrated effort to stop the tremor, and fatigue. In such cases the worsening of tremor may be due to enhanced physiologic tremor rather than enhanced essential tremor. The distinction is important in considering treatment options.

Essential tremor is generally lifelong.

DIAGNOSIS. Essential tremor in children is often mistaken for cerebellar dysfunction because it occurs with action (intention). The two are easily differentiated because essential tremor is rhythmic and not dysmetric (does not become worse at the endpoint) and because it is not associated with other signs of cerebellar dysfunction.

The distinction between essential tremor and enhanced physiologic tremor may be more difficult because the two are often concurrent. Enhanced physiologic tremor is always circumstantial, whereas essential tremor remains even when the patient is alone and relaxed.

TREATMENT. Not all patients with essential tremor require treatment. Medication should be reserved for situations in which tremor impairs function. Propranolol, 1 to 2 mg/kg/day, and primidone, 2 to 10 mg/kg/day, are each effective drugs to control tremor in approximately 70% of cases. Propranolol has fewer side effects and should be the first drug chosen.

Essential tremor is also relieved by alcohol ingestion. This treatment should be discouraged as the incidence of alcoholism may be increased in adults with essential tremor.

PAROXYSMAL DYSTONIC HEAD TREMOR

CLINICAL FEATURES. Paroxysmal dystonic head tremor is an uncommon, nonfamilial syndrome of unknown cause (Hughes et al, 1991). The major feature is attacks of horizontal head tremor (frequency 5 to 8 Hz), as if the person were saying "no." Onset occurs in adolescence, and two reported patients as well as three adolescents in my own practice were male. The attacks vary from 1 to 30 minutes, are not provoked by any single stimulus, and cannot be suppressed. My patients also had a head tilt that had predated the onset of tremor by 5 to 10 years (Davis et al, 1995). The attacks are reported to continue for more than 10 years but do not progress to other neurologic symptoms. Results of the examination are otherwise normal.

DIAGNOSIS. Imaging studies of the brain show no abnormalities. In an infant, the combination of head nodding and head tilt would be diagnosed as spasmus nutans even in the absence of nystagmus (see Chapter 15), and perhaps the underlying mechanism is similar.

TREATMENT. Daily clonazepam reduces the frequency and severity of attacks, but the head tilt may persist.

REFERENCES

Bain PG, Findley LJ, Thompson PD, et al. A study of hereditary essential tremor. Brain 1994;117:805-824.

Barron TF, Younkin DP. Propranolol therapy for shuddering attacks. Neurology 1992;42:258-259.

Beall SS, Patten BM, Mallette L, et al. Abnormal systemic metabolism of iron, porphyrin, and calcium in Fahr's syndrome. Ann Neurol 1989;26:569-575.

Bressman SB, de Leon D, Kramer PL, et al. Dystonia in Ashkenazi Jews: Clinical characterization of a founder mutation. Ann Neurol 1994;36:771-777.

Calne DB. Dopa-responsive dystonia. Ann Neurol 1994;35: 381-382.

Cohen HA, Nussinovitch M, Ashkenazi A, et al. Benign paroxysmal torticollis in infancy. Pediatr Neurol 1993;9: 488-490.

Cohen LG, Meer J, Tarkka I, et al. Congenital mirror movements. Abnormal organization of motor pathways in two patients. Brain 1991;114:381-403.

Davis TL, Charles PD, Burns RS. Clonazepam sensitive intermittent dystonic tremor. South Med J, 1995;88:1069-1071.

Dhuna A, Pascuel-Leone A, Talwar D. Exacerbation of partial

seizures and onset of nonepileptic myoclonus with carbamazepine. Epilepsia 1991;32:275-278.

Dobyns WB, Ozelius LJ, Kramer PL, et al. Rapid-onset dystonia-parkinsonism. Neurology 1993;43:2596-2602.

Feinberg TE, Cianci CD, Morroe JS, et al. Diagnostic tests for choreoacanthocytosis. Neurology 1991;41:1000-1006.

Fletcher NA, Harding AE, Marsden CD. A genetic study of idiopathic torsion dystonia in the United Kingdom. Brain 1990;113:379-395.

Goldenberg JN, Brown SB, Weiner WJ. Coprolalia in younger patients with Gilles de la Tourette syndrome. Movement Dis 1994;9:622-625.

Greene PE, Fahn S. Baclofen in the treatment of idiopathic dystonia in children. Movement Dis 1992;7:48-52.

Hardie RJ, Pullon HWH, Harding AE, et al. Neuroacanthocytosis. A clinical, haematological and pathological study of 19 cases. Brain 1991;114:13-49.

Hughes AJ, Lees AJ, Marsden CD. Paroxysmal dystonic head tremor. Movement Dis 1991;6:85-86.

Jankovic J, Brin MF. Therapeutic uses of botulinum toxin. N Engl J Med 1991;324:1186-1194.

Koller WC, Busenbark K, Miner K, et al. The relationship of essential tremor to other movement disorders: Report on 678 patients. Ann Neurol 1994;35:717-723.

Kurlan R, Eapen V, Stern J, et al. Bilineal transmission in Tourette's syndrome families. Neurology 1994;44:2336-2342.

Kyllerman M, Skjeldal OH, Lundberg M, et al. Dystonia and dyskinesia in glutaric aciduria Type I: Clinical heterogeneity and therapeutic considerations. Movement Dis 1994;9:22-30.

Leuzzi V, Bertini E, De Negri AM, et al. Bilateral striatal necrosis, dystonia and optic atrophy in two siblings. J Neurol Neurosurg Psychiatry 1992;55:16-19.

Manyam BV, Bhatt MH, Moore WD, et al. Bilateral striatopallidodentate calcinosis. Cerebrospinal fluid, imaging, and electrophysiological studies. Ann Neurol 1992;31:379-384.

Medlock MD, Cruse RS, Winek SJ, et al. A 10-year experience with postpump chorea. Ann Neurol 1993;34:820-826.

Meirleir LD, Seneca S, Lissens W, et al. Bilateral striatal necrosis with a novel point mutation in the mitochondrial ATPase gene. Pediatr Neurol 1995;13:242-246.

Mizuguchi M, Usuda I, Yoneyama A, et al. Infantile bilateral striatal necrosis: Chronic and acute manifestations in a single case. Brain Dev 1994;16:61-64.

Nigro MA, Martens ME, Awerbuch GI, et al. Partial cytochrome b deficiency and generalized dystonia. Pediatr Neurol 1990;6:407-410.

Nygaard TG, Marsden CD, Fahn S. Dopa-responsive dystonia: Long-term treatment response and prognosis. Neurology 1991;41:174-181.

Orrell RW, Amrolia PJ, Heald A, et al. Acanthocytosis, retinitis pigmentosa, and pallidal degeneration: A report of three patients, including the second reported case with hypoprebetalipoproteinemia (HARP syndrome). Neurology 1995;45:487-492.

Petrukhin K, Gilliam TC. Genetic disorders of copper metabolism. Curr Opin Pediatr 1994;6:698-701.

Pranzatelli MR, Albin RL, Cohen BH: Acute dyskinesias in young asthmatics treated with theophylline. Pediatr Neurol 1991;7:216-219.

Prayer L, Wimberger D, Kramer J, et al. Cranial MRI in Wilson's disease. Neuroradiology 1990;32:211-214.

Rasmussen P. Persistent mirror movements: A clinical study of 17 children, adolescents and young adults. Dev Med Child Neurol 1993;35:699-707.

Roig M, Calopa M, Rovira A, et al. Bilateral striatal lesions in childhood. Pediatr Neurol 1993;9:349-358.

Rosemberg S, Amaral LC, Kliemann, et al. Acute encephalopathy with bilateral striatal necrosis: A distinctive clinicopathologic condition. Neuropediatr 1992;23:310-315.

Saint Hilaire M-H, Burke RE, Bressman SB, et al. Delayed-onset dystonia due to perinatal or early childhood asphyxia. Neurology 1991;41:216-222.

Schaffert DA, Johnsen SD, Johnsen PC, et al. Magnetic resonance imaging in pathologically proven Hallervorden-Spatz disease. Neurology 1989;39:440-442.

Shannon KM, Fenichel GM. Pimozide treatment of Sydenham's chorea. Neurology 1990;40:186.

Shintani S, Shiozawa Z, Tsunoda S, et al. Paroxysmal choreoathetosis precipitated by movement, sound and photic stimulation in a case of arterio-venous malformation of the parietal lobe. Clin Neurol Neurosurg 1991;93:237-239.

Singer HS, Walkup JT. Tourette syndrome and other tic disorders: Diagnosis, pathophysiology, and treatment. Medicine 1991;70:15-32.

Swaiman KF: Hallervorden-Spatz syndrome and brain iron metabolism. Arch Neurol 1991;48:1285-1293.

Swedo SE. Sydenham's chorea: A model for childhood autoimmune neuropsychiatric disorders. JAMA 1994;272:1788-1791.

Swedo SE, Leonard HL, Schapiro MB, et al. Sydenham's chorea: Physical and psychological symptoms of St. Vitus dance. Pediatrics 1993;91:706-713.

Tanaka H, Endo K, Tsuji S, et al. Ann Neurol 1995;37:405-408.

Traill Z, Pike M, Byrne J. Sydenham's chorea: A case showing reversible striatal abnormalities on CT and MRI. Dev Med Child Neurol 1995;37:270-273.

Walters AS, Picchietti DL, Ehrenberg BL, et al. Restless legs syndrome in childhood and adolescence. Pediatr Neurol 1994;11:241-245.

Wheeler PG, Weaver DD, Dobyns WB. Benign hereditary chorea. Pediatr Neurol 1993;9:337-340.

15
Disorders of Ocular Motility

The maintenance of binocular vision by conjugate movement of the eyes is perhaps the most delicate feat of muscular coordination achieved by the nervous system. Disorders of the visual sensory system, ocular muscles, ocular motor nerves, neuromuscular transmission, or gaze centers of the central nervous system may disturb ocular motility. This chapter deals with nonparalytic strabismus, paralytic strabismus (ophthalmoplegia), gaze palsies (supranuclear palsies), ptosis, and nystagmus. Visual disorders and disorders of the pupil are discussed in Chapter 16.

 Nonparalytic Strabismus

Strabismus (squint), or abnormal ocular alignment, affects 3% to 4% of preschool children. Many individuals have a latent tendency for ocular misalignment, *heterophoria,* which becomes apparent only under stress or fatigue. During periods of misalignment the child may have diplopia or headache. Constant ocular misalignment is called *heterotropia.* Children with heterotropia suppress the image from one eye to avoid diplopia. If only one eye is used for fixation, visual acuity may be permanently lost in the other (developmental amblyopia).

In nonparalytic strabismus the amount of deviation in different directions of gaze is relatively constant (comitant). Each eye moves through a normal range when tested separately (ductions), but the eyes are disconjugate when used together (versions). Many children with chronic brain damage syndromes, such as malformations or perinatal asphyxia, have nonparalytic strabismus. This is caused by faulty fusion or control of conjugate gaze mechanisms by the abnormal brain. In neurologically normal children, the most common cause of nonparalytic strabismus is either a genetic influence or an intraocular disorder. Ocular alignment in the newborn is usually poor, with transitory shifts of alignment from convergence to divergence. Constant ocular alignment usually begins after 3 months of age. Approximately 2% of newborns exhibit tonic downward deviation of the eyes during the waking state. The eyes assume a normal position during sleep and are able to move upward reflexively.

Esotropia

Esotropia is an inward deviation (convergence) of the eyes. Early-onset or infantile esotropia is noted before 1 year of age, and accommodative esotropia is usually noted between 2 and 3 years but may be delayed until adolescence.

CLINICAL FEATURES. Children with infantile esotropia often alternate fixation between eyes and may cross-fixate, that is, look to the left with the right eye and to the right with the left eye. The misalignment is sufficient to be noticed by family members. Some children fixate almost entirely with one eye and are at risk for permanent loss of visual acuity, *amblyopia,* in the other.

Accommodative esotropia occurs when accommodation is used to correct hyperopia. Accommodation causes the blurred hyperopic image to be more sharply focused. Because accommodation is accompanied by convergence, the eyes turn inward. Some children with accommodative esotropia cross-fixate so that both eyes are used. However, if one eye is more hyperopic than the other, the better eye may be used exclusively for fixation, and the unused eye has a considerable potential for amblyopia.

DIAGNOSIS. The eyes should be examined with a retinoscope by an ophthalmologist to determine whether hyperopia is present.

TREATMENT. Hyperopic errors should be corrected with eyeglasses. Early-onset esotropia in which only one eye is used for fixation is treated with alternate patching of the eyes. Early corrective surgery is required for persistent esotropia. A recently introduced alternative to surgery is chemodenervation of overactive muscles by injection of botulinum toxin. The technique has proved effective in research trials but is not yet approved for regular use.

Exotropia

Exotropia is an outward deviation of the eyes. It may be intermittent or constant.

CLINICAL FEATURES. Intermittent exotropia is a relatively common condition that begins before 4 years of age. It is most often evident when the child is fatigued and fixating on a far object or in bright sunlight. The natural history of the condition is unknown.

Constant exotropia may be congenital but can also be caused by poor vision in the outward-turning eye.

DIAGNOSIS. The eyes must be examined for intraocular disease.

TREATMENT. In children with intermittent exotropia, the decision to perform corrective surgery depends on the frequency and degree of the abnormality. When exotropia is constant, treatment depends on the underlying cause of visual loss.

Ophthalmoplegia (Paralytic Strabismus)

Ophthalmoplegia can be due to disorders of the ocular motor nerves, the ocular muscles, or neuromuscular transmission. The muscles, the nerves, and their functions are summarized in

■ TABLE 15–1
The Extraocular Muscles

OCULAR MUSCLES	INNERVATION	FUNCTIONS
Lateral rectus	Abducens	Abduction
Medial rectus	Oculomotor	Adduction
Superior rectus	Oculomotor	Elevation, intorsion, adduction
Inferior rectus	Oculomotor	Depression, extorsion, adduction
Inferior oblique	Oculomotor	Extorsion, elevation, abduction
Superior oblique	Trochlear	Intorsion, depression, abduction

Table 15-1. The eye appears to deviate in a direction opposite to the field of action of the paralyzed ocular muscle, and diplopia is experienced. Strabismus and diplopia are made worse when the child gazes in the direction of action of the paralyzed muscle.

CONGENITAL OPHTHALMOPLEGIA

Ophthalmoplegia in the newborn is often missed because eye movements are infrequently tested. It is common for strabismus to remain unnoticed for several months and then to be discounted as transient esotropia. Therefore, congenital ophthalmoplegia should be considered even when there is no history of ophthalmoplegia at birth.

Oculomotor Nerve Palsy

CLINICAL FEATURES. Congenital oculomotor nerve palsy usually is unilateral and complete. Pupillary reflex paralysis is variable. Other cranial nerve palsies, especially abducens, may be associated (Ing et al, 1992). The palsy often is not recognized at birth. An occasional case is familial or due to trauma of the orbit at birth, but most are idiopathic. The affected eye is exotropic and usually amblyopic. Aberrant regeneration may be evidenced by lid retraction on attempted adduction or downward gaze.

DIAGNOSIS. Magnetic resonance imaging (MRI) is indicated to exclude the possibility of an intracranial mass compressing the nerve. Exophthalmos suggests an orbital tumor. A dilated pupil excludes the diagnosis of myasthenia gravis, but an edrophonium chloride (Tensilon) test is indicated if the pupil is normal (see "Myasthenia Gravis," later on).

TREATMENT. Extraocular muscle surgery may improve the cosmetic appearance but does not improve ocular motility or visual function.

Trochlear Nerve Palsy

CLINICAL FEATURES. Congenital superior oblique palsy is unilateral in 94% of cases. Birth trauma is often suspected but is rarely established. Most congenital cases are idiopathic.

The head is tilted away from the paralyzed side to keep the eyes in alignment and avoid diplopia. The major ocular features are noncomitant hypertropia, greatest in the nasal field of the involved eye; underaction of the paretic superior oblique and overaction of the inferior oblique muscle; and increased hypertropia when the head is tilted to the paralyzed side (positive Bielschowsky test).

DIAGNOSIS. Head tilt, or *torticollis* (see Chapter 14), is a constant feature. Once a superior oblique palsy is confirmed by examination, important etiologic considerations other than congenital ones include trauma, myasthenia gravis, and brainstem glioma.

TREATMENT. Most patients require surgery. Several procedures are available to restore balance between the superior and inferior oblique muscles.

Abducens Nerve Palsy

CLINICAL FEATURES. Congenital abducens nerve palsy may be unilateral or bilateral and is sometimes associated with other cranial nerve palsies. Lateral movement of the affected eye(s) is limited partially or completely. Most infants use cross-fixation and thereby retain vision in both eyes. In the few reported cases of congenital palsy with pathologic correlation the abducens nerve is absent and its nucleus is hypoplastic.

Möbius syndrome is the association of congenital facial diplegia and bilateral abducens nerve palsies (see Chapter 17). *Duane syndrome* is aplasia of one or both nuclei of the abducens nerve with innervation of the atrophic lateral rectus by fibers of the oculomotor nerve. It is characterized by a lateral rectus palsy, some limitation of adduction, and narrowing of the palpebral fissure because of globe retraction on attempted adduction. Other ocular, ear, and systemic malformations may be associated.

DIAGNOSIS. MRI is indicated to exclude the possibility of an intracranial mass lesion. Hearing should be tested, and if there is facial weakness, electromyography (EMG) of the face may be useful to determine facial nerve function.

TREATMENT. Surgical procedures may be useful to correct head turn and to provide binocular vision, but they do not restore ocular motility.

Brown Syndrome

Brown syndrome consists of mechanical limitation of elevation in adduction as a result of congenital shortening of the superior oblique muscle or tendon (Kaban et al, 1993). Only one eye may be involved.

CLINICAL FEATURES. Elevation is limited to adduction but normal in abduction. Passive elevation (forced duction) is also restricted. Other features include widening of the palpebral fissure on adduction and backward head tilt.

DIAGNOSIS. Brown syndrome must be differentiated from acquired shortening of the superior oblique muscle caused by juvenile rheumatoid arthritis, trauma, and inflammatory processes affecting the top of the orbit (see "Orbital Pseudotumor" later in this chapter).

TREATMENT. Surgical procedures that extend the superior oblique muscle can be useful in congenital cases.

Congenital Myasthenia Gravis

Several clinical syndromes of myasthenia gravis occur in the newborn (see Chapter 6). Congenital myasthenia gravis is the only one with ophthalmoplegia as the primary clinical feature. It is probably transmitted by autosomal recessive inheritance and may be caused by several underlying defects, including abnormal acetylcholine resynthesis or immobilization, reduced endplate acetylcholinesterase, and impaired function of the acetylcholine receptor.

CLINICAL FEATURES. Although these disorders are transmitted by autosomal recessive inheritance, a male-to-female bias of 2:1 exists. Symmetric ptosis and ophthalmoplegia are noted at birth or shortly thereafter. Mild facial weakness may be present but is not severe enough to impair feeding. If partial at birth, the ophthalmoplegia becomes complete during infancy or childhood. Generalized weakness sometimes develops.

DIAGNOSIS. The diagnosis should be suspected in any newborn with bilateral ptosis or limitation of eye movement. Intramuscular injection of edrophonium chloride produces a transitory improvement in ocular motility. Repetitive nerve stimulation of the limbs at a frequency of 3 Hz may evoke a decremental response, reversible with edrophonium chloride. This suggests that the underlying defect, although producing symptoms only in the eyes, is already generalized at birth.

TREATMENT. There is no evidence for an immunopathy or a rational basis for immunosuppressive therapy. Thymectomy and corticosteroids are ineffective. Anticholinesterases may decrease facial paralysis, but they have little or no effect on ophthalmoplegia. 3,4-diaminopyridine, an agent that releases acetylcholine, is beneficial in some children (Palace et al, 1991).

Congenital Ptosis

CLINICAL FEATURES. Congenital drooping of one or both lids is relatively common, and the drooping is unilateral in 70%. The cause is unknown, but the condition is rarely familial. Congenital ptosis is often unnoticed until early childhood or even adult life and then is thought to be an "acquired" ptosis. Miosis is sometimes an associated feature and suggests the possibility of a Horner syndrome, except that the pupil responds normally to pharmacologic agents. Some patients have a synkinesis between the oculomotor and the trigeminal nerves, so that jaw movements produce opening of the eye *(Marcus-Gunn phenomenon)*.

DIAGNOSIS. The differential diagnosis of ptosis is listed in Table 15–2. Distinguishing congenital ptosis from acquired ptosis is essential. This is best accomplished by examining baby pictures. If miosis is present, the eye must be tested with pharmacologic agents to determine whether sympathetic hypersensitivity is present.

■ TABLE 15–2
Causes of Ptosis

Congenital
Fibrosis of extraocular muscles
Horner syndrome
Myasthenia
Oculomotor nerve palsy
Acquired
Lid inflammation
Mitochondrial myopathies (see Chapter 8)
Myasthenia gravis
Oculomotor nerve palsy
Oculopharyngeal dystrophy (see Chapter 17)
Ophthalmoplegic migraine
Orbital cellulitis
Trauma

Concurrent paralysis of extraocular motility is evidence against congenital ptosis.

TREATMENT. Corrective surgery is useful in elevating the lid to improve appearance or when ptosis impairs vision.

Fibrosis of Extraocular Muscles

Fibrosis of extraocular muscles is an ill-defined entity with partial or complete paralysis of ocular motility at birth. It is caused by maldevelopment of the ocular muscles, which are represented as fibrous bands. In some cases, the underlying cause may be hypoplasia of the ocular motor nerves.

CLINICAL FEATURES. The only clinical feature is restricted ocular motility, which is usually bilateral although unilateral occurrence has been reported. Ptosis is almost always present.

DIAGNOSIS. Other causes of congenital ophthalmoplegia must be excluded. MRI shows the fibrotic muscles, but biopsy provides the more definitive diagnosis.

TREATMENT. Surgery offers some cosmetic benefit and relieves ptosis but does not correct the disturbed motility.

ACUTE UNILATERAL OPHTHALMOPLEGIA

The causes of acquired ophthalmoplegia are summarized in Table 15–3. Many of the conditions are discussed in other chapters.

Acute ophthalmoplegia is defined as reaching maximum intensity within 1 week of onset. It may be partial or complete (Table 15–4). Generalized increased intracranial pressure is always an important consideration in patients with unilateral or bilateral abducens palsy (see Chapter 4).

Aneurysm

Arterial aneurysms are discussed fully in Chapter 4, because the important clinical feature in children is hemorrhage rather than nerve compression. This section deals only with possible ophthalmoplegic features.

CLINICAL FEATURES. Aneurysms at the junction of the internal carotid and posterior communicating arteries are an important cause of unilateral oculomotor palsy in adults, but are a rare cause in children (Gabianelli et al, 1989). The palsy is attributed to compression of the nerve by expansion of the aneurysm. Intense

■ T A B L E   1 5 – 3
Causes of Acquired Ophthalmoplegia

Brainstem
Brainstem encephalitis (see Chapter 10)
Intoxication
Multiple sclerosis (see Chapter 10)
Subacute necrotizing encephalopathy (see Chapter 10)
Tumor
    Brainstem glioma
    Craniopharyngioma (see Chapter 16)
    Leukemia
    Lymphoma
    Metastases
    Pineal region tumors
Vascular
    Arteriovenous malformation
    Hemorrhage
    Infarction
    Migraine
    Vasculitis

Nerve
Familial recurrent cranial neuropathies (see Chapter 17)
Increased intracranial pressure (see Chapter 4)
Infectious
    Diphtheria
    Gradenigo syndrome
    Meningitis (see Chapter 4)
    Orbital cellulitis
Inflammatory
    Sarcoid
    Tolosa-Hunt syndrome
Postinfectious
    Idiopathic (postviral)
    Miller Fisher syndrome (see Chapter 10)
    Polyradiculoneuropathy (see Chapter 7)
Trauma
    Head
    Orbital
Tumor
    Cavernous sinus hemangioma
    Orbital tumors
    Sellar and parasellar tumors (see Chapter 16)
    Sphenoid sinus tumors
Vascular
    Aneurysm
    Carotid-cavernous fistula
    Cavernous sinus thrombosis
    Migraine

Neuromuscular Transmission
Botulism (see Chapter 7)
Myasthenia gravis

Myopathies
Fiber-type disproportion myopathies (see Chapter 6)
Kearns-Sayres syndrome
Mitochondrial myopathies (see Chapter 8)
Oculopharyngeal dystrophy (see Chapter 17)
Orbital inflammatory disease
Thyrotoxicosis
Vitamin E deficiency

■ T A B L E   1 5 – 4
Causes of Acute Unilateral Ophthalmoplegia

Aneurysm*†
Brain tumors
    Brainstem glioma
    Parasellar tumors (see Chapter 16)
    Tumors of pineal region (see Chapter 4)
Brainstem stroke*
Cavernous sinus fistula
Cavernous sinus thrombosis
Gradenigo syndrome
Idiopathic cranial nerve palsy*
Increased intracranial pressure (see Chapter 4)
Multiple sclerosis* (see Chapter 10)
Myasthenia gravis*
Ophthalmoplegic migraine*†
Orbital inflammatory disease*†
Orbital tumor†
Recurrent familial* (see Chapter 17)
Tolosa-Hunt syndrome*†
Trauma
    Head
    Orbital

*May be recurrent.
†May be associated with pain.

pain in and around the eye is frequently experienced at the time of hemorrhage. Because the parasympathetic fibers are at the periphery of the nerve, mydriasis is an almost constant feature of ophthalmoplegia caused by aneurysms of the posterior communicating artery. However, pupillary involvement may develop several days after onset of an incomplete ophthalmoplegia. A normal pupil with complete ophthalmoplegia effectively excludes the possibility of aneurysm.

The superior branch of the oculomotor nerve is sometimes affected earlier and more severely than the inferior branch. Ptosis may precede the development of other signs by hours or days.

DIAGNOSIS. Most aneurysms can be identified by contrast-enhanced MRI and magnetic resonance angiography (MRA).

TREATMENT. Surgical clipping is the treatment of choice whenever technically feasible. Oculomotor function often returns to normal after the aneurysm is removed.

Brainstem Glioma

CLINICAL FEATURES. Symptoms begin between 2 and 13 years of age with a peak between ages 5 and 8 (Maria et al, 1993). The period from onset of symptoms to diagnosis is less than 6 months. Cranial nerve palsies, usually abducens and facial, are the initial features in most cases. Later contralateral hemiplegia and ataxia, dysphagia, and hoarseness develop. Hemiplegia at

□ FIGURE 15-1 Brainstem glioma. MRI shows a large lesion infiltrating the brainstem.

onset is associated with a more rapid course. With time, cranial nerve and corticospinal tract involvement may become bilateral. Increased intracranial pressure is not an early feature, but vomiting may be caused by direct irritation of the brainstem emetic center. Intractable hiccough, facial spasm, personality change, and headache are early symptoms in occasional patients.

Brainstem gliomas carry the worst prognosis of any childhood tumor. The course is one of steady progression with median survival times of 9 to 12 months.

DIAGNOSIS. MRI delineates the tumor well and differentiates tumor from inflammatory and vascular disorders (Figure 15-1).

TREATMENT. Radiation therapy is the treatment of choice. Several chemotherapeutic programs are undergoing experimental trials, but none is established as beneficial.

Brainstem Stroke

The causes of stroke in children are summarized in Table 11-2. Small brainstem hemorrhages resulting from emboli, leukemia, or blood dyscrasias have the potential to cause isolated ocular motor palsies, but this is not the rule. Other cranial nerves are also involved, and hemiparesis, ataxia, and decreased consciousness are typical associated features.

Cavernous Sinus Fistula

CLINICAL FEATURES. Arteriovenous communications between the carotid artery and the cavernous sinus may be congenital but are usually caused by trauma. The injury may be closed or penetrating. The carotid artery or one of its branches ruptures into the cavernous sinus, increasing pressure in the venous system. The results are a pulsating proptosis, redness and swelling of the conjunctiva, and ophthalmoplegia. A bruit, heard over the eye, is reduced in volume by compression of the ipsilateral carotid artery.

DIAGNOSIS. Computed tomography (CT) of the head and orbit is usually the first study in patients with the acute onset of proptosis. It often shows an enlarged superior ophthalmic vein. Intra-arterial digital subtraction angiography shows early filling of the cavernous sinus and retrograde filling of the superior ophthalmic vein.

TREATMENT. Several surgical procedures are recommended, including carotid ligation, injection of fibrin glue through the superior ophthalmic vein, transcavernous electrocoagulation, and intra-arterial occlusion with a balloon catheter.

Cavernous Sinus Thrombosis

Cavernous sinus thrombosis may produce either unilateral or bilateral ophthalmoplegia. It is almost always caused by anterograde spread of infection from the mouth, face, or nose.

CLINICAL FEATURES. A typical history is the development of fever, malaise, and frontal headache following dental infection. These are followed by proptosis, orbital congestion, ptosis, external ophthalmoplegia, and sometimes pupillary paralysis and blindness. The infection begins in one cavernous sinus and spreads to the other. If untreated, it may extend to the meninges. Even with vigorous antibiotic treatment the mortality rate is 15%.

DIAGNOSIS. The ocular signs may suggest orbital cellulitis or orbital pseudotumor. The cerebrospinal fluid is normal early in the course. A mixed leukocytosis develops, and the protein concentration is moderately elevated even in the absence of meningitis. Once the meninges are involved, the pressure becomes elevated, the leukocytosis increases, and the glucose concentration falls.

Cranial CT may show clouding of infected paranasal sinuses. MRA shows decreased or absent flow in the cavernous portion of the carotid artery (Berge et al, 1994).

TREATMENT. The infection must be vigorously treated with intravenous antibiotics as if the child had meningitis. Surgical drainage of infected paranasal sinuses is sometimes necessary.

Gradenigo Syndrome

CLINICAL FEATURES. The abducens nerve lies adjacent to the medial aspect of the petrous bone before entering the cavernous sinus. Infections of the middle ear sometimes extend to the petrous bone and cause thrombophlebitis of the inferior petrosal sinus. The infection involves not only the abducens nerve but also the facial nerve and the trigeminal ganglion. The resulting syndrome is characterized by ipsilateral paralysis of abduction, facial palsy, and facial pain.

DIAGNOSIS. The combination of unilateral abducens and facial palsy can also be seen after closed head injuries. The diagnosis of Gradenigo syndrome requires the demonstration of middle-ear infection. Radiographs of the mastoid bone and lumbar puncture are indicated in all patients in whom the syndrome is suspected.

TREATMENT. Antibiotic therapy must be initiated early to prevent permanent nerve damage.

Idiopathic Cranial Nerve Palsy

CLINICAL FEATURES. The sudden onset of a single cranial neuropathy without apparent cause is frequently attributed to a viral infection occurring during the previous month. The condition is thought to be immunologically mediated. However, a cause-and-effect relationship between viral infection and ocular motor palsies is not established.

The abducens nerve is more commonly affected than either the oculomotor or the trochlear nerve. Bilateral involvement is unusual. The complaints are of painless diplopia and paralytic strabismus. Girls are affected more often than boys, and the left eye more often than the right. Full motility is restored within 6 months, but shorter duration recurrences occur in half of children (Cohen et al, 1993).

DIAGNOSIS. Other causes of isolated nerve palsy must be excluded. Examination of the cerebrospinal fluid and MRI of the head and orbit are warranted in every case to exclude tumor and infection. Tumors in and around the orbit are sometimes difficult to demonstrate, and if ophthalmoplegia persists, a repeat MRI may be necessary. Myasthenia gravis is always a consideration, and an edrophonium chloride test should be performed even though myasthenia gravis is less likely when there is a fixed single nerve deficit.

TREATMENT. Corticosteroids are not recommended. In children less than 9 years of age, intermittent patching of the normal eye may be necessary if the affected eye is not used for fixation.

Myasthenia Gravis

Some neonatal forms of myasthenia are discussed in Chapter 6; congenital myasthenia is included in the section "Congenital Ophthalmoplegia," earlier in this chapter; and limb-girdle myasthenia is discussed in Chapter 7. This section describes the immune-mediated form of myasthenia that is encountered from late infancy through adult life. Two clinical forms are recognized: *ocular myasthenia,* in which the eye muscles are primarily or exclusively affected but facial and limb muscles may also be mildly involved, and *generalized myasthenia,* in which weakness of bulbar and limb muscles is moderate to severe.

The term *juvenile myasthenia* is sometimes used to denote immune-mediated myasthenia gravis in children, but because the disease is similar in children and adults, the term should be discarded.

CLINICAL FEATURES. The first symptoms do not appear until after 6 months of age; 75% of children first have symptoms after age 10. Prepubertal onset is associated with a male bias, only ocular symptoms, and seronegativity for acetylcholine receptor antibodies; whereas postpubertal onset is associated with a strong female bias, generalized myasthenia, and seropositivity (Andrews et al, 1993). In general, boys have lesser disease severity than girls (Andrews et al, 1994).

The initial features of both the ocular and the generalized form are usually ptosis, diplopia, or both. Myasthenia is the most common cause of unilateral or bilateral acquired ptosis. Pupillary function is normal. Between 40% and 50% of patients have weakness of other bulbar muscles or limb weakness at the time of onset. Ocular motor weakness is generally not constant initially, and the specific muscles affected may change from examination to examination. Usually both eyes are affected, but one more than the other.

Children with ocular myasthenia may have mild facial weakness and easy fatigability of the limbs. However, they do not have respiratory distress or difficulty speaking or swallowing. The subsequent courses of ocular myasthenia may be characterized by steady progression to complete ophthalmoplegia, or by relapses and remissions. The relapses are of varying severity and last for weeks to years. At least 20% of patients have permanent remissions. Prepubertal onset is more commonly associated with spontaneous remission than postpubertal onset.

Children with generalized myasthenia have generalized weakness within 1 year of the initial ocular symptoms. Dysarthria, dysphagia, difficulty chewing, and limb muscle fatigability are observed. Spontaneous remissions are unusual. As many as 40% of patients experience respiratory insufficiency, or *myasthenic crises,* if not treated.

Children with generalized myasthenia, but not those with ocular myasthenia, have a higher than expected incidence of other autoimmune disorders, especially thyroiditis and collagen vascular diseases. Thymoma is present in 15% of adults with generalized myasthenia but occurs in less than 5% of children (Lanska, 1991).

DIAGNOSIS. The edrophonium chloride test has been used as a standard of diagnosis for both the ocular and generalized forms of myasthenia gravis but has limitations. Edrophonium chloride is a short-acting anticholinesterase that is administered intravenously at a dose of 0.15 mg/kg. Before the test is initiated, an endpoint for the study must be determined. The best endpoint is the resolution of ptosis or the restoration of ocular motility and test results are difficult to evaluate in their absence. Ptosis generally responds better to edrophonium chloride than does ocular motor paralysis.

Some patients with myasthenia are supersensitive to edrophonium chloride, and fasciculations and sometimes respiratory arrest develop when a full dose is administered. For this reason a test dose of one-tenth the full dose is injected first. Unfortunately, respiratory embarrassment sometimes develops in response to the test dose and a hand ventilator should be readily available before any drug is given. Atropine is an effective antidote to the muscarinic side effects of edrophonium chloride but does not counteract the nicotinic effects on the motor endplate that result in paralysis of the skeletal muscles.

After the test dose is given, the remainder should be injected one third at a time (approximately 0.05/mg/kg), allowing up to 1 minute after each injection to test the response. Interpretation may be difficult. The judgment of improved strength is always subjective and may be influenced by examiner bias. The test becomes more objective when combined with electrophysiologic studies.

Repetitive nerve stimulation studies are abnormal in 66% of children when proximal nerves are stimulated but in only 33% when distal nerves are studied (Afifi and Bell, 1993). Abnormal repetitive nerve studies are unusual in children with ocular myasthenia but are the rule in children with generalized myasthenia. In patients with mild myasthenia a decremental response is recorded at low rates of stimulation (2 to 5/sec), but not at high rates (50/sec). In severe myasthenia a decremental response is recorded at both low and high rates of stimulation.

The clinical features of myasthenia gravis are attributed to the presence of antibodies against the acetylcholine receptor protein. Elevated concentrations of the antibody, greater than 10 nmol/L, are detected in the sera of 90% of patients with generalized myasthenia. Patients with ocular myasthenia may be seronegative or have low antibody concentrations. Early-onset, seronegative cases of immune-mediated ocular myasthenia are difficult to distinguish from genetic myasthenia. The distinction is important because one responds to immunotherapy and the other does not. A trial of plasma exchange may determine the usefulness of immunotherapy (Andrews et al, 1993).

TREATMENT. The treatment selected depends on whether the child has ocular or generalized myasthenia. Children with ocular myasthenia have a reasonable hope of spontaneous remission, but those with generalized disease do not. Anticholinesterase therapy is the treatment of choice for ocular myasthenia. The initial dose of neostigmine is 0.5 mg/kg every 4 hours in children younger than 5 years of age and 0.25 mg/kg in older children, not to exceed 15 mg in any child. The equivalent dose of pyridostigmine is four times greater. After treatment is initiated, the dose is slowly increased as tolerated. Diarrhea and gastrointestinal cramps are the usual limiting factors. Edrophonium chloride should not be administered to determine whether the child would benefit from higher oral doses of anticholinesterases. It is not an accurate guide and may cause cholinergic crisis in children with generalized myasthenia.

Ocular myasthenia is difficult to treat. The response to anticholinesterase is often transitory and the addition of corticosteroids is usually without benefit. The efficacy of any drug regimen in ocular myasthenia is difficult to assess because of the fluctuating course of the disease.

Children with generalized myasthenia and increased concentrations of antibody against the acetylcholine receptor should undergo thymectomy as soon as possible after diagnosis. While the efficacy of thymectomy is not established by controlled clinical trials, experience indicates that most children will be in remission within 3 years if thymectomy is performed early in the course of disease. Corticosteroids should be started immediately after surgery, preferably while the patient is still in the surgical intensive care unit. An equivalent dosage to prednisone, 1.5 mg/kg/day (not to exceed 100 mg), is given parenterally until the patient can take oral medication. After 5 days, an alternate-day regimen is used for the remainder of the month. The prednisone dose is then tapered by 10% each month until a dose is reached that keeps the patient symptom free. Withdrawal of prednisone should be attempted after the child has been free of symptoms for 1 year (Miano et al, 1991). High-dose corticosteroids may make the patient weaker at first. For this reason, treatment is initiated while the patient is still in hospital. Improvement usually begins after the first week and continues in the months that follow.

Anticholinesterase medication need not be given concurrently with corticosteroids at first but may be used later if the patient weakens on the alternate days that corticosteroids are not taken.

The clinical characteristics and response to treatment of individuals with generalized myasthenia who are seronegative do not differ from those who are seropositive, except that seronegative patients are unlikely to show thymic abnormalities and show only a modest improvement after thymectomy (Verma and Oger, 1992).

Plasmapheresis or intravenous immunoglobulin is useful as an acute intervention in patients who have respiratory insufficiency or are so weak that strength must be restored prior to thymectomy.

Ophthalmoplegic Migraine

CLINICAL FEATURES. Transitory ocular motor palsy, lasting sometimes as long as 4 weeks, may occur as part of a migraine attack in children and adults. The palsy affects the oculomotor nerve alone in 83% of cases and all three nerves in the remainder. Ptosis usually precedes ophthal-

moplegia. Partial or complete pupillary involvement is present in 60%. The average age at onset is 15 years, but the onset may be as early as infancy. In infants recurrent painless ophthalmoplegia or ptosis may be the only feature of the migraine attack. In older children ophthalmoplegia usually occurs during the headache phase and is ipsilateral to the headache.

The mechanism of ophthalmoplegia is not established. Although migraine is hereditary, the tendency for ophthalmoplegia is not.

DIAGNOSIS. The diagnosis is obvious when ophthalmoplegia occurs during a typical migraine attack in a child previously known to have migraine. Diagnostic uncertainty is greatest when an infant has transitory strabismus or ptosis as an isolated sign. In such cases a family history of migraine is essential for diagnosis. Even so, most infants with a first episode of ophthalmoplegia should be studied with MRI of the head and orbit to exclude other causes. The transitory nature of the palsy is comforting and indicates that a structural abnormality is unlikely.

TREATMENT. Children with ophthalmoplegic migraine should be treated in the same manner as other children with migraine (see Chapter 3).

Orbital Inflammatory Disease (Pseudotumor)

The term *orbital inflammatory disease* encompasses a group of nonspecific inflammatory conditions involving the orbit. Some experts include the Tolosa-Hunt syndrome as part of the spectrum. Inflammation may be diffuse or localized to specific tissues within the orbit *(orbital myositis)*.

CLINICAL FEATURES. The disorder is unusual before age 20 years but may occur as early as 3 months of age. Males and females are affected equally. Acute and chronic forms are described.

The main features are pain, ophthalmoplegia, proptosis, and lid edema evolving over several days or weeks. One eye or both eyes may be involved. Ocular motility is disturbed in part by the proptosis, but mainly by myositis. Some patients have only myositis, whereas others have inflammation in other orbital structures. Vision is initially preserved, but loss of vision is a threat if the condition remains untreated.

DIAGNOSIS. The development of unilateral pain and proptosis in a child should suggest an orbital tumor. This possibility must be excluded by MRI of the orbit. Bilateral proptosis suggests thyroid myopathy.

Imaging studies of the orbit show a soft tissue

mass without sinus involvement or bone erosion. This radiographic appearance may also be seen with orbital involvement by lymphoma or leukemia. The extraocular muscles may appear enlarged.

TREATMENT. Orbital inflammatory disease has a self-limited course but must be treated to prevent vision loss or permanent ophthalmoplegia. Prednisone, 1 mg/kg/day, should be administered for at least 1 month and then tapered. If the disorder recurs during the tapering, the full dose should be reinitiated.

Orbital Tumors

CLINICAL FEATURES. The initial feature of intraorbital tumors is proptosis, ophthalmoplegia, or ptosis. When the globe is displaced forward, the palpebral fissure is widened and it may not be possible to close the eye fully. As a consequence, the exposed portion of the eye becomes erythematous and may suffer exposure keratitis. The direction of displacement of the globe is the best clue to the tumor's position. Ophthalmoplegia may occur because the globe is displaced forward and causing direct pressure on one or more ocular nerves or muscles.

DIAGNOSIS. The differential diagnosis of proptosis in children includes infection and inflammation, hemorrhage and other vascular disorders, orbital tumors, hyperthyroidism and other metabolic disorders, developmental anomalies, and Hand-Schüller-Christian disease and related disorders; some are idiopathic. The most common orbital tumors are dermoid cyst, hemangioma, metastatic neuroblastoma, optic glioma, and rhabdomyosarcoma.

TREATMENT. Treatment varies with tumor type. Surgical resection is indicated for many.

Tolosa-Hunt Syndrome

Tolosa-Hunt syndrome is a painful ophthalmoplegia attributed to an idiopathic granulomatous disease of the cavernous sinus or superior orbital fissure. No other structure is involved.

CLINICAL FEATURES. The pain is described as steady and penetrating, involving the entire hemicranium but centered around or behind the eye. It may precede the ophthalmoplegia by several days, may occur concurrently, or may appear later. The oculomotor nerve is ordinarily involved first and more severely than the two others, but all three ocular motor nerves, as well as the first and second divisions of the trigeminal nerve, may be affected. Vision may be diminished; the pupil is usually small and may be reactive or nonreactive. Symptoms last for days or months. Spontaneous remissions occur, but partial neurologic deficits may persist.

DIAGNOSIS. Tolosa-Hunt syndrome is easily confused with ophthalmoplegic migraine. The major clinical points of differentiation are that patients with ophthalmoplegic migraine also have nonophthalmoplegic migraine attacks, that they have a family history of migraine, and that the trigeminal nerve is not involved.

Tolosa-Hunt syndrome is differentiated from orbital inflammatory disease by the absence of proptosis and the presence of trigeminal nerve involvement. Other diseases of the cavernous sinus, such as tumor or thrombosis, may resemble the Tolosa-Hunt syndrome.

The erythrocyte sedimentation rate is elevated in most patients. MRI shows alterations of shape and signal of the cavernous sinus that are almost diagnostic (Rousseaux et al, 1993).

TREATMENT. Prednisone, 1 mg/kg/day, is both diagnostic and therapeutic. If pain subsides within 2 days of initial administration, the diagnosis is likely but not certain. Other lesions in the cavernous sinus or orbit may also respond to corticosteroids. Ophthalmoplegia may subside, but can take several days or weeks to clear completely. If prednisone fails to relieve the pain, the diagnosis of Tolosa-Hunt syndrome can be excluded and another cause must be identified.

Trauma

Trauma accounts for 40% of isolated acquired ocular motor nerve palsies, and 55% of multiple nerve palsies in children (Kodsi and Younge, 1992). Hemorrhage and edema into the nerves or muscles may occur from closed head injuries even in the absence of direct orbital injury (Baker and Epstein, 1991). When orbital fracture is present, the nerves and muscles may be lacerated, avulsed, or entrapped by bone fragments.

CLINICAL FEATURES. Superior oblique palsy, caused by trochlear nerve damage, is a relatively common consequence of closed head injuries (Keane, 1993). Usually the trauma is severe, often causing loss of consciousness, but it may be mild. The palsy is more often unilateral than bilateral. Patients with unilateral superior oblique palsy have a marked hypertropia in primary position and a compensatory head tilt to preserve fusion; 65% of cases resolve spontaneously. When bilateral involvement is present, the hypertropia is milder and alternates between the two eyes; spontaneous recovery occurs in only 25% of cases.

Transient lateral rectus palsy is rare in newborns and has been attributed to birth trauma. The palsy is unilateral and clears completely within 6 weeks.

DIAGNOSIS. Direct injuries to the orbit with associated hemorrhage and swelling do not pose a diagnostic dilemma. CT of the head with orbital views shows the extent of fracture so the need for surgical intervention can be determined. CT may also show a lateral midbrain hemorrhage as the cause of a trochlear nerve palsy.

A greater problem of diagnosis is caused by a delay between the time of injury and the onset of ophthalmoplegia. The possible mechanisms of delayed ophthalmoplegia following trauma to the head include progressive local edema in the orbit; progressive brainstem edema; progressive increased intracranial pressure; development of meningitis, mastoiditis or petrous osteomyelitis; venous sinus or carotid artery thrombosis; and carotid cavernous fistula.

TREATMENT. Local trauma and fracture of the orbit may require surgical repair. Permanent ocular motor nerve palsies following head injury are sometimes improved by surgery directed at rebalancing the extraocular muscles.

ACUTE BILATERAL OPHTHALMOPLEGIA

Many of the conditions that cause acute unilateral ophthalmoplegia (Table 15-4) may also cause acute bilateral ophthalmoplegia. The conditions listed in Table 15-5 are marked by a high incidence of bilateral involvement. Thyrotoxicosis could be added to this list, but it is discussed with the chronic conditions because progression of ophthalmoplegia is likely to occur over a period greater than 1 week.

Botulism

Botulism is caused by a toxin elaborated by several strains of the bacterium *Clostridium botulinum*. The infantile form of botulism causes ptosis but not ophthalmoplegia and is discussed in Chapter 6. This section deals with cases of later onset.

CLINICAL FEATURES. Botulism is most often caused by ingestion of toxin in home-canned food. This is most likely when canning is done at

■ TABLE 15–5
Causes of Acute Bilateral Ophthalmoplegia

Basilar meningitis (see Chapter 4)
Botulism
Brainstem encephalitis (see Chapter 10)
Carotid-cavernous fistula
Cavernous sinus thrombosis
Diphtheria
Intoxication
Miller Fisher syndrome (see Chapter 10)
Myasthenia gravis
Polyradiculoneuropathy (see Chapter 7)
Subacute necrotizing encephalomyelopathy (see
   Chapter 5)
Tick paralysis (see Chapter 7)

high altitudes, where the boiling temperature is too low to destroy spores. Because *C. botulinum* spores are ubiquitous in soil, infection may also follow burns and wounds. Blurred vision, diplopia, dizziness, dysarthria, and dysphagia begin in 12 to 36 hours after ingestion of toxin. The pupillary response is usually normal. The early symptoms are followed by an ascending paralysis that suggests the Guillain-Barré syndrome and may lead to death from respiratory paralysis. Patients remain conscious and alert throughout. Most patients make a complete recovery within 2 to 3 months, but those with severe involvement may not return to normal for a year.

DIAGNOSIS. The presence of ophthalmoplegia and normal findings of a spinal fluid examination distinguish botulism from the Guillain-Barré syndrome. EMG is useful in the diagnosis. The motor and sensory nerve conduction velocities are normal, evoked muscle action potentials are usually reduced in amplitude, and a decremental response is not ordinarily present at low rates of stimulation, although facilitation may be present at high rates of stimulation.

The diagnosis is established by showing the organism or the toxin in food, stool, or wound.

TREATMENT. The administration of antitoxin, 20,000 to 40,000 units 2 or 3 times a day, is recommended. The stomach and intestines should be emptied. 3,4-diaminopyridine is effective in some patients and should be used for those with potential respiratory failure. Mechanical respiratory support must be made available to every patient as soon as the diagnosis is suspected.

Intoxications

CLINICAL FEATURES. Anticonvulsants, tricyclic antidepressants, and many other psychoactive drugs selectively impair ocular motility at toxic blood concentrations. The overdose may be accidental or intentional. A child is found unconscious and brought to the emergency department. The state of consciousness varies from obtundation to stupor, but the eyes cannot be made to move either by rapidly rotating the head laterally or with ice water irrigation of the ears. Complete ophthalmoplegia may be expected in a comatose child if brainstem function is otherwise impaired (see Chapter 2), but if it occurs in a noncomatose child with otherwise intact brainstem function, ingestion of a drug that selectively impairs ocular motility should be suspected.

DIAGNOSIS. The family should be questioned about drugs available in the household, and the blood and urine should be screened for toxic substances.

TREATMENT. Specific treatment depends on the drug ingested; in most cases supportive care is sufficient.

CHRONIC BILATERAL OPHTHALMOPLEGIA

The conditions responsible for bilateral ophthalmoplegia developing over a period longer than 1 week are listed in Table 15-6. Most are discussed in previous sections of this chapter or in other chapters.

Graves Ophthalmopathy

It is not clear whether the association of ophthalmopathy with hyperthyroidism is causal or the two are associated autoimmune diseases (Feldon, 1990). One hypothesis suggests the presence of a cross-reacting antigen in thyroid and orbital tissues.

CLINICAL FEATURES. Disorders of ocular motility are present in the majority of patients with hyperthyroidism and may precede systemic features of nervousness, heat intolerance, diaphoresis, weight loss, tachycardia, tremulousness, and weakness. The major pathologic conditions in the orbit is a myopathy of the extraocular muscles. They become inflamed, swollen with interstitial edema, and finally fibrotic. If the two eyes are affected equally, the patient may not complain of diplopia despite considerable limitation of ocular motility. Staring or lid retraction (Dalrymple sign) occurs in more than 50% of cases, lid lag on downward gaze (von Graefe sign) in 30% to 50%, and proptosis

■ TABLE 15-6
Causes of Chronic Bilateral Ophthalmoplegia

Brainstem glioma
Chronic meningitis (see Chapter 4)
Chronic orbital inflammation
Graves ophthalmopathy
Kearns-Sayre syndrome
Myasthenia gravis
  Congenital
  Juvenile
Myopathies
  Fiber-type disproportion myopathy (see Chapter 6)
  Mitochondrial myopathies (see Chapter 8)
  Myotubular myopathy (see Chapter 6)
  Oculopharyngeal muscular dystrophy (see Chapter 17)
Subacute necrotizing encephalomyelopathy (see Chapter 5)
Vitamin E deficiency

(exophthalmos) in almost 90%. Severe exophthalmos is due to edema and infiltration of all orbital structures.

DIAGNOSIS. Thyroid disease should be considered in any child with evolving ophthalmoplegia. CT of the orbit shows enlargement of the extraocular muscles. This finding must be followed by direct measurement of plasma thyroxine, triiodothyronine, and thyroid-stimulating hormone concentrations. If these are normal but the diagnosis remains suspect, a thyroid-releasing hormone stimulation test and a measure of the concentration of thyroid-stimulating immunoglobulin may confirm the diagnosis.

TREATMENT. Meticulous control of hyperthyroidism provides the best relief of the ophthalmopathy but is not necessarily curative (Prummel et al, 1990). Hypothyroidism must be avoided. If the exophthalmos progresses even after the patient is euthyroid, corticosteroids may prevent further proptosis, but surgical decompression is indicated if optic nerve compression persists.

Kearns-Sayre Syndrome

Kearns-Sayre syndrome is caused by deletions of mitochondrial DNA (Moraes et al, 1989). Variability in the clinical syndrome reflects variability in the size of the deletion and the specific respiratory complex affected (see Chapter 8). Most cases are sporadic.

CLINICAL FEATURES. The invariable features of the disease are onset before 20 years of age, progressive external ophthalmoplegia, and pigmentary degeneration of the retina. At least one of three other features must also be present for diagnosis: heart block, cerebrospinal fluid protein greater than 100 mg/dl, and cerebellar dysfunction.

DIAGNOSIS. Diagnosis is based on the major clinical criteria. Electrocardiographic monitoring for cardiac arrhythmia and examination of the cerebrospinal fluid are essential.

TREATMENT. Treatment with vitamins or coenzyme Q, depending on the specific respiratory complex defect, may be beneficial in some patients (Phillips and Gosden, 1991). A cardiac pacemaker may be lifesaving.

 Gaze Palsies

This section deals with supranuclear palsies. To verify that a palsy is supranuclear and not due to an abnormality of the ocular motor nuclei or nerves, ocular muscles, or myasthenia, the examiner must show that the eyes move normally in response to brainstem reflexes, such as the doll's head maneuver, caloric testing, and the Bell phenomenon. The differential diagnosis of gaze palsies is listed in Table 15–7.

APRAXIA OF HORIZONTAL GAZE

Ocular motor apraxia is a deficiency in voluntary horizontal lateral fast eye movements (saccades) with retention of slow pursuit movements. Jerking movements of the head are used to bring the eyes to a desired position. The rapid phase of optokinetic nystagmus is absent.

Congenital Ocular Motor Apraxia

CLINICAL FEATURES. Although ocular motor apraxia is present at birth, it is usually not detected until late infancy. Blindness may be suspected because of failure of fixation. Overshooting head thrusts, often accompanied by blinking of the eyes, are used for refixation. When the head is held immobile, the child makes no effort at initiating horizontal eye movements.

Many children with ocular motor apraxia have other signs of cerebral abnormality, such as psychomotor retardation, learning disabilities, and clumsiness. When hypotonia is present, the child may have difficulty in making the head movements needed for refixation. Agenesis of the corpus callosum and agenesis of the cerebellar vermis are concurrent conditions in some patients with congenital ocular motor apraxia.

■ T A B L E   1 5 – 7
Gaze Palsies

Apraxia of Horizontal Gaze
Ataxia telangiectasia (see Chapter 10)
Ataxia-ocular motor apraxia (see Chapter 10)
Brainstem glioma
Congenital ocular motor apraxia
Huntington disease (see Chapter 5)

Internuclear Ophthalmoplegia
Brainstem stroke
Brainstem tumor
Exotropia (Pseudo-internuclear ophthalmoplegia [INO])
Multiple sclerosis
Myasthenia gravis (pseudo-INO)
Toxic-metabolic

Vertical Gaze Palsy
Aqueductal stenosis (see Chapter 18)
Congenital vertical ocular motor apraxia
Gaucher disease (see Chapter 5)
Hydrocephalus (see Chapters 4 and 18)
Miller Fisher syndrome (see Chapter 10)
Niemann-Pick disease, type C (see Chapter 5)
Tumor (see Chapter 4)
    Midbrain
    Pineal region
    Third ventricle
Vitamin B_{12} deficiency

Horizontal Gaze Palsy
Adversive seizures (see Chapter 1)
Brainstem tumors
Destructive lesions of the frontal lobe (see Chapter 11)
Familial horizontal gaze palsy

Convergence Paralysis
Head trauma
Idiopathic
Multiple sclerosis (see Chapter 10)
Pineal region tumors (see Chapter 4)

The association does not indicate that the malformations are responsible for ocular motor apraxia.

DIAGNOSIS. The possibility of ocular motor apraxia must be considered in any infant referred for evaluation of blindness. Once the presence of apraxia is established, MRI is indicated to search for other cerebral malformations, and tests for ataxia-telangiectasia (see Chapter 10) and lysosomal storage diseases (see Chapter 5) should be performed.

TREATMENT. No treatment is available.

INTERNUCLEAR OPHTHALMOPLEGIA

The medial longitudinal fasciculus (MLF) contains fibers that connect the abducens nucleus to the contralateral oculomotor nucleus for the purpose of performing horizontal conjugate lateral gaze. Unilateral lesions in the MLF disconnect the two nuclei, so that when the patient attempts lateral gaze, the adducting eye ipsilateral to the abnormal MLF is unable to move medially but the abducting eye is able to move laterally. Nystagmus (actually *overshoot dysmetria*) is often present in the abducting eye. This symptom complex, which may be unilateral or bilateral, is called *internuclear ophthalmoplegia* (INO). Unilateral INO is usually caused by vascular occlusive disease, and bilateral INO by demyelinating disease or toxic-metabolic causes.

Patients with myasthenia gravis sometimes have ocular motility dysfunction that resembles an INO except that nystagmus is usually lacking. The disorder is referred to as pseudo-INO because the MLF is intact. Pseudo-INO can also be caused by exotropia. When the normal eye is fixating in full abduction, there is no visual stimulus to bring the paretic eye into full adduction. Nystagmus is not present in the abducting eye.

The combination of an INO in one direction of lateral gaze and a complete gaze palsy in the other is called *one-and-a-half syndrome*. The syndrome is caused by a unilateral lesion in the dorsal pontine tegmentum affecting the pontine lateral gaze center and the adjacent MLF. It is most often due to multiple sclerosis but may be caused by brainstem glioma, infarction, or myasthenia gravis.

Toxic-Metabolic Disorders

CLINICAL FEATURES. Toxic doses of several drugs may produce the clinical syndrome of INO. The patient is usually found comatose and may have complete ophthalmoplegia that evolves into a bilateral INO, or a bilateral INO may be present at onset. The drugs reported to produce INO include amitriptyline, barbiturates, carbamazepine, doxepin, phenothiazine, and phenytoin. INO may also occur during hepatic coma.

DIAGNOSIS. Drug intoxications are always a consideration in children who were previously well and then show decreased consciousness. The presence of an INO following drug ingestion limits the possibilities to anticonvulsant and psychotropic drugs.

TREATMENT. The INO resolves as the blood concentration of the drug falls.

VERTICAL GAZE PALSY

Children with supranuclear vertical gaze palsies are unable to look upward or downward fully, but they retain reflex eye movements such as the Bell phenomenon. Disorders of upward gaze in children are generally due to lesions in the region of the dorsal midbrain and are almost always caused by tumors in the pineal region or aqueductal stenosis. The usual features are impaired upward and downward gaze, eyelid retraction, occasional disturbances in horizontal movement, convergence, and skew deviation. Mydriasis with light-near dissociation is an early feature of extrinsic compression of the dorsal midbrain. Isolated paralysis of upward gaze may be the initial feature of the Miller Fisher syndrome and of vitamin B_{12} or B_1 deficiency.

Isolated disturbances of downward gaze are caused by bilateral lesions in the midbrain reticular formation. They are rare in children but may occur in neurovisceral lipid storage disease.

Congenital Vertical Ocular Motor Apraxia

CLINICAL FEATURES. Congenital vertical ocular motor apraxia is a rare syndrome similar to congenital horizontal ocular motor apraxia, except for the direction of gaze palsy. At rest the eyes are fixed in either an upward or a downward position with little random movement. Head flexion or extension is used initially to fixate in the vertical plane; later, the child learns to use head thrusts. The Bell phenomenon is present.

DIAGNOSIS. Vertical gaze palsy suggests intracranial tumor, and MRI must be performed. Low-density lesions on both sides of the posterior third ventricle were shown in one child (Ebner et al, 1990). However, the presence of a gaze palsy from birth without the development of other neurologic signs usually indicates a nonprogressive process. Bilateral restriction of upward eye movement resulting from muscle fibrosis must also be considered. However, in children with ocular motor apraxia the eyes can move upward reflexively or by forced ductions; in children with muscle fibrosis, the eyes will not move upward by any means.

HORIZONTAL GAZE PALSY

Inability to look to one side is generally caused by a lesion in the contralateral frontal or ipsilateral pontine gaze center. Immediately after frontal lobe lesions the eyes are tonically deviated toward the side of the lesion and contralateral hemiplegia is often present. The eyes can be made to move horizontally by stimulation of the brainstem gaze center with ice water caloric techniques.

In contrast, an irritative frontal lobe lesion, such as an epileptic seizure, generally causes the eyes to deviate in a direction opposite to the side with the seizure focus. Movements of the head and eyes during a seizure are called *adversive seizures* (see Chapter 1). The initial direction of eye movement reliably predicts a contralateral focus, especially if the movement is forced and sustained in a unilateral direction. Later movements that are mild and unsustained are not predictive.

CONVERGENCE PARALYSIS

Convergence paralysis, inability to adduct the eyes to focus on a near object in the absence of medial rectus palsies, can be caused by a pineal region tumor; in such cases, however, other signs of midbrain compression are usually present. Convergence paralysis is sometimes factitious or due to lack of motivation or attention; this can be identified by the absence of pupillary constriction when convergence is attempted.

Convergence insufficiency is frequently encountered after closed head injuries (Waltz and Lavin, 1993). The head injury need not be severe. Diplopia, headache, or eyestrain during reading or other close work is reported. Convergence insufficiency also occurs in the absence of prior head injury. The onset often follows a change in study time or intensity, poor lighting in the workplace, or the use of new

contact lenses or eyeglasses. Treatment consists of convergence exercises or prisms.

 Nystagmus

Nystagmus is an involuntary, rhythmic oscillation of the eyes in which at least one phase is slow. With *pendular nystagmus,* the movements in each direction are slow. The oscillations of congenital pendular nystagmus are in the horizontal plane even on vertical gaze. On lateral gaze the oscillations may change to jerk nystagmus.

Jerk nystagmus is characterized by movements of unequal speed. An initial slow component in one direction is followed by a fast component with saccadic velocity in the other direction. Oscillation may be horizontal or vertical. The direction of jerk nystagmus is named for the fast (saccadic) component. Nystagmus intensity increases in the horizontal plane when gaze is in the direction of the fast phase.

Table 15–8 describes other eye movements that cannot be classified as nystagmus but that have diagnostic significance. *Opsoclonus* consists of conjugate, rapid, chaotic movements in all directions of gaze, often referred to as "dancing eyes." It occurs in infants with neuroblastoma or with idiopathic encephalopathy (see Chapter 10). *Ocular flutter* is a brief burst of conjugate horizontal saccadic eye movements that interrupt fixation. It occurs in the recovery phase of opsoclonus or in association with cerebellar disease. *Ocular dysmetria* is either an overshoot or an undershoot of the eyes during refixation or an oscillation before the eyes come to rest on a new fixation target. *Ocular bobbing* is not downbeat nystagmus, but rather a sudden downward movement of both eyes with a slow

■ TABLE 15–8
Abnormal Eye Movements

MOVEMENT	APPEARANCE	PATHOLOGY
Nystagmus	Rhythmic oscillation	Variable
Opsoclonus	Nonrhythmic, chaotic conjugate movements	Neuroblastoma, encephalitis
Ocular flutter	Intermittent bursts of rapid, horizontal, oscillations during fixation	Cerebellar/brainstem disease
Ocular dysmetria	Overshooting or oscillation on refixation	Cerebellar disease
Ocular bobbing	Intermittent, rapid downward movement	Pontine lesions
Periodic alternating gaze	Cyclic conjugate lateral eye deviations, alternating from side to side	Posterior fossa

drift back to midposition. It is most often seen in comatose patients with pontine dysfunction.

Congenital nystagmus and acquired nystagmus are discussed separately because their differential diagnoses are different (Table 15–9).

PHYSIOLOGIC NYSTAGMUS

A high-frequency (1 to 3 Hz), low-amplitude oscillation of the eyes occurs normally when lateral gaze is sustained to the point of fatigue. A jerk nystagmus, present at the endpoint of lateral gaze, is also normal. A few beats are usual, but even sustained nystagmus occurring at the endpoint should be considered normal unless it is associated with other signs of neurologic dysfunction or is distinctly asymmetric.

CONGENITAL NYSTAGMUS

Although congenital nystagmus is present at birth, it may not be noticed until infancy or childhood and then is misdiagnosed as acquired

nystagmus. One reason that it may not be noticed is that the *null point,* the angle of ocular movement at which the nystagmus is minimal, may be very wide. Often the nystagmus is observed but is mistaken for normal movement.

The cause of congenital nystagmus is thought to be a defect in the gaze-holding mechanism. In the past, it was thought that loss of visual acuity before the age of 2 years, regardless of cause, could produce nystagmus and that the nystagmus could be reversed by correction of the visual disturbance. It is now accepted by neurologists, but not all ophthalmologists, that the visual defect is not causal, but associated, and intensifies the underlying defect in neural control.

Congenital nystagmus is sometimes inherited. The pattern of inheritance may be autosomal recessive, autosomal dominant, or X linked.

CLINICAL FEATURES. Congenital nystagmus is almost always horizontal in plane but may be either pendular or jerk in character. It is generally diminished by convergence and increased by fixation. Because a null zone exists where nystagmus is minimal, the head may be held to one side, or tilted, or both to improve vision. Periodic head turning may accompany periodic alternating nystagmus.

Two forms of head oscillation are associated with congenital nystagmus. One is involuntary and does not improve vision. The other, also seen in spasmus nutans, is opposite in direction to the nystagmus but not phase locked, and improves vision. Many children have impaired vision from the nystagmus in the absence of a primary disturbance in visual acuity.

DIAGNOSIS. Determination that the nystagmus was present at birth is important, but not always possible. The eyes must be carefully examined for abnormalities in the sensory system that may be accentuating nystagmus. If the neurologic findings are otherwise normal, MRI is unnecessary.

TREATMENT. Nystagmus may be reduced by correcting a visual defect, particularly with contact lenses rather than eyeglasses, and by the use of prisms or surgery to move the eyes into the null zone without the head's turning.

SPASMUS NUTANS

Spasmus nutans is difficult to classify as either a congenital or an acquired nystagmus. It is probably never present at birth; the onset is early in infancy. The clinical entity of spasmus nutans is characterized by nystagmus, head nodding, and abnormal head positioning.

CLINICAL FEATURES. Onset typically occurs between 6 and 12 months of age. Nystagmus is characteristically binocular (but may be monocular), has a high frequency and a low amplitude, is often dysconjugate, and can be horizontal, vertical, or torsional in direction. The head is held in a tilted position and titubates in a manner that resembles nodding. Head tilt and movement may be more prominent than nystagmus, and torticollis is often the first complaint (see Chapter 14). The syndrome usually lasts 1 to 2 years, sometimes as long as 5, and then resolves spontaneously.

DIAGNOSIS. Spasmus nutans is ordinarily a transitory, benign disorder of unknown cause. On rare occasions, the syndrome may be mimicked by a glioma of the anterior visual pathways (Newman, 1990), or by subacute necrotizing encephalopathy (see Chapter 10). Tumor should be considered if the nystagmus is monocular, the optic nerve is pale, or the onset is after 1 year of age. I do not image the head and orbit in typical cases, although others have recommended this (Gottlob et al, 1990).

TREATMENT. Treatment is not needed.

ACQUIRED NYSTAGMUS

Pendular Nystagmus

Pendular nystagmus may be either congenital or acquired. In adults, the usual causes of acquired pendular nystagmus are brainstem infarction and multiple sclerosis. In children, pendular nystagmus in the absence of other neurologic signs is either congenital or the first sign of spasmus nutans. However, the development of optic atrophy in a child with pendular nystagmus indicates a glioma of the anterior visual pathway.

Vertical pendular nystagmus is unusual and sometimes occurs in association with rhythmic vertical oscillations of the palate (*palatal myoclonus* or *tremor*). This syndrome of oculopalatal oscillation is encountered in some spinocerebellar degenerations and ischemic disorders of the deep cerebellar nuclei and central tegmental tract.

Jerk Nystagmus

Drug-Induced Nystagmus

CLINICAL FEATURES. Many psychoactive drugs, including tranquilizers, antidepressants, anticonvulsants, and alcohol, produce nystagmus at high therapeutic or toxic blood concentrations. The nystagmus is horizontal or horizontal-rotary and is augmented by lateral gaze. Vertical nystagmus may be present on upward, but rarely on downward, gaze. Phenytoin and carbamazepine occasionally produce primary-position downbeat nystagmus as well.

DIAGNOSIS. Drug-induced nystagmus is common and should be considered in any patient taking psychoactive drugs. Drug overdose should be suspected in patients with nystagmus and decreased consciousness. A drug screen and measurement of drug blood concentrations are indicated.

TREATMENT. Nystagmus resolves when the blood concentration of the drug falls.

Ictal Nystagmus

CLINICAL FEATURES. Nystagmus as a seizure manifestation is binocular. It can be jerk, pendular, or rotary; and it may occur alone or in association with other ictal manifestations. Pupillary oscillations synchronous with the nystagmus may be observed. As a rule, concurrent epileptiform discharges are focal, contralateral to the fast phase of nystagmus, and frontal, parieto-occipital, or occipital. However, individual cases of nystagmus accompanying generalized 3-Hz spike-wave discharges, ipsilateral focal discharges, and periodic lateralized epileptiform discharges are reported.

DIAGNOSIS. Other seizure manifestations that identify the nature of the nystagmus are usually present. The electroencephalogram confirms the diagnosis by the presence of epileptiform activity concurrent with nystagmus.

TREATMENT. Ictal nystagmus responds to anticonvulsant drug therapy (see Chapter 1).

Vestibular Nystagmus

Vestibular nystagmus occurs with disorders of the labyrinth, vestibular nerve, vestibular nuclei of the brainstem, or cerebellum.

CLINICAL FEATURES. Labyrinthine disease (especially labyrinthitis) is usually associated with severe vertigo, nausea, and vomiting (see Chapter 17). Deafness or tinnitus is often present as well. The symptoms are enhanced by movement of the head, and motion may be more critical to the mechanism of nystagmus than the position obtained. Nystagmus is usually horizontal and torsional, with an initial linear slow phase followed by a rapid return. It is worse when gaze is in the direction of the fast phase. Fixation reduces nystagmus and vertigo.

Vertigo and nausea are mild when nystagmus is of central origin. Nystagmus is constantly present and is not affected by head position. It may be horizontal or vertical and does not improve with fixation. Other neurologic disturbances referable to the brainstem or cerebellum are frequently associated features.

DIAGNOSIS. Vestibular nystagmus is readily identified by observation and is identical to the nystagmus provoked by caloric stimulation or rotation. Labyrinthine disorders in children are almost always infectious, sometimes viral, and sometimes a result of otitis media. Central causes of vestibular nystagmus include spinocerebellar degeneration, brainstem glioma or infarction, subacute necrotizing encephalomyelitis, and demyelinating disorders.

TREATMENT. Vertigo and nausea associated with labyrinthine disease are appreciably improved by several different classes of drugs. Diazepam is especially effective. Other useful drugs include scopolamine, antihistamines, and tranquilizers.

Downbeat Nystagmus

CLINICAL FEATURES. In primary position the eyes drift slowly upward and then spontaneously beat downward. The intensity of the nystagmus is usually greatest when the eyes are directed slightly downward and laterally. Downbeat nystagmus should be distinguished from *downward-beating nystagmus,* in which the nystagmus is present only on downward gaze. Down-ward-beating nystagmus is usually caused by toxic doses of anticonvulsant and sedative drugs, whereas downbeat nystagmus indicates a structural abnormality of the brainstem, especially the cervicomedullary junction or cerebellum.

Patient complaints include dizziness, oscillopsia, blurred vision, and difficulty reading. Approximately one third of patients are asymptomatic. Cerebellar ataxia is present in about half of patients and usually is the only associated neurologic sign.

DIAGNOSIS. Cerebellar degenerations, both congenital and acquired, are the most common identifiable cause. The Chiari malformation must be considered as well. Metabolic disturbances include thiamine deficiency, phenytoin toxicity, and hypomagnesemia resulting from either dietary depletion or the use of lithium salts.

A congenital hereditary downbeat nystagmus

was described in a mother and son. It was noted in the boy at birth, and by infancy he needed to keep his chin down to look at people. He had no other neurologic abnormalities, but the nystagmus caused difficulty in learning to read. His mother had a subclinical downbeat nystagmus evident only in oblique downward gaze.

TREATMENT. Oscillopsia and acuity can be improved in some individuals by the use of clonazepam. A single test dose of 1 to 2 mg can be tried to determine whether long-term therapy will be useful. Trihexyphenidyl may prove effective when clonazepam fails. Prisms that increase convergence may also be useful.

Upbeat Nystagmus

CLINICAL FEATURES. In primary position the eyes drift slowly downward and then spontaneously beat upward. Upward gaze accentuates the nystagmus. A large- and a small-amplitude type are described. Large-amplitude nystagmus increases in intensity during upward gaze and indicates a lesion in the anterior vermis of the cerebellum or an abnormality in the anterior visual pathway. Anterior visual pathway abnormalities include Leber congenital amaurosis, bilateral optic nerve hypoplasia, and congenital cataract (see Chapter 16). Small-amplitude nystagmus decreases in intensity during upward gaze and when present suggests an intrinsic lesion of the medulla.

DIAGNOSIS. Upbeat nystagmus is usually an acquired disorder caused by vascular lesions or tumors of the brainstem or cerebellar vermis. Therefore, cranial MRI is indicated in every child with a normal anterior visual pathway. Upbeat nystagmus is also reported with impairment of smooth pursuit movements in a familial cerebellar vermian atrophy transmitted by autosomal dominant inheritance.

TREATMENT. No specific treatment is available.

Dissociated Nystagmus

Divergence Nystagmus

Divergence nystagmus is a rare condition in which each eye beats outward simultaneously. The mechanism is poorly understood, but the condition suggests an abnormality in the posterior fossa and may be seen with spinocerebellar degenerations.

Monocular Nystagmus

Monocular nystagmus may be congenital or acquired. The most important diagnostic considerations in children are spasmus nutans and chiasmal tumors. Although no clinical feature consistently differentiates the two groups, optic nerve abnormalities, especially optic hypoplasia, are sometimes found in children with tumors but not in those with spasmus nutans.

A coarse pendular vertical nystagmus may develop in an amblyopic eye years after the visual loss. The nystagmus is noted in the blind eye when distance fixation is attempted with the sighted eye and is inhibited by convergence.

See-Saw Nystagmus

See-saw nystagmus is the result of two different oscillations. One is a pendular vertical oscillation, the other a torsional movement in which one eye rises and intorts while the other falls and extorts. It may be congenital or acquired. The congenital form is sometimes associated with a horizontal pendular nystagmus. Acquired cases are usually due to tumors of the sellar and parasellar regions and are associated with bitemporal hemianopia.

REFERENCES

Afifi AK, Bell WE. Tests for juvenile myasthenia gravis: comparative diagnostic yield and prediction of outcome. J Child Neurol 1993;8:403-411.

Andrews PI, Massey JM, Howard JF, et al. Race, sex, and puberty influence onset, severity, and outcome in juvenile myasthenia gravis. Neurology 1994;44:1208-1214.

Andrews PI, Massey JM, Sanders DB. Acetylcholine receptor antibodies in juvenile myasthenia gravis. Neurology 1993; 43:977-982.

Baker RS, Epstein AD. Ocular motor abnormalities from head trauma. Surv Ophthalmol 1991;35:245-267.

Berge J, Louail C, Calle JM. Cavernous sinus thrombosis diagnostic approach. J Neuroradiol 1994;21:101-117.

Cohen HA, Nussinovitch M, Ashkenazi A, et al. Benign abducens nerve palsies of childhood. Pediatr Neurol 1993;9:394-395.

Ebner R, Lopez L, Ochoa S, et al. Vertical ocular motor apraxia. Neurology 1990;40:712-713.

Feldon SE: Graves' ophthalmopathy. Is it really a thyroid disease? Arch Intern Med 1990;150:948-950.

Gabianelli EB, Klingele TG, Burden RM. Acute oculomotor nerve palsy in children: Is arteriography necessary? J Clin Neuro Ophthalmol 1989;9:33-36.

Gottlob I, Zubcov A, Catalano RA, et al. Signs distinguishing spasmus nutans (with and without central nervous system lesions) from infantile nystagmus. Ophthalmology 1990;97: 1166-1175.

Ing EB, Sullivan TJ, Clarke MP, et al. Oculomotor nerve palsies in children. J Pediatr Ophthalmol Strabismus 1992; 29:331-336.

Kaban TJ, Smith K, Orton RB, et al. Natural history of presumed congenital Brown syndrome. Arch Ophthalmol 1993;111:943-946.

Keane JR. Fourth nerve palsy: Historical review and study of 215 inpatients. Neurology 1993;43:2439-2443.

Kodsi SR, Younge BR. Acquired oculomotor, trochlear, and abducens cranial nerve palsies in pediatric patients. Am J Ophthalmol 1992;114:568-574.

Lanska DJ. Diagnosis of thymoma in myasthenics using antistriated muscle antibodies: Predictive value and gain in diagnostic certainty. Neurology 1991;41:520-524.

Maria BL, Rehder K, Eskin TA, et al. Brainstem glioma: I. Pathology, clinical features, and therapy. J Child Neurol 1993;8:112-128.

Miano MA, Bosley TM, Heiman-Patterson TD, et al. Factors influencing outcome of prednisone dose reduction in myasthenia gravis. Neurology 1991;41:919-921.

Moraes CT, DiMauro S, Zeviani M, et al. Mitochondrial DNA deletions in progressive external ophthalmoplegia and Kearns-Sayre syndrome. N Engl J Med 1989;320:1293-1299.

Newman SA. Spasmus nutans—or is it? Surv Ophthalmol 1990;34:453-456.

Palace J, Wiles CM, Newsom-Davis J. 3,4-diaminopyridine in the treatment of congenital (hereditary) myasthenia. J Neurol Neurosurg Psychiatry 1991;54:1069-1072.

Phillips CI, Gosden CM. Leber's hereditary optic neuropathy and Kearns-Sayre syndrome: Mitochondrial DNA mutations. Surv Ophthalmol 1991;35:463-472.

Prummel MF, Wiesinga WM, Mourits MP, et al. Effect of abnormal thyroid function on the severity of Graves' disease. Arch Intern Med 1990;150:1098-1101.

Rousseaux P, Peruzzi P, Schaison-Cusin M. Should Tolosa-Hunt syndrome still be an exclusion diagnosis. Rev Neurol 1993;149:315-319.

Verma Pk, Oger JJ-F. Seronegative generalized myasthenia gravis: Low frequency of thymic pathology. Neurology 1992;42:586-589.

Waltz K, Lavin PJM. Accommodative insufficiency, In Margo CE, Hamed RN, eds: Diagnostic Problems in Clinical Ophthalmology. WB Saunders, Philadelphia, 1993;862-866.

16

Disorders of the Visual System

L ess than 1 child in 100,000 suffers serious visual loss (Robinson and Jan, 1993). Both congenital blindness and acquired visual loss in childhood are often associated with neurologic disorders. The most common causes of visual impairment in children are refractive errors, congenital cataracts, and genetic disorders. Two conditions that cause visual impairment are increasing in frequency: retrolental fibroplasia as a consequence of improved survival of premature babies, and retinal hemorrhage caused by child abuse.

 ## Assessment of Visual Acuity

The assessment of visual acuity in preverbal children relies mainly on assessing fixation and following, and observation of the way an infant or young child interacts with the environment.

CLINICAL ASSESSMENT

The pupillary light reflex is an excellent test of the functional integrity of the afferent and efferent pathways and is reliably present after 31 weeks' gestation. A blink response to light develops at about the same time, and the lid may remain closed for as long as light is present, (*the dazzle reflex*). The blink response to a threat may not be present until 5 months of age. These responses are integrated in the brain stem and do not provide information on the cognitive (cortical) aspects of vision.

Fixation and following are the principal means to assess visual function in newborns and infants. The human face, at a distance of approximately 30 cm, is the best target for fixation. After fixation is obtained, the examiner slowly moves from side to side to test the following response.

Visually directed grasping is present in normal children by 3 months of age. It is difficult to test before 6 months of age, and its absence may indicate a motor rather than a visual disturbance.

Optokinetic nystagmus can show fixation in infants when observation alone is inconclusive. The stimulus must be compelling, filling the visual field. Small hand-held tapes or drums may not be satisfactory. When such small stimuli are used, the demonstration of optokinetic nystagmus is clear evidence of visual function, but its absence does not establish that an abnormality is present. Visual fields can be evaluated in infants and young children by eliciting a refixation reflex when a stimulus is moved in the peripheral field.

Clues to visual impairment are structural abnormalities (i.e., microphthalmia, cloudy cornea), absent or asymmetric pupillary response to light, dysconjugate gaze, nystagmus, and failure to fixate or follow.

Visual Evoked Response

The visual evoked response to strobe light is an excellent technique for showing the anatomic integrity of subcortical visual pathways without patient cooperation. A positive "cortical" wave with a peak latency of 300 ms is first demonstrated at 30 weeks' gestation. The latency linearly declines at a rate of 10 ms each week throughout the last 10 weeks of gestation. In the newborn the morphology of the visual evoked response is variable during wakefulness and active sleep and is best studied just after the child goes to sleep. By 3 months of age, the morphology and latency of the visual evoked response are mature.

 Congenital Blindness

Cortical blindness is the most common cause of congenital blindness among children referred to a neurologist. The causes are numerous and include prenatal and perinatal disturbances. Optic nerve dysplasia, with or without other ocular malformations, is second in frequency, followed by congenital cataracts and corneal opacities. Corneal abnormalities usually do not cause visual loss unless clouding is extensive. Such extensive clouding may occur in the mucopolysaccharidoses and Fabry disease. Table 16–1 lists those conditions in which corneal clouding is present during childhood.

CONGENITAL CATARACT

For the purpose of this discussion, congenital cataract includes cataracts discovered within the first 3 months. The differential diagnosis is listed in Table 16–2.

In previous studies, approximately one third of congenital cataracts were attributed to intrauterine infection. That percentage has declined with prevention of rubella embryopathy by immunization. Genetic and chromosomal disorders account for at least one third and cause

■ T A B L E   1 6 – 1
Corneal Clouding in Childhood

Cerebrohepatorenal syndrome (Zellweger syndrome)
Congenital syphilis
Fabry disease (ceramide trihexosidosis)
Familial high-density lipoprotein deficiency (Tangier Island disease)
Generalized (GM$_1$) gangliosidosis
Juvenile metachromatic dystrophy
Marinesco-Sjögren disease
Mucolipidosis
Mucopolysaccharidoses
Pelizaeus-Merzbacher disease

---

cannot be determined in half of cases (Lloyd et al, 1992). When cataract is the only hereditary abnormality, genetic transmission is usually by autosomal dominant inheritance; when hereditary cataracts are associated with other features composing a syndrome, the mode of genetic transmission varies. In many hereditary syndromes cataracts can be either congenital or delayed in appearance until infancy, childhood, or even adulthood. Several of these syndromes are associated with dermatoses: *incontinentia pigmenti* (irregular skin pigmentation), *Marshall syndrome* (anhidrotic ectodermal dysplasia), *Schafer syndrome* (follicular hyperkeratosis), *congenital ichthyosis,* and *Siemens syndrome* (cutaneous atrophy).

Congenital cataracts occur in approximately 10% of children with trisomy 13 and trisomy 18 and in most children with trisomy 21. Cataracts develop by puberty in up to 40% of children with Turner syndrome. The association of congenital cataract and lactic acidosis or cardiomyopathy indicates a mitochondrial disorder (van Ekeren et al, 1993).

CLINICAL FEATURES. Small cataracts do not impair vision and may be difficult to detect by direct ophthalmoscopy. Large cataracts appear as a white mass in the pupil and, if left in place, lead to loss of vision. The initial size of a cataract does not predict its course; congenital cataracts may remain stationary or become more dense, but they never improve spontaneously.

Other congenital ocular abnormalities, aniridia, coloboma, and microphthalmos, occur in 40% to 50% of newborns with congenital cataracts.

DIAGNOSIS. Large cataracts are obvious on inspection. Smaller cataracts distort the normal red reflex when the direct ophthalmoscope is held at a distance from the eye and a +12 to +20 lens is used.

Genetic disorders and maternal drug exposure should be considered when cataracts are the only abnormality. Intrauterine disturbances, such as maternal illness and fetal infection, are usually associated with growth retardation and other malformations. Chromosome analysis should be performed for all children with dysmorphic features. Galactosemia is suspected in children with hepatomegaly and milk intolerance (see Chapter 5), but cataracts may be present even before the development of systemic features.

TREATMENT. Early recognition and removal of cataracts before age 3 months is important to prevent developmental amblyopia. Urgent

■ TABLE 16-2
Lens Abnormalities in Childhood

Congenital Cataract	Acquired Cataract
Chromosomal aberrations	Drug induced
Trisomy 13	Corticosteroids
Trisomy 18	Long-acting miotics
Trisomy 21*	Genetic
Turner syndrome*	Autosomal dominant inheritance (Alport syndrome)
Drug exposure during pregnancy	Autosomal recessive inheritance
Chlorpromazine	Cockayne disease
Corticosteroids	Hepatolenticular degeneration (Wilson disease)
Sulfonamides	Laurence-Moon-Biedl syndrome
Galactosemia	Rothmund-Thompson syndrome
Galactokinase deficiency	Werner syndrome
Galactose-1-phosphate uridyltransferase deficiency	X-linked inheritance (Pseudo-pseudohypopara-thyroidism)
Genetic	Chromosomal (Prader-Willi syndrome)
Autosomal dominant inheritance	Metabolic
Hereditary spherocytosis*	Cretinism
Incontinentia pigmenti*	Hypocalcemia
Marshall syndrome*	Hypoparathyroidism
Myotonic dystrophy*	Juvenile diabetes
Schafer syndrome*	Pseudohypoparathyroidism
Without other anomalies	Trauma
Autosomal recessive inheritance	Varicella (postnatal)
Congenital ichthyosis*	**Dislocated Lens**
Congenital stippled epiphyses (Conradi disease)	Crouzon syndrome
Marinesco-Sjögren syndrome*	Ehlers-Danlos syndrome
Siemens syndrome*	Homocystinuria
Smith-Lemli-Opitz syndrome	Hyperlysinemia
X-linked inheritance (oculocerebrorenal syndrome)*	Marfan syndrome
Idiopathic	Sturge-Weber syndrome
Intrauterine infection*	Sulfite oxidase deficiency
Mumps	
Rubella	
Syphilis	
Maternal factors	
Diabetes	
Radiation	
Malnutrition	
Prematurity	
Syndromes of uncertain etiology	
Hallerman-Streiff syndrome	
Pseudo-Turner syndrome*	
With oxycephaly	
With polydactyly	

*Cataracts may not be noted until infancy or childhood.

referral to a pediatric ophthalmologist is warranted.

CONGENITAL OPTIC NERVE HYPOPLASIA

Optic nerve hypoplasia is a developmental defect in the number of optic nerve fibers and may result from excessive regression of retinal ganglion cell axons (Zeki and Dutton, 1990). Hypoplasia may be bilateral or unilateral and varies in severity. It may occur as an isolated defect and cause astigmatism, or it may be associated with intracranial anomalies (Brodsky and Glasier, 1993). The most common association is with midline defects of the septum pellucidum and hypothalamus (*septo-optic dysplasia*).

CLINICAL FEATURES. When hypoplasia is severe, the child is blind and attention is drawn to the eyes at birth because of strabismus and nystagmus. Ophthalmoscopic examination reveals a small, pale nerve head (Figure 16-1). A pigmented area surrounded by a yellowish mottled halo is sometimes present at the edge of the disk margin, giving the appearance of a double ring. The degree of hypothalamic-pituitary involvement varies (Costello and Gluck-man, 1988). Possible symptoms include neo-natal hypoglycemia and seizures, recurrent hy-poglycemia in childhood, growth retardation, diabetes insipidus, and sexual infantilism. Some combination of mental retardation, cerebral palsy, and epilepsy is often present and indicates malformations in other portions of the brain.

DIAGNOSIS. Cranial magnetic resonance im-aging (MRI) of the head and an assessment of endocrine status should be performed on all infants with ophthalmoscopic evidence of optic nerve hypoplasia. The common findings on MRI are absence of the septum pellucidum, posterior pituitary ectopia, and hemispheric migration anomalies (Brodsky and Glasier, 1993). Endo-crine studies should include assays of growth hormone, antidiuretic hormone, and the integ-rity of hypothalamic-pituitary control of the thyroid, adrenal, and gonadal systems. Infants with hypoglycemia usually have growth hor-mone deficiency.

TREATMENT. No treatment is available for optic hypoplasia, but endocrine abnormalities respond to replacement therapy.

CONGENITAL COLOBOMA

Congenital coloboma is a defect in embryo-genesis that may affect only the disk or may include the retina, iris, ciliary body, and chor-

☐ FIGURE 16–1 Optic nerve hypoplasia. The optic nerve is small and pale, but the vessels are of normal size.

oid. Colobomas isolated to the nerve head appear as deep excavations. They may be unilateral or bilateral. The causes of congenital coloboma are genetic (monogenic and chromo-somal) and intrauterine disease (toxic and infec-tious) (Warburg, 1993). Retinochoroidal colobo-mas are glistening white or yellow defects inferior or inferonasal to the disk. The margins are distinct and surrounded by pigment. *Morn-ing glory disk,* a form of coloboma, is an enlarged dysplastic disk with a white excavated center surrounded by an elevated annulus of pigmentary change. Retinal vessels enter and leave at the margin of the disk, giving the appearance of a morning glory flower.

LEBER CONGENITAL AMAUROSIS

Leber congenital amaurosis is an hereditary generalized retinal degeneration that is present at birth or in early infancy and is transmitted by autosomal recessive inheritance. The term was used in the past to include some peroxisomal disorders, and for that reason the disorder was thought to have genetic heterogeneity (Lambert et al, 1993).

CLINICAL FEATURES. Blindness is present at birth or shortly thereafter and may be associated with pendular nystagmus, upbeat nystagmus, and photophobia. Ophthalmoscopy of the retina shows no abnormality in infancy and early childhood, but with time, progressive retinal stippling and pallor of the disk appear. Mental retardation and other neurologic disturbances may be associated (Steinberg et al, 1992).

DIAGNOSIS. The disease is seldom diagnosed in infancy because the retina appears normal. Electroretinography is the primary method for detecting the widespread retinal degeneration. Other disorders that may be mistaken for Leber congenital amaurosis are Zellweger syndrome, infantile Refsum disease, and several varieties of infantile-onset progressive retinal degeneration.

TREATMENT. No treatment is available.

 ## Acute Monocular or Binocular Blindness

The differential diagnoses of acute and pro-gressive blindness show a considerable overlap. Although older children recognize sudden visual loss, slowly progressive ocular disturbances may produce an asymptomatic decline until vision is severely disturbed. When finally noticed, the

■ TABLE 16-3
Causes of Acute Loss of Vision

Carotid Dissection (see Chapter 11)
Cortical Blindness
Anoxic encephalopathy (see Chapter 2)
Benign occipital epilepsy (see Chapter 1)
Hydrocephalus
Hypoglycemia
Hypertension (malignant or accelerated)
Hyperviscosity
Hypotension
Migraine (see Chapter 3)
Occipital metastatic disease
Post-traumatic transient cerebral blindness
Systemic lupus erythematosis
Toxic (cyclosporin, etc.)
Trauma
Hysteria
Optic Neuropathy
Demyelinating
  Idiopathic optic neuritis
  Multiple sclerosis (see Chapter 10)
  Neuromyelitis optica (see Chapter 12)
Ischemic
Toxic
Traumatic
Pituitary Apoplexy
Pseudotumor Cerebri (see Chapter 4)
Retinal Disease
Central retinal artery occlusion
Migraine
Trauma

■ TABLE 16-4
Causes of Progressive Loss of Vision

Compressive Optic Neuropathies
Aneurysm (see Chapters 4 and 15)
Arteriovenous malformations (see Chapters 4, 10, and 11)
Craniopharyngioma
Hypothalamic and optic tumors
Pituitary adenoma
Pseudotumor cerebri (see Chapter 4)
Disorders of the Lens (see Table 16-3)
Cataract
Dislocation of the lens
Hereditary Optic Atrophy
Dominant optic neuropathy
Infantile Refsum disease
Leber hereditary optic neuropathy
Wolfram syndrome
Intraocular Tumors
Tapetoretinal Degenerations
Abnormal carbohydrate metabolism
  Mucopolysaccharidosis (see Chapter 5)
  Primary hyperoxaluria
Abnormal lipid metabolism
  Abetalipoproteinemia (see Chapter 10)
  Hypobetalipoproteinemia (see Chapter 10)
  Multiple sulfatase deficiency (see Chapter 5)
  Neuronal ceroid lipofuscinosis (see Chapter 5)
  Niemann-Pick disease (see Chapter 5)
  Refsum disease (see Chapter 7)
Other syndromes of unknown etiology
  Cockayne syndrome
  Laurence-Moon-Biedl syndrome
  Refsum disease (see Chapter 7)
  Usher syndrome (see Chapter 17)

child's loss of visual acuity seems to be recent. Slowly progressive visual disturbances are often noted first by a teacher or parent rather than by the child. Table 16-3 lists conditions in which visual acuity is normal and then suddenly lost. Table 16-4 lists disorders in which the underlying pathologic process is progressive; in most of these conditions the patient quickly perceives the visual loss. Therefore, both tables should be consulted in the differential diagnosis of "acute blindness."

The duration of transient monocular blindness suggests the underlying cause: seconds indicates disk swelling; minutes, emboli; hours, migraine; and days, optic neuritis.

CORTICAL BLINDNESS

Cortical blindness in children may be permanent or transitory depending on the cause (Wong, 1991). Transitory cortical blindness in childhood can be caused by migraine (see Chapter 3), mild head trauma, brief episodes of hypoglycemia or hypotension, and benign oc-

cipital epilepsy (see Chapter 1). Acute and sometimes permanent blindness may occur following anoxia; as a result of massive infarction of, or hemorrhage into, the visual cortex; and when multifocal metastatic tumors or abscesses are located in the occipital lobes.

The main feature of cortical blindness is loss of vision with preservation of the pupillary light reflex. The results of ophthalmoscopic examination are normal.

Hypoglycemia

Repeated episodes of acute cortical blindness may occur at the time of mild hypoglycemia in children with glycogen storage diseases and following insulin overdose in diabetic children.

CLINICAL FEATURES. Sudden blindness is associated with clinical evidence of hypoglycemia (sweating and confusion). Ophthalmoscopic and neurologic findings are normal. Recovery is complete in 2 to 3 hours.

DIAGNOSIS. During an episode of cortical blindness caused by hypoglycemia, electroencephalography (EEG) shows high-voltage slowing over both occipital lobes. Afterward the EEG returns to normal.

TREATMENT. Glucose can be given during the attack, but treatment may not be needed.

Transient Post-traumatic Cerebral Blindness

CLINICAL FEATURES. Transient post-traumatic cerebral blindness is a benign syndrome that most often occurs in children with a history of migraine or seizures (Rodriguez et al, 1993). The spectrum of visual disturbance is broad, but a juvenile and an adolescent pattern have been delineated. In children younger than 8 years, the precipitating trauma is usually associated with either a brief loss of consciousness or a report that the child was "stunned." Blindness is noted almost immediately on recovery of consciousness and lasts for an hour or less. During the episode the child may be lethargic and irritable but is usually coherent. Recovery is complete, and the child may not recall the event.

In older children, the syndrome is characterized by blindness, confusion, and agitation several minutes or hours after trivial head trauma. Consciousness is not lost. All symptoms resolve after several hours, and the child has complete amnesia for the event. These episodes share many features with acute confusional migraine and are probably a variant of that disorder (see Chapter 2).

DIAGNOSIS. Children with transitory blindness and a normal neurologic examination following head trauma do not need brain imaging studies. Those with persistent blindness require MRI to exclude injury to the occipital lobes. Occipital intermittent rhythmic delta suggests migraine as the underlying cause. Recognition of the syndrome can spare the trouble and expense of other studies. Family history should be scrutinized for the possibility of migraine or epilepsy. The rapid and complete resolution of all symptoms confirms the diagnosis.

TREATMENT. Treatment is not needed. Symptoms resolve spontaneously.

HYSTERICAL BLINDNESS

A claim of complete binocular blindness is easily identified as spurious. A pupillary response to light indicates that the anterior pathway is intact and only cerebral blindness is a possibility. Visual function can be assessed by using a full-field optokinetic stimulus tape or by moving a large mirror in front of the patient to stimulate matching eye movements. When monocular blindness is claimed, the same tests can be performed with a patch covering the good eye.

Spurious claims of partial visual impairment are more difficult to challenge. Helpful tests include failure of acuity to improve linearly with increasing test size, inappropriate ability to detect small test objects on tangent screen, and constricted (tunnel) visual fields to confrontation.

OPTIC NEUROPATHIES

Demyelinating Optic Neuropathy

Demyelination of the optic nerve (optic neuritis) may occur as an isolated finding affecting one or both eyes, or it may be associated with demyelination in other portions of the nervous system. *Neuromyelitis optica* (Devic syndrome), the syndrome combining optic neuritis and transverse myelitis, is discussed in Chapter 12, and multiple sclerosis in Chapter 10. MRI is a useful technique for surveying the central nervous system for demyelinating lesions (see Figure 10-3). The incidence of later multiple sclerosis among children with optic neuritis is 15% or less if the child has no evidence of more diffuse involvement when brought to medical attention (Kriss et al, 1988), but is almost 100% when diffuse involvement is present or when relapse of optic neuritis occurs within 1 year (Riikonen et al, 1988). Unilateral optic neuritis has a higher incidence of later multiple sclerosis than does bilateral optic neuritis.

CLINICAL FEATURES. Monocular involvement is the rule in adults, but binocular involvement occurs in more than half of children. Binocular involvement may be concurrent or sequential, sometimes occurring over a period of weeks. The initial feature in some children is pain in the eye, but for most it is blurred vision, progressing within hours or days to partial or complete blindness. Visual acuity is reduced to less than 20/200 in almost all patients within 1 week. A history of a preceding "viral" infection or immunization is often presented, but no evidence has shown a cause-and-effect relationship between optic neuritis and either of these events.

Results of ophthalmoscopic examination may be normal at the onset of symptoms, if neuritis

☐ FIGURE 16–2 Neuroretinitis. The optic disk is swollen with peripapillary nerve fiber layer opacification. Exudates surround the macula in a star pattern. (Courtesy of Patrick Lavin, M.D.)

is primarily retrobulbar. However, most children have papillitis rather than retrobulbar neuritis, and the nerve head is swollen and hemorrhagic, resembling papilledema. The two are readily distinguished because optic neuritis is characterized by early and severe visual loss with afferent pupillary defect and papilledema is not.

Neuritis of the peripapillary nerve fiber layer of the retina is called *neuroretinitis*. Ophthalmoscopic examination shows disk swelling, peripapillary retinal detachment, and a macular star (Figure 16-2). Neuroretinitis suggests the possibility of conditions other than idiopathic optic neuritis.

In the absence of myelitis, the prognosis in children with bilateral optic neuritis is good; complete recovery occurs in 90%.

DIAGNOSIS. Optic neuritis must be considered when monocular or binocular blindness develops suddenly in a child. The diagnosis is often established by ophthalmoscopic or slit-lamp examination. Further confirmation, when necessitated by the suspicion of malingering or hysteria, can be accomplished by testing the visual evoked response. In children with optic neuritis, the latency of the major negative wave that ordinarily appears at 100 ms is invariably prolonged. Once optic neuritis is confirmed, MRI of the head is indicated to search for diffuse encephalomyelitis or paranasal sinusitis because these findings influence therapy. Pe-

roneal stimulated somatosensory evoked responses and MRI of the spine are indicated if the history or physical findings suggest spinal dysfunction.

Examination of the cerebrospinal fluid is unnecessary. Such examination sometimes shows a leukocytosis and an increased concentration of protein but does not provide information about etiology or prognosis.

TREATMENT. Oral corticosteroids had been widely used in the treatment of optic neuritis, but a controlled study in adults has shown that intravenous methylprednisolone, 250 mg every 6 hours for 3 days, followed by oral prednisone, 1 mg/kg/day for 14 days, speeds the recovery of visual loss, and may reduce the rate of development of multiple sclerosis over a 2 year period (Beck et al, 1993).

Ischemic Optic Neuropathy

Infarction of the anterior portion of the optic nerve is rare in children and is usually associated with systemic vascular disease or hypotension.

CLINICAL FEATURES. Ischemic optic neuropathy usually occurs as a sudden segmental loss of vision in one eye, but slow or step-wise progression over several days is possible. Recurrent episodes are unusual except with migraine and some idiopathic cases.

DIAGNOSIS. Altitudinal visual field defects are present in 70% to 80% of patients. Color vision loss is roughly equivalent in severity to visual acuity loss, whereas in demyelinating optic neuritis, color vision is affected more than visual acuity. Ophthalmoscopic examination reveals diffuse or partial swelling of the optic disk. When swelling is diffuse, it gives the appearance of papilledema and flame-shaped hemorrhages may be present adjacent to the disk margin. After acute swelling subsides, optic atrophy follows.

TREATMENT. Treatment depends on the underlying disease that causes the ischemia.

Toxic-Nutritional Optic Neuropathies

Drugs, toxins, and nutritional deficiencies alone or in combination may cause an acute or progressive optic neuropathy. These factors may cause optic neuropathy by inducing mitochondrial changes, perhaps in susceptible populations with mitochondrial DNA (mtDNA) mutations (Johns and Sadun, 1994).

CLINICAL FEATURES. Implicated drugs include barbiturates, antibiotics (chloramphenicol, isoniazid, streptomycin, sulfonamides), chemotherapeutic agents, chlorpropamide, digitalis, ergot, halogenated hydroxyquinolines, penicillamine, and quinine. Nutritional deficiencies that may cause such optic neuropathies include folic acid vitamins B_1, B_2, B_6, and B_{12}.

Symptoms vary with the specific drug, but progressive loss of central vision is typical. In some cases, visual loss is rapid and develops as acute binocular blindness that may be asymmetric at onset, suggesting monocular involvement. Many of the drugs produce optic neuropathy by interfering with the action of folic acid or vitamin B_{12} and thereby causing a nutritional deficiency.

DIAGNOSIS. Drug toxicity should be suspected whenever central and paracentral scotomas develop during the course of drug treatment. Optic nerve hyperemia with small paracentral hemorrhages may be an early feature. Later, the disk becomes pale.

TREATMENT. Drug-induced optic neuropathy is dose related. Dosage reduction may be satisfactory in some cases, especially if concurrent treatment with folic acid or vitamin B_{12} reverses the process. Some drugs must be discontinued completely.

Traumatic Optic Neuropathies

Trauma to the head may cause an indirect optic neuropathy in one or both eyes (Wolin and Lavin, 1990). The nerve is tethered along its course and therefore subject to shearing forces when the skull suddenly accelerates or decelerates. Possible consequences include acute swelling, hemorrhage, or tear. This is particularly common in children who sustain bicycle injuries when not wearing a helmet.

CLINICAL FEATURES. Loss of vision is usually immediate. Delayed visual loss caused by a hematoma or by edema may respond to corticosteroids and has a better prognosis. Traumatic optic neuropathy is readily distinguished from cortical blindness because the pupillary response is diminished or absent. Prognosis for recovery is best if there is a brief delay between the time of injury and the onset of blindness.

DIAGNOSIS. The loss of vision and pupillary light response immediately following a head injury should suggest the diagnosis. Peripapillary hemorrhages may be seen by ophthalmoscopic examination.

TREATMENT. Corticosteroids and surgical decompression of the nerve are suggested.

PITUITARY APOPLEXY

Pituitary apoplexy is a rare, life-threatening condition caused by hemorrhagic infarction of the pituitary gland (Rolih and Ober, 1993).

CLINICAL FEATURES. Pituitary infarction occurs most often when there is a pre-existing pituitary tumor but may also occur in the absence of tumor.

Several different clinical features are possible depending on which structures are affected by the swollen gland. These include any of the following, alone or in combination: monocular or binocular blindness, visual field defects, ophthalmoplegia, chemical meningitis, cerebrospinal fluid rhinorrhoea, and shock from hypopituitarism. Leakage of blood and necrotic material into the subarachnoid space causes a chemical meningitis associated with headache, meningismus, and loss of consciousness.

DIAGNOSIS. MRI of the head with views of the pituitary gland establishes the diagnosis. Endocrine testing may show a deficiency of all pituitary hormones.

TREATMENT. Patients deteriorate rapidly and may die within a few days if corticosteroids are not administered promptly. Other hormones must also be replaced, but are not lifesaving. In patients who continue to do poorly, as evidenced by loss of consciousness, hypothalamic instability, or loss of vision, require urgent surgical decompression of the expanding pituitary mass.

RETINAL DISEASE

Central Retinal Artery Occlusion

Migraine and coagulopathies are the main predisposing disorders among children with retinal artery obstruction. Others are sickle cell disease, cardiac disorders, vasculitis, and pregnancy. Congenital heart disease is the usual pre-existing condition causing emboli to the central retinal artery in young people. Mitral valve prolapse is a potential cause but is more likely to produce transient cerebral ischemia than transient monocular blindness.

CLINICAL FEATURES. Most affected children have an abrupt loss of monocular vision of variable intensity without premonitory symptoms. Some describe spots, a shadow, or a descending veil before the loss of vision. Bilateral retinal artery occlusion is uncommon in children.

DIAGNOSIS. The diagnosis of retinal artery obstruction is usually based on the clinical history and ophthalmoscopic examination. The posterior pole of the retina becomes opacified except in the foveal region, where a cherry-red spot is seen. The peripheral retina appears normal. Visual field examination and fluorescein angiography help confirm the diagnosis in some cases. Once the diagnosis is established, the underlying causes must be found. Evaluation should include auscultation of the heart, radiographs of the chest, echocardiography in selected cases, complete blood cell count with sedimentation rate, cholesterol and triglyceride screening, coagulation studies, hemoglobin electrophoresis, and lupus anticoagulant and antiphospholipid antibodies (Brey et al, 1990).

TREATMENT. Treatment is determined by underlying cause. The management of idiopathic occlusion of the retinal artery in adults is controversial, with some authorities recommending the use of corticosteroids. In children, giant cell arteritis is not a consideration and corticosteroids are not indicated. Visual acuity is more likely to improve when the obstruction is in a branch artery than in the central retinal artery.

Retinal Migraine

CLINICAL FEATURES. Visual symptoms are relatively common during an attack of classic migraine (see Chapter 3). The typical scintillating scotomas, or "fortification spectra," are field defects caused by altered neuronal function in the occipital cortex. The affected field is contralateral to the headache.

Transient monocular blindness is caused by retinal ischemia. It is not associated with stroke in children, who usually have migraine as the underlying cause (Tippin et al, 1989). The visual loss is sudden in most cases, may be partial or complete, and often precedes and is ipsilateral to the headache. Recurrences are usually in the same eye, and attacks may occur without headache.

Typical patients have a long history of migraine with aura in which both field defects and monocular blindness are experienced separately or together. The visual aberrations are often described as a mosaic or jigsaw pattern of scotomas that clear within minutes. Permanent monocular blindness is unusual and occurs mainly in adolescent and adult women. Many patients with persistent blindness have other risk factors for vascular disease, such as the use of oral contraceptives or vasculitis.

DIAGNOSIS. The diagnosis can be considered when there is a history of migraine with aura. Ophthalmoscopic findings may be normal initially and then include retinal edema with scattered hemorrhages. Several patterns of retinal vaso-occlusive disease may be observed by fluorescein angiography: branch retinal artery, central retinal artery, central retinal vein, and cilioretinal artery.

TREATMENT. Children who have retinal ischemia during migraine attacks should be treated with agents that prevent further episodes. Propranolol remains the most effective drug against migraine despite the theoretical, but unproven, fear that it might enhance vasospasm.

Retinal Trauma

Direct blunt injury to the orbit causes visual impairment by retinal contusion, tear, or detachment. All three are characterized by a diminished pupillary response. Contusion is associated with retinal edema. Although visual loss is immediate, the retina appears normal for the first few hours and only later becomes white and opaque. The severity of visual loss varies, but complete recovery is the rule.

Retinal tear is often associated with vitreous hemorrhage. Visual loss is usually immediate and easily diagnosed by ophthalmoscopic appearance. Recovery is spontaneous unless there is detachment, for which cryotherapy is required.

⇒ Progressive Loss of Vision
COMPRESSIVE OPTIC NEUROPATHY

Compression of one or both optic nerves often occurs in the region of the chiasm. Visual loss may be confined to one eye or to a visual field. In children with tumors in and around the diencephalon, the most constant feature is growth failure. This may not be recognized until other symptoms develop.

Craniopharyngioma

CLINICAL FEATURES. The initial features of craniopharyngioma in children are growth retardation, visual disturbances, endocrinopathies, and failure of sexual maturation. Field defects are frequently asymmetric or unilateral. Bitemporal hemianopsia is present in 50% of children, with craniopharyngioma and homonymous hemianopsia in 10% to 20%. Visual acuity is always diminished in one or both eyes.

Approximately 25% of children have hydrocephalus that causes headache and papilledema. Hypothalamic involvement may produce diabetes insipidus or the *hypodipsia-hyponatremia syndrome,* characterized by lethargy, confusion, and hypotension. Other features depend on the direction of tumor growth. Anterior extension may compress the olfactory tract, causing anosmia, whereas lateral extension may compress the third and fifth nerves.

DIAGNOSIS. Craniopharyngiomas are readily visualized by MRI.

TREATMENT. Subtotal resection followed by radiation therapy is the accepted standard of treatment (Hetelekidis et al, 1993). The extent of resection remains an issue, but total resection is discouraged. Hormone replacement therapy is needed.

Hypothalamic and Optic Gliomas

Gliomas of the hypothalamus and optic nerves are difficult to distinguish by histologic criteria and share many clinical features. Optic gliomas represent 3% to 5% of childhood brain tumors. More than half of children with optic gliomas have neurofibromatosis type 1 (NF1). Among children with optic pathways tumors, precocious puberty is a common initial feature in those with NF1, and is not found in children without NF1 (Listernick et al, 1995). The subsequent course is similar whether or not neurofibromatosis is present, except that recurrences are more common in children with neurofibromatosis.

CLINICAL FEATURES. Initial symptoms depend on location, but hypothalamic tumors eventually affect the optic chiasm and optic chiasm tumors affect the hypothalamus. In children younger than 3 years, tumors of the hypothalamus or optic chiasm may produce the *diencephalic syndrome.* This syndrome is characterized by marked loss of subcutaneous fat and total body weight with maintenance or acceleration of long bone growth. Despite the appearance of cachexia, the infant is mentally alert and does not seem as sick as the appearance suggests. Pendular nystagmus is usually associated. The precise endocrine mechanism of the diencephalic syndrome has never been clarified. Hamartomas of the tuber cinereum, astrocytomas, ependymomas, ectopic pinealomas, and craniopharyngiomas are also associated with the diencephalic syndrome. Precocious puberty,

☐ F I G U R E 1 6 – 3 Optic nerve glioma identified by MRI (*arrow*).

rather than the diencephalic syndrome, can be the initial feature of hypothalamic tumors in infants and children.

Slowly progressive loss of vision is the most common early feature in children. Monocular visual loss suggests optic nerve involvement but also may occur with tumors of the chiasm. Binocular involvement suggests involvement of the optic chiasm or tract. Visual field deficits vary. Tumors in or near the orbit may produce proptosis, optic disk swelling in which blurring of the disk resembles papilledema, and central loss of vision. Ophthalmoplegia is unusual.

Increased intracranial pressure suggests extension of tumor from the chiasm to the hypothalamus. When this is the initial feature, the site of tumor origin is difficult to determine.

DIAGNOSIS. MRI is the preferred imaging modality because it permits visualization of the hypothalamus in several different planes and identification of brainstem extension of tumor (Figure 16-3).

Optic nerve gliomas usually produce an enlarged, tubular appearance of the nerve and chiasm. Sometimes the tumors are globular and suprasellar and appear to compress the chiasm.

Intrinsic gliomas of the hypothalamus are

identified by MRI as high-density signals on T_2-weighted studies.

TREATMENT. Stereotaxic-guided biopsy of hypothalamic tumors should be performed before treatment to identify histologic type. The combination of radiation therapy and chemotherapy provides 5- and 10-year survivals of 93% and 74%, respectively (Rodriguez et al, 1990). Oral etoposide is beneficial in children with recurrent tumors (Chamberlain, 1995).

Management of optic gliomas is a greater problem. Half of these tumors grow slowly and have a relatively benign course (Dutton, 1994). Unfortunately, slowly growing tumors are difficult to differentiate from aggressive tumors at the onset.

Biopsy of tumors to identify tissue type is recommended. Several other tumors may mimic optic nerve gliomas at both the orbit and the chiasm. Children with hydrocephalus require a ventricular shunt to relieve symptoms of hydrocephalus. Surgical excision of the optic nerve to remove the tumor completely should be considered if vision is already negligible. This is most easily accomplished when the tumor is intraorbital. Patients with chiasmatic tumors causing hypothalamic dysfunction require partial excision and radiation therapy with doses greater than 4,500 rads.

Because radiation has serious adverse effects on the developing brain, progressive chiasmatic and hypothalamic tumors in children less than 5 years of age have been treated with chemotherapy (actinomycin D and vincristine) without radiation therapy (Packer et al, 1988). Chemotherapy may prevent disease progression without shrinking tumor size and delay radiation therapy until the child is older.

Pituitary Adenoma

Pituitary adenomas represent only 1% to 2% of intracranial tumors of childhood. The sexes are affected equally.

CLINICAL FEATURES. The initial diagnosis is usually during adolescence. Amenorrhea is usually the first symptom in girls with prolactin-secreting tumors. Galactorrhea may also be present. In boys, the initial features are growth retardation, delayed puberty, and headache.

Papilledema is rare, but optic atrophy is present in 10% to 20% of cases. Visual field defects may be unilateral temporal, bitemporal, or occasionally homonymous.

DIAGNOSIS. Visualization of the tumor and identification of its extrasellar extent are best accomplished by MRI. Measurement of hormone production is useful in distinguishing tumor type. Increased concentration of prolactin is recorded in 60% of adenomas, growth hormone in 15%, and adrenocorticotropic hormone in 12%; 12% of adenomas are nonfunctioning.

TREATMENT. The tumor can be totally resected when restricted to the sella. In such cases, the outcome is generally good, the recurrence rate is low, and hormone replacement therapy is not always required. Radiation therapy should be used in patients with partial excision or recurrence.

HEREDITARY OPTIC ATROPHY

Hereditary optic neuropathies may affect only the visual system, or the visual system and central nervous system, or multisystems. Multisystem disease is usually caused by mitochondrial dysfunction (Huber, 1994). These disorders can cause acute, subacute, or chronic decline in visual acuity. Diagnosis relies on family history and DNA analysis.

Dominant Optic Neuropathy

CLINICAL FEATURES. The onset of visual disturbances is insidious, but most patients date the onset to the first decade, usually 4 to 8 years of age (Glaser, 1990). The progressive reduction in visual acuity occurs equally in both eyes and may be mild, with vision remaining between 20/40 and 20/200. Considerable asymmetry between the eyes is common. In some cases the disease is identified only because other family members are affected.

Visual fields show central, paracentral, or cecocentral scotomas, which are best delineated with red test objects. Optic atrophy primarily affects the temporal portion of the disk, which appears pale. Additional neurologic abnormalities are unusual.

DIAGNOSIS. Family history of the defect is critical for diagnosis. It is distinguished from Leber hereditary optic neuropathy by the absence of microangiopathy.

TREATMENT. No treatment is available.

Infantile Refsum Disease

Infantile Refsum disease is a generalized peroxisomal disorder that is closely related to the oculocerebrorenal syndrome and neonatal adrenoleukodystrophy (see Chapter 6). It is probably different from the later onset Refsum disease, described in Chapter 7. Autosomal recessive inheritance is suspected.

CLINICAL FEATURES. The initial features are early acquired blindness and deafness. These are usually detected during infancy and may be congenital. Subsequent features are slow neurologic deterioration characterized by dementia, ataxia, hypotonia, and nystagmus (Torvik et al, 1988). Hepatomegaly and growth retardation are common features. Death ordinarily occurs in the second decade.

DIAGNOSIS. The concentration of protein in the spinal fluid is elevated, and EEG may show epileptiform activity. Liver transaminase levels are elevated, as is the serum concentration of bile acids. An elevated concentration of serum phytannic acid is essential to the diagnosis.

TREATMENT. No treatment is available.

Leber Hereditary Optic Neuropathy

Leber hereditary optic neuropathy (LHON) is a multisystem mitochondrial disease caused by one or more mutations of the mtDNA at positions 11778, 3460, and 4484 (Riordan-Eva et al, 1995). The point mutation at position 11778 is the most common and accounts for about half of cases of LHON. It causes abnormalities in respiratory complex chain I. Similar phenotypes are produced by mutations in complexes III and IV. Intrafamily phenotypic variability may be caused by the ratio of mutant to normal mtDNA within an individual, but interfamily variability is probably caused by alternative mutations.

CLINICAL FEATURES. Less than half of patients have a family history of similar disease. The characteristic early symptoms is rapid loss of vision in young, otherwise healthy men. Onset is usually between 18 and 23 years, but children younger than 10 years of age may be affected. Age at onset may vary by several decades within a kindred.

The initial complaint is usually painless blurred central vision in one eye, described as fogging of vision or central fading of color. The other eye ordinarily shares the symptoms within days or weeks but may remain unimpaired for several years. Examination of the visual fields reveals first central and then cecocentral scotomas.

The characteristic changes in the ocular fundus include circumpapillary telangiectatic microangiopathy, edema of the nerve fiber layer around the disk, and absence of peripapillary

staining on fluorescein angiography. However, some patients never have these characteristic features even at the time of acute visual loss. Telangiectatic microangiopathy may be observed in presymptomatic maternal family members. As the patient's symptoms develop, the nerve fiber layer becomes swollen; retinal vessels on and around the disk become dilated, tortuous, and telangiectatic; and hemorrhages appear in the nerve fiber layer. Atrophy first appears in the papillomacular bundle and then involves the rest of the retina. The vascular bed involutes, leaving a pale retina and optic atrophy.

Visual improvement occurs in perhaps 20% of patients within 1 to 5 years after vision is lost. This occurs mainly in the 14484 mutation; recovery in the more common 11778 mutation is rare. Ten percent are reported to regain full vision. Once vision is restored, relapses do not occur.

Although visual loss is the only symptom in most families, neurologic impairment may be an associated feature in some. Commonly associated disturbances include dystonia, spastic paraplegia, and ataxia. Some family members may have neurologic impairment without optic atrophy, and some have optic atrophy without neurologic impairment.

Childhood-onset cases have the greatest likelihood of regaining vision.

DIAGNOSIS. LHON should be suspected in every kindred with optic neuropathy or with progressive neurologic impairment in which transmission is restricted to the maternal line. The optic fundus changes, especially the microangiopathy, are the basis for diagnosis in the context of a compatible family history. Fluorescein angiography shows the development and involution of the telangiectatic microangiopathy and is useful in the diagnosis before symptoms occur.

TREATMENT. No treatment is available.

Wolfram Syndrome

The major features of Wolfram syndrome are juvenile diabetes mellitus, optic atrophy, and bilateral neurosensory hearing loss (Aldenhovel et al, 1991). Autosomal recessive inheritance is the presumed pattern of genetic transmission, but most cases are sporadic in occurrence.

CLINICAL FEATURES. The onset of diabetes is usually in the first decade. Insulin therapy is required soon after diagnosis. Visual loss progresses rapidly in the second decade but does not lead to complete blindness. Diabetes is not thought to cause optic atrophy. It is more likely that all clinical features result from a progressive neurodegenerative process. The sensorineural hearing loss affects high frequencies first and progresses slowly, rarely leading to severe hearing loss. Features reported in some patients include anosmia, autonomic dysfunction, ptosis, external ophthalmoplegia, tremor, ataxia, nystagmus, seizures, central diabetes insipidus, and endocrinopathies.

DIAGNOSIS. Diagnosis depends on the combination of juvenile-onset diabetes mellitus and optic atrophy. Wolfram syndrome is distinguished from infantile Refsum disease by the concurrence of diabetes mellitus and a later age at onset. MRI shows diffuse atrophy that correlates with the clinical syndrome (Rando et al, 1992). A family history of the syndrome is not always present.

TREATMENT. Each of the clinical features is treated symptomatically.

INTRAOCULAR TUMORS

Although retro-orbital tumors generally cause strabismus and proptosis, intraocular tumors always diminish visual acuity. Retinoblastoma is the most common malignant intraocular tumor. Its prompt recognition can be lifesaving.

The typical features of intraocular tumor in a young child are an abnormal appearance of the eye, loss of vision, and strabismus. Monocular blindness is usually unrecognized by parents. Older children may complain of visual blurring and floaters. Ocular pain is uncommon.

Leukokoria, a white pupillary reflex, is the initial feature in most children with retinoblastoma. This is first noted in bright sunlight or in a flash photograph; the pupil does not constrict and has a white color. Strabismus occurs when visual acuity is impaired. The sighted eye is used for fixation, and the other remains deviated outward in all directions of gaze.

Most children with intraocular tumors are referred directly to an ophthalmologist. A neurologist may be the primary consulting physician when the tumor is part of a larger syndrome that includes mental retardation. Such syndromes include retinoblastoma associated with deletion of the long arm of chromosome 13, retinal astrocytoma associated with tuberous sclerosis, choroidal hemangioma associated with Sturge-Weber disease, and optic nerve glioma in children with neurofibromatosis.

TAPETORETINAL DEGENERATIONS

Most tapetoretinal degenerations are hereditary and due to inborn errors of lipid or carbohydrate metabolism. These disorders also cause dementia, peripheral neuropathy, and ataxia as initial features, and are discussed in several chapters. The conditions discussed here are less common, but other neurologic features are not prominent initial complaints.

Cockayne Syndrome

Cockayne syndrome, like xeroderma pigmentosum (see Chapter 5), is a disorder of DNA repair (Broughton et al, 1995). It is believed to be transmitted by autosomal recessive inheritance with a male-to-female bias of 3:1.

CLINICAL FEATURES. Primary pigmentary degeneration of the retina occurs during infancy. Affected children appear cachectic, and a disproportionate dwarfism develops in which the limbs are large compared with the trunk. The characteristic facies includes lack of subcutaneous fat with prominence of facial bones, enophthalmos, a beaklike nose, and large ears. Mental deficiency and microcephaly are constant features. Neurologic signs may include cerebellar ataxia, involuntary movements, spasticity, peripheral neuropathy, sensorineural hearing loss, and ocular motor apraxia.

DIAGNOSIS. The constellation of clinical signs suggests the diagnosis. Hyperbetaglobulinemia, hyperinsulinemia, and hyperlipoproteinemia are present in some cases.

TREATMENT. No treatment is available, but ultraviolet light exposure must be avoided.

Laurence-Moon-Biedel Syndrome

Lawrence-Moon-Biedel syndrome comprises a heterogeneous group of disorders that share similar ocular and systemic features. It is transmitted by autosomal recessive inheritance.

CLINICAL FEATURES. Pigmentary retinopathy usually is manifested in the second decade. It may be characterized by salt-and-pepper retinopathy, macular pigmentation, or macular degeneration. In some patients, the retina appears normal, but the electroretinogram always shows abnormalities. Other cardinal features include hypogenitalism, obesity, polydactyly, and mental retardation. Less common associated features are sensorineural deafness, cataract, external ophthalmoplegia, and diabetes mellitus.

DIAGNOSIS. Diagnosis depends on recognition of the clinical constellation of symptoms and signs.

TREATMENT. No treatment is available for the underlying defect.

Disorders of the Pupil

In the awake state the size of the pupil is constantly changing in response to light and autonomic input. This pupillary unrest is called *hippus*. An isolated disturbance of pupillary size is not evidence of intracranial disease.

Essential Anisocoria

Between 20% and 30% of healthy people have an observable difference in the size of their pupils. Like congenital ptosis, it may go unnoticed until late childhood or adult life and then it is thought to be a new finding. The difference is constant at all levels of illumination but may be greater in darkness. The absence of other pupillary dysfunction or disturbed ocular motility suggests essential anisocoria, but old photographs are invaluable to confirm the diagnosis.

Tonic Pupil Syndrome (Adie Syndrome)

CLINICAL FEATURES. Tonic pupil syndrome is caused by a defect in the orbital ciliary ganglion. The onset usually occurs after childhood but has been reported as early as 5 years. Women are affected more often than men.

The defect is usually monocular and is manifested as anisocoria or photophobia. The abnormal pupil is slightly larger in bright light but changes little, if at all, with alteration in illumination. In a dark room the normal pupil dilates and then is larger than the tonic pupil. With attempted accommodation, which may also be affected, the pupil constricts slowly and incompletely and redilates slowly afterward.

Binocular tonic pupils are seen in children with dysautonomia and are also seen in association with diminished tendon reflexes (*Holmes-Adie syndrome*).

DIAGNOSIS. The tonic pupil is supersensitive to parasympathomimetic agents; constriction is achieved with 0.125% pilocarpine.

TREATMENT. The condition is benign and seldom needs treatment.

Fixed Dilated Pupil

CLINICAL FEATURES. A fixed dilated pupil is an ominous sign in unconscious patients because it suggests transtentorial herniation (see Chapter 4). However, a dilated pupil that does not respond to light or accommodation in a child who is otherwise well and has no evidence of ocular motor dysfunction can result only from the application of a pharmacologic agent or from a ruptured sphincter. The application may be accidental, as when a drug or chemical is inadvertently wiped from hand to eye. Many cosmetics contain chemicals that can induce mydriasis. A careful history must be obtained.

Factitious application of mydriatics is a relatively common attention-seeking device, and convincing parents that the problem is self-inflicted may be difficult.

DIAGNOSIS. Pilocarpine 1% should be instilled in both eyes, using the normal eye as a control. Parasympathetic denervation produces prompt constriction. A slow or incomplete response indicates pharmacologic dilation.

TREATMENT. Most pharmacologic agents are long acting, and their affects cannot be rapidly reversed.

Horner Syndrome

Horner syndrome is characterized by sympathetic denervation; it may be congenital or acquired. When acquired, it may occur at birth as part of a brachial plexus injury, during infancy from neuroblastoma, or in childhood from tumors or injuries affecting the superior cervical ganglion or the carotid artery.

CLINICAL FEATURES. Unilateral Horner syndrome consists of the following ipsilateral features: mild to moderate ptosis (ptosis of the lower lid in one third); miosis, which is best appreciated in dim light so that the normal pupil dilates; anhidrosis of the face, heterochromia, and apparent enophthalmos when the syndrome is congenital.

DIAGNOSIS. Horner syndrome may be caused by disruption of the sympathetic system anywhere from the hypothalamus to the eye. Brainstem disturbances from stroke are common in adults, but peripheral lesions are more common in children. Topical instillation of 1% hydroxyamphetamine produces pupillary dilation after 30 minutes when postganglionic denervation is present. Ten percent cocaine solution produces little or no dilatation regardless of the site of abnormality.

TREATMENT. Treatment depends on the underlying cause.

Argyll Robertson Pupil

Argyll Robertson pupil is associated with tertiary syphilis and is almost never seen in children. Both pupils are irregularly shaped and miotic. Iris atrophy may be present. The pupils respond poorly to light, but response to near fixation is present (light-near dissociation).

Aniridia

Hypoplasia of the iris may occur as a solitary abnormality or may be associated with mental retardation, genitourinary abnormalities, and Wilms tumor. About two thirds of cases are genetic and transmitted as an autosomal dominant trait. One third of sporadic cases are associated with Wilms tumor. In some cases, the short arm of chromosome 11 is abnormal.

REFERENCES

Aldenhovel HBG, Gallenkamp U, Suelemana CA. Juvenile onset diabetes mellitus, central diabetes insipidus and optic atrophy (Wolfram syndrome)—neurological findings and prognostic implications. Neuropediatrics 1991;22:103-106.

Beck RW, Cleary, PA, Trobe JD, et al. The effect of corticosteroids for acute optic neuritis on the subsequent development of multiple sclerosis. N Engl J Med 1993;329: 1764-1769.

Brey RL, Hart RG, Sherman DG, et al. Antiphospholipid antibodies and cerebral ischemia in young people. Neurology 1990;40:1190-1196.

Brodsky MC, Glasier CM. Optic nerve hypoplasia: Clinical significance of associated central nervous system abnormalities on magnetic resonance imaging. Arch Ophthalmol 1993;111:66-74.

Broughton BC, Thompson AF, Harcourt SA, et al. Molecular and cellular analysis of the DNA repair defect in a patient in xeroderma pigmentosum complementation group D who has the clinical features of xeroderma pigmentosum and Cockayne syndrome. Am J Hum Genet 1995;56:167-174.

Chamberlain MC. Recurrent chiasmatic-hypothalamic glioma treated with oral etoposide. Arch Neurol 1995;52: 509-513.

Costello JM, Gluckman PD. Neonatal hypopituitarism: A neurological perspective. Dev Med Child Neurol 1988;30: 190-199.

Dutton JJ. Gliomas of the anterior visual pathways. Surv Ophthalmol 1994;38:427-452.

Glaser JS. Topical diagnosis: Prechiasmal visual pathways. In Glaser JS (ed): Neuroophthalmology, 2nd edition. JB Lippincott, Philadelphia, 1990; 108.

Hetelekidis S, Barnes PD, Tao ML, et al. 20-year experience in childhood craniopharyngioma. Int J Radiat Oncol Biol Phys 1993;27:189-195.

Huber A. Genetic diseases of vision. Curr Opin Neurol 1994;7:65-68.

Johns DR, Sadun AA. Cuban epidemic optic neuropathy: Mitochondrial DNA analysis. J Neuroophthalmol 1994;14: 130-134.

Kriss A, Francis DA, Cuendet F, et al. Recovery after optic neuritis in childhood. J Neurol Neurosurg Psychiatry 1988;51:1253-1258.

Lambert SR, Sherman S, Taylor D, et al. Concordance and recessive inheritance of Leber congenital amaurosis. Am J Med Genet 1993;46:275-277.

Listernick R, Darling C, Greenwald M, et al. Optic pathway tumors in children: The effect of neurofibromatosis type 1 on clinical manifestations and natural history. J Pediatr 1995;127:718-722.

Lloyd IC, Goss-Sampson, Jeffrey BG, et al. Neonatal cataract: Aetiology, pathogenesis and management. Eye 1992;6: 184-196.

Packer RJ, Sutton LN, Bilaniuk LT, et al. Treatment of chiasmatic/hypothalamic gliomas of childhood with chemotherapy: an update. Ann Neurol 1988;23:79-85.

Rajan B, Ashley S, Gorman C, et al. Craniopharyngioma— long term results following limited surgery and radiotherapy. Radiother Oncol 1993;26:1-10.

Rando TA, Horton JC, Layzer RB. Wolfram syndrome: Evidence of a diffuse neurodegenerative disease by magnetic resonance imaging. Neurology 1992;42:1220-1224.

Riikonen R, Donner M, Erkkila H. Optic neuritis in children and its relationship to multiple sclerosis: A clinical study of 21 children. Dev Med Child Neurol 1988;30:349-359.

Riordan-Eva P, Sanders MD, Govan GG, et al. The clinical features of Leber's hereditary optic neuropathy defined by the presence of a pathogenic mitochondrial DNA mutation. Brain 1995;118:319-337.

Robinson GC, Jan JE. Acquired ocular visual impairment in children: 1969-1989. Am J Dis Child 1993;147:325-328.

Rodriguez A, Lozano JA, del Pozo D, et al. Post-traumatic transient cortical blindness. Int Ophthalmol 1993;17: 277-283.

Rodriguez LA, Edwards MSB, Levin VA. Management of hypothalamic gliomas in children: An analysis of 33 cases. Neurosurgery 1990;26:242-246.

Rolih CA, Ober KP. Pituitary apoplexy. Endocrinol Metab Clin North Am 1993;22:291-302.

Steinberg A, Ronen S, Zlotogorski Z, et al. Central nervous system involvement in Leber congenital amaurosis. Hum Mut 1992;1:478-485.

Tippin J, Corbett JJ, Kerber RE, et al. Amaurosis fugax and ocular infarction in adolescents and young children. Ann Neurol 1989;26:69-77.

Torvik A, Torp S, Kase BF, et al. Infantile Refsum's disease: A generalized peroxisomal disorder. Case report with postmortem examination. J Neurol Sci 1988;85:39-53.

van Ekeren GJ, Stadhouders AM, Smeitink JA, et al. A retrospective study of patients with the hereditary syndrome of congenital cataract, mitochondrial myopathy of heart and skeletal muscle and lactic acidosis. Eur J Pediatr 1993;152:255-259.

Warburg M. Classification of microphthalmus and coloboma. J Med Genet 1993;30:664-669.

Wolin MJ, Lavin PJM. Spontaneous visual recovery from traumatic optic neuropathy after blunt head injury. Am J Ophthalmol 1990;109:430-435.

Wong VC. Cortical blindness in children: A study of etiology and prognosis. Pediatr Neurol 1991;7:178-185.

Zeki SM, Dutton GH. Optic nerve hypoplasia in children. Br J Ophthalmol 1990;76:300-304.

17

Lower Brainstem and Cranial Nerve Dysfunction

This chapter considers disorders causing dysfunction of the seventh through twelfth cranial nerves. Many such disorders also disturb extraocular motility, and are discussed in Chapter 15. The chapter assignment is based on the usual initial clinical feature. For example, myasthenia gravis is discussed in Chapter 15 because diplopia is a more common initial complaint than dysphagia.

An acute isolated cranial neuropathy, such as facial palsy, is usually a less ominous sign than multiple cranial neuropathies and is likely to have a self-limited course. However, an isolated cranial neuropathy may be the first sign of progressive cranial nerve dysfunction. Therefore conditions causing isolated and multiple cranial neuropathies are discussed together because they may not be separable at onset.

Facial Weakness and Dysphagia
ANATOMIC CONSIDERATIONS
Facial Movement

The motor nucleus of the facial nerve is a column of cells in the ventrolateral tegmentum of the pons. Nerve fibers leaving the nucleus take a circuitous path in the brainstem before emerging close to the pontomedullary junction, where they enter the internal auditory meatus with the acoustic nerve. After bending forward and downward around the inner ear, the facial nerve traverses the temporal bone in the facial canal and exits the skull at the stylomastoid foramen. Extracranially, the facial nerve passes into the parotid gland, where it divides into several branches and is distributed to all muscles of facial expression except the levator palpebrae superioris.

Sucking and Swallowing

The sucking reflex requires the integrity of the trigeminal, facial, and hypoglossal nerves. Stimulation of the lips produces coordinated movements of the face, jaw, and tongue. The automatic aspect of the reflex disappears after infancy but returns in bilateral disease of the cerebral hemispheres.

The afferent arc of the swallowing reflex is formed by fibers of the trigeminal and glossopharyngeal nerves that end in the nucleus solitarius. The efferent arc is formed by the motor root of the trigeminal nerve, glossopharyngeal and vagus fibers from the nucleus ambiguus, and the hypoglossal nerves. A swallowing center that coordinates the reflex is located in the lower pons and upper medulla. A bolus of food stimulates the pharyngeal wall or back of the tongue, and food is moved into the esophagus by

■ TABLE 17-1
Causes of Congenital Facial Weakness

Aplasia of facial muscles
Birth injury
Congenital myotonic dystrophy (see Chapter 6)
Congenital bilateral perisylvian syndrome
Fiber-type disproportion myopathies (see Chapter 6)
Myasthenic syndromes
   Congenital myasthenia (see Chapter 15)
   Familial infantile myasthenia (see Chapter 6)
   Transitory neonatal myasthenia (see Chapter 6)

■ TABLE 17-2
Causes of Postnatal Facial Weakness

Autoimmune and Postinfectious
Bell palsy
Idiopathic cranial polyneuropathy
Miller Fisher syndrome (see Chapter 10)
Myasthenia gravis (see Chapter 15)
Genetic
Muscular disorders
   Facioscapulohumeral syndrome, infantile form
   Facioscapulohumeral syndrome (see Chapter 7)
   Fiber-type disproportion myopathies (see Chapter 6)
   Myotonic dystrophy (see Chapter 7)
   Oculopharyngeal dystrophy
Myasthenic syndromes
   Congenital myasthenia (see Chapter 15)
   Familial infantile myasthenia (see Chapter 6)
Recurrent facial palsy
   Melkersson syndrome
   Multiple cranial neuropathies
Hypertension
Infectious
Diphtheria
Herpes zoster oticus
Infectious mononucleosis
Lyme disease (see Chapter 2)
Otitis media
Sarcoidosis
Tuberculosis
Juvenile Progressive Bulbar Palsy (Fazio-Londe Disease)
Metabolic Disorders
Hyperparathyroidism
Hypothyroidism
Osteopetrosis (Albers-Schönberg disease)
Multiple Sclerosis (see Chapter 10)
Syringobulbia
Toxins
Trauma
Delayed
Immediate
Tumor
Glioma of brainstem (see Chapter 15)
Histiocytosis X
Leukemia
Meningeal carcinoma
Neurofibromatosis

action of the tongue, palatine arches, soft palate, and pharynx.

APPROACH TO DIAGNOSIS

Weakness of facial muscles may be caused by supranuclear palsy (pseudobulbar palsy), intrinsic brainstem disease, or disorders of the motor unit: facial nerve, neuromuscular junction, and facial muscles (Tables 17-1 and 17-2). The differential diagnosis of dysphagia is similar (Table 17-3) except that isolated dysfunction of the nerves that enable swallowing is very uncommon.

Pseudobulbar Palsy

Because the corticobulbar innervation of most cranial nerves is bilateral, pseudobulbar palsy occurs only when hemispheric disease is bilateral. Many children with pseudobulbar palsy have a progressive degenerative disorder of gray or white matter. Most of these disorders are discussed in Chapter 5 because dementia is usually the initial feature. Bilateral stroke, simultaneous or in sequence, causes pseudobulbar palsy in children; the usual causes are coagulation defects, leukemia, and trauma (see Chapter 11). Pseudobulbar palsy is a major feature of the *congenital bilateral perisylvian syndrome*, discussed in this chapter.

Pseudobulbar palsy is characterized by inability to use bulbar muscles in voluntary effort, whereas reflex movements initiated at a brainstem level are performed normally. Extraocular motility is unaffected. The child can reflexly suck, chew, and swallow but cannot coordinate these reflexes for eating; movement of a food bolus from the front of the mouth to the back has a volitional component. Emotionally derived facial expression occurs but facial movements do not occur on command. Severe dysarthria is often present. Affected muscles do not show atrophy or fasciculations. The gag reflex and jaw jerk are usually exaggerated, and emotional volatility is often an associated feature.

Newborns with familial dysautonomia have difficulty in feeding, despite normal sucking and swallowing, because they fail to coordinate the two reflexes (see Chapter 6). The differential diagnosis of feeding difficulty in an alert newborn is summarized in Table 6-8. Children with cerebral palsy often have a similar disturbance in

■ TABLE 17–3
Neurologic Causes of Dysphagia

Autoimmune/Postinfectious
Dermatomyositis (see Chapter 7)
Guillain-Barré syndrome (see Chapter 7)
Idiopathic cranial polyneuropathy
Myasthenia gravis (see Chapter 15)
Transitory neonatal myasthenia gravis (see Chapter 6)

Congenital or Perinatal
Aplasia of brainstem nuclei
Cerebral palsy (see Chapter 5)
Chiari malformation (see Chapter 10)
Congenital bilateral perisylvian syndrome
Syringobulbia

Genetic
Degenerative disorders (see Chapter 5)
Familial dysautonomia (see Chapter 6)
Familial infantile myasthenia (see Chapter 6)
Fiber-type disproportion myopathies (see Chapter 6)
Myotonic dystrophy (see Chapters 6 and 7)
Oculopharyngeal dystrophy

Glioma of Brainstem

Infectious
Botulism (see Chapters 6 and 7)
Diphtheria
Poliomyelitis (see Chapter 7)

Juvenile Progressive Bulbar Palsy

---

the coordination of chewing and swallowing, and feeding is impaired.

Motor Unit Disorders

Disorders of the facial nuclei and nerves always cause ipsilateral facial weakness and atrophy, but associated features vary with site of abnormality:

1. Motor nucleus: Hyperacusis is present, but taste, lacrimation, and salivation are normal.

2. Facial nerve between the pons and the internal auditory meatus: Taste is spared, but lacrimation and salivation are impaired and hyperacusis is present.

3. Geniculate ganglion: Taste, lacrimation, and salivation are impaired, and hyperacusis is present.

4. Facial nerve from the geniculate ganglion to the stapedius nerve: Taste and salivation are impaired and hyperacusis is present, but lacrimation is normal.

5. Facial nerve from the stapedius nerve to the chorda tympani: Taste and salivation are impaired, hyperacusis is not present, and lacrimation is normal.

■ TABLE 17–4
Causes of Recurrent Cranial Neuropathies/Palsy

Familial
  Isolated facial palsy
  Melkersson syndrome
Hypertensive facial palsy
Myasthenia gravis
Sporadic multiple cranial neuropathies
Toxins

---

6. Facial nerve below the exit of the chorda tympani nerve: Only facial weakness is present.

Disturbances of cranial nerve nuclei seldom occur in isolation; they are often associated with other features of brainstem dysfunction (bulbar palsy). Usually some combination of dysarthria, dysphagia, and diplopia is present. Examination may show strabismus, facial diplegia, loss of gag reflex, atrophy of bulbar muscles, and fasciculations of the tongue.

The weakness of myasthenia gravis and facial myopathies is almost always bilateral, whereas brainstem disorders usually begin on one side but eventually cause bilateral impairment. Facial nerve palsies are usually unilateral. The differential diagnosis of recurrent facial palsy or dysphagia is limited to disorders of the facial nerve and neuromuscular junction (Table 17–4).

CONGENITAL BILATERAL PERISYLVIAN SYNDROME

This syndrome is a migrational disorder of unknown cause that results in pachygyria of the sylvian and rolandic regions (Kuzniecky et al, 1993).

CLINICAL FEATURES. All affected children have a pseudobulbar palsy that causes failure of speech development and dysphagia. Mental retardation and seizures are present in approximately 85% of cases. The retardation varies from mild to severe and the seizures, which begin between 4 and 12 years, may be atypical absence, atonic/tonic, partial, or generalized tonic-clonic.

DIAGNOSIS. Magnetic resonance imaging (MRI) shows bilateral perisylvian gyral malformations, pachygyria, and polymicrogyria (Figure 17–1). Postmortem studies have confirmed the MRI impression.

TREATMENT. The seizures are usually difficult to control and corpus callosotomy has been useful in some cases with intractable drop attacks (Kuzniecky et al, 1994). Speech therapy does not overcome the speech disorder and sign language should be taught to children of near-normal intelligence.

CONGENITAL FACIAL ASYMMETRY

Most facial asymmetries observed at birth are caused by congenital aplasia of muscle and are not traumatic. Facial diplegia, whether complete or incomplete, suggests the Möbius syndrome or other congenital muscle aplasia. Complete unilateral palsies are likely to be traumatic in origin, whereas partial unilateral palsies may be either traumatic or aplastic. The term *neonatal facial asymmetry* is probably more accurate than *facial nerve palsy* to denote partial or complete unilateral facial weakness in the newborn and emphasizes the difficulty in differentiating traumatic nerve palsies from congenital aplasias.

Aplasia of Facial Muscles

CLINICAL FEATURES. The Möbius syndrome is the best-known congenital aplasia of facial nerve nuclei and facial muscles. Whether nerve or muscle aplasia is the primary event has not

☐ F I G U R E   1 7 – 1 Perisylvian syndrome (MRI). This child has lissencephaly and schizencephaly. Bilateral disturbances in the perisylvian region caused a pseudobulbar palsy.

been established. Facial diplegia may occur alone, with bilateral abducens palsies, or with involvement of several cranial nerves (D'Cruz et al, 1993). Congenital malformations elsewhere in the body—dextrocardia, talipes equinovarus, absent pectoral muscle, and limb deformities—may be associated features.

DIAGNOSIS. Congenital facial diplegia is by definition a Möbius syndrome. MRI of the brain is indicated in all such cases to determine whether other cerebral malformations are present. Causes other than primary malformation must be considered as well. Some cases are due to intrauterine toxins or structural disturbances of the brainstem, such as vascular malformation or infarction.

Electromyography (EMG) can help determine the timing of injury. Denervation potentials are present only if the facial nuclei or nerves were injured 2 to 6 weeks before the study. Facial muscles that are aplastic as a result of Möbius syndrome or nerve injury occurring early in gestation do not show active denervation.

TREATMENT. No treatment is available.

Depressor Anguli Oris Muscle Aplasia

CLINICAL FEATURES. Isolated unilateral weakness of the depressor anguli oris muscle (DAOM) is the most common cause of facial asymmetry at birth. One corner of the mouth fails to move downward when the child cries. All other facial movements are symmetric. The lower lip on the paralyzed side feels thinner to palpation, even at birth, suggesting antepartum hypoplasia.

DIAGNOSIS. Traumatic lesions of the facial nerve would not selectively injure nerve fibers to the DAOM and spare all other facial muscles. Electrodiagnostic studies aid in differentiating aplasia of the DAOM from traumatic injury. In aplasia the conduction velocity and latency of the facial nerve are normal. Fibrillations are not present at the site of the DAOM. Instead, motor unit potentials are absent or decreased in number.

TREATMENT. No treatment is available or needed. The DAOM is not a significant component of facial expression in older children and adults, and its absence is not noticed.

Birth Injury

Perinatal traumatic facial palsy is a disorder of large term newborns delivered vaginally after a prolonged labor. The palsy is more often caused by nerve compression against the sacrum during labor than by misapplication of forceps. Children with forceps injuries, an unusual event, have forceps marks on the cheeks.

CLINICAL FEATURES. The clinical expression of complete unilateral facial palsy in the newborn can be subtle and may not be apparent immediately after birth. Failure of eye closure on the affected side is the first noticeable evidence of weakness. Only when the child cries does flaccid paralysis of all facial muscles become obvious. The eyeball rolls up behind the open lid, the nasolabial fold remains flat, and the corner of the mouth droops during crying. The normal side, which appears to pull and distort the face, may be thought to be paralyzed, and the paralyzed side normal.

When paralysis of the facial nerve is partial, the orbicularis oculi is the muscle most frequently spared. In these injuries the compression site is usually over the parotid gland with sparing of nerve fibers that course upward just after leaving the stylomastoid foramen.

DIAGNOSIS. Facial asymmetry is diagnosed by observation of the crying newborn. The facial skin must be carefully examined for laceration. Otoscopic examination is useful to establish the presence of hemotympanum. EMG does not alter the management of the palsy.

TREATMENT. Prospective studies regarding the natural outcome of perinatal facial nerve injuries are not available. Most authors are optimistic and indicate a high rate of spontaneous recovery. The optimism may be warranted, but it is based on anecdotal experience alone. In the absence of data on long-term outcome, the efficacy of suggested therapeutic measures cannot be evaluated. Most newborns should not be subjected to surgical intervention unless the nerve is lacerated at delivery. In that event the best response is to reconstitute the nerve if possible or at least to allow the proximal stump a clear pathway toward regeneration by debridement of the wound.

CONGENITAL DYSPHAGIA

Congenital dysphagia is usually associated with infantile hypotonia and is therefore discussed in Chapter 6. Because the neuroanatomic substrates of swallowing and breathing are contiguous, congenital dysphagia and dyspnea are often concurrent (Alvord and Shaw, 1989). Isolated aplasia of cranial nerve nuclei subserving swallowing has not been documented, but I have seen one infant in whom the clinical syndrome was consistent with isolated aplasia.

AUTOIMMUNE AND POSTINFECTIOUS DISORDERS

Most cases of acute unilateral facial neuritis (Bell palsy) or bilateral facial neuritis are attributed to postinfectious demyelination of the nerve (Keane, 1994). A bilateral Bell palsy is distinguished from the Guillain-Barré syndrome (acute inflammatory demyelinating polyneuropathy) mainly on the basis that in Bell palsy the tendon reflexes are preserved in the limbs. The Guillain-Barré syndrome is discussed in Chapter 7.

Bell Palsy

Bell palsy is an acute idiopathic paralysis of the face caused by dysfunction of the facial nerve. In adults, the pathogenesis is considered to be immune-mediated demyelination or vascular insufficiency. Childhood cases are almost always considered to be immune mediated. The annual incidence is approximately 3/100,000 in the first decade, 10/100,000 in the second decade, and 25/100,000 in adults. Only 1% of cases have clinical evidence of bilateral involvement but most have electrophysiologic abnormalities on the unaffected side.

CLINICAL FEATURES. A history of viral infection, usually upper respiratory, is recorded in many cases, but the frequency is not significantly greater than expected by chance. The initial feature of neuritis is often pain or tingling in the ear canal ipsilateral to the subsequent facial palsy. Sensory symptoms, when present, are usually mild and do not demand medical attention.

The palsy has an explosive onset and becomes maximal within hours. It may be noticed first by the child or the parents. The palsy affects all muscles on one side of the face. Half the face sags, enlarging the palpebral fissure. Weakness of the levator palpebrae muscle prevents closure of the lid. Efforts to use muscles of expression cause the face to pull to the normal side. Eating and drinking become difficult, and the dribbling of liquids from the weak corner of the mouth causes embarrassment.

The most commonly affected portion of the nerve is within the temporal bone; taste, lacrimation, and salivation are impaired, and hyperacusis is present. However, examination of all facial nerve functions in small children is difficult and precise localization is not critical to diagnosis or prognosis.

The muscles remain weak for 2 to 4 weeks and then strength returns spontaneously. The natural history of Bell palsy in children has not been studied, but experience indicates that almost all patients recover completely.

DIAGNOSIS. Every child with acute unilateral facial weakness must be fully examined to determine whether the palsy is an isolated abnormality. Mild facial weakness on the other side or the absence of tendon reflexes in the limbs suggests the possibility of Guillain-Barré syndrome. Such children must be watched carefully for the development of progressive limb weakness.

Possible underlying causes (e.g., hypertension, infection, trauma) of facial nerve palsy should be excluded before the diagnosis of Bell palsy is considered satisfactory. The ear ipsilateral to the facial palsy should be examined for herpetic lesions (see later discussion of herpes zoster oticus). *Cranial computed tomography (CT) or MRI is not indicated for every child with acute, isolated facial palsy.* A more reasonable approach is to watch the child and recommend an imaging study if other neurologic disturbances develop or if the palsy does not begin to resolve within 1 month.

TREATMENT. If the blink reflex is absent, the cornea must be protected. The eye should be patched when the child is outside the home or at play, and artificial tears should be applied several times a day to keep the cornea moist.

The use of corticosteroids has been advocated in adults, but has no scientific basis in children because their prognosis for complete spontaneous recovery is excellent. The clinician who elects to use corticosteroid therapy must first exclude hypertension or infection as an underlying cause.

Idiopathic Cranial Polyneuropathy

As the name implies, idiopathic cranial neuropathy is of uncertain nosology. A postinfectious basis is presumed, and some consider it to be an abortive form of the Guillain-Barré syndrome.

CLINICAL FEATURES. Onset is usually in adults, and most childhood cases occur in adolescence. Similar cases had been described in infants, but because many subsequently developed limb weakness, infantile botulism was the more likely diagnosis (see Chapter 6).

Constant, aching facial pain usually precedes weakness by hours or days. The pain is often localized to the temple or frontal region but can be anywhere in the face. Weakness may develop all in a day or may evolve over several weeks. Extraocular motility is usually affected. Facial and trigeminal nerve disturbances occur in half of cases, but lower cranial nerve involvement is uncommon. Occasional patients have transitory visual disturbances, ptosis, pupillary abnormalities, and tinnitus. Tendon reflexes in the limbs remain active.

Recurrent idiopathic cranial neuropathies occur as sporadic cases in adults but are usually familial in children.

DIAGNOSIS. The differential diagnosis includes the Guillain-Barré syndrome, infant and childhood forms of botulism, brainstem glioma, juvenile progressive bulbar palsy, pontobulbar palsy with deafness, and the Tolosa-Hunt syndrome. Preservation of tendon reflexes in idiopathic cranial polyneuropathy is the major feature distinguishing it from the Guillain-Barré syndrome. Botulism can be separated clinically by its prominent autonomic dysfunction and limb weakness (see Chapters 6 and 7). Cranial nerve dysfunction in patients with brainstem glioma, juvenile progressive bulbar palsy, and pontobulbar palsy with deafness usually evolves over a longer period. The Tolosa-Hunt syndrome of painful ophthalmoplegia and idiopathic cranial polyneuropathy shares many features and may be a variant of the same disease process (see Chapter 15).

All laboratory findings are normal. MRI of the brainstem should be performed in all cases to exclude the possibility of a brainstem glioma. Examination of the cerebrospinal fluid occasionally reveals a mild elevation of protein concentration and a lymphocyte count of 5 or 6/mm^3.

TREATMENT. The disease is self-limited, and full recovery is expected 2 to 4 months from onset. Corticosteroids are used routinely and are believed to relieve facial pain and shorten the course. The relief of pain may be dramatic, but evidence documenting a shortened course is lacking.

GENETIC DISORDERS

Facioscapulohumeral Syndrome

The facioscapulohumeral (FSH) syndrome (see Chapter 7) sometimes begins during infancy as facial diplegia (Brouwer et al, 1995). All forms of the disease are transmitted by autosomal dominant inheritance with the genetic defect on chromosome 4p.

CLINICAL FEATURES. The onset of infantile FSH is usually during infancy and no later than age 5. Facial diplegia, the first feature, is often misdiagnosed as congenital aplasia of facial muscles when the onset is in infancy. Later, nasal speech and sometimes ptosis develop. Progressive proximal weakness begins 1 to 2 years after onset, first affecting the shoulders and then the pelvis. Pseudohypertrophy of the calves may be present. Tendon reflexes are depressed and then absent in weak muscle. Progression of weakness is often rapid and unrelenting, leading to disability and death from respiratory insufficiency before age 20, but may also stabilize for long intervals and not cause severe disability until adult life.

Retinal telangiectasia and high-frequency hearing loss occur in about of half of affected families (Padberg et al, 1995). Both conditions are progressive and may not be symptomatic in early childhood.

DIAGNOSIS. The diagnosis should be suspected in any child with progressive facial diplegia. A family history of FSH syndrome cannot always be obtained because the defect may be only minimally expressed in the affected parent.

Myasthenia gravis and brainstem glioma must be considered in infants with progressive facial diplegia. The serum concentration of creatine kinase is helpful in differentiating these disorders. It is usually elevated in the infantile FSH syndrome and is normal in myasthenia gravis and brainstem glioma.

Electrophysiologic studies show brief, small-amplitude polyphasic potentials in weak muscles and a normal response to repetitive nerve stimulation.

TREATMENT. No treatment is available.

Oculopharyngeal Muscular Dystrophy

Oculopharyngeal muscular dystrophy is usually transmitted by autosomal dominant inheritance. It is most often described in families of French-Canadian descent but is not restricted to any ethnic group (Hardiman et al, 1993). Most cases that are not clearly transmitted by autosomal dominant inheritance will prove to be mitochondrial myopathies (Schröder et al, 1995).

CLINICAL FEATURES. Onset is usually in the fourth decade but may be as early as adolescence. The initial features are ptosis and dyspha-

gia, followed by proximal weakness in the legs and external ophthalmoplegia. Eventually all skeletal muscle is affected, but smooth muscle and cardiac muscle are spared.

Many patients with oculopharyngeal muscular dystrophy also have EMG or biopsy evidence of denervation in the limbs. The neurogenic features may be attributed to neuronopathy rather than neuropathy suggesting that this disorder is actually a spinal (bulbar) muscular atrophy.

DIAGNOSIS. Myasthenia gravis must be excluded by an edrophonium chloride (Tensilon) test and repetitive nerve stimulation. The serum concentration of creatine kinase is normal, but EMG of affected muscles shows brief, small-amplitude polyphasic potentials, as well as prolonged polyphasic potentials and fibrillations. The presence of ragged-red fibers on histologic examination of muscle indicates an underlying mitochondrial myopathy.

TREATMENT. Therapy is directed at the symptoms. Ptosis can be corrected by levator palpebrae shortening, and dysphagia may be helped by constrictor or cricopharyngeal myotomy.

Melkersson Syndrome

As many as 7% of facial palsies are recurrent (Keane, 1994). Autosomal dominant inheritance with variable expression is suspected in many cases. Some members of a kindred may have only recurrent facial nerve palsy, whereas others have recurrent neuropathies of the facial and ocular motor nerves.

The Melkersson syndrome may be genetically distinct from other recurrent facial palsies but could also represent the concurrence of several linked genetic errors such as recurrent facial palsy, lingua plicata (deeply furrowed tongue), and migraine.

CLINICAL FEATURES. Melkersson syndrome is a rare disorder characterized by the triad of recurrent facial palsy, lingua plicata, and facial edema. Attacks of facial palsy usually begin in the second decade, but the deeply furrowed tongue is present from birth.

The first attack of facial weakness is indistinguishable from Bell palsy except that it may be preceded by a migraine-like headache. Subsequent attacks are associated with facial edema, which is soft, painless, nonerythematous, and nonpruritic. The edema is most often asymmetric, involving only the upper lip on the paralyzed side, but may affect the cheek and eyelid of one or both sides. Attacks of facial swelling may be precipitated by cold weather or emotional stress and are not coincident with attacks of facial palsy.

Lingua plicata is present in 30% to 50% of cases. Furrowing and deep grooving on the dorsal surface of the tongue are permanent from birth. This feature is transmitted by autosomal dominant inheritance and occurs as an isolated finding in some families.

DIAGNOSIS. Melkersson syndrome can be diagnosed when two features of the triad are present. It should be considered in any child with a personal or family history of recurrent facial palsy or recurrent facial edema. The presence of lingua plicata in any member of the kindred confirms the diagnosis.

TREATMENT. This disease has no established treatment. Corticosteroids have not proved beneficial.

HYPERTENSION

Unilateral facial palsy may be a feature of malignant hypertension in children. The palsy is caused by swelling and hemorrhage into the facial canal.

CLINICAL FEATURES. The course of the facial paralysis is indistinguishable from that in Bell palsy. The nerve is compressed in its proximal segment, impairing lacrimation, salivation, and taste. The onset coincides with a rise in blood pressure to greater than 120 mm Hg, and recovery begins when pressure is reduced. The duration of palsy varies from days to weeks. Recurrences are associated with repeated episodes of hypertension.

DIAGNOSIS. The occurrence of facial palsy in a child with known hypertension suggests that the hypertension is out of control. Blood pressure should be measured in every child thought to have Bell palsy.

TREATMENT. Control of hypertension is the only effective treatment.

INFECTION

The facial nerve is sometimes involved when bacterial infection spreads from the middle ear to the mastoid. External otitis may lead to facial nerve involvement by spread of infection from the tympanic membrane to the chorda tympani.

Diphtheria may cause single or multiple cranial neuropathies from a direct effect of its toxin. Facial palsy, dysarthria, and dysphagia are potential complications. Basilar meningitis, from tuberculosis or other bacterial infections, causes inflammation of cranial nerves as they leave the brain and enter the skull. Multiple and bilateral cranial nerve involvement is usually progressive.

Herpes Zoster Oticus (Ramsay Hunt Syndrome)

Herpes zoster oticus is caused by herpes zoster infection of the geniculate ganglion.

CLINICAL FEATURES. The initial feature is pain in and behind the ear. This pain is often more severe and persistent than that expected with Bell palsy. Unilateral facial palsy, which cannot be distinguished from Bell palsy by appearance, follows. However, examination of the ipsilateral ear, especially in the fossa of the helix and behind the lobule, shows a vesicular eruption characteristic of herpes zoster.

DIAGNOSIS. The only historical feature distinguishing herpes zoster oticus from Bell palsy is the severity of ear pain. Examination of the ear for vesicles is critical to the diagnosis.

TREATMENT. Herpes zoster infections are self-limited but painful. Oral acyclovir, 800 mg, five times a day, has been found beneficial in adults to shorten the course of disease and reduce pain.

Sarcoidosis

Cranial nerve dysfunction is the most common neurologic complication of sarcoidosis. It is usually caused by basilar granulomatous meningitis, but the facial nerve may also be involved when parotitis is present.

CLINICAL FEATURES. Onset is usually in the third decade but may be as early as adolescence. Neurologic complications occur in only 5% of patients with sarcoidosis but when present, they are often an early feature of the disease. Facial nerve palsy, unilateral or bilateral, is the single most common feature. Visual impairment or deafness is next in frequency. Single cranial neuropathies are present in 73%, and multiple cranial neuropathies in 58%. Any cranial nerve except the accessory nerve may be involved. Systemic features of sarcoidosis occur in almost every case: intrathoracic involvement is present in 81% and ocular involvement is present in 50%.

Uveoparotitis is an uncommon manifestation of sarcoidosis. The patient ordinarily comes to medical attention because of visual impairment and a painful eye. The mouth is dry and the parotid gland swollen. Facial nerve compression and palsy are present in 40% of cases.

DIAGNOSIS. Sarcoidosis should be considered in any patient with single or multiple cranial neuropathies. The suspicion is confirmed by documentation of multisystem disease. Radiographs of the chest either establish or are compatible with the diagnosis in almost all patients with neurologic manifestations.

Increased serum concentrations of serum angiotensin-converting enzyme (ACE) are detected in approximately 75% of patients with active pulmonary disease, and patients with neurosarcoidosis may have elevated cerebrospinal fluid concentrations of ACE. Biopsy of lymph nodes or other affected tissues provides histologic confirmation.

TREATMENT. Prednisone, 0.5 to 1 mg/kg/day, should be maintained until a clinical response is evident and then tapered at a slow enough rate to prevent relapse. The prognosis for neurologic complications of sarcoidosis is good without treatment, but corticosteroids appear to hasten recovery.

JUVENILE PROGRESSIVE BULBAR PALSY

Juvenile progressive bulbar palsy, also known as *Fazio-Londe disease,* is a motor neuron disease limited to bulbar muscles. Most cases are sporadic and autosomal recessive inheritance is suspected. However, two reports of affected mothers and sons suggest the existence of a rare autosomal dominant subtype (McShane et al, 1992).

CLINICAL FEATURES. Two clinical patterns are described. Stridor is the initial feature in early-onset cases (ages 1 to 5 years). Progressive bulbar palsy occurs and respiratory compromise causes death within 2 years of onset. Respiratory symptoms are less common in later-onset cases (ages 6 to 20 years). The initial feature may be facial weakness, dysphagia, or dysarthria. Eventually, all the lower motor cranial nerve nuclei are affected, but the ocular motor nerve nuclei are spared. Fasciculations and atrophy of the arms are reported in some cases, but limb strength and tendon reflexes are usually spared despite severe bulbar palsy.

DIAGNOSIS. The major diagnostic considerations are myasthenia gravis and brainstem glioma. MRI of the brainstem is needed to exclude brainstem tumors, and EMG is useful to show active denervation of facial muscles with sparing of the limbs and normal repetitive stimulation of nerves.

Children with rapidly progressive motor neuron disease affecting the face and limbs should be considered to have a childhood form of amyotrophic lateral sclerosis.

TREATMENT. The disorder is often devastating. A previously normal child is no longer able to speak intelligibly or swallow. Feeding gastrostomy is soon required. The child needs considerable psychological support. No treatment is available for the underlying disease.

METABOLIC DISORDERS

Hyperparathyroidism

The most common neurologic features of primary hyperparathyroidism are headache and confusion (see Chapter 2). Occasionally, hyperparathyroidism is associated with a syndrome that is similar to amyotrophic lateral sclerosis and includes ataxia and internuclear ophthalmoplegia. Dysarthria and dysphagia are prominent features.

Hypothyroidism

Cranial nerve abnormalities are unusual in hypothyroidism. Deafness is the most common feature, but acute facial nerve palsy resembling Bell palsy is also described.

Osteopetrosis (Albers-Schönberg Disease)

The term *osteopetrosis* encompasses at least three hereditary skeletal disorders of increased bond density (Shapiro, 1993). The most common form is transmitted by autosomal recessive inheritance.

The calvarium becomes thickened, and cranial nerves are compressed and compromised as they pass through the bone. Deafness and facial diplegia are common features. Treatment with high-dose calcitrol is effective in reducing the sclerosis and preventing many neurologic complications.

SYRINGOBULBIA

Syringobulbia is usually the medullary extension of a cervical syrinx (see Chapter 12), but may also originate in the medulla. The syrinx usually involves the nucleus ambiguus and the spinal tract and motor nucleus of the trigeminal nerve. Symptoms in order of frequency are headache, vertigo, dysarthria, facial parasthesias, dysphagia, diplopia, tinnitus, and palatal palsy (Morgan and Williams, 1992).

TOXINS

Most neurotoxins produce either diffuse encephalopathy or peripheral neuropathy. Only ethylene glycol, trichlorethylene, and chlorocresol exposure cause selective cranial nerve toxicity. Ethylene glycol is used as an antifreeze. Ingestion causes facial diplegia, hearing impairment, and dysphagia. Trichlorethylene intoxication can cause multiple cranial neuropathies but has a predilection for the trigeminal nerve and was previously used in the treatment of tic douloureux.

Chlorocresol, a compound used in the industrial production of heparin, was reported to cause recurrent unilateral facial palsy in an exposed worker. Inhalation of the compound caused tingling of one side of the face followed by weakness of the muscles. The neurologic disturbance was brief, relieved by exposure to fresh air, and could be reproduced experimentally.

TRAUMA

Facial palsy following closed head injury is usually associated with bleeding from the ear and fracture of the petrous bone.

CLINICAL FEATURES. The onset of palsy may be immediate or may be delayed for as long as 3 weeks after injury. In most cases the interval is between 2 and 7 days. The mechanism of delay is unknown.

DIAGNOSIS. Electrophysiologic studies are helpful in prognosis. If the nerve is intact but shows a conduction block, recovery usually begins within 5 days and is complete. The majority of patients with partial denervation recover full facial movement but have evidence of aberrant reinnervation. Full recovery is not expected when denervation is complete.

TREATMENT. The management of traumatic facial palsy is controversial. Some authors have recommended surgical decompression and corticosteroids, but no evidence supporting either mode of therapy is available.

TUMORS

Tumors of the facial nerve are rare in children. The major neoplastic cause of facial palsy is brainstem glioma (see Chapter 15), followed by

tumors that infiltrate the meninges, such as leukemia, meningeal carcinoma, and histiocytosis X. Acoustic neuromas are unusual in childhood and are limited to children with neurofibromatosis type 2. These neuromas cause hearing impairment before facial palsy and are discussed in the next section.

 Hearing Impairment and Deafness

ANATOMIC CONSIDERATIONS

Sound is mechanically funneled through the external auditory canal to the tympanic membrane, causing it to vibrate. The vibrations are transmitted by ossicles to the oval window of the cochlea, the sensory organ of hearing. The air-filled space from the tympanic membrane to the cochlea is the middle ear. The membranous labyrinth within the osseous labyrinth is the principal structure of the inner ear. It contains the cochlea, the semicircular canals, and the vestibule. The semicircular canals and vestibule are the sensory organs of vestibular function. The cochlea consists of three fluid-filled canals wound into a snail-like configuration.

The organ of Corti is the transducer within the cochlea that converts mechanical to electrical energy. Impulses are transmitted in the auditory portion of the eighth nerve to the ipsilateral cochlear nuclei of the medulla. The cochlear nuclei on each side transmits information to both superior olivary nuclei, causing bilateral representation of hearing throughout the remainder of the central pathways. From the superior olivary nuclei, impulses are transmitted by the lateral lemniscus to the inferior colliculus. Further cross-connections occur in collicular synapses. Rostrally directed fibers from the inferior colliculi ascend to the medial geniculate and auditory cortex of the temporal lobe.

SYMPTOMS OF AUDITORY DYSFUNCTION

The major symptoms of disturbance in the auditory pathways are hearing impairment, tinnitus, and hyperacusis. Hearing impairment is characterized in infants by failure to develop speech (see Chapter 5), and in older children by inattentiveness and poor school performance.

Fifty percent of infants use words with meaning by 12 months and join words into sentences by 24 months. Failure to accomplish these tasks by 21 months and 3 years, respectively, is always abnormal. A hearing loss of 25 to 30 dB is sufficient to interfere with normal acquisition of speech (Nadol, 1993).

Hearing Impairment

Hearing impairment is classified as conductive, sensorineural (perceptive), or central.

Conductive hearing impairment is caused by disturbances in the external or middle ear; the mechanical vibrations that make up the sensory input of hearing are not faithfully delivered to the inner ear because the external canal is blocked or the tympanic membrane or ossicles are abnormal. The major defect in conductive hearing loss is sound amplification. Patients with conductive hearing impairment are better able to hear loud speech in a noisy background than soft speech in a quiet background.

Sensorineural hearing impairment is caused by disturbances of the cochlea or auditory nerve. The frequency content of sound is improperly analyzed and transduced. High frequencies may be selectively lost. Individuals with sensorineural hearing impairment have difficulty discriminating speech when there is background noise.

Central hearing impairment results from disturbance of the cochlear nuclei or their projections to the cortex. Brainstem lesions usually cause bilateral hearing impairment. Cortical lesions lead to difficulty in processing information. Pure-tone audiometry is normal, but speech discrimination is impaired by background noise or competing messages.

Thirty percent of childhood deafness is clearly genetic in origin, 40% is acquired, and the remaining 30% is idiopathic. Many of the idiopathic cases are probably genetic as well (Beighton, 1990).

Tinnitus

Tinnitus is the illusion of noise in the ear. The noise is usually high pitched and constant. In most cases tinnitus is caused by disturbances of the auditory nerve, but it may occur as a simple partial seizure originating from the primary auditory cortex. Sounds generated by the cardiovascular system (heartbeat and bruit) are sometimes audible, especially while a person is lying down, but should not be confused with tinnitus.

Hyperacusis

Hyperacusis is caused by failure of the stapedius muscle to dampen sound by its effect on the ossicles. This occurs when the chorda tympani branch of the facial nerve is damaged (see the discussion of Bell palsy earlier in this chapter).

APPROACH TO THE PATIENT

Hearing assessment in the office is satisfactory for severe hearing impairment but is unsatisfactory for detecting loss of specific frequency bands. The speech and hearing handicap generated by a high-frequency hearing impairment should not be underestimated.

When testing an infant, the physician should stand behind the patient and provide interesting sounds to each ear. Such sounds could be produced by bells, chimes, rattles, or a tuning fork. Dropping a large object and watching the infant and parents startle from the noise is not a test of hearing. Once the infant sees the source of the interesting sound or hears it several times, interest is lost. Therefore, different high-frequency and low-frequency sounds should be used for each ear. The normal responses of the infant are to become alert and to attempt to localize the source of the sound.

Older children can be tested by observing their response to spoken words at different intensities and with tuning forks that provide pure tones of different frequencies. The *Rinne test* compares air conduction (conductive plus sensorineural hearing) with bone conduction (sensorineural hearing). A tuning fork is held against the mastoid process until the sound fades and is then held 1 inch from the ear. Normal children hear the vibration produced by air conduction twice as long as that produced by bone conduction. Impaired air conduction with normal bone conduction indicates a conductive hearing loss.

The *Weber test* compares bone conduction in the two ears. It is based on the principle that signals transmitted by bone conduction are localized to the better-hearing ear or the ear with the greater conductive deficit. A tuning fork is placed at the center of the forehead, and the patient is asked whether sound is perceived equally in both ears. A normal response is to hear the sound in the center of the head. If bone conduction is normal in both ears, sound is localized to an ear with impaired air conduction because the normal blocking response of air conduction is lacking. If a sensorineural hearing impairment is present in one ear, bone conduction is perceived in the good ear.

Otoscopic examination is imperative in every child with hearing problems or tinnitus. The cause may be seen through the speculum in the form of impacted wax, otitis media, perforated tympanic membrane, or cholesteatoma.

TESTS OF HEARING

The usual battery of audiologic tests include pure-tone air and bone conduction testing, and measures of speech threshold and word discrimination.

Pure-Tone Audiometry

Selected frequencies are presented by earphones (air conduction) or by a vibrator applied to the mastoid (bone conduction), and the subject is asked to determine the minimum level perceived for each frequency. Normal hearing levels are defined by an international standard. The test can be performed adequately only in children old enough to cooperate. With conductive hearing impairment, air conduction is abnormal and bone conduction is normal; with sensorineural hearing impairment, both are abnormal; and with central hearing impairment, both are normal.

Speech Tests

The *speech reception threshold* measures the intensity at which a subject can repeat 50% of presented words. The *speech discrimination test* measures the subject's ability to understand speech at normal conversational levels. Both tests are abnormal out of proportion to pure-tone loss with auditory nerve disease, abnormal in proportion to pure-tone loss with cochlear disease, and normal with conductive and central hearing loss.

Special Tests

Cochlear lesions may cause *diplacusis* and *recruitment.* Auditory nerve lesions produce *tone decay.* Diplacusis is a distortion of pure tones so that the subject perceives a mixture of tones. With recruitment the sensation of loudness increases at an abnormally rapid rate as the intensity of sound is increased. Tone decay is diminished perception of a suprathreshold tone with time.

Brainstem Auditory Evoked Response

The brainstem auditory evoked response (BAER) is used to test hearing and the integrity of the brainstem auditory pathways in infants and small children. No cooperation is required, and sedation improves the accuracy of results.

When each ear is stimulated with repetitive clicks and simultaneous recordings are made from an electrode over the ipsilateral mastoid referenced to the forehead, five waves are recorded. Wave I is generated by the acoustic nerve, wave II by the cochlear nerve, wave III by the superior olivary complex, wave IV by the lateral lemniscus, and wave V by the inferior colliculus.

The BAER first appears at a conceptional age of 26 to 27 weeks. The absolute latencies of waves I and V and V-I interpeak interval decline progressively with advancing conceptional age. The latency of wave V bears an inverse relationship to the intensity of the stimulus and can be used to test hearing.

An initial test is performed with a stimulus intensity of 70 dB. If wave V is not produced, hearing is impaired and the test should be repeated at higher intensities until a response threshold is found. If wave V is present, the test is repeated at sequential reductions of 10 dB until the lowest intensity capable of producing wave V—the hearing threshold—is established. Because the latency of wave V is proportional to the intensity of the stimulus, a latency-intensity curve can be drawn. In normal newborns, the latency of wave V will decrease by 0.24 to 0.44 ms for each 10 dB in sound intensity between 70 and 110 dB.

In children with conductive hearing impairment, the time required to transmit sound across the middle ear and activate the cochlea is prolonged and the total amount of sound energy is reduced. As a consequence the latency of wave I is prolonged and the latency-intensity curve of wave V shifts to the right by an amount equivalent to the hearing impairment, without any alteration in the slope of the curve.

In children with sensorineural hearing impairment, the latency-intensity curve of wave V is shifted to the right because of the hearing impairment and in addition the slope of the curve becomes steeper, exceeding 0.55 ms/dB.

CONGENITAL DEAFNESS

Congenital deafness is often missed in the newborn unless there is an obvious deformity of the external ear or a family history of genetic hearing loss. Congenital ear malformations are present in approximately 2% of newborns with congenital deafness. Genetic factors account for about one third of all congenital deafness and half of profound deafness (Table 17-5).

Aplasia of Inner Ear

Inner ear aplasia is always associated with auditory nerve abnormalities. The three main types are (1) the *Michel defect,* complete absence of the otic capsule and eighth cranial nerve; (2) the *Mondini defect,* incomplete development of the bony and membranous labyrinths and dysgenesis of the spiral ganglion; and (3) the *Scheibe defect,* dysplasia of the membranous labyrinth and atrophy of the eighth nerve.

Chromosome Disorders

Hearing impairment is relatively uncommon in children with chromosomal disorders. Abnormalities of chromosome 18 are often associated with profound sensorineural hearing loss and malformations of the external ear.

Genetic Disorders

Isolated Deafness

Isolated deafness in newborns and infants is usually genetic and may be transmitted by autosomal dominant, autosomal recessive, or X-linked inheritance. In many sporadic cases the hearing loss proves to be transmitted by autosomal recessive inheritance.

The association of congenital deafness and external ear deformities is often caused by genetic disorders transmitted by autosomal dominant inheritance, but chromosomal disorders and fetal exposure to drugs and toxins must be considered as well. Maternal use of heparin during pregnancy produces an embryopathy characterized by skeletal deformities, flattening of the nose, cerebral dysgenesis, and deafness.

In the absence of external malformation, a sporadic case of deafness may not be suspected until the infant fails to develop speech. Intrauterine infection with cytomegalovirus is an important cause of congenital deafness (see Chapter 5). Nearly 1% of newborns in the United States are infected with cytomegalovirus, and sensorineural hearing loss develops in approximately 10% (Raynor, 1993). Rubella embryopathy was once an important cause of deafness, but it has been almost eliminated in the United States by mass immunization.

■ TABLE 17-5
Hearing Impairment and Deafness

Congenital
Aplasia of inner ear
 Michel defect
 Mondini defect
 Scheibe defect
Chromosome disorders
 Trisomy 13
 Trisomy 18
 18q-syndrome
Genetic disorders
 Isolated deafness
 Pendred syndrome
 Usher syndrome
 Waardenburg syndrome
Intrauterine viral infection (see Chapter 5)
Maternal drug use

Drugs
Antibiotics
Beta-blockers
Chemotherapy

Genetic Neurologic Disorders
Facioscapulohumeral dystrophy (see Chapter 7)
Familial spastic paraplegia (see Chapter 12)
Hereditary motor sensory neuropathies (see Chapter 7)
Hereditary sensory autonomic neuropathies (see Chapter 9)
Infantile Refsum disease (see Chapter 16)
Neurofibromatosis type 2 (see "Acoustic Neuroma")
Pontobulbar palsy with deafness
Mitochondrial disorders (see Chapter 8)
Spinocerebellar degenerations (see Chapter 10)
Xeroderma pigmentosum (see Chapter 5)

Infectious Diseases
Bacterial meningitis
Otitis media (see "Vertigo")
Sarcoidosis (see "Facial Weakness")
Viral encephalitis (see Chapter 2)
Viral exanthems

Metabolic Disorders
Hypothyroidism
Ménière disease (see "Vertigo")

Skeletal Disorders
Apert acrocephalosyndactyly
Cleidocranial dysostosis
Craniofacial dysostosis (Crouzon disease)
Craniometaphyseal dysplasia (Pyle disease)
Klippel-Feil syndrome
Mandibulofacial dysostosis (Treacher Collins syndrome)
Osteogenesis imperfecta
Osteopetrosis (Albers-Schönberg disease)

Trauma (see "Vertigo")

Tumor
Acoustic neuroma
Cholesteatoma (see "Vertigo")

Pendred Syndrome

Pendred syndrome is a genetic defect in thyroxine synthesis transmitted by autosomal recessive inheritance. It is characterized by goiter and sensorineural hearing impairment (Kabakkaya et al, 1993).

CLINICAL FEATURES. Sensorineural hearing impairment is present at birth and is severe in 50% of cases. Milder hearing impairment may not be detected until the child is 2 years of age. Vestibular function may also be impaired.

A diffuse, non-nodular goiter becomes apparent during the first decade, often in infancy. No clinical signs of hypothyroidism are present. Growth and intelligence are usually normal.

DIAGNOSIS. The laboratory method for assessing iodide organification is the perchlorate discharge test. It is a measure of thyroidal radioactive iodine content following the administration of potassium perchlorate. A decline of 10% or more from baseline levels of thyroidal radioactive iodine is considered a positive result.

TREATMENT. Goiter is best treated medically and not surgically. Exogenous hormone decreases production of thyroid-stimulating hormone with subsequent reduction in goiter size. Hearing loss is not reversible.

Usher Syndrome

The Usher syndrome, characterized by congenital deafness and retinitis pigmentosa, is transmitted by autosomal recessive inheritance, but genetic heterogeneity exists.

CLINICAL FEATURES. Bilateral severe sensorineural deafness is present at birth. Slowly progressive loss of vision caused by retinitis pigmentosa begins during the second decade and leads to blindness in the fifth decade or later. Vestibular responses to caloric testing are absent, and mild ataxia may be present. Mental retardation is present in 25% of cases.

DIAGNOSIS. The combination of retinitis pigmentosa and hearing impairment is also present in other syndromes: *Alstrom syndrome,* obesity and diabetes mellitus; *Cockayne syndrome* (see Chapter 16); *Laurence-Moon-Biedl syndrome,* mental deficiency, hypogonadism, obesity; and *Refsum disease* (see Chapter 7). Usher syndrome is the only one in which profound deafness is present at birth.

TREATMENT. Deafness is too profound to be corrected with hearing aids. No treatment is available.

Waardenburg Syndrome

The Waardenburg syndrome is clinically and genetically heterogeneous. It is transmitted by autosomal dominant inheritance and is caused by deletions within a segment of chromosome 2q35-37 (Pasteris et al, 1993).

CLINICAL FEATURES. The Waardenburg syndrome is relatively easy to recognize because of its cutaneous features: a white forelock, eyes of different colors (usually different shades of blue), hypertelorism, and depigmented dermal patches. Phenotypic variability is the rule and deafness is not a constant feature.

DIAGNOSIS. The diagnosis is established by the family history and the cutaneous features. DNA analysis is not commercially available.

TREATMENT. No treatment is available.

ACQUIRED HEARING IMPAIRMENT

Drug-Induced Impairment

Antibiotics are the most commonly used class of drugs with potential ototoxicity in children. The incidence of toxic reactions is greatest with amikacin, furosemide, and vancomycin and only a little less with kanamycin and neomycin. Permanent damage is unusual with any of these drugs. The characteristic syndrome consists of tinnitus and high-frequency hearing impairment. Vancomycin produces hearing loss only when blood concentrations exceed 45 μg/ml.

By contrast, aminoglycosides may cause irreversible cochlear toxicity, which begins as tinnitus, progresses to vertigo and high-frequencyhearing impairment, and finally impairs all frequencies. This is of special concern in sick preterm newborns who are given aminoglycosides for periods of 15 days or longer.

Beta-adrenoceptor blocking drugs are a rare cause of hearing impairment and tinnitus. Cessation of therapy reverses symptoms. Cisplatin, an anticancer drug, has ototoxic effects in 30% of recipients. Tinnitus is the major feature. Hearing impairment occurs at frequencies above those used for speech.

Salicylates tend to concentrate in the perilymph of the labyrinth and are ototoxic. Tinnitus and high-frequency hearing impairment result from long-term exposure to high doses.

Genetic Neurologic Disorders

Several of the disorders listed in Table 17–5 are discussed in other chapters. Sensorineural hearing impairment occurs as part of several spinocerebellar degenerations, hereditary motor sensory neuropathies, and sensory autonomic neuropathies. It is a major feature of Refsum disease (hereditary motor sensory neuropathy type IV) and can be controlled by dietary measures to reduce serum concentrations of phytanic acid.

Pontobulbar Palsy with Deafness

Pontobulbar palsy with deafness is a rare hereditary motor neuron disorder. The mode of transmission is not established (Hawkins et al, 1990). It shares many clinical features with juvenile progressive bulbar palsy, and some cases may be variant expressions of the same genetic error.

CLINICAL FEATURES. Onset most often occurs during the second decade. Progressive sensorineural hearing loss is the initial symptom and may affect first one ear and then the other. Deafness is accompanied or quickly followed by facial weakness and dysphagia. Tongue atrophy occurs in most cases, but masseter and ocular motor palsies are uncommon.

Approximately half of patients have evidence of pyramidal tract dysfunction, such as extensor plantar responses, and half have atrophy and fasciculations of limb muscle. Loss of tendon reflexes is an early feature of most cases.

Respiratory insufficiency is a common feature and a frequent cause of death.

DIAGNOSIS. The presence of deafness and areflexia distinguishes pontobulbar palsy from juvenile progressive bulbar palsy, but can also suggest a hereditary motor sensory neuropathy if symptoms of bulbar palsy are delayed. The diagnosis depends on the clinical features and cannot be confirmed by laboratory tests. MRI of the brainstem should be performed to exclude the possibility of tumor.

TREATMENT. A feeding gastrostomy is needed in most patients. No treatment is available for the underlying disease.

Infectious Diseases

Otitis media is a common cause of reversible conductive hearing impairment in children, but only rarely does suppurative infection spread to the inner ear (see "Vertigo" later in this chapter). Hearing impairment is a relatively common symptom of viral encephalitis (see Chapter 2) and may be an early feature. Sudden hearing loss

may also accompany childhood exanthems (chickenpox, mumps, measles), and in such cases virus can be isolated from the cochlear and auditory nerves.

The overall incidence of persistent unilateral or bilateral hearing loss in children with acute bacterial meningitis is 10%. The risk can be reduced by early treatment with dexamethasone (see Chapter 4). *Streptococcus pneumoniae* meningitis is also associated with a 20% incidence of persistent dizziness, gait ataxia, and other neurologic deficits.

The site of disease is probably the inner ear or auditory nerve. Organisms may gain access to the inner ear from the subarachnoid space. Otitis media is the source of meningitis in many children and produces a transitory conductive hearing loss, but it has not been proved to cause a permanent sensorineural hearing loss. It is common in many centers to screen all children hospitalized for treatment of acute bacterial meningitis with BAER audiometry prior to discharge.

Metabolic Disorders

Ménière disease is characterized by vertigo, tinnitus, and hearing impairment. Vertigo is often the presenting feature (see later discussion of vertigo).

Tinnitus and decreased hearing are common features of hypothyroidism and are reversible by thyroid replacement therapy.

Skeletal Disorders

The combination of hearing impairment and skeletal deformities almost always indicates a genetic disease. Skeletal disorders may be limited, usually to the face and digits, or generalized. Almost all are transmitted by autosomal dominant inheritance with variable expression. The exceptions are osteopetrosis, which is transmitted by autosomal recessive inheritance; craniometaphyseal dysplasia, which has both a dominant and a recessive form; and the Klippel-Feil anomaly, for which the pattern of transmission is uncertain.

Trauma

Acute auditory and vestibular injuries occur with fractures of the petrous portion of the temporal bone. Vestibular function is more likely to be impaired than auditory function (see "Vertigo" later in this chapter).

Tumor

Acoustic neuroma and cholesteatoma are the tumors most likely to impair children's hearing. Other cerebellopontine angle tumors are extremely rare before the third or fourth decade. Cholesteatoma is discussed in the section on vertigo.

Acoustic Neuroma

Acoustic neuromas are more properly classified as schwannomas of the eighth nerve. Only 6% of acoustic neuromas come to medical attention in the second decade, and even fewer are seen in the first decade. Children with acoustic neuroma almost always have *neurofibromatosis type 2 (NF2)*, a genetic disease distinct from neurofibromatosis type 1 (see Chapter 5). NF2 is transmitted by autosomal dominant inheritance with the locus on chromosome 22 (National Institutes of Health, 1990). It is characterized by bilateral acoustic neuromas, and the later development of other cerebral tumors such as meningioma, glioma, schwannoma, and juvenile posterior subcapsular lenticular opacity. Café au lait spots may be present on the skin but are fewer than five in number.

CLINICAL FEATURES. Deafness or tinnitus is the usual initial complaint. Approximately one third of patients have nonaudiologic symptoms, such as facial numbness or paresthesia, vertigo, headache, and ataxia. Hearing impairment is present in almost every patient; ipsilateral diminished corneal reflex occurs in half; and ataxia, facial hypesthesia or weakness, and nystagmus are found in 30% to 40%. Large tumors cause obstructive hydrocephalus with symptoms of increased intracranial pressure and brainstem compression.

DIAGNOSIS. Every child with progressive hearing impairment or tinnitus should be carefully examined for café au lait spots on the skin. The family history should be explored for acoustic neuroma or other neurologic disturbance.

Abnormalities in pure-tone audiometry and in the BAER are present in almost every patient. Audiometry is consistent with a sensorineural hearing impairment. Small tumors cause ipsilateral prolongation of the V-I interval or absence of wave I of the BAER; large tumors cause absence of waves on the ipsilateral side and prolongation of the V-III interval on the contralateral side as a result of brainstem compression.

Gadolinium-enhanced MRI is the test of choice to visualize tumors in the cerebellopontine angle (Figure 17–2).

☐ F I G U R E   1 7 – 2   CT of acoustic neuroma. A large tumor (*arrow*) is pressing on and displacing the brainstem.

TREATMENT. Acoustic neuromas must be resected, either by surgery or the photon (gamma ray) knife. Surgery often sacrifices residual hearing and sometimes causes a facial palsy. The superiority of the photon knife to standard surgery is not yet established.

Vertigo

Vertigo is the sensation of rotation or spinning. It can terrify small children. Balance is lost, and posture is difficult to maintain, giving the appearance of ataxia (see Chapter 10). Nausea and nystagmus are often associated features. When nystagmus is present, the fast phase is in the same direction as the perceived rotation. All symptoms are exacerbated by movement of the head.

ANATOMIC CONSIDERATIONS

The semicircular canals and the vestibule, within the labyrinth, are the sensory organs of the vestibular system. The stimulus for excitation of the semicircular canals is rotary motion of the head; for the vestibule it is gravity. Information from the sensory organs is transmitted by the vestibular portion of the eighth cranial nerve to the vestibular nuclei in the brainstem and the cerebellum. The vestibular nuclei have extensive connections with the cerebellum and medial longitudinal fasciculus. Cortical projections terminate in the superior temporal gyrus and frontal lobe.

APPROACH TO VERTIGO

History and Physical Examination

Children often complain of dizziness or lightheadedness but rarely complain of vertigo (Tusa et al, 1994). Those who complain of dizziness or lightheadedness must be carefully questioned about the sensation of rotation. Whether the subject or the environment is perceived to rotate is irrelevant. The illusion of rotation separates vertigo from presyncope, ataxia, and other disturbances of balance and localizes the disturbance to the vestibular system. Vertigo implies dysfunction of the labyrinth or vestibular nerve (peripheral vertigo) or the brainstem or temporal lobe (central vertigo).

Important historical points to document include the course of vertigo (acute, recurrent, chronic), precipitating events (trauma, infection, position change), association of hearing impairment and tinnitus, drug exposure, cardiovascular disease, and family history of migraine.

Acute, episodic attacks of vertigo, not induced by motion, are most often caused by migraine or epilepsy, with migraine as the more common of the two. A single, prolonged attack of vertigo, especially when combined with nausea and vomiting, is usually due to infection of the labyrinth or vestibular nerve. Chronic vertigo often waxes and wanes and may seem intermittent rather than chronic. Both central and peripheral causes of vertigo must be considered (Table 17-6), but the two are readily distinguished by their clinical and laboratory features (Table 17-7).

Special Tests

Caloric and audiometric testing is indicated for most children with chronic vertigo. Caloric testing is described in this section and audiometric testing in the section on hearing impairment. The Nylen-Hallpike test is useful to define position-induced vertigo.

Caloric Testing

The simplest method of caloric testing is to instill small quantities of cool water into the ex-

ternal auditory canal with a rubber-tipped syringe. The canal must first be inspected to determine whether there is clear passage to an intact tympanic membrane. A sufficient quantity of water is used, depending on the child's size, to keep the tympanic membrane cooled for 20 seconds. The eyes are then observed for nystagmus. A normal response is slow deviation of the eyes to the side stimulated, followed by a fast component to the opposite side. If stimulation with cool water fails to produce a response, the procedure is repeated with ice water. Absence of nystagmus indicates absence of peripheral vestibular function. Partial dysfunction of one vestibular apparatus results in asymmetry of response *(directional preponderance)*.

Electronystagmography

Electronystagmography is a technique that allows better quantification of caloric testing. A standard caloric stimulus is delivered into the ear, and the duration and velocity of nystagmus are recorded on paper by a machine designed for this purpose.

Nylan-Hallpike Test

In the Nylan-Hallpike test, the patient is tilted backward from the sitting position to the supine

■ TABLE 17-6
Causes of Vertigo

Drugs and toxins
Epilepsy
Complex partial seizures
Simple partial seizures
Infectious
Otitis media
Vestibular neuronitis
Ménière disease
Migraine
Basilar migraine (see Chapter 10)
Benign paroxysmal vertigo (see Chapter 10)
Motion sickness
Multiple sclerosis (see Chapter 10)
Psychogenic
Hyperventilation syndrome (see Chapter 1)
Panic attacks
Trauma
Migraine
Post-traumatic neurosis
Temporal bone fracture
Vestibular concussion
Whiplash injury

■ TABLE 17–7
Distinguishing Peripheral and Central Vertigo

Peripheral Vertigo

CLINICAL FEATURES

Hearing loss, tinnitus, and otalgia may be associated features.
Past pointing and falling in direction of unilateral disease occur.
Ataxia occurs with eyes closed in bilateral disease.
Vestibular and positional nystagmus is present.

LABORATORY FEATURES

Caloric testing reveals vestibular paresis, directional preponderance, or both.
Pure tone audiometry reveals sensorineural hearing loss.
Recruitment is present with end-organ disease and tone decay with nerve disease.

Central Vertigo

CLINICAL FEATURES

Cerebellar and cranial nerve dysfunction are frequently associated.
Hearing is intact.
Loss of consciousness may be associated.

LABORATORY FEATURES

Pure tone audiometry and speech discrimination are normal.
Comprehension of competing messages is impaired.
Caloric testing may reveal directional preponderance but not vestibular paresis.
Brainstem evoked response, EEG, CT, or MRI may be abnormal.

position so that the head hangs down below the level of the examining table. The head is then turned 45 degrees to the right, and the eyes are observed for position-induced nystagmus. Several minutes later, the maneuver is repeated with the head turned 45 degrees to the left, then repeated again with the head tilted 45 degrees backward.

CAUSES OF VERTIGO

Drugs

Many drugs that disturb vestibular function also disturb auditory function. This section deals only with drugs affecting vestibular function more than auditory function. Toxic doses of anticonvulsants and neuroleptics produce ataxia,

incoordination, and measurable disturbances of vestibular function, but patients do not ordinarily complain of vertigo.

Antibiotics are the main class of drugs with vestibular toxicity. Streptomycin, minocycline, and aminoglycosides have a high incidence of toxic reactions, and sulfonamides have a low incidence.

Streptomycin disturbs vestibular function but has little effect on hearing. A toxic milligram-per-kilogram dose can not be established because of variation in individual susceptibility. However, the vestibular toxicity of streptomycin is so predictable at high doses that the drug has been used to destroy vestibular function in patients with severe Ménière disease. Dihydrostreptomycin affects auditory function and spares vestibular function. It is so ototoxic that its use has been abandoned.

Minocycline produces nausea, vomiting, dizziness, and ataxia at standard therapeutic doses. Symptoms begin 2 to 3 days after treatment is started and cease 2 days after it is stopped. Gentamicin and other aminoglycosides have an adverse effect on both vestibular and auditory function. Some disturbance is noted in 2% of patients treated with gentamicin. Vestibular dysfunction, either alone or in combination with auditory dysfunction, occurs in 84% of cases, whereas auditory dysfunction alone occurs in only 16%. Ototoxic effects develop when the total dose exceeds 17.5 mg/kg.

Epilepsy

Vertigo can be the only feature of a simple partial seizure or the initial feature of a complex partial seizure. Between 10% and 20% of patients with complex partial seizures experience vertigo as an aura.

CLINICAL FEATURES. When vertigo is followed by a complex partial seizure, it is readily recognized as an aura. Diagnosis is more problematic when vertigo is the only feature of a simple partial seizure. The child ceases activity, becomes pale, appears frightened, and then recovers. Unsteadiness and nausea may be associated features.

DIAGNOSIS. Electroencephalography (EEG) is indicated in children with unexplained brief attacks of vertigo, especially when vestibular and auditory function is normal between attacks. Ambulatory EEG or 24-hour video monitoring may be needed to capture an attack if interictal EEG is normal.

TREATMENT. Management of simple and complex partial seizures is discussed in Chapter 2.

Infectious

Bacterial Infection

Otitis media and meningitis are leading causes of vestibular and auditory impairment in children. Acute suppurative labyrinthitis resulting from extension of bacterial infection from the middle ear has become uncommon since the introduction of antibiotics. However, even without direct bacterial invasion, bacterial toxins may cause serous labyrinthitis.

Chronic otitic infections cause labyrinthine damage by the development of *cholesteatoma*. A cholesteatoma is a sac containing keratin, a silvery-white debris shed by squamous epithelial cells. Such cells are not normal constituents of the middle ear but gain access from the external canal when the eardrum is repeatedly perforated by infection. Cholesteatomas erode surrounding tissues, including bone, and produce a fistula between the perilymph and the middle ear.

CLINICAL FEATURES. Acute suppurative or serous labyrinthitis is characterized by the sudden onset of severe vertigo, nausea, vomiting, and unilateral hearing loss. Meningismus may also be present. Chronic otitis causes similar symptoms. Fistula formation is identified when severe vertigo is provoked by sneezing, coughing, or merely applying pressure on the external canal. Otoscopic examination reveals evidence of otitis media and tympanic membrane perforation, and allows visualization of cholesteatoma.

DIAGNOSIS. When vestibular dysfunction develops in children with otitis media, radiographs or CT scans of the skull are needed to visualize erosion of bone or mastoiditis. The presence of meningismus or increased intracranial pressure (see Chapter 4) necessitates CT to exclude the possibility of abscess and then examination of cerebrospinal fluid to exclude meningitis.

TREATMENT. Vigorous antibiotic therapy and drainage of the infected area are required in every case. Myringotomy and mastoidectomy may be needed for drainage. Cholesteatomas are progressive and must be surgically excised.

Viral Infections

Viral infections may affect the labyrinth or vestibular nerve. The two are difficult to differentiate by clinical features, and the term *vestibular neuritis* or *neuronitis* is used to describe acute peripheral vestibulopathies. Vestibular neuritis may be part of a systemic viral infection, such as mumps, measles, and infectious mononucleosis, or it may occur in epidemics without an identifiable viral agent, or as part of a postinfectious cranial polyneuritis. The incidence in children is low, accounting for less than 7% of all cases (Sekitani et al, 1993).

CLINICAL FEATURES. The main feature is the acute onset of vertigo. Any attempt to move the head is met with severe exacerbation of vertigo, nausea, and vomiting. Nystagmus is present on fixation and increased by head movement. The patient is unable to maintain posture and lies motionless in bed. Recovery begins after 3 days. Spontaneous nausea diminishes, and nystagmus on fixation ceases. During the second week, vertigo decreases in severity but positional nystagmus is still present. Recovery is usually complete within 3 weeks.

DIAGNOSIS. The diagnosis is usually established on the basis of clinical features alone. Caloric testing shows unilateral vestibular paresis. Hearing is normal.

TREATMENT. During the acute phase the child must be kept in bed and provided with vestibular sedation. Diazepam or dimenhydrinate is given orally. Transdermal scopolamine should not be used in children, but may be used in adolescents. As recovery progresses, activity is gradually increased and sedation reduced.

Methylprednisolone may shorten the attack (Ariyasu et al, 1990).

Ménière Disease

Ménière disease is believed to be an overaccumulation of endolymph resulting in rupture of the labyrinth. It is uncommon in children.

CLINICAL FEATURES. The clinical features of hearing impairment, tinnitus, and vertigo are attributed to rupture of the labyrinth. Hearing impairment fluctuates and may temporarily return to normal when the rupture heals. Tinnitus may be ignored, but vertigo demands attention and is often the complaint that brings the disorder to attention.

A typical attack consists of disabling vertigo and tinnitus lasting 1 to 3 hours. The vertigo may be preceded by tinnitus, fullness in the ear, or increased loss of hearing. Tinnitus becomes worse during the attack. Pallor, sweating, nausea, and vomiting are often associated features.

Afterward, the patient is tired and sleeps. Attacks occur at unpredictable intervals for years and then subside, leaving the patient with permanent hearing loss. Bilateral involvement is present in 20% of cases.

Nystagmus is present during an attack. At first the fast component is toward the abnormal ear (irritative); later, as the attack subsides, the fast component is away (paralytic). Between attacks the results of examination are normal with the exception of unilateral hearing impairment.

DIAGNOSIS. Pure tone audiometry shows threshold fluctuation. Speech discrimination is preserved, and recruitment is present on the abnormal side. Caloric stimulation demonstrates unilateral vestibular paresis or directional preponderance.

TREATMENT. The underlying disease cannot be reversed. Treatment is directed at management of the acute attack and attempts to increase the interval between attacks. The acute attack is treated with bed rest, sedation, and antiemetics. Maintenance therapy usually consists of a low-salt diet and diuretics; neither provides substantial benefit.

Migraine

Seventeen percent of migraineurs report vertigo at the time of an attack. Such individuals have no difficulty in recognizing vertigo as a symptom of migraine. Another 10% experience vertigo in the interval between attacks and may have difficulty relating vertigo to migraine.

Brief (minutes), recurrent episodes of vertigo in infants and small children are recognized as a migraine equivalent, despite the absence of headache, because the attacks later evolve into classic migraine. Affected children appear ataxic, and for this reason the disorder is discussed in Chapter 10 (see "Benign Paroxysmal Vertigo").

Motion Sickness

Motion sickness is induced by unfamiliar body accelerations or a mismatch in information provided to the brain by the visual and vestibular systems during acceleration of the body. It is inhibited when motion in the visual field is in opposition to actual body movement. Therefore, looking out the window when driving reduces motion sickness. Small children in the back seat, where the only visual input is the car interior, are at the greatest risk for motion

sickness. The minivan, which allows children access to a window probably reduces the incidence of car sickness.

The prevalence of motion sickness depends on how violent the movement is and approaches 100% in the worst case. Twenty-five percent of a ship's passengers become sick during a 2- to 3-day Atlantic crossing, and 0.5% of commercial airline passengers are affected.

The first symptom is pallor, which is followed by nausea and vomiting. Because nausea usually precedes vomiting there is time to prevent vomiting in some situations. Stopping the motion is the best way to abort an attack. Early attacks may be inhibited by watching the environment move opposite the direction of body movement. Individuals with known susceptibility to motion sickness should take an antihistamine, diazepam, or scopolamine before travel.

Trauma

Fifty percent of children complain of dizziness and headache during the first 3 days after a closed head injury, with or without loss of consciousness. One third have persistent vertigo without hearing loss. This group may be separated into patients with direct trauma to the labyrinth *(vestibular concussion)* and those in whom the vestibular apparatus is not injured (whiplash injury, migraine, and vertiginous seizures). Children with post-traumatic neurosis complain of dizziness or giddiness but do not experience the illusion of rotation.

Vestibular Concussion

CLINICAL FEATURES. Vestibular concussion follows blows to the parieto-occipital or temporoparietal region of the skull. Severe vertigo is present immediately after injury. The child is unsteady and sways toward the affected side. Symptoms persist for several days and then resolve completely, but recurrent episodes of vertigo and nausea lasting 5 to 10 seconds are precipitated by specific movements of the head *(paroxysmal positional vertigo).*

DIAGNOSIS. Radiography of the skull is indicated in all children with vertigo following head injury. Special attention should be paid to fractures through the petrous pyramid. Bleeding from the ear or a facial palsy should raise suspicion of such a skull fracture.

Positional nystagmus is induced by the Nylen-

Hallpike technique when the injured ear is moved down. Caloric testing or electronystagmography shows a reduced response from the injured ear.

TREATMENT. Immediately after injury the patient should be treated with an antihistamine and diazepam until the acute phase is over.

Individuals with paroxysmal positional vertigo are treated with *fatigue therapy.* The patient is tilted to a position that reproduces symptoms. The patient remains in that position until the vertigo subsides for at least 30 seconds, then sits up for 30 seconds. The procedure is repeated four times. This exercise is performed several times each day until the patient is no longer sensitive to positional change.

Whiplash Injury

Whiplash injuries are frequently associated with vestibular and auditory dysfunction. Symptoms are probably caused by basilar artery spasm.

CLINICAL FEATURES. Vertigo may be present immediately after injury and subsides within a few days. Brief attacks of vertigo and tinnitus, sometimes associated with headache or nausea, may develop months later in children who appear fully recovered from the injury. Many features of the attacks suggest basilar artery migraine (see Chapter 10) and probably represent a post-traumatic migraine.

DIAGNOSIS. During the acute phase, vertigo may be induced by the Nylen-Hallpike technique and unilateral dysfunction is documented by caloric testing. Vestibular function may also be abnormal in children who are experiencing basilar artery migraine, especially at the time of attack. EEG often shows occipital intermittent rhythmic delta activity (see Figure 10–2).

REFERENCES

Alvord EC Jr, Shaw C-M. Congenital difficulties with swallowing and breathing associated with maternal polyhydramnios: Neurocristopathy or medullary infarction? J Child Neurol 1989;4:299-306.

Ariyasu L, Byl FM, Sprague MS, et al. The beneficial effects of methylprednisolone in acute vestibular vertigo. Arch Otolaryngol Head Neck Surg 1990;116:700-703.

Beighton P. Hereditary deafness. In Emery AE, Rimoin DA (eds): Principles and Practice of Medical Genetics, 2nd edition. Churchill Livingstone, London, 1990; 733.

Brouwer OF, Padberg GW, Bakker E. Early onset facioscapulohumeral muscular dystrophy. Muscle Nerve 1995;Suppl 2:S67-S72.

D'Cruz OF, Swisher CN, Jaradeh S, et al. Möbius syndrome: Evidence for a vascular etiology. J Child Neurol 1993; 8:260-265.

Hardiman O, Halperin JJ, Shapiro BE, et al. Neuropathological findings in oculopharyngeal muscular dystrophy: A report of seven cases and a review of the literature. Arch Neurol 1993;50:481-488.

Hawkins SA, Nevin NC, Harding AE. Pontobulbar palsy and neurosensory deafness (Brown-Vialetto-Van Laere syndrome) with possible autosomal dominant inheritance. J Med Genet 1990;27:176-179.

Kabakkaya Y, Bakan E, Yigitoglu MR, et al. Pendred's syndrome. Ann Otol Rhinol Laryngol 1993;102:285-288.

Keane JR. Bilateral seventh nerve palsy: Analysis of 43 cases and review of the literature. Neurology 1994;44:1198-1202.

Kuzniecky R, Andermann F, Guerrini R, et al. Congenital bilateral perisylvian syndrome: Study of 31 patients. Lancet 1993;341:608-612.

Kuzniecky R, Andermann F, Guerrini R, et al. The epileptic spectrum in the congenital bilateral perisylvian syndrome. Neurology 1994;44:379-385.

McShane MA, Boyd S, Harding B, et al. Progressive bulbar paralysis of childhood: A reappraisal of Fazio-Londe disease. Brain 1992;115:1889-1900.

Morgan D, Williams B. Syringobulbia: A surgical appraisal. J Neurol Neurosurg Psychiatry 1992;55:1132-1141.

Nadol JB Jr. Hearing loss. N Engl J Med 1993;329:1092-1102.

National Institutes of Health Conference. Neurofibromatosis 1 (Recklinghausen Disease) and neurofibromatosis 2 (bilateral acoustic neurofibromatosis): An update. Ann Intern Med 1990;113:39-52.

Padberg GW, Brouwer OF, de Keizer RJW, et al. On the significance of retinal vascular disease and hearing loss in facioscapulohumeral muscular dystrophy. Muscle Nerve 1995;Suppl 2:S73-S80.

Pasteris NG, Trask BJ, Sheldon S, et al. Discordant phenotype of two overlapping deletions involving the PAX3 gene in chromosome 2q35. Hum Mol Genet 1993;2:953-959.

Raynor BD. Cytomegalovirus infection in pregnancy. Semin Perinat 1993;17:394-402.

Schröder JM, Krabbe B, Weis J. Oculopharyngeal muscular dystrophy: Clinical and morphological follow-up study reveals mitochondrial alterations and unique nuclear inclusions in a severe autosomal recessive type. Neuropath Appl Neurobiol 1995;21:68-73.

Sekitani T, Imate Y, Noguchi T, et al. Vestibular neuronitis: Epidemiological survey by questionnaire in Japan. Acta Otolaryngol Suppl (Stockh) 1993;503:9-12.

Shapiro F. Osteopetrosis. Current clinical considerations. Clin Orthop Rel Res 1993;294:34-44.

Tusa ARJ, Saada AA Jr, Niparko JK. Dizziness in childhood. J Child Neurol 1994;9:261-274.

18

Disorders of Cranial Volume and Shape

During infancy, the size of the skull is determined by the volume of the three compartments that fill the calvarium: brain, cerebrospinal fluid, and blood. Expansion of one compartment is at the expense of another so that intracranial volume and pressure remain constant (see Chapter 4). The extracerebral spaces (epidural, subdural, and subarachnoid) may expand with blood and significantly affect cranial volume. Less important factors contributing to head size are the thickness of the skull bones and the rate of their fusion.

The skull's shape is determined in part by its content, but external forces on the skull and the rate at which individual skull bones fuse are even more important factors.

 Measuring Head Size

Head circumference is determined by measuring the greatest occipitofrontal circumference. The accuracy of the measurement in estimating cranial volume is influenced by fluid in and beneath the scalp and by head shape. The scalp can be thickened from edema or blood following a prolonged and difficult delivery, and cephalohematoma may be present as well. Fluid that infiltrates from a scalp infusion can markedly increase head circumference.

A round head has a larger intracranial volume than an oval head of equal circumference. A head with a relatively large occipitofrontal diameter has a larger volume than a head with a relatively large biparietal diameter.

Head circumference measurements are most informative when plotted over time. The head sizes of male and female infants are different, and head growth charts that provide median values for both sexes should not be used. The rate of head growth in premature infants is considerably faster than in full-term newborns (Figure 18-1). For this reason, head circumference must always be charted by conceptional age and not by postnatal age.

 Macrocephaly

Macrocephaly means a large head, larger than 2 standard deviations from the normal distribution. Thus, 2% of the "normal" population has macrocephaly. Investigation of such individuals may show an abnormality that has caused macrocephaly, but many are normal, often with a familial tendency for a large head. *When asked to evaluate a large head in an otherwise normal child, first ask the parents for their hat sizes.*

The causes of a large head include *hydrocephalus,* or excessive volume of cerebrospinal fluid in the skull; *megalencephaly,* or enlargement of the brain; thickening of the skull; and hemorrhage into the subdural or epidural spaces. Hydrocephalus is traditionally *communicating*

☐ FIGURE 18–1 Normal growth of head circumference in boys. The rate of growth in premature infants is greater than in full-term infants.

(nonobstructive) or *noncommunicating* (obstructive), depending on whether cerebrospinal fluid communicates between the ventricles and subarachnoid space (Table 18-1). Hydrocephalus is the only cause of macrocephaly at birth in which intracranial pressure is increased.

The causes of megalencephaly are anatomic and metabolic. The anatomic disorders are primary megalencephaly and neurocutaneous disorders (Table 18-2). Children with anatomic megalencephaly are often macrocephalic at birth but have normal intracranial pressure. Children with metabolic megalencephaly are usually normocephalic at birth and develop megalencephaly from cerebral edema during the neonatal period.

Macrocephaly caused by increased thickness of the skull bones is not present at birth or in the newborn period, but develops during infancy. The conditions associated with increased skull growth are summarized in Table 18-3 but are not discussed in the text. Intracranial hemorrhage in the newborn is discussed in Chapter 1, and intracranial hemorrhage in older children is discussed in Chapter 2.

■ TABLE 18–1
Causes of Hydrocephalus

Communicating

Achondroplasia
Basilar impression (see Chapter 10)
Benign enlargement of subarachnoid space
Choroid plexus papilloma (see Chapter 4)
Meningeal malignancy
Meningitis (see Chapter 4)
Posthemorrhagic (see Chapter 4)

Noncommunicating

Aqueductal stenosis
  Infectious
  X-linked
Chiari malformation (see Chapter 10)
Dandy-Walker malformation
Klippel-Feil syndrome
Mass lesions
  Abscess (see Chapter 4)
  Hematoma (see Chapters 1 and 2)
  Tumors and neurocutaneous disorders
  Vein of Galen malformation
Warburg syndrome

Hydranencephaly

Holoprosencephaly
Massive hydrocephalus
Porencephaly

*Modified from DeMyer W. Pediatr Neurol 2:321, 1986.

■ TABLE 18–2
Causes of Megalencephaly

Anatomic Megalencephaly

Genetic megalencephaly
Megalencephaly with achondroplasia
Megalencephaly with gigantism (Sotos syndrome)
Megalencephaly with a neurologic abnormality
Neurocutaneous disorders
   Hypomelanosis of Ito
   Incontinentia pigmenti (see Chapter 1)
   Linear nevus sebaceus syndrome
   Neurofibromatosis (see Chapter 5)
   Tuberous sclerosis (see Chapter 5)

Metabolic Megalencephaly

Alexander disease (see Chapter 5)
Canavan disease (see Chapter 5)
Galactosemia: transferase deficiency (see Chapter 5)
Gangliosidosis (see Chapter 5)
Globoid leukodystrophy (see Chapter 5)
Glutaric aciduria type I (see Chapter 14)
Leukencephalopathy with a mild clinical course
Maple syrup urine disease (see Chapter 1)
Metachromatic leukodystrophy (see Chapter 5)
Mucopolysaccharidoses (see Chapter 5)

■ TABLE 18–3
Conditions with a Thickened Skull Causing Macrocephaly*

Anemia
Cleidocranial dysostosis
Craniometaphyseal dysplasia of Pyle
Epiphyseal dysplasia
Hyperphosphatemia
Leontiasis ossea
Orodigitofacial dysostosis
Osteogenesis imperfecta
Osteopetrosis
Pyknodysostosis
Rickets
Russell dwarfism

COMMUNICATING HYDROCEPHALUS

Communicating hydrocephalus is usually caused by impaired absorption of cerebrospinal fluid secondary to meningitis or subarachnoid hemorrhage. Meningeal malignancy, usually caused by leukemia or primary brain tumor, is a less common cause. The excessive production of cerebrospinal fluid by a choroid plexus papilloma rarely causes communicating hydrocephalus because the potential rate of cerebrospinal reabsorption far exceeds the productive capacity of the choroid plexus (see Chapter 4). Such tumors more commonly cause hydrocephalus by obstructing one or more ventricles.

Achondroplasia

Achondroplasia is a genetic disorder, transmitted as an autosomal dominant trait, that causes skeletal deformities resulting in dwarfism.

CLINICAL FEATURES. The main features of achondroplasia are macrocephaly and rhizomelic shortening of the limbs: the proximal portion of the limbs is shorter than the distal portion. Enchondral bone formation at the skull base and in the face is stunted, causing the typical recessed facial appearance.

Affected newborns have megalencephaly but do not have hydrocephalus. The ventricles start enlarging during infancy because increased venous pressure impairs the reabsorption of cerebrospinal fluid. Venous return from the brain is probably obstructed because of narrowed venous sinuses in the small posterior fossa.

Despite considerable, and sometimes alarming, enlargement of head circumference, achondroplastic dwarfs seldom show clinical evidence of increased intracranial pressure or progressive dementia. Respiratory disturbances are common. Dyspnea is sometimes caused by cervicomedullary compression, but more often the cause is a primary pulmonary disorder, such as a small thoracic cage or an obstructed airway. Other features of cervicomedullary compression are hyperreflexia, spasticity, and sensory disturbances of the limbs.

DIAGNOSIS. The diagnosis of achondroplasia is established by clinical examination. The mutation rate is high and no other family member may be affected. Computed tomography (CT) shows a small posterior fossa and enlargement of the sphenoid sinuses. Basilar impression is sometimes present. Ventricular size varies from normal in newborns and young infants to moderate or severe dilation in older children and adults.

TREATMENT. Ventricular size, after initial dilatation, usually remains stable, and surgical diversion of cerebrospinal fluid is rarely needed. Decompressive surgery is required in children with evidence of progressive cervicomedullary compromise.

Benign Enlargement of Subarachnoid Space

Benign enlargement of the subarachnoid space is described under several names in the literature: *external hydrocephalus, extraventricular hydrocephalus, benign subdural effusions,* and *benign extracerebral fluid collec-*

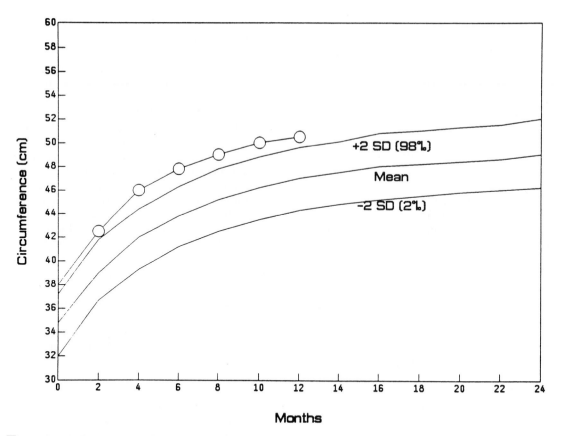

☐ F I G U R E   1 8 – 2   Benign enlargement of subarachnoid space. Head circumference is already large at birth, grows to exceed the 98th percentile, and then parallels the curve.

tions. It is a relatively common cause of macrocephaly in infants, a fact not fully appreciated before the widespread use of CT to investigate large head size. A genetic cause of this condition is likely in some cases, with the infant's father often having a large head.

CLINICAL FEATURES. The condition occurs more commonly in males than females. A large head circumference is the only feature. An otherwise normal infant is brought to medical attention because serial head circumference measurements show an enlarging head size. Circum- ference is usually above the 90th percentile at birth, grows to exceed the 98th percentile, and then parallels the normal curve (Figure 18-2). The anterior fontanelle is large but soft. Neurologic findings and developmental status are normal.

DIAGNOSIS. Cranial CT shows an enlarged frontal subarachnoid space, widening of the sylvian fissures and other sulci, and normal or minimally enlarged ventricular size (Figure 18-3). Normal ventricular size distinguishes this condition from cerebral atrophy. In infants, the upper limit of normal size for the frontal subarachnoid space is 5.7 mm and for the sylvian fissure is 7.6 mm.

TREATMENT. Most affected infants develop normally and do not require ventricular shunts. Head circumference measurements should be plotted monthly for the next 6 months after diagnosis to be certain that growth is paralleling the normal curve. Repeat CT is not needed unless head growth deviates upward from the normal curve, neurologic findings become abnormal, or development is delayed.

Meningeal Malignancy

Tumors that infiltrate the meninges and subarachnoid space impair the reabsorption of cerebrospinal fluid and cause communicating hydrocephalus. The primary site of tumor is usually established before its meningeal spread, but hydrocephalus may be the initial feature of diffuse meningeal gliomatosis.

CLINICAL FEATURES. Tumors that infiltrate the meninges are usually aggressive, causing a rapid progression of symptoms. Headache and vomiting are the initial features and are followed by lethargy and personality change. Meningismus and papilledema are common features and may suggest a bacterial meningitis. Multifocal neurologic disturbances may be present.

DIAGNOSIS. Magnetic resonance imaging (MRI) shows dilatation of the entire ventricular system but not of the subarachnoid space, which may appear obliterated except for a layer of enhancement. The pressure of the cerebrospinal fluid is increased, as is its protein concentration. The glucose concentration may be depressed or normal. Tumor cell identification in the cerebrospinal fluid is essential for early diagnosis and treatment, although it is rarely accomplished unless large volumes are examined. Meningeal biopsy is required for tissue diagnosis in many cases.

TREATMENT. A ventricular shunt is necessary to relieve symptoms of increased intracranial pressure. Radiation therapy and chemotherapy provide palliation and extend life in some cases, but the outcome is generally poor.

NONCOMMUNICATING HYDROCEPHALUS

Complete obstruction of the egress of cerebrospinal fluid from the ventricles to the sub-

☐ F I G U R E   1 8 – 3 Benign enlargement of subarachnoid space. CT reveals an enlarged frontal subarachnoid space, prominent sulci, and normal ventricular size.

arachnoid space causes increased pressure and dilatation of all ventricles proximal to the obstruction.

Noncommunicating hydrocephalus is the most common form of hydrocephalus in fetuses. Aqueductal stenosis is the usual cause of congenital hydrocephalus in the absence of other associated cerebral malformations. It becomes less common during infancy but increases in frequency again during childhood. Childhood onset is usually caused by mass lesions.

Children with congenital hydrocephalus who have seizures usually have other cerebral malformations. Such children have a higher incidence of mental retardation (Noetzel and Blake, 1992).

Congenital Aqueductal Stenosis

At birth, the mean length of the cerebral aqueduct is 12.8 mm and its smallest cross-sectional diameter is usually 0.5 mm. The small lumen of the cerebral aqueduct, in relation to its length, makes it especially vulnerable to internal compromise from infection and hemorrhage and to external compression by tumors and venous malformations.

Congenital atresia or stenosis of the cerebral aqueduct can occur as a solitary malformation, but a familial form transmitted by X-linked inheritance accounts for 2% of all cases of congenital hydrocephalus.

CLINICAL FEATURES. Hydrocephalus is present at birth. Head circumference ranges from 40 to 50 cm and may cause cephalopelvic disproportion and poor progress of labor. The forehead is bowed, the scalp veins are dilated, the skull sutures are widely separated, and the fontanelles are large and tense. These signs are exaggerated when the child cries but are also present in the quiet state. The eyes are deviated downward so that the sclera shows above the iris (*setting-sun sign*), and abducens palsies may be present.

Adduction and flexion of the thumbs are seen in approximately 20% of newborns with X-linked aqueductal stenosis. The thumb position was thought to be an associated malformation but probably represents a nonspecific sign of corticospinal tract compression by the dilated lateral ventricles.

DIAGNOSIS. Antenatal diagnosis is accomplished by intrauterine sonography. When macrocephaly is present in the fetus, alpha-fetoprotein should be assayed in the amniotic fluid for the detection of neural tube defects (see Chapter 12) and chromosomal analysis should be performed. Information concerning the in-

☐ FIGURE 18-4 Aqueductal stenosis. CT demonstrates marked enlargement of the third ventricle (*arrow*) and the lateral ventricles.

tegrity of the fetal nervous system is needed to develop a management plan.

The postpartum diagnosis of aqueductal stenosis is readily accomplished with CT. The lateral and third ventricles are markedly enlarged, as is the cephalic end of the cerebral aqueduct. The remainder of the cerebral aqueduct and the fourth ventricle cannot be visualized (Figure 18-4).

TREATMENT. Congenital hydrocephalus caused by aqueductal stenosis is severe, does not respond to medical therapy directed at decreasing the volume of cerebrospinal fluid, and progresses to a stage that harms the brain. Diversion of the cerebrospinal fluid from the ventricular system to an extracranial site is the only effective method of management.

The management of fetal hydrocephalus depends on the presence of other malformations. Between 70% and 80% of patients have other abnormalities, usually spina bifida. Many pregnancies with an affected fetus are terminated voluntarily.

Ventriculoperitoneal shunt is generally considered the procedure of choice for newborns and small infants with aqueductal stenosis. It is easier to revise and better tolerated than ventriculoatrial shunt. Mechanical obstruction and infection are the most common complications of shunt placement in infancy (see Chapter 4).

The relief of hydrocephalus increases the potential for normal development, even when the cerebral mantle appears very thin preoperatively, but does not necessarily result in a normal child. The growth of intelligence is often uneven, with better development of verbal skills than of nonverbal skills. Associated anomalies may cause motor deficits and seizures.

Dandy-Walker Malformation

The Dandy-Walker malformation consists of partial or complete agenesis of the cerebellar vermis, cystic dilatation of the posterior fossa communicating with the fourth ventricle, and hydrocephalus (Bordarier and Aicardi, 1990). The hydrocephalus may not be present at birth and more often develops during childhood or even later. The size of the lateral ventricles does not correlate with the size of the cyst in the fourth ventricle. Other malformations are present in 68% of patients. The most common associated malformation is agenesis of the corpus callosum. Other malformations are heterotopia, abnormal gyrus formation, dysraphic states, aqueductal stenosis, and congenital tumors.

CLINICAL FEATURES. The diagnosis is made at birth in only 25% of cases, and by 1 year in 75% (Pascual-Castroviejo et al, 1991). Macrocephaly is the usual initial feature. Bulging of the skull, when present, is more prominent in the occipital than in the frontal region. The rapidity of head growth is considerably slower than with aqueductal stenosis. Compression of posterior fossa structures leads to neurologic dysfunction; including apneic spells, nystagmus, truncal ataxia, cranial nerve palsies, and hyperreflexia in the legs.

DIAGNOSIS. CT or MRI is usually ordered because of macrocephaly or ataxia. Either study shows cystic dilatation of the posterior fossa and partial or complete agenesis of the cerebellar vermis (Figure 18-5). MRI is more useful because it also identifies other cerebral abnormalities such as heterotopia. Incomplete vermian agenesis may be difficult to differentiate from an enlarged cisterna magna.

The Dandy-Walker malformation is part of the spectrum of anomalies associated with trisomy 9, and karyotyping is suggested (Golden and Schoene, 1993).

TREATMENT. Decompression of the cyst alone provides immediate relief of symptoms; however, hydrocephalus recurs and ventricular shunting is required in two thirds of affected children. Shunting of the lateral ventricle alone provides immediate relief of hydrocephalus but fails to relieve brainstem compression. The procedure of choice is a dural shunt of both the lateral ventricle and the posterior fossa cyst.

Even after successful shunt placement, many children have transitory episodes of lethargy, personality change, and vomiting. Shunt failure is suspected but cannot be substantiated. The mechanism of such episodes, which may prove fatal, is unknown.

Klippel-Feil Syndrome

Klippel-Feil syndrome is a malformation of the craniocervical skeleton that may be associated with the Chiari malformation and with basilar impression. Hydrocephalus is caused by obstruction of the egress of cerebrospinal fluid from the fourth ventricle to the subarachnoid space. The malformation is classified into three types: I, extensive fusion of thoracic and upper cervical vertebrae; II, one or two interspace fusions with hemivertebrae and occipitoatlantal fusion; and III, cervical and lower thoracic or lumbar fusion. Type II is the most common form.

CLINICAL FEATURES. The essential features of the Klippel-Feil syndrome are a low posterior hairline, a short neck, and limitation of neck movement. Head asymmetry, facial asymmetry, scoliosis, and mirror movements of the hands are common. Unilateral or bilateral failure of

☐ F I G U R E 1 8 – 5 Dandy-Walker malformation. CT demonstrates cystic dilatation of the fourth ventricle and partial agenesis of the cerebellar vermis.

downward migration of the scapula (Sprengel deformity) is present in 25% to 35% of patients. Malformations of the genitourinary system and deafness are associated features.

Hydrocephalus affects the fourth ventricle first and then the lateral ventricles. This results in symptoms of posterior fossa compression: ataxia, apnea, and cranial nerve dysfunction.

DIAGNOSIS. The characteristic fusion and malformations of vertebrae is seen on radiographs of the spine. MRI may show an associated Chiari malformation and dilatation of the ventricles.

TREATMENT. Children with unstable cervical vertebrae require cervical fusion to prevent myelopathy. Those with symptoms of obstructive hydrocephalus require a ventriculoperitoneal shunt to relieve pressure in the posterior fossa.

Congenital Brain Tumors

Congenital brain tumors and congenital brain malformations are both disorders of cellular proliferation. A noxious agent active during early embryogenesis might stimulate either or both abnormalities. The relative oncogenicity or teratogenicity depends on the virulence of the agent, the timing of the insult, the duration of exposure, and the genetic background and health of the fetus.

The most common tumors of infancy are astrocytoma, medulloblastoma, teratoma, and choroid plexus papilloma.

CLINICAL FEATURES. Congenital tumors are more often supratentorial than infratentorial and more often in the midline than situated laterally. Newborns with hemispheric gliomas and teratomas may develop hydrocephalus in utero or in the first days or weeks postpartum. The point of obstruction is usually at the cerebral aqueduct (see Chapter 4). Choroid plexus papillomas are usually located in one lateral ventricle and usually become symptomatic during infancy rather than in the perinatal period. They produce hydrocephalus either by obstruction of the foramen of Monro or by excessive production of cerebrospinal fluid (see Chapter 4). Medulloblastomas are located in the posterior fossa and obstruct the fourth ventricle and cerebral aqueduct (see Chapter 10).

The clinical features of all congenital tumors are those of increasing intracranial pressure: enlarging head size, separation of the sutures, lethargy, irritability, difficult feeding, and vomiting. Seizures are unusual. Because of its posterior fossa location, medulloblastoma also produces nystagmus, downward deviation of the eyes, opisthotonos, and apnea.

DIAGNOSIS. All congenital tumors are readily visualized by CT or MRI performed to investigate hydrocephalus. Some have been identified by uterine sonography.

TREATMENT. Complete resection of congenital brain tumors is unusual with the exception of choroid plexus papilloma. The management of individual tumors is discussed in Chapters 4 and 10.

Vein of Galen Malformation

Arteriovenous malformations of the cerebral circulation may become symptomatic during infancy and childhood (see Chapters 4 and 10), but the one associated with congenital hydrocephalus is the vein of Galen malformation (Lasjaunias et al, 1989). The vein of Galen is just above the quadrigeminal plate and, when dilated, compresses the cerebral aqueduct and causes dilatation of the lateral ventricles. The increased blood volume in the skull also causes macrocrania.

CLINICAL FEATURES. Eighty percent of newborns with vein of Galen malformations are males. The usual initial feature is either high-output cardiac failure or an enlarging head size. Hemorrhage almost never occurs early in the course. A cranial bruit is invariably present. Unexplained, persistent hypoglycemia has been noted in some children.

Large midline arteriovenous malformations produce a hemodynamic stress in the newborn because of the large quantities of blood shunted from the arterial to the venous system. The heart enlarges in an effort to keep up with the demands of the shunt, but high-output cardiac failure ensues. Affected newborns often come to the attention of a pediatric cardiologist first because congenital heart disease is suspected. The intracranial malformation is then diagnosed during cardiac catheterization.

When the hemodynamic stress is not severe and cardiac compensation is possible, symptoms are delayed until infancy or early childhood. In such a case, the initial feature of the malformation is obstructive hydrocephalus because it compresses the tegmentum and aqueduct. Symptoms usually begin before age 5 and always before age 10. The lateral ventricles enlarge, causing headache, lethargy, and vomiting. In infants, the head enlarges and the fontanelle feels full.

□ FIGURE 18-6 Vein of Galen malformation. The malformation is visible on contrast-enhanced CT as a large aneurysmal sac compressing the midbrain and producing obstructive hydrocephalus.

DIAGNOSIS. Vein of Galen malformations are readily visualized by contrast-enhanced CT (Figure 18-6) or MRI. The lateral and third ventricles are dilated behind the compressed cerebral aqueduct. Radiographs of the chest in newborns with high-output cardiac failure show an enlarged heart that has a normal shape.

TREATMENT. The overall results of direct surgical approaches are poor; the mortality rate is high, as is neurologic morbidity in survivors. Embolization has become the treatment of choice, but the long-term results are not established.

Warburg Syndrome

The Warburg syndrome is characterized by cerebral and ocular abnormalities. Hydrocephalus is a constant feature. The combination of Warburg syndrome and congenital muscular dystrophy is called *cerebro-ocular dysplasia* (see Chapter 6).

The risk of recurrence among siblings exceeds 50%, but the syndrome is not transmitted from one generation to the next. Some believe that this is a genetic disease transmitted by autosomal recessive inheritance; others think that it is caused by an acquired agent transmitted transplacentally through consecutive pregnancies.

CLINICAL FEATURES. Hydrocephalus is usually present at birth. It may be caused by aqueductal stenosis or the Dandy-Walker malformation. Most children with both a Dandy-Walker malformation and ocular abnormalities have the Warburg syndrome. Some children are born with microcephaly, yet have enlarged ventricles.

Severe neurologic abnormalities are caused by partial or total agyria (lissencephaly) resulting from failure of neuronal migration. The pattern of architectural abnormalities throughout the neuraxis suggests a disruption of cerebral maturation in the fourth conceptional month.

Several ocular abnormalities may be present, usually in combination: hypoplasia of the iris, abnormal anterior chamber, microphthalmos, cataracts, persistence of primary vitreous, optic disk coloboma, retinal detachment, retinal dysplasia, and hypoplasia of the optic nerve.

In addition to having hydrocephalus and blindness, affected infants are hypotonic and have difficulty feeding. Seizures are uncommon. Most children with Warburg syndrome die during the neonatal period or early infancy.

DIAGNOSIS. The diagnosis is based on the characteristic combination of cerebral and ocular abnormalities. Congenital infections may produce similar disturbances and must be excluded, but multisystem disease (visceromegaly and disturbed hematopoiesis), an expected feature of most intrauterine infections, is lacking in the Warburg syndrome.

Cerebro-ocular abnormalities at birth are also encountered in septo-optic dysplasia (see Chapter 16) and the oculocerebrorenal syndrome (see Chapter 6), but hydrocephalus is not a component of either syndrome.

TREATMENT. Hydrocephalus can be managed by ventricular shunt, but the outcome is poor because of the concomitant severe cerebral malformations.

HYDRANENCEPHALY

The term *hydranencephaly* encompasses several conditions that result in the extensive replacement of brain by cerebrospinal fluid. This may be caused by failure of normal brain development or from an intrauterine disorder that destroys the brain parenchyma. Progressive obstructive hydrocephalus may cause hydranencephaly if left untreated. Excessive pressure within the lateral ventricles destroys the midline structures and reduces the cerebral mantle to a thin membrane.

Head circumference at birth is large when hydranencephaly is caused by obstructive hydrocephalus, is small when the condition is caused by intrauterine diseases, and may be large or small with primary malformations.

PORENCEPHALY

Porencephaly is a term used loosely in the literature. It was originally used to describe defects in the final stage of prosencephalization resulting in a hemispheric cyst that communicated with the subarachnoid space and the lateral ventricle. The term is now used broadly for any hemispheric cyst; most are caused by intrauterine or perinatal infarction or trauma. The injured immature brain loses neurons, glia, and supporting structures. A fluid-filled cyst is formed in the injured area and may not communicate with either the ventricular system or the subarachnoid space. Pressure within the cyst often becomes excessive, causing compression of adjacent structures and macrocrania.

Congenital Midline Porencephaly

Congenital midline porencephaly is a distinct malformation characterized by congenital hydrocephalus, alopecia or encephalocele in the parietal midline, and a midline defect in the posterior cerebral mantle. Midline porencephaly differs from holoprosencephaly, because the forebrain divides into two separate hemispheres. It may be caused by early hydrocephalus with upward outpouching and destruction of adjacent structures, including the corpus callosum, cerebral mantle, skull, and scalp.

CLINICAL FEATURES. The head is large in utero and may cause cephalopelvic disproportion at delivery. Possible defects in the parietal midline range from a small round area of alopecia to an encephalocele. Affected children are severely retarded and blind. Most die during infancy or early childhood.

DIAGNOSIS. A large dorsal cyst that has destroyed the septum pellucidum and corpus callosum is seen on CT or MRI. The cyst communicates with enlarged lateral ventricles and extends through a skull defect to produce an encephalocele.

TREATMENT. Shunting the cyst may ease child care by reducing the size of the head or encephalocele, but it does not prevent severe neurologic impairment from the underlying cerebral malformation.

ANATOMIC MEGALENCEPHALY

Anatomic megalencephaly includes conditions in which the brain is enlarged because the number or size of cells increases. There is no evidence of metabolic disease or acute encephalopathy.

Genetic Megalencephaly

CLINICAL FEATURES. The term *genetic megalencephaly* describes a familial condition in which neurologic and mental function is normal but head circumference is larger than the 98th percentile. Head circumference may not be large at birth but increases during infancy, usually to between 2 and 4 cm above the 98th percentile. Body size is normal, and no physical deformities are present.

DIAGNOSIS. The enlargement is indistinguishable by physical examination from benign enlargement of the subarachnoid space but the two can be distinguished by CT, the results of which are normal in genetic megalencephaly.

TREATMENT. No treatment is required.

Megalencephaly with a Neurologic Disorder

The term *megalencephaly with a neurologic disorder* is used to encompasses all disorders, other than neurocutaneous syndromes, in which the head is large and the child is neurologically abnormal.

CLINICAL FEATURES. Head circumference may be large at birth or may become large during infancy. It is generally 2 to 4 cm greater than the 98th percentile. Results of neurologic tests are normal, but the children have learning disabilities, mental deficiency, or seizures. Neurologic status remains stable.

DIAGNOSIS. The skin of the patient and other family members must be carefully examined to exclude the possibility of a neurocutaneous disorder. Ophthalmoscopic examination of family members should be carried out.

Results of CT or MRI may be normal or may show mild dilatation of the ventricular system. Agenesis of the corpus callosum is the only abnormality found in some families with macrocrania and borderline intelligence.

TREATMENT. Seizures often respond to anticonvulsant drugs. Special education is usually required. No treatment is available for the underlying disorder.

Megalencephaly with Gigantism

Megalencephaly with gigantism is also termed *cerebral gigantism* or *Sotos syndrome*. It probably encompasses several disorders, most of them sporadic and some clearly genetic, transmitted by autosomal recessive or dominant inheritance. Chromosome studies are normal.

CLINICAL FEATURES. Affected children are in 75th to 90th percentile at birth and grow at an excessive rate in height, weight, head circumference, and bone age up to the age of 3. Afterward, the rate of growth is normal. All children with the syndrome are large as adults, but they are not usually giants.

Prominent forehead, high arched palate, and hypertelorism are present in almost every case. Several other dysmorphic features are reported in small numbers of patients. Approximately 80% of patients have some degree of mental retardation.

DIAGNOSIS. Cranial CT is usually normal except for mild ventricular widening. Extensive studies of endocrine function have failed to show a consistent abnormality other than glucose intolerance. Plasma somatomedin levels are elevated during the first year in some infants and fall below normal during early childhood.

TREATMENT. Girls may benefit from high doses of estrogens to curtail excessive growth, but no treatment is available for the underlying disorder.

Neurocutaneous Disorders

Seizures (see Table 1–8) and mental retardation (see Chapter 5) are the common features of most neurocutaneous disorders (Pascual-Castroviejo et al, 1988). The cutaneous features may be present at birth (incontinentia pigmenti) or during infancy (neurofibromatosis, tuberous sclerosis). Macrocrania is caused by either hydrocephalus or megalencephaly. Hemimegalencephaly, hemihypertrophy of the body, or hypertrophy of a single limb should always suggest the possibility of a neurocutaneous disorder.

Hypomelanosis of Ito

Hypomelanosis of Ito, also called *incontinentia pigmenti achromians,* is a rare syndrome believed to be transmitted by autosomal dominant inheritance. Some patients have been reported to have trisomy 18 and a balanced translocation between chromosomes 2 and 8.

CLINICAL FEATURES. The cutaneous feature is a large hypopigmented area that has a whorled or streaked appearance. It is a negative image of the hyperpigmented lesions of incontinentia pigmenti (see Chapter 1). Other cutaneous features are café au lait spots, angiomatous nevi, heterochromia of the iris or hair, and other nevi. Mental capacity is retarded or borderline in 80%, and seizures are present in half. Spastic diplegia may also be present. These symptoms are caused by disturbances of neuronal migration. Megalencephaly occurs in approximately 25% of cases.

About one third of patients have skeletal and eye anomalies, including limb hypertrophy or atrophy, facial hemiatrophy, poorly formed ears, dysplastic teeth, hypertelorism, strabismus, and corneal opacities.

DIAGNOSIS. The characteristic cutaneous lesions are critical to the diagnosis and should be sought in the parents and siblings as well as the child. Chromosome studies are indicated in the child and parents.

TREATMENT. Treatment is directed at the symptoms.

Linear Nevus Sebaceous Syndrome

Linear nevus sebaceous syndrome is sporadic, and is also called the *organoid nevus syndrome* and the *epidermal nevus syndrome*.

CLINICAL FEATURES. A unilateral linear nevus is present on the skin of the face or scalp. It may not be visible at birth but darkens during infancy and becomes verrucous. Hemihypertrophy of the face, head, and limbs ipsilateral to the nevus may be present at birth or may develop during infancy (Cavenagh et al, 1993).

The spectrum of neurologic disability is considerable. Developmental delay and seizures are expected. The head may be enlarged generally or unilaterally. Focal neurologic deficits, such as hemiplegia and hemianopia, contralateral to the nevus are relatively common. Eye abnormalities, such as microphthalmia and coloboma, occur in one third of children.

DIAGNOSIS. Diagnosis relies on recognition of the linear nevus. Electroencephalography (EEG) usually shows unilateral slowing and epileptiform discharges ipsilateral to the nevus. Hypsarrhythmia is seen on EEG when infantile spasms are the initial feature (see Chapter 1). Hemihypsarrhythmia may also occur.

CT shows asymmetry of the cranial vault with enlargement of one hemisphere. The abnormal hemisphere may have porencephaly or an enlarged lateral ventricle and a simplified convolutional pattern.

TREATMENT. Seizures may respond to standard anticonvulsant therapy (see Chapter 1), but no treatment is available for the underlying cerebral malformation.

Metabolic Megalencephaly

Several inborn errors of metabolism produce megalencephaly by storage of abnormal substances or by producing cerebral edema (Table 18-2). They are discussed elsewhere in the text because the initial features are usually developmental regression (see Chapter 5) or seizures (see Chapter 1). Two exceptions are glutaric aciduria type I caused by deficiency of glutaryl-coenzyme A dehydrogenase (see Chapter 14) and *leukoencephalopathy with a mild clinical course*. Infants with glutaric aciduria type I are normal for up to 3 years, except for macrocephaly, and then develop an acute encephalitic illness that resembles encephalitis (Hoffmann et al, 1991).

Most infants with metabolic megalencephaly have a normal head circumference at birth. Head enlargement parallels neurologic regression and clinical evidence of increased intracranial pressure. The ventricles are often small.

Leukoencephalopathy with a Mild Clinical Course

Leukoencephalopathy with a mild clinical course is a newly recognized syndrome (van der Knaap et al, 1995). The metabolic defect has not been established, but autosomal recessive inheritance is suspected because of an affected sibling pair and instances of parental consanguinity.

CLINICAL FEATURES. Age at onset is 3 months to 3 years. The initial feature is abnormal head enlargement in a child whose development is either normal or only mildly delayed. The subsequent course is characterized by very slowly progressive ataxia and spasticity. Seizures and mild mental deterioration may occur late in the course.

DIAGNOSIS. MRI shows a severe leukoencephalopathy that suggests a demyelinating white matter disorder. The hemispheres appear swollen, with cyst-like spaces in the frontoparietal and anterior temporal areas. The occipital white matter is relatively spared.

TREATMENT. No treatment is available.

➔ Microcephaly

Microcephaly means a head circumference that is smaller than 2 standard deviations below the normal distribution. The standard for head circumference varies among different ethnic groups. A small head circumference indicates a small brain. Most full-term newborns whose head circumferences are smaller than 2 standard deviations, but who are neurologically normal, will have normal intelligence at age 7, but a head circumferences smaller than 3 standard deviations usually indicates later mental retardation (Dolk, 1991).

A small head circumference at birth establishes the antepartum timing of brain damage, but does not distinguish primary from secondary microcephaly (Table 18–4). *Primary microcephaly* encompasses conditions in which the brain is small and never formed properly because of genetic or chromosomal abnormalities. *Secondary microcephaly* implies that the brain was forming normally but a disease process impaired further growth. Normal head circumference at birth, followed by failure of normal head growth, usually indicates a secondary microcephaly. Chromosomal disorders are an exception to that rule unless they cause defective prosencephalization or cellular migration.

Perinatal brain damage does not cause a recognizable decrease of head circumference until 3 to 6 months postpartum. Failure of normal brain growth removes the force keeping the cranial bones separated, and they fuse prematurely. A primary disorder of the skull (craniostenosis) may cause premature closure of the cranial sutures even though the brain is attempting to grow normally. The distinction between the two is relatively simple: craniostenosis is always associated with an abnormal skull shape and heaping up of bone along the cranial sutures; failure of brain growth produces a relatively normal-shaped skull with some overlapping of skull bones.

Cranial MRI may be informative in distinguishing primary from secondary microcephaly. In most children with primary microcephaly, either MRI results are normal or a recognizable pattern of cerebral malformation is present. In those with secondary microcephaly, the brain image is usually abnormal, characterized by one or more of the following features: ventricular enlargement, cerebral atrophy, and porencephaly.

TABLE 18–4
Conditions Causing Microcephaly

Primary Microcephaly
Microcephaly vera (genetic)
Chromosomal disorders
Defective neurolation
  Anencephaly
  Encephalocele
Defective prosencephalization
  Agenesis of the corpus callosum
  Holoprosencephaly (arhinencephaly)
Defective cellular migration
Secondary Microcephaly
Intrauterine disorders
  Infection
  Toxins
  Vascular
Perinatal brain injuries
  Hypoxic-ischemic encephalopathy
  Intracranial hemorrhage
  Meningitis and encephalitis
  Stroke
Postnatal systemic diseases
  Chronic cardiopulmonary disease
  Chronic renal disease
  Malnutrition

PRIMARY MICROCEPHALY

Many cerebral malformations are of uncertain cause and cannot be classified as primary or secondary. Morphogenetic errors, although lacking in the traditional stigmata of tissue injury, could result from exposure of the embryo to a noxious agent during the first weeks after conception. At this early stage, the delicate sequencing of neuronal development could be disorganized at a time when the brain is incapable of generating a cellular response.

Microcephaly Vera (Genetic)

Microcephaly vera is a term applied to genetic defects that decrease bulk growth of the brain. The defect may be transmitted as an autosomal dominant or as an autosomal recessive trait.

CLINICAL FEATURES. The autosomal dominant form is less disabling than the recessive form. Intelligence ranges from normal to mildly retarded. Learning disabilities are a common feature. The face is not usually dysmorphic, although some children have a receding forehead, upslanting of the palpebral fissures, and large prominent ears. Physical stature is normal. Seizures may be present during childhood but tend to disappear by adult life.

Children with the autosomal recessive form of microcephaly vera are usually short and have a characteristic disproportion in size between the face and the skull. The forehead slants backward, and the reduced size of the skull causes the scalp to wrinkle in the occipital region. The chin is small, and the ears and nose are prominent. Mental retardation is moderate to severe, and other neurologic abnormalities, such as spastic diplegia and seizures, may be present.

DIAGNOSIS. A family history of microcephaly is critical to the diagnosis in the autosomal dominant form but is often lacking in the autosomal recessive form. Results of brain imaging are normal.

TREATMENT. No treatment is available.

Chromosomal Disorders

Chromosomal disorders are not usually a cause of microcephaly at birth unless cerebral aplasia, such as holoprosencephaly, is part of the syndrome. Hypotonia and dysmorphism are the prominent features of chromosomal disorders in the newborn (see Chapter 5), and microcephaly becomes evident during infancy.

Defective Neurulation

At the end of the first week, a rostrocaudal axis appears on the dorsal aspect of the embryo. This axis is responsible for the subsequent induction of a neural plate, the anlage of the nervous system. The neural plate is converted into a closed neural tube during the third and fourth weeks. Defects in closure are called *dysraphic states.* The most rostral portion of the neural tube, the anterior neuropore, closes at about the 24th day.

Anencephaly

Anencephaly is the result of defective closure of the anterior neuropore, just as myelomeningocele is the result of defective closure of the posterior neuropore (see Chapter 12). The rate of each is declining. The cause of the malformations and the reason for their decline in prevalence are unknown.

CLINICAL FEATURES. Less than half of anencephalics are born alive, and those who are rarely survive the first month. The scalp is absent, and the skull is open from the vertex to the foramen magnum. The brain, appearing hemorrhagic and fibrotic, is exposed to view. It consists mainly of the hindbrain and parts of the diencephalon; the forebrain is completely lacking.

The orbits are shallow, and the eyes protrude. The neck is held in retroflexion, and the proximal portion of the arms seem overgrown compared with the legs. The overall appearance of the anencephalic newborn is grotesque and described as "toadlike."

DIAGNOSIS. Following the birth of a child with a neural tube defect, the chance of anencephaly or myelomeningocele in subsequent pregnancies increases twofold to fivefold. After two affected children have been born, the chance of having another affected child doubles again. The prenatal diagnosis of dysraphic states is discussed in the section on myelomeningocele (see Chapter 12).

TREATMENT. No effort to prolong life should be attempted.

Encephalocele

An encephalocele is a protrusion of cortex and meninges, covered by skin, through a defect in the skull. Encephaloceles may occur in any location; however, most are midline-occipital, except in Asians, in whom the defects are usually midline-frontal.

CLINICAL FEATURES. The size of the encephalocele may range from a small protrusion to a cyst as big as the skull. When the protrusion is large, the skull is likely to be microcephalic. No conclusion can be drawn concerning the contents of the mass by its size, but an encephalocele with a sessile base is more likely to contain cerebral tissue than is one with a pedunculated base.

Encephaloceles rarely occur as a solitary cerebral malformation and are usually associated with abnormalities of the cerebral hemispheres, cerebellum, and midbrain.

DIAGNOSIS. Cranial MRI is reasonably accurate in defining the contents of the encephalocele. Despite its midline location, the protruded material is usually derived from one hemisphere that is smaller than the other and is displaced across the midline by the larger hemisphere.

TREATMENT. The desire to remove the encephalocele surgically should be tempered by its contents and the extent of associated anomalies. Occipital meningocele, in which the sac contains no neural tissue, should be surgically removed, and the outcome is often excellent. Children with protruded brain material and associated malformations usually die during infancy.

Defective Prosencephalization

The forebrain develops between 25 and 30 days' gestation from a midline vesicle that is generated from the closed anterior neuropore. Between 30 and 40 days' gestation, bilateral cerebral vesicles are formed by the cleavage and outpouching of the midline vesicle. The midline vesicle is the primordium of the third ventricle, and the bilateral cerebral vesicles are the primordia of the lateral ventricles.

Holoprosencephaly

A spectrum of malformations has been described as resulting from defective cleavage of the embryonic forebrain. The term *arhinencephaly* is often used to refer to the full spectrum of abnormalities, but *holoprosencephaly* is a more accurate term.

Total failure of cleavage produces a small brain with a midline vesicle covered by a horseshoe of limbic cortex. With less severe defects, the third ventricle and diencephalon differentiate, and the hemispheres are partial cleaved in the occipital lobe. The corpus callosum is hypoplastic or absent. The minimal defect (arhinencephaly) is the unilateral or bilateral absence of the olfactory bulbs and tracts associated with some degree of rhinic lobe aplasia. Hemispheric cleavage is complete, the ventricles are normal, and the corpus callosum is present in part or in total.

Chromosomal abnormalities are often demonstrable in newborns with holoprosencephaly. Trisomy, deletions, and rings of chromosome 13 account for most of the chromosomal abnormalities. The remainder are composed of trisomy, deletions, and rings of chromosome 18 and partial trisomy of chromosome 7.

CLINICAL FEATURES. Craniofacial dysplasia is almost always associated and malformations in other organs are common. The facial deformities are primarily in the midline (cyclopia or ocular hypotelorism, flat nose, cleft lip, cleft palate) and their severity is often predictive of the severity of the brain malformation (Müller and O'Rahilly, 1989). Associated malformations include congenital heart defects, clubbing of the hands or feet, polydactyly and syndactyly, hypoplasia of the genitourinary system, accessory spleen and liver, and malrotation of the intestine.

Most children with severe defects in cleavage of the forebrain are stillborn or die in the neonatal period. Microcephaly, hypotonia, apnea, and seizures are prominent features. Hypotonia is especially severe when the defect is associated with a chromosomal abnormality. Infants who survive have severe intellectual, motor, and sensory impairment.

Children with only arhinencephaly may appear physically normal and may display minor disturbances in neurologic function such as learning disabilities and seizures.

DIAGNOSIS. Holoprosencephaly should be suspected in every child with midline facial deformities, especially when malformations are present in other organs. Excellent visualization of the malformation is provided by MRI.

TREATMENT. Considering the multiplicity of malformations, measures to extend life are inappropriate.

Agenesis of the Corpus Callosum

Anomalous development of the three telencephalic commissures—the corpus callosum, the anterior commissure, and the hippocampal commissure—is an almost constant feature of defective prosencephalization, but it also occurs in association with many other malformations, with some metabolic defects (see "Glycine Encephalopathy" in Chapter 1), and as a solitary genetic defect (Bodensteiner et al, 1994). When only the corpus callosum is absent, the anterior and hippocampal commissures may be normal or enlarged.

Callosal agenesis is part of the Aicardi syndrome (see Chapter 1), *Andermann syndrome* (autosomal recessive callosal agenesis, mental deficiency, and peripheral neuropathy), and trisomies 8, 11, and 13.

CLINICAL FEATURES. Solitary agenesis of the corpus callosum is clinically inapparent except for subtle disturbances in the interhemispheric transfer of information, for which special testing is needed. Mental retardation or learning disabilities occur in most cases, and epilepsy usually indicates concurrent focal heterotopia.

DIAGNOSIS. Neuroimaging shows lateral displacement of the lateral ventricles and upward displacement of the third ventricle. Intraventricular pressure is normal.

TREATMENT. No treatment is available.

Defective Cellular Migration

When neurons that should form the superficial layers of the cerebral cortex are unable to pass through the already established deeper layers of neurons, the results are a simplification of the cortical convolutional pattern (*agyria*) and an abnormal accumulation of neurons in the white matter (*heterotopia*). Complete absence of gyri causes a smooth cerebral surface (*lissencephaly*), whereas incomplete gyral formation causes the existing convolutions to be reduced in number and enlarged (*pachygyria*).

Lissencephaly is divided into two types (Kurlemann et al, 1993). Type I affects only the cerebral cortex and type II affects the cerebellum and brainstem as well. Facial dysmorphism may be associated with either type. The *Miller-Dieker syndrome* is a familial type I lissencephaly characterized by microcephaly and a peculiar facies that include micrognathia, high forehead, thin upper lip, short nose with anteverted nares, and low-set ears. A microdeletion at the 17p13.3 locus occurs in most patients with Miller-Dieker syndrome and deletions on chromosome 17 are also shown in other lissencephaly syndromes (Dobyns et al, 1993).

Lissencephaly is also transmitted as an X-linked dominant trait (Pinard et al, 1994) and as a component of several neurocutaneous disorders.

CLINICAL FEATURES. Most children with agyria-pachygyria are referred for evaluation of developmental delay or intractable myoclonic seizures. Many initially exhibit muscular hypotonia that later evolves into spasticity and opisthotonos. Microcephaly is not always present, but all have mental retardation, epilepsy, and cerebral palsy (Aicardi, 1993). Isolated heterotopia is an important cause of intractable epilepsy in an otherwise normal child (see Chapter 1).

DIAGNOSIS. EEG findings are characteristic, but not specific. Fast, high-voltage dysrhythmic activity dominates the background. It does not react to eye opening or photic stimulation and resembles a fast hypsarrhythmia.

The diagnosis is based on MRI abnormalities: a smooth cortical surface except for rudimentary sulci (agyria) may be limited to the parietal or frontal regions or encompass the whole brain; the sylvian fissure is broad and triangular; the interhemispheric fissure is widened; and nests of gray matter are present within the white matter. The ventricles may be enlarged, and the corpus callosum absent. Chromosome analysis should be done in most cases.

TREATMENT. Seizures are usually intractable but may be partially controlled by standard drugs for the management of infantile spasms or myoclonic seizures (see Chapter 1). Death often occurs during infancy, but long survival is possible.

SECONDARY MICROCEPHALY

Intrauterine Disorders

Intrauterine infection is an established cause of microcephaly. Cytomegalovirus infection (see Chapter 5) can be manifest as microcephaly, without any features of systemic disease. Because maternal infection is asymptomatic, such cases are difficult to identify as being caused by cytomegalovirus disease. However, surveys of cytomegalovirus antibody demonstrate a higher rate of seropositive individuals among microcephalic than normocephalic children. This suggests that such cases do exist.

Efforts to identify environmental toxins that produce cerebral malformation have had only limited success. Drugs of abuse and several pharmaceutical agents have been implicated, but the evidence is rarely compelling. The only absolute conclusion that can be derived from an abundance of studies is that a negative impact occurs on fetuses of women whose lifestyle includes some combination of heavy alcohol or drug use, poor nutrition, and inadequate health care. This negative impact is usually expressed as intrauterine growth retardation, dysmorphic features, and microcephaly.

Aplasia of major cerebral vessels is a rare malformation of unknown cause. Brain tissue that should have been supplied by the aplastic vessels either never forms or is infarcted and replaced by calcified cystic cavities. The cavities are present at birth, and the CT appearance suggests an intrauterine infection except that the cysts conform to a vascular distribution.

Perinatal Brain Injuries

Perinatal brain injuries are an important cause, but not the only cause, of failure of brain growth during infancy when head circumference is normal at birth. The initial feature of this group of disorders is neonatal encephalopathy and seizures (see Chapter 1). Children with microcephaly and mental retardation from perinatal brain injuries always have cerebral palsy and often have epilepsy. Microcephaly and mental retardation in the absence of motor impairment are always of prenatal origin.

Postnatal Systemic Disease

Infants who are chronically ill and malnourished fail to thrive. All growth is retarded; however, as a rule, head circumference is maintained better than length and weight.

Therefore, if body size is below the third percentile, head circumference might be at the fifth or tenth percentile. If the systemic disturbance is not corrected, brain injury generally occurs, brain growth slows, and head circumference falls into the microcephalic range.

 ## Abnormal Head Shape

Whereas the size of the skull is determined almost exclusively by its contents, the shape of the skull is the result of forces acting from within and without, and of the time of closure of the cranial sutures.

INTRACRANIAL FORCES

The shape of the brain contributes to the shape of the skull by influencing the time of closure of cranial sutures. Temporal lobe agenesis results in a narrower calvarium, and cerebellar agenesis results in a small posterior fossa. Hydrocephalus produces characteristic changes in skull shape. Large lateral ventricles cause bowing of the forehead, and the Dandy-Walker malformation causes bowing of the occiput. In infants with subdural hematomas, bitemporal widening may be seen because of separation of the sagittal suture.

EXTRACRANIAL FORCES

Head shape may be influenced in utero by constricting forces, such as a bicornuate uterus or multiple fetuses. Physical constraint of the skull in utero may contribute to premature closure of a cranial suture, but perinatal and postnatal constraints do not. Molding of the skull is common during a prolonged vaginal delivery, but the closure of cranial sutures is unaffected and eventual head shape is not influenced by the molding.

In premature infants, *scaphocephaly* (Table 18-5) often develops because the poorly mineralized skull becomes flattened on one side and then the other as the child is turned back and forth. The shape of the skull becomes normal with maturity.

Plagiocephaly or occipital flattening is a frequent finding in hypotonic infants. This is caused by constantly lying in the same position. The hair over the flattened portion of skull is usually sparse from rubbing against the bed

■ TABLE 18-5
Terms That Describe Head Shapes

Acrocephaly	High, tower-like head with vertical forehead
Brachycephaly	Broad head with recessed lower forehead
Oxycephaly	Pointed head
Plagiocephaly	Flattening of one side of head
Scaphocephaly (dolicocephaly)	Abnormally long and narrow head
Trigonocephaly	Triangular head with prominent vertical ridge in the midforehead

surface. A normal head shape is resumed if the infant's lying position can be changed.

CRANIOSTENOSIS

Craniostenosis and *craniosynostosis* are terms used for premature closure of one or more cranial sutures that results in an abnormal skull shape. These terms should be applied only to infants in whom the sutures close while the brain is growing. Early closure of sutures in infants with microcephaly is not premature because the intracranial pressure required to keep sutures apart is lacking.

Most cases of craniostenosis are sporadic and of uncertain etiology. Autosomal dominant and recessive forms of single-suture closure are reported (Cohen et al, 1990). Autosomal dominant inheritance is more common than autosomal recessive inheritance but is also more easily identified as hereditary. Many sporadic cases could represent autosomal recessive inheritance.

Craniostenosis may be one feature of a larger recognized syndrome of chromosomal or genetic abnormality. Genetic disorders are often associated with syndactyly or polydactyly (see "Acrocephalosyndactyly," later on in this chapter), whereas chromosomal disorders are usually characterized by other limb malformations and growth retardation.

Craniostenosis is also reported in association with other disorders (Table 18-6). Some of these associations are coincidental, but a cause-and-effect relationship probably does exist with metabolic disorders of bone.

CLINICAL FEATURES. The first, and usually the only, clinical feature is an abnormal head shape. Normal bone growth is impaired in a plane perpendicular to the fused suture, but is able to grow in a parallel plane. Scaphocephaly is caused by premature fusion of the sagittal suture, brachycephaly by fusion of both coronal sutures, plagiocephaly by fusion of one coronal or one lambdoid sutures, trigonocephaly by fusion of the metopic suture, and oxycephaly by fusion of all sutures.

When several sutures close prematurely, the growing brain is constricted and symptoms of increased intracranial pressure develop. Hydrocephalus occurs more frequently in children with craniostenosis than in normal children. Several different forms of communicating and noncommunicating hydrocephalus are described. It seems more likely that both are caused by a common underlying factor rather than one causing the other.

Sagittal synostosis accounts for almost 60% of all cases of craniostenosis and occurs primarily in males. Coronal synostosis accounts for approximately 20% of cases and occurs primarily in females.

DIAGNOSIS. Visual inspection of the skull and palpation of the sutures are sufficient for diagnosis in most cases of single-suture craniostenosis. Radiography of the skull shows a band of increased density at the site of the prematurely closed suture. CT is indicated in all children with craniostenosis of multiple sutures and in children with craniostenosis of a single suture if hydrocephalus is suspected.

TREATMENT. The two indications for surgery to correct craniostenosis are to improve the appearance of the head and to relieve increased intracranial pressure. The cosmetic indication should be used sparingly and only to make severe deformities less noticeable.

Acrocephalosyndactyly

Acrocephalosyndactyly is characterized by the combination of craniostenosis and fusion of

■ TABLE 18–6
Disorders Associated with Craniostenosis

Ataxia-telangiectasia
Familial hypophosphatemia
Hyperthyroidism
Idiopathic hypercalcemia
Mucopolysaccharidoses
Polycythemia vera
Rickets
  Renal rickets
  Vitamin D deficient
  Vitamin D resistant
Sickle cell disease
Thalassemia major

---

fingers and toes. Some degree of mental retardation is often present. Several different syndromes with this basic combination have been described (Cohen et al, 1990).

Apert syndrome is characterized by syndactyly and premature closure of the coronal suture resulting in brachycephaly. The forehead is high and prominent, and the face is similar to but less severely deformed than the face in Crouzon disease. Most cases are sporadic, but autosomal dominant inheritance is suspected. Agenesis of the corpus callosum and limbic structures may be an associated feature.

Carpenter syndrome differs from Apert syndrome because it is transmitted by autosomal recessive inheritance and the patient has polydactyly as well as syndactyly, premature closure of all sutures, obesity, and hypogonadism. Approximately 75% of patients are retarded secondary to cerebral malformations that are demonstrable on MRI (Taravath and Tonsgard, 1993).

Chotzen syndrome is similar to Carpenter syndrome but is transmitted by autosomal dominant inheritance and also is marked by a low-set frontal hairline, ptosis, and a deviated nasal septum.

Crouzon Disease (Craniofacial Dysostosis)

Crouzon disease is the combination of premature closure of any or all cranial sutures and maldevelopment of facial bones. It is transmitted by autosomal dominant inheritance.

CLINICAL FEATURES. The facial deformity is present at birth and becomes worse during infancy. The skull is usually widened anteriorly as a result of premature closure of the coronal suture. The eyes are widely separated and prominent, but the lower face appears recessed because of maxillary hypoplasia and prognathism. Adding to the deformity are a beaklike nose and a large protuberant tongue. Intracranial pressure is often increased because several cranial sutures are usually involved.

DIAGNOSIS. The typical facies and genetic pattern of inheritance are diagnostic. Cranial CT is indicated in every case to follow the progression of cerebral compression.

TREATMENT. A sequential neurosurgical and plastic surgical approach has been successful in opening the sutures to relieve intracranial pressure and in advancing the facial bones forward to improve cosmetic appearance.

REFERENCES

Aicardi J. Disorders of neuronal migration: A spectrum of cortical abnormalities. Int Pediatr 1993;8:162-170.

Bodensteiner J, Schaefer GB, Breeding L, et al. Hypoplasia of the corpus callosum: A study of 445 consecutive MRI scans. J Child Neurol 1994;9:47-49.

Bordarier C, Aicardi J. Dandy-Walker syndrome and agenesis of the cerebellar vermis: Diagnostic problems and genetic counselling. Dev Med Child Neurol 1990;32:285-294.

Cavenagh EC, Hart BL, Rose D. Association of linear sebaceous nevus syndrome and unilateral megalencephaly. Am J Neurol Radiol 1993;14:405-408.

Cohen MM Jr, Fraser FC, Gorlin RJ. Craniofacial disorders. In Emery AE, Rimoin DA (eds): Principles and Practice of Medical Genetics, 2nd edition, Churchill Livingstone, London, 1990;749.

Dobyns WB, Reiner O, Carrozzo R, et al. Lissencephaly: A human brain malformation associated with deletion of the LIS 1 gene located at chromosome 17p13. JAMA 1993;270: 2838-2842.

Dolk H. The predictive value of microcephaly during the first year of life for mental retardation at seven years. Dev Med Child Neurol 1991;33:974-983.

Golden JA, Schoene WC. Central nervous system malformations in trisomy 9. J Neuropathol Exp Neurol 1993;52: 71-77.

Hoffmann GF, Trefz FK, Barth PG, et al. Macrocephaly: An important indication for organic acid analysis. J Inher Metab Dis 1991;14:329-332.

Kurlemann G, Schuierer G, Kuchelmeister K, et al. Lissencephaly syndromes: Clinical aspects. Child Nerv Syst 1993;9:380-386.

Lasjaunias P, Rodesch G, Pruvost P, et al. Treatment of vein of Galen malformation. J Neurosurg 1989;70:746-750.

Müller F, O'Rahilly R. Mediobasal prosencephalic defects, including holoprosencephaly and cyclopia, in relation to the development of the human forebrain. Am J Anat 1989;185:391-414.

Noetzel MJ, Blake JN. Seizures in children with congenital hydrocephalus: Long-term outcome. Neurology 1992;42: 1277-1281.

Pascual-Castroviejo I, Lopez-Rodriguez L, de la Cruz Medina M, et al. Hypomelanosis of Ito. Neurological complications in 34 cases. Can J Neurol Sci 1988;15:124-129.

Pascual-Castroviejo I, Velez A, Pascual-Pascual SI, et al. Dandy-Walker malformation: Analysis of 38 cases. Child Nerv Syst 1991;7:88-97.

Pinard J-M, Motte J, Chiron C, et al. Subcortical laminar heterotopia and lissencephaly in two families: a single X linked dominant gene. J Neurol Neurosurg Psychiatry 1994;57:914-920.

Taravath S, Tonsgard JH. Cerebral malformations in Carpenter syndrome. Pediatr Neurol 1993;9:230-234.

van der Knaap MS, Barth PG, Stroink H, et al. Leukoencephalopathy with swelling and a discrepantly mild clinical course in eight children. Ann Neurol 1995;37:324-334.

Index

Note: Page numbers in italics refer to illustrations; those followed by t refer to tables.

A

Abducens nerve, aplasia of, in Duane syndrome, 312
  in increased intracranial pressure, 94
  palsy of, 312
    in Mobius syndrome, 312
Abetalopoproteinemia, 246–247
Abscess(es), epidural, and paraplegia/quadriplegia, 274–275
  of brain, from increased intracranial pressure, 111–112
Absence seizure(s), 26-28, *27*
  myoclonic, 29-30
Absence status, and acute hemiplegia, 263
Abuse, of children, shaking as, 72–73
Acanthyocytosis, hypoprebetaliproteinemia, retinitis pigmentosa, and pallidal degeneration with, 299
ACE (angiotensin-converting enzyme), in sarcoidosis, 352
Acetazolamide-responsive ataxia, 233–234
Acetylcholine, and continuous motor unit activity, 206
Achondroplasia, and macrocephaly, 367
Acid maltase deficiency, 173
  and progressive proximal weakness, 187
Acidemia, argininosuccinic, 9–11, *10*, 10t
  in newborns, methylmalonic, 12
    propionic, 11-12
  isovaleric, in newborns, 11
Acidosis, lactic, with mitochondrial encephalopathy, and stroke, 260-261
Acoustic neuroma(s), 359, *359*
Acquired epileptiform aphasia, 31
Acquired nystagmus. See *Nystagmus, acquired.*
Acquired ophthalmoplegia. See *Ophthalmoplegia, acquired.*
Acquired ptosis, etiology of, 313t
Acrocephalosyndactyly, and abnormal head shape, 381
Acrocephaly, 380t
Acyl-coenzyme A dehydrogenase deficiency, very-long-chain, and exercise intolerance, 213–214
Addison disease, cramps in, 208
Additive(s), in food, and headaches, 85–86
Adenoma(s), pituitary, and progressive vision loss, 339
ADH (antidiuretic hormone). See *Antidiuretic hormone (ADH).*
Adhalin, in limb-girdle dystrophy, 183

Adie syndrome, 342
Adrenal gland, disorders of, and altered consciousness, 64
  and progressive proximal weakness, 188
Adrenoleukodystrophy, and paraplegia/quadriplegia, 268
  neonatal, 158
Adrenomyeloneuropathy, and paraplegia/quadriplegia, 268
Agitation, etiology of, 47, 48t
Agyria, 378
Albers-Schönberg disease, and facial weakness/dysphagia, 352
Alcohol abuse, 71
  jerk nystagmus from, 326
Algodystrophy, 227
Alice-in-Wonderland syndrome, 80
Alpha-fetoprotein, in myelomeningocele, 271
Alstrom syndrome, hearing impairment/deafness in, 357
Alternating gaze, periodic, 324t
Alternating hemiplegia, 255
Amaurosis, leber congenital, and blindness, 332
Amikacin, and hearing impairment/deafness, 357
  intravenous, for meningitis, 110, 110t
Aminoacidopathy, in newborns, 8–11, *9–10*, 10t
Aminoglycoside(s), and hearing impairment/deafness, 357
  and vertigo, 361
Amitroptyline, and internuclear ophthalmoplegia, 323
Ammonia, in ischemic exercise test, 210–211, *212*
  metabolism of, in neonatal urea cycle disturbances, *10*, 10t
Amnesia, transient global, 69
Amphotericin B, for coccidioidal meningitis, 114, 114t
Ampicillin, intravenous, for meningitis, 108, 109t, 110, 110t
Amyloid polyneuropathy, familial, 226
Amyotrophic lateral sclerosis, juvenile, 189
Amyotrophy, asthmatic, and monoplegia, 286
Analgesic rebound headache(s), 85
Anaplastic tumor(s), 99–100, *100*
Anatomic megalencephaly. See *Megalencephaly, anatomic.*
Anemia, sickle cell, and acute hemiplegia, 261-262
Anencephaly, and microcephaly, 377
Anesthetic(s), and malignant hyperthermia, 217-218
Aneurysm(s), and acute unilateral opthalmoplegia, 313-314
  arterial, and intracranial hemorrhage, 105-106
Angiitis, of central nervous system, and acute hemiplegia, 262

ISBN 0-7216-6852-6